PET

Springer
New York
Berlin
Heidelberg
Hong Kong
London
Milan
Paris
Tokyo

PET

MOLECULAR IMAGING AND ITS BIOLOGICAL APPLICATIONS

With 243 Illustrations, 46 in Full Color

Michael E. Phelps, PhD

Norton Simon Professor
Chair, Department of Molecular and Medical Pharmacology
Director, Institute for Molecular Medicine
Director, Crump Institute for Molecular Imaging
University of California School of Medicine
Los Angeles, California

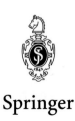

Springer

Michael E. Phelps, PhD
Norton Simon Professor
Chair, Department of Molecular and Medical Pharmacology
Director, Institute for Molecular Medicine
Director, Crump Institute for Molecular Imaging
University of California School of Medicine
Los Angeles, CA 90095, USA

Library of Congress Cataloging-in-Publication Data
PET : molecular imaging and its biological applications / [edited by] Michael E. Phelps.
     p. ; cm.
   Includes index.
   ISBN 0-387-40359-0 (h/c : alk. paper)
     1. Tomography, Emission.   I. Title: Positron emission tomography.   II. Phelps, Michael E.
   [DNLM: 1. Tomography, Emission-Computed—methods.   2. Brain Mapping—methods.
   3. Heart Diseases—diagnosis.   4. Neoplasms—diagnosis.   WN 206 P477 2003]
RC78.7.T62P465 2003
616.07′575—dc21   2003052958

ISBN 0-387-40359-0   Printed on acid-free paper.

Printed in China.

9 8 7 6 5 4 3 2 1   SPIN 10937013

www.springer-ny.com

Springer-Verlag New York Berlin Heidelberg
A member of BertelsmannSpringer Science+Business Media GmbH

CONTENTS

PREFACE

This book is written as both a text and a reference book. It contains numerous images from the biological sciences and clinical practice, tables, graphs, and figures, as well as exercises that are worked out to aid the reader in understanding principles or solving problems. In some cases, derivations are placed in appendices so as not to break up the flow of the subject matter in the text.

The book is intended for a broad audience interested in molecular imaging with positron emission tomography (PET). It is expected that the readers will range from undergraduate, graduate, and medical students to residents, physicians, and scientists with backgrounds from various physical, biological, and medical specialty areas. Each chapter presents material in a straightforward manner that is well illustrated and explained. Because of the diverse audience for the book, certain chapters or sections of chapters will be of more interest than others to certain segments of the readership.

Chapter 1 introduces the fundamental physics upon which PET imaging systems is based and discusses in detail the technologies and methods used to produce PET images. The chapter starts out by reviewing the physics of positron emission and annihilation and explains how positron range and photon noncolinearity in coincidence detection place certain limits on spatial resolution.

Next, detector technologies suitable for detecting 511 keV annihilation photons are introduced and the geometries for typical PET scanner configurations discussed. The corrections needed to achieve quantitative images, namely detector normalization, detector dead-time correction, attenuation correction, and correction for scattered and accidental coincidences are explained. The various types of algorithms used to reconstruct the data recorded by the PET scanner into tomographic images are described.

Finally, methods for assessing the performance of PET imaging systems are presented. The PET systems described range from human PET and PET/CT scanners to those used for small animal imaging.

Chapter 2 presents molecular imaging assays as a central theme to using PET as a fundamental tool for dissecting molecular events that constitute biological processes. The assay developer must integrate information from all the other chapters of the book in order to produce quantitative tracer kinetic models and biological assays. A knowledge of tracer kinetics also guides the development of new molecular imaging probes.

The fundamental requirements of quantitative PET data for tracer kinetic modeling are initially discussed followed by defining the central principles underlying tracer kinetic modeling including compartmental models, perfusion, volume of distribution, rate constants, rate coefficients, and flux. The "tracer thought experiment" is used to help the reader visualize the movement of a tracer throughout the body in order to build an understanding of how to develop a comprehensive tracer kinetic model and assay.

Specific examples of various PET tracer kinetic models including the ^{18}F-fluorodeoxyglucose three-compartment model, ^{13}N-ammonia and ^{15}O-water perfusion models, and receptor–ligand models are presented. The fundamental nature of the input function, tissue time–activity curve, and differential equations governing various models are described. In addition, the approach to structuring new models for imaging PET reporter gene expression are presented in detail to highlight the step-by-step process of building a model. Model validation and fitting of PET data to a given model are also detailed. The translation of PET assays from animal models to human subjects is examined.

Numerous work sets and systematic guidelines, reinforced with specific examples, provide the reader with an intuitive and fundamental understanding of PET assay development.

Chapter 3 describes the concept of the "electronic generator" for preparing PET molecular imaging probes. An electronic generator represents the integration of a small cyclotron with an automated molecular imaging probe synthesizer operating under the control of a personal computer. This technology, revolutionized by joint efforts between academia and industry, enables production of multiple doses of various PET molecular imaging probes by a technician for clinical and research applications.

Discussed in this chapter are the fundamental principles behind positive, and negative-ion cyclotrons and the advantages of the latter for the automated production of positron emitting isotopes for PET. A description of the relevant parameters that determine the course of nuclear reactions and a conceptual design of a cyclotron target body appropriate for the production of positron emitting isotopes are also provided. A number of numerical examples are included to accentuate and facilitate understanding of all these basic concepts and the mathematical relationships defining them.

Important ^{15}O-, ^{13}N-, ^{11}C- and ^{18}F-labeled precursors that are currently used in the synthesis of labeled molecular imaging probes for PET are summarized. Representative examples of low-energy small cyclotrons, target systems, and automated radiosynthesis modules are also discussed from the standpoint of the genesis and future of electronic generators.

Finally, the crucial role of the recent FDA legislative action, namely, FDAMA '97, on PET radiopharmacies and their impact on the emerging clinical PET are addressed.

Chapter 4 describes the fundamental principles of molecular imaging probe design as a biochemical tool to reveal the molecular basis of normal biological processes and those of disease. Emphasis is given to the ultimate objective of the molecular imaging determination, namely, how properly designed molecular probes are used to select out and quantify the target process to be measured. Specific examples illustrate the main concepts and their extension to the development of other imaging probes.

Molecular imaging probes (diagnostics) and drugs (therapeutics) share common concepts in structural design and common biochemical targets of enzymes, receptors, neurotransmitter systems, RNA, DNA, and pathological depositions. Application of molecular imaging to aid in drug development (e.g., receptor occupancy determinations, pharmacokinetics, surrogate markers, the development of combinatorial radiolabeled drug libraries) is discussed. The concept of making molecular imaging probes available to physicians and researchers via distribution centers is also illustrated.

Chapter 5 focuses on the integration of PET imaging with ^{18}F-fluorodeoxyglucose (FDG) into the care of patients with cancer. PET has now been incorporated into diagnostic algorithms for many cancers, and the number of PET studies performed in the United States is approaching a million per year in 2003 and is increasing at a rate of about 50%/year. A similar magnitude and rate of growth is occurring for the rest of the world.

The chapter reviews the clinical role and accuracy of FDG-PET for diagnosing, staging, and detecting recurrent disease in various cancers in the context of other diagnostic imaging modalities. In addition, the role of PET for monitoring various cancer treatments is discussed. Further, the prognostic value, cost-effectiveness, and impact on patient management with FDG-PET are reviewed.

New concepts for molecular imaging of cancer with PET are introduced. These include the emergence of combined PET/CT imaging devices and the development of new tracers that target specific biological properties of cancer cells including ^{11}C-acetate and ^{18}F-fluoroethylcholine for lipid synthesis and ^{18}F-fluorothymidine (FLT) for assessing DNA replication and cell proliferation.

Chapter 6 examines the principles, methods, and applications of PET to the study and characterization of the cardiovascular system. The chapter proceeds from studies of normal cardiac function to its failure in disease. The impact of the heart's anatomical and functional properties on PET images of the cardiovascular system are examined. Approaches are presented for deriving qualitative and, more importantly, quantitative information on regional molecular imaging probe tissue concentrations. Since quantitative information is fundamental to the application tracer kinetic principles to the heart, it is reviewed in considerable detail together with a description of how this information can be employed for the determination of regional rates of blood flow, oxygen consumption, and substrate metabolism in the myocardium. PET-derived estimates of these processes for the normal human heart are summarized in several tables together with data established through invasive techniques.

The chapter then explores the value of PET for diagnosing and characterizing coronary artery disease by utilizing measurements of myocardial blood flow and its response to physiological and pharmacological stresses. The use of these types of studies for detecting pre-clinical coronary artery disease, as well as for monitoring responses to lifestyle and pharmacological risk factor modification, are also described.

Alterations of myocardial substrate metabolism as observed with PET in non-coronary cardiac disease are then reviewed. This is followed by an extensive description of the utility of PET for the assessment of myocardial viability in cardiac disease. Underlying pathophysiological mechanisms are examined and related to alterations in blood flow and substrate metabolism as observed with PET.

Relevant to the clinician, the chapter then discusses clinical implications of viability assessments with PET, especially in the severely symptomatic patient with end-stage coronary artery disease. The chapter concludes by reviewing current and future clinical applications of PET in patients with cardiovascular disease.

Chapter 7 covers the ways in which imaging studies with PET have advanced our understanding of the brain through in vivo assessment of diverse aspects of neurobiology and biochemistry. In vivo measurements of cerebral glucose metabolism, blood flow, enzyme activities, neurotransmitter synthesis, and receptor binding are described, along with the ways in which such parameters are affected by normal development and by a host of neurological and psychiatric disorders.

The properties and actions of the molecular imaging probes used in studying the brain are integral to understanding the measurements of cerebral function made with PET. This knowledge of molecular imaging probes is discussed alongside the kinds of investigations in which the probes are employed.

Since the synthesis of over 95% of the adenosine triphosphate (ATP) molecules that are hydrolyzed to fuel cerebral function originates from metabolism of glucose, PET imaging of glucose metabolism with FDG provides an excellent way to evaluate the distributed function of the brain. Studies of various normal and disease states of the brain are presented to illustrate this approach to mapping cerebral function and providing an accurate disease diagnosis.

Studies are presented to show how the anatomical pattern of blood flow imaged with diffusible tracers such as ^{15}O-water closely parallels that of the cerebral metabolic rate for glucose throughout much of the normal brain. Examples are also shown where under certain pathologic circumstances the normal coupling between glucose metabolism and blood flow is disturbed.

PET provides a unique window through which to view neurotransmitter systems in the brain with a continuing goal in PET research to design molecular imaging probes and tracer kinetic models that provide detailed assessments of neurotransmitter system function in vivo. PET methods have been developed to assess occupancy of receptors by pharmacologic doses of drugs and the effects of drugs on neurotransmitter release. As studies on other neurotransmitter systems have largely mimicked approaches used for the dopamine system, a detailed presentation of dopaminergic PET probes and their applications are first presented, followed by probes used in studying serotonergic, cholinergic, GABAergic, and opioid neurotransmitter systems.

Phenomena that had previously been studied at only the psychological level, such as human mood states, pain perception, and substance abuse, are explored in terms of their underlying neuroanatomical and neurochemical substrates, in living human beings. Many diseases that show no gross structural abnormalities on CT and MRI have been revealed with molecular imaging studies with PET. Disorders in which PET is used to examine biological abnormalities in human brain that are detailed in the text include Alzheimer's, Parkinson's, and other neurodegenerative diseases, epilepsy, cerebrovascular disease, pain syndromes, depression, obsessive–compulsive disorder, schizophrenia, and addiction. In addition, related work conducted with PET in non-human primates and rodents is highlighted.

Finally, this chapter looks at some of the future directions of PET in the study of the biological basis of both normal and abnormal states of the brain.

MICHAEL E. PHELPS, PhD

ACKNOWLEDGMENTS

PET continues to mature as a molecular imaging technology for the scientific exploration and for molecular diagnostics of the biological basis of cellular function in vivo through great ideas from great people.

Joining in this effort have been dedicated members of Congress and the administration such as Senators Stevens, Kennedy, and their colleagues; Liz Connell of Senator Stevens' staff, HHS Secretaries Shalala and Thompson; and Dr. Sean Tunis of CMS. The Biological and Environmental Research Division of the Department of Energy supported PET in that most difficult period, "In the Beginning," and has continued to do so, under the direction of Dr. Ari Patrinos, along with the National Institutes of Health, under the direction of Alias Zerhouni.

I am most appreciative of the faculty, students, technologists, and staff at UCLA who have stood with me through the good times and the difficult ones. They have always remained enthusiastic and passionate about doing their part to make PET successful through the long days and nights of this journey. The UCLA faculty and staff have trained a large percentage of the people in PET throughout the world and this has been our privilege.

I am appreciative that my university, UCLA, has provided so many resources to my program and has put up with so many demands that I have placed on them. I have posed awkward situations for them at times but I have always tried to make up for this by also being productive.

The chapter authors have labored for two years to write this book. They have gone through many re-writes and debates with me that have at times been challenging to our relationship. We surfaced from all this as we began—great colleagues and friends who are proud of what we accomplish together.

Norton Simon deserves special recognition as the greatest teacher I ever had. He was also my friend. Before he passed away in 1993 he gave me a precious present in a simple saying, "Life has a natural curve. You go up, plateau and go down. The only way to deal with this is to be constantly starting new curves and in this way always remain in a state of becoming."

This guiding statement and Norton will always be a part of my life.

MICHAEL E. PHELPS, PHD

CONTRIBUTORS

Jorge R. Barrio, PhD
Professor, Department of Molecular
and Medical Pharmacology, David
Geffen School of Medicine,
University of California, Los
Angeles, Los Angeles, CA 90095-
1735, USA.

Simon R. Cherry, PhD
Professor, Biomedical Engineering,
University of California, Davis,
Davis, CA 95616, USA.

Johannes Czernin, MD
Associate Professor, Department of
Molecular and Medical
Pharmacology, Chief, Ahmanson
Biological Imaging Division,
David Geffen School of Medicine,
University of California, Los Angeles,
Los Angeles, CA 90095-1735, USA.

Magnus Dahlbom, PhD
Associate Professor, Department of
Molecular and Medical
Pharmacology/Nuclear Medicine,
David Geffen School of Medicine,
University of California, Los
Angeles, Los Angeles, CA 90095-
1735, USA.

Sanjiv Sam Gambhir, MD, PhD
Director, Molecular Imaging
Program at Stanford (MIPS), Head,
Division of Nuclear Medicine,
Professor, Department of Radiology
and Bio-X Program, Stanford
University School of Medicine,
Stanford, CA 94305-5427, USA.

William P. Melega, PhD
Associate Professor, Department of
Molecular and Medical
Pharmacology, David Geffen School
of Medicine, University of
California, Los Angeles,
Los Angeles, CA 90095-1735, USA.

Nagichettiar Satyamurthy, PhD
Professor, Department of Molecular
and Medical Pharmacology,
David Geffen School of Medicine,
University of California, Los
Angeles, Los Angeles, CA 90095-
1735, USA.

Heinrich R. Schelbert, MD, PhD
George V. Taplin Professor,
Department of Molecular and
Medical Pharmacology, David
Geffen School of Medicine,
University of California, Los
Angeles, Los Angeles, CA 90095-
1735, USA.

Daniel H.S. Silverman, MD, PhD
Assistant Professor, Department of
Molecular and Medical
Pharmacology/Nuclear Medicine,
David Geffen School of Medicine,
University of California, Los
Angeles, Los Angeles, CA 90095-
1735, USA.

CHAPTER 1

PET: Physics, Instrumentation, and Scanners

Simon R. Cherry and Magnus Dahlbom

Positron emission tomography (PET) is a nuclear imaging technique that uses the unique decay characteristics of radionuclides that decay by positron emission. These radionuclides are produced in a cyclotron and are then used to label compounds of biological interest. The labeled compound (typically 10^{13}–10^{15} labeled molecules) is introduced into the body, usually by intravenous injection, and is distributed in tissues in a manner determined by its biochemical properties. When the radioactive atom on a particular molecule decays, a positron is ejected from the nucleus, ultimately leading to the emission of high-energy photons that have a good probability of escaping from the body. A PET scanner consists of a set of detectors that surround the object to be imaged and are designed to convert these high-energy photons into an electrical signal that can be fed to subsequent electronics. In a typical PET scan, 10^6 to 10^9 events (decays) will be detected. These events are corrected for a number of factors and then reconstructed into a tomographic image using mathematical algorithms. The output of the reconstruction process is a three-dimensional (3-D) image volume, where the signal intensity in any particular image voxel* is proportional to the amount of the radionuclide (and, hence, the amount of the labeled molecule to which it is attached) in that voxel. Thus, PET images allow the spatial distribution of radiolabeled tracers to be mapped quantitatively in a living human. By taking a time sequence of images, the tissue concentration of the radiolabeled molecules as a function of time is measured, and with appropriate mathematical modeling, the rate of specific biological processes can be determined (Chapter 2).

This chapter is designed to give the reader a solid understanding of the physics and instrumentation aspects of PET, including how PET data are collected and formed into an image. The chapter begins with a review of the basic physics underlying PET and discusses in detail the detector technology used in modern PET scanners. The manner in which PET data are acquired is described, and the many correction factors that must be applied to ensure that the data are

---

*A voxel is a volume element in a three-dimensional image array. It is analogous to a pixel in a two-dimensional image array.

quantitative are introduced. The methods by which PET data are reconstructed into a three-dimensional image volume are explained, along with some of the approaches that are used to analyze and quantify the resultant images. Finally, a variety of modern PET imaging systems are discussed, including those designed for clinical service and research and small-animal imaging, along with methods for evaluating the performance of these systems.

PHYSICS OF POSITRON EMISSION AND ANNIHILATION

Basic nuclear physics and positron emission

The nucleus of an atom is composed of two different types of *nucleons*, known as *protons* and *neutrons*. These particles have similar masses but differ in that a proton has positive charge, whereas a neutron is uncharged. A cloud of negatively charged *electrons* surrounds the nucleus. In an uncharged atom, the number of electrons equals the number of protons. The basic properties of protons, electrons, and neutrons are listed in Table 1-1. The number of protons in an atom is known as the *atomic number* (often denoted as Z) and defines the element to which the atom belongs. The total number of nucleons is known as the *mass number*, often denoted by A. Atoms with the same Z, but different values of A, are *isotopes* of the element corresponding to atomic number Z. Nuclei usually are defined by the following notation:

$$^{A}_{Z}X \; or \; ^{A}X \tag{1-1}$$

where X is the one- or two-letter symbol for the element with atomic number Z (e.g., Fe for iron and C for carbon), and A is the mass number. For example, ^{18}F is an isotope of fluorine and consists of 9 protons (because it is fluorine) and 9 neutrons. Sometimes, this isotope will also be written as F-18 or fluorine-18.

> **EXAMPLE 1-1**
> How many neutrons and protons are in the nucleus of ^{13}N?
>
> **ANSWER**
> Consulting a periodic table of the elements reveals that nitrogen has an atomic number of 7 and therefore, 7 protons. The mass number of this isotope is 13, so the number of neutrons must be $(13 - 7) = 6$.
>
> **EXAMPLE 1-2**
> How would an atom with 29 protons and 35 neutrons be written in the notation of Equation 1-1?
>
> **ANSWER**
> Referring to a periodic table of the elements shows that the element corresponding to Z = 29 is copper (symbol Cu). The total number of nucleons is $(29 + 35) = 64$. Therefore, this nucleus is ^{64}Cu.

The nucleus is held together by two opposing forces. The strong force is an attractive force between nucleons and is balanced by the repulsive coulomb (elec-

TABLE 1-1. Mass and Charge Properties of Nucleons, Electrons, and Positrons

	Proton (p)	Neutron (n)	Electron (e$^-$)	Positron (e$^+$)
Mass	1.67×10^{-27} kg	1.67×10^{-27} kg	9.1×10^{-31} kg	9.1×10^{-31} kg
Charge	$+1.6 \times 10^{-19}$ C	0	-1.6×10^{-19} C	$+1.6 \times 10^{-19}$ C

Based on data from Handbook of Physics and Chemistry, 71st Edition, Ed: D.R. Lide, CRC Press, Boca Raton, FL, 1991.

trical) force between the positively charged protons. If a nucleus has either an excess number of protons or neutrons, it is unstable and prone to radioactive decay, leading to a change in the number of protons or neutrons in the nucleus and a more stable configuration. Nuclei that decay in this manner are known as *radionuclides*. For a specific element with atomic number Z, isotopes that are unstable and which undergo radioactive decay are known as *radioisotopes* of that element.

One common method by which nuclei with an excess of protons may decay is through *positron emission* (also known as β^+ or *beta-plus decay*). Essentially, a proton in the nucleus of the atom is converted into a neutron (n) and a positron (e$^+$). The positron is the antiparticle to the electron with the same mass but opposite electric charge (see Table 1-1). The positron is ejected from the nucleus, along with a neutrino (ν) that is not detected. An example of a radionuclide that decays by positron emission is ^{11}C:

$$^{11}C \rightarrow {}^{11}B + e^+ + \nu \tag{1-2}$$

The net energy released during positron emission is shared between the daughter nucleus, the positron, and the neutrino. Positrons are therefore emitted with a range of energies, from zero up to a maximum *endpoint energy* E$_{max}$. This endpoint energy is determined by the difference in atomic masses between the parent atom and the daughter atom, taking into account gamma-ray emission from excited states that may occur if the transition is not between the ground states of the two nuclei. The mean kinetic energy of the emitted positrons is approximately $0.33 \times E_{max}$. Decay by positron emission is the basis for PET imaging.

Proton-rich radionuclides also can decay by a process known as *electron capture*. Here, the nucleus captures an orbital electron and converts a proton into a neutron, thus decreasing the atomic number Z by one. Once again, a neutrino is released. An example of electron capture would be the decay of ^{125}I:

$$^{125}I \rightarrow {}^{125}Te + \nu \tag{1-3}$$

Electron capture decay can lead to emission of x-rays (filling of the orbital vacancy created by the captured electron) or gamma-rays (electron capture leaves the nucleus in an excited state with further decay to the ground state by emission of one or more gamma-rays). These emissions may also be used for in vivo imaging but do not share the unique properties of decay by positron emission which are explained in the section on Annihilation (p. 5). Decay by electron capture and positron emission compete with one another, with positron emission usually being the dominant process in low Z nuclei, and electron capture being more likely in higher Z nuclei. Radionuclides that decay predominantly by positron emission are preferred for PET imaging.

TABLE 1-2. Select List of Radionuclides That Decay by Positron Emission and Are Relevant to PET Imaging

Radionuclide	Half-life	$E_{max}(Mev)$	β^+ Branching Fraction
^{11}C	20.4 min	0.96	1.00
^{13}N	9.97 min	1.20	1.00
^{15}O	122 s	1.73	1.00
^{18}F	109.8 min	0.63	0.97
^{22}Na	2.60 y	0.55	0.90
^{62}Cu	9.74 min	2.93	0.97
^{64}Cu	12.7 h	0.65	0.29
^{68}Ga	67.6 min	1.89	0.89
^{76}Br	16.2 h	Various	0.56
^{82}Rb	1.27 min	2.60, 3.38	0.96
^{124}I	4.17 d	1.53, 2.14	0.23

Based on data from Table of Nuclides: www2.bnl.gov/ton (accessed October 17th, 2002)

Many radionuclides decay by positron emission. Table 1-2 presents a selection of these radionuclides that are commonly encountered in relation to PET imaging. The production of these positron-emitting radionuclides for medical use is discussed in Chapter 3. Included in the table are the maximum kinetic energy of the emitted positrons, E_{max}, and the fraction of decays that occur by positron emission. The energy of the emissions from radioactive decay are normally given in units of electron volts (eV), which is a more convenient unit than standard Système International (SI) energy units for handling the relatively small energies involved. One electron volt is defined as being equal to the energy acquired by an electron when it is accelerated through a potential difference of one volt. The conversion to joules, the SI unit for energy is:

$$1 \text{ eV} = 1.6 \times 10^{-19} \text{ J} \tag{1-4}$$

For PET imaging, units of kiloelectron volts (1 keV $= 10^3$ eV) and megaelectron volts (1 MeV $= 10^6$ eV) are commonly used.

Table 1-2 also lists the half-life of the radionuclides. A sample of identical radioactive atoms will decay in an exponential fashion, and the half-life is the time required for half the atoms in the sample to decay. The relationship between the activity A of a sample at time t, and the half-life, $T_{1/2}$, is given by:

$$A(t) = A(0)\exp(-\ln2 \times t/T_{1/2}) \tag{1-5}$$

where A(0) is the activity of the sample at time 0. Activity is measured in units of the number of disintegrations per second:

$$1 \text{ bequerel (Bq)} = 1 \text{ disintegration per second} \tag{1-6}$$

In the United States, traditional units of the curie (Ci) and millicurie (1 mCi $= 10^{-3}$ Ci) are still frequently used. The conversion is:

$$1 \text{ mCi} = 37 \times 10^6 \text{ Bq} = 37 \text{ MBq} \tag{1-7a}$$

or

$$1 \text{ MBq} = 27 \times 10^{-6} \text{ Ci} = 27 \text{ } \mu\text{Ci} \tag{1-7b}$$

For more information on the physics of positron emission, see the textbook by Evans.[1]

EXAMPLE 1-3

A sample of ^{18}F is measured at 10:40 AM and has an activity of 30 MBq. It is injected into a patient at 11:30 AM. How much activity was injected?

ANSWER

From Table 1-2, the half-life of ^{18}F is 109.8 minutes. The time elapsed between measurement of the sample and injection is 50 minutes. Using Equation 1-5, the activity at the time of injection is:

$$A(t) = 30 \text{ MBq} \times \exp(-0.693 \times 50/109.8) = 21.9 \text{ MBq}$$

Annihilation

The positron that is ejected following β^+ decay has a very short lifetime in electron-rich material such as tissue. It rapidly loses its kinetic energy in inelastic interactions with atomic electrons in the tissue, and once most of its energy is dissipated (typically within 10^{-1} to 10^{-2} cm, depending on its energy), it will combine with an electron and form a hydrogen-like state known as *positronium*. In the analogy to hydrogen, the proton that forms the nucleus in a hydrogen atom is substituted by a positron. This state lasts only about 10^{-10} seconds before a process known as *annihilation* occurs, where the mass of the electron and the positron is converted into electromagnetic energy. Because the positron and electron are almost at rest when this occurs, the energy released comes largely from the mass of the particles and can be computed from Einstein's mass-energy equivalence as:

$$E = mc^2 = m_e c^2 + m_p c^2 \qquad (1\text{-}8)$$

where m_e is the mass of the electron, m_p is the mass of the positron, and c is the speed of light (3×10^8 m/s). Inserting the values from Table 1-1, and using Equation 1-8 and the conversion in Equation 1-4, the energy released can be shown to be 1.022 MeV.

The energy is released in the form of high-energy photons. As the positron and electron are almost at rest when the annihilation occurs, the net momentum is close to zero. Because momentum as well as energy must be conserved, it is not in general possible for annihilation to result in the emission of a single photon; otherwise, a net momentum would occur in the direction of that photon. Instead, two photons are emitted simultaneously in opposite directions (180° apart), carrying an energy equal to 1.022 MeV/2, or 511 keV, ensuring that both energy and momentum are conserved. This process is shown schematically in Figure 1-1. Higher order annihilation, in which more than 2 photons are emitted, is also possible, but only occurs in about 0.003% of the annihilations.

The annihilation process has a number of very important properties that are advantageous for imaging and lead directly to the concept of PET. First, the annihilation photons are very energetic (they fall in the gamma-ray region of the electromagnetic spectrum and are roughly a factor of ten higher in energy than diagnostic x-rays), which means they have a good chance of escaping the body for external detection. It is, therefore, the annihilation photons that are detected in PET imaging, not the positrons (which are absorbed locally). Second, two photons are emitted with a precise geometric relationship. If both photons can

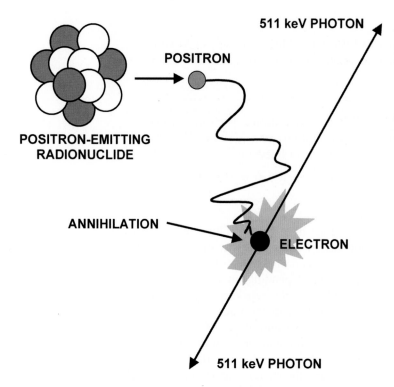

511 keV PHOTON

POSITRON

POSITRON-EMITTING RADIONUCLIDE

ANNIHILATION

ELECTRON

511 keV PHOTON

FIGURE 1-1. The process of positron emission and subsequent positron-electron annihilation results in two 511 keV annihilation photons emitted 180° apart. The site of annihilation is usually very close to the point of positron emission because the emitted positrons rapidly lose their energy in tissue (see Figure 1-5).

be detected and localized externally, the line joining the detected locations passes directly through the point of annihilation (Figure 1-2A). This was originally referred to as *electronic collimation.*[2] Because the point of annihilation is very close to the point of positron emission, this also gives a good indication (again to within a line) of where the radioactive atom was in the body. Contrast this with radioactive decay schemes that result in emission of a single photon. Although a single detector can be used, the detection and localization of a single photon tells nothing about where it came from in the body (Figure 1-2B). The direction of the photon can only be determined by the using a form of absorptive collimation, which only allows photons emitted in a certain direction to impinge on the detector (Figure 1-2C). This reduces the number of events that are detected for a given amount of radioactivity in the body by at least 1 to 2 orders of magnitude compared with electronic collimation. Electronic collimation also allows events to be collected from many different directions simultaneously leading to the capability of rapid tomographic imaging (see Image Reconstruction, p. 70). Third, all positron-emitting radionuclides, independent of the element involved, or the energy of the emitted positrons, ultimately lead to the emission of two back-to-back 511 keV photons; that is, a PET scanner can be designed and optimized for imaging all positron-emitting radionuclides at this single energy. One drawback to this, however, is that it is not possible to perform dual-radionuclide studies with PET and distinguish between the radionuclides based on the energy of the emissions. Because the annihilation photons fall in the gamma-ray region of the electromagnetic spectrum, the terms photons and gamma-rays are often used interchangeably when referring to the annihilation photons. Annihilation photons is technically the correct term because the radiation does not

FIGURE 1-2. (A) Radionuclides that decay by positron emission result in two annihilation photons emitted 180° apart. If both photons are detected, the detection locations define (to within the distance traveled by the positron prior to annihilation) a line along which the decaying atom was located. (B) Radionuclides that decay by emitting single photons provide no positional information, as a detected event could originate from anywhere in the sample volume. (C) For single photon imaging, physical collimation can be used to absorb all photons except those that are incident on the detector from one particular direction (in this case perpendicular to the detector face), defining a line of origin just like the coincident 511-keV photons do following positron emission. To achieve this localization, however, the radiation from the majority of decays has been absorbed and does not contribute to image formation, leading to the detection of many fewer events for a given amount of radioactivity in the object. Absorptive collimation of this kind is the approach used in planar nuclear medicine imaging and in single photon emission computed tomography (SPECT).

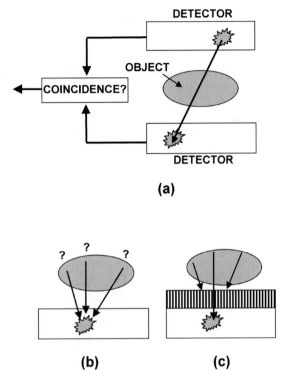

arise directly from the nucleus. However, the properties of annihilation photons are absolutely identical to a 511-keV gamma-ray—the difference in terminology reflects their different origins.

The annihilation process forms the basis for PET imaging. A PET scanner is designed to detect and localize the simultaneous back-to-back annihilation photons that are emitted following decay of a radionuclide by positron emission (Figure 1-3). In a typical PET scan, many millions of these photon pairs will be detected from a compound that is tagged with a positron-emitting radionuclide and which has been injected into the body.

As described above, the detection of the annihilation photons only localizes the location of the radioactive atom to within a line joining the detecting positions. Two approaches can then be used to form an image that reflects the actual locations of the radioactive atoms and, therefore, the compound to which it is attached. The first approach is conceptually the most simple, but is rarely used. It involves measuring the difference in arrival time of the two photons at the detectors. Obviously, if an annihilation occurs closer to detector 1 than detector 2, then the annihilation photon directed towards detector 1 will arrive at that detector earlier than the annihilation photon directed towards detector 2. The relationship between the difference in arrival time of the two annihilation photons, Δt, and the location d of the annihilation with respect to a point exactly half-way between the two detectors, is given by:

$$d = \frac{\Delta t \times c}{2} \tag{1-9}$$

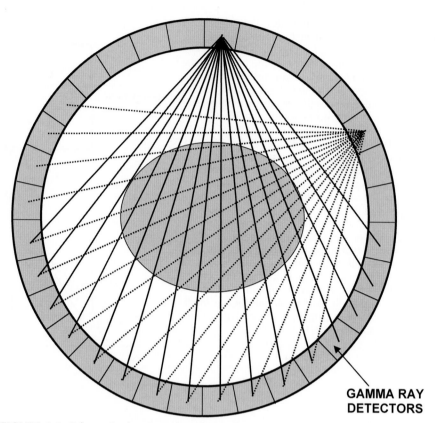

**GAMMA RAY
DETECTORS**

FIGURE 1-3. Schematic drawing of a PET scanner consisting of a ring of high-energy photon (gamma-ray) detectors. A ring geometry is shown, but other possibilities include polygonal assemblies of panels and opposing rotating planar detectors. The detectors are designed to record as many of the annihilation photons as possible and to locate the line along which the decay occurred by determining the two interaction vertices. Each detector is in electronic coincidence with a fan of detectors on the opposite side of the ring, so the object is simultaneously sampled from many different angles. For clarity, the measured lines of response for just two detectors are shown in this figure. Typically, 10^6 to 10^9 events (detections of annihilation photon pairs) are needed in a PET scan to reconstruct a statistically meaningful image of the distribution of radioactivity in the body.

where c is the speed of light (30 cm/ns). In practice, this method, known as *time of flight*, is very difficult and costly to implement because of the very small time differences involved. Even a timing resolution as fine as 100 ps would only yield a positional resolution of $\sim$1.5 cm. With currently available detector technology, the best timing resolution that can be achieved is on the order of a few hundred picoseconds. Therefore, time-of-flight approaches do not yield the desired accuracy of a few millimeters, and no PET scanners are currently manufactured using this technique. The approach that is used almost universally involves the concept of *computed tomography*. By measuring the total radioactivity along lines that pass at many different angles through the object, mathematical algorithms can be used to compute cross-sectional images that reflect the concentration of the positron-emitting radionuclide in tissues throughout the body. This is discussed in Image Reconstruction (p. 70).

Positron range and noncolinearity

There are two effects in PET imaging systems that lead to errors in determining the line along which a positron-emitting radionuclide is to be found. These effects place some finite limits on the spatial resolution attainable with PET and manifest themselves as a blurring of the reconstructed images.

The first of these effects is positron range. As shown in Figure 1-4 (top), this is the distance from the site of positron emission to the site of annihilation. A PET scanner detects the annihilation photons which define the line along which the annihilation takes place, not the line along which the decaying atom is located. Because the positrons follow a tortuous path in tissue, undergoing multiple direction-changing interactions with electrons prior to annihilation, the total path length the positron travels is considerably longer than the positron range. From the perspective of PET imaging, it is the perpendicular distance from the emission site to the line defined by the annihilation photons that matters and which causes mispositioning.

As described earlier, radionuclides differ in the energy of emitted positrons. Some radionuclides emit, on average, higher energy positrons than others, making the positron range effect radionuclide-dependent. Figure 1-5 shows the annihilation locations for positron emission from a point source emitter located at the center of a block of tissue-equivalent material. Notice the broader distribution for oxygen-15 (a high energy positron emitter with $E_{max} = 1.72$ MeV) compared to fluorine-18 ($E_{max} = 0.64$ MeV). Profiles through these distributions reveal that they are nonGaussian in nature and are best fitted by exponential functions. Several groups have either measured,[3] computed,[4] or simulated[5] these distributions. Although the trends are similar, some disagreement between these studies is noted on the exact width and shape of the distribution. The blurring effect on the final PET image, however, clearly ranges from a few tenths of a millimeter up to several millimeters, depending on the radionuclide and its E_{max}.

Positron range limits the ultimate resolution attainable by PET. Studies have shown the ability to reduce positron range, particularly in radionuclides with large E_{max}, by using strong magnetic fields.[6–8] However, this is not currently practical to implement in the complex setting of a PET system. The positron range distribution may also in theory be deconvolved from the PET image.[9,10] In practice, the data rarely, if ever, have the statistical quality (sufficient number of events) to make this advantageous, as deconvolution leads to noise amplification. A better approach may be to incorporate positron range distribution information into iterative reconstruction algorithms (Iterative Reconstruction Methods, p. 86), which should lead to improvements in image resolution that are consistent with the statistical quality of the data when using positron-emitters with a high E_{max}. To put this discussion in perspective, it should also be pointed out that positron range is not a major limiting factor in PET imaging at the present time, except perhaps in animal studies of the very highest resolution using positron emitters with relatively high values (> 1.5 MeV) of E_{max}.

The second effect comes from the fact that the positron and electron are not completely at rest when they annihilate. The small net momentum of these particles means that the annihilation photons will not be at exactly 180° and will, in fact, be emitted with a distribution of angles around 180°. This is known as

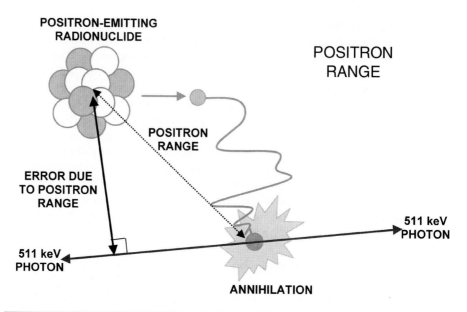

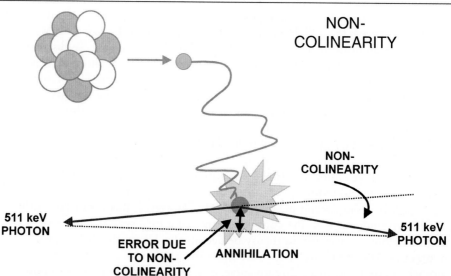

FIGURE 1-4. Error in determining the location of the emitting nucleus due to positron range (top) and noncolinearity (bottom). The positron range error is dependent on the energy of the emitted positrons. Noncolinearity is independent of radionuclide, and the error is determined by the separation of the detectors. The deviation from noncolinearity is highly exaggerated in the figure; the average angular deviation from 180° is about ± 0.25°. (Reproduced with permission from Cherry SR, Sorenson JA, Phelps ME. *Physics in Nuclear Medicine*, W.B. Saunders, New York, 2003.)

FIGURE 1-5. A: Simulations for several PET radionuclides showing the distribution of positron annihilation sites in water for positrons emitted at the center of the image (position 0.0 mm). B: Profiles through the simulated distributions showing measured FWHM and FWTM of the distributions. Abbreviations: FWHM, full width at half maximum; FWTM, full width at tenth maximum. (Reproduced with permission from Levin C, Hoffman EJ. *Phys Med Biol* 1999, 44: 781–799.)

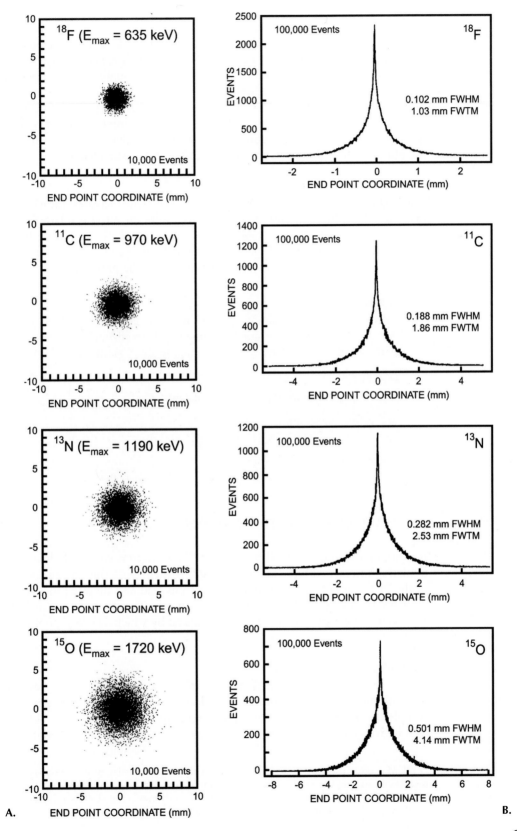

A.

B.

11

noncolinearity. This effect is independent of radionuclide because the positrons must lose most of their energy before they can annihilate; hence, the initial energy is irrelevant. The distribution of emitted angles is roughly Gaussian in shape, with a full width at half maximum (FWHM)* of ~0.5°. After detecting the annihilation photons, PET assumes that the emission was exactly back to back, resulting in a small error in locating the line of annihilation (Figure 1-4 bottom). Assuming a Gaussian distribution and using the fact that the angles are small, the blurring effect due to noncolinearity, Δ_{nc}, can be estimated as:

$$\Delta_{nc} = 0.0022 \times D \qquad\qquad (1\text{-}10)$$

where D is the diameter of the PET scanner. The error increases linearly as the diameter of the PET scanner increases. Once again, the effect is relatively small compared with the detector resolution in most clinical PET scanners. In PET scanners used for animals, D generally is small, and as illustrated in Example 1-4, noncolinearity is not a major limiting factor at the present time.

EXAMPLE 1-4
Calculate the blurring due to photon noncolinearity in an 80-cm diameter PET scanner designed for imaging humans and in a 15-cm diameter PET scanner designed for imaging small animals.

ANSWER
From Equation 1-10, the blurring is calculated as:

80-cm human scanner:
$$\Delta_{nc} = 0.0022 \times D = 0.0022 \times 800 \text{ mm} = 1.76 \text{ mm}$$

15-cm small-animal scanner:
$$\Delta_{nc} = 0.0022 \times D = 0.0022 \times 150 \text{ mm} = 0.33 \text{ mm}$$

---

511 keV PHOTON INTERACTIONS IN MATTER

It is important to understand how the 511-keV photons emitted following annihilation interact with the tissue surrounding them, with the detector material of the PET scanner, and with materials such as lead and tungsten that may be used for shielding or slice collimation purposes. The *photoelectric effect* and *Compton scattering* are two major mechanisms by which 511-keV photons interact with matter.

Photoelectric interactions
Figure 1-6 summarizes interaction by the photoelectric effect. A 511-keV photon will interact with an atom as a whole in the surrounding medium and is completely absorbed by transferring its energy to an orbital electron. This electron is given enough energy to escape the atom but is quickly absorbed in solids

---

*FWHM is often used to characterize a distribution that is Gaussian or nearly Gaussian and involves measuring the width of the distribution at the point where it reaches half the maximum amplitude. A related measure, full width at tenth maximum (FWTM), identifies the width of the distribution where it reaches one tenth of its maximum amplitude.

FIGURE 1-6. Schematic representation of the photoelectric effect. The incident photon transfers all of its energy to an electron which is ejected from the atom but which is itself absorbed by material nearby. (Reproduced with permission from Cherry SR, Sorenson JA, Phelps ME. *Physics in Nuclear Medicine*, W.B. Saunders, New York, 2003.)

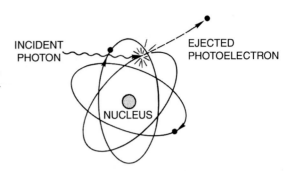

and liquids. An x-ray with an energy equal to the binding energy of the electron is also generated as the vacancy in the electron shell of the atom is filled. These x-rays typically have energies of tens of keV and are also quickly absorbed in the medium. The net result of a photoelectric interaction in a reasonably dense liquid or solid is the complete absorption of the original photon with all 511 keV of energy deposited locally (within a sphere of a few hundred microns in diameter) in the material. The probability of photoelectric absorption per unit distance in a medium strongly depends on the atomic number of the medium in which the photon is propagating. At 511 keV, it is roughly proportional to $Z^{3,4}$.

Compton scattering interactions

Compton scattering interactions are shown in Figure 1-7. Here, the 511-keV photon scatters off a free or loosely bound electron in the medium, transferring some of its energy to the electron and changing direction in the process. Imposing conservation of momentum and energy leads to a simple relationship[1] between the energy of the original photon (E), the energy of the scattered photon (E_{sc}) and the angle through which it is scattered, θ:

$$E_{sc} = \frac{m_e c^2}{\dfrac{m_e c^2}{E} + 1 - \cos\theta} \qquad (1\text{-}11)$$

In this equation, m_e is the mass of the electron and c is the speed of light (2.998×10^8 m/s). Using units of electron volts for energy, the term $m_e c^2$ is equal to 511

FIGURE 1-7. Schematic representation of Compton scattering in which the incident photon transfers part of its energy to an electron, causing it to change direction. The scattered photon carries considerable energy and can have a long range in materials such as tissue. (Reproduced with permission from Cherry SR, Sorenson JA, Phelps ME. *Physics in Nuclear Medicine*, W.B. Saunders, New York, 2003.)

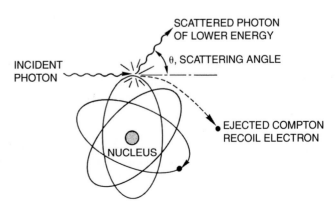

keV. In PET, the incoming photon of interest has an energy level of 511 keV; the equation, therefore, reduces further to:

$$E_{sc}(\text{keV}) = \frac{511}{2 - \cos\theta} \tag{1-12}$$

The recoil energy that is transferred to the electron, E_{re}, which is dissipated in the medium, is equal to $E - E_{sc}$:

$$E_{re} = E - E_{sc} = E \times \frac{(1 - \cos\theta)}{\left(\dfrac{m_e c^2}{E} + 1 - \cos\theta\right)} \tag{1-13}$$

Again substituting $E = 511$ keV, this reduces to:

$$E_{re}(\text{keV}) = 511 \times \frac{1 - \cos\theta}{2 - \cos\theta} \tag{1-14}$$

The maximum energy that can be imparted to the electron (and, therefore, the medium) occurs when the photon is scattered through 180°. The probability of Compton scattering per unit length of absorbing medium is linearly proportional to the atomic number of the medium.

EXAMPLE 1-5
Calculate the minimum energy of a 511-keV photon after it has undergone Compton scattering. What is the energy given up to the recoil electron?

ANSWER
The minimum energy will occur when the maximum energy is given to the electron. This occurs for a scattering angle of 180°. From Equation 1-12, the energy of the scattered photon will be:

$$E_{sc} = 511 \text{ keV} / (2 - \cos 180°) = 170 \text{ keV}$$

The energy given to the electron is simply $E - E_{sc} = 511$ keV $- 170$ keV $= 340$ keV.

The angular distribution of the scattered photons is given by the Klein–Nischina equation.[1] It is independent of the scattering medium but strongly dependent on the energy of the photons. The angular distribution for a range of energies is shown in Figure 1-8.

Interaction cross-sections in various materials
The interaction (absorption or scattering) of 511-keV photons by matter can be described with a simple exponential relationship:

$$I(x) = I(0)\exp(-\mu x) \tag{1-15}$$

where $I(0)$ is the 511-keV photon flux impinging on the medium, x is the thickness of the medium, and $I(x)$ is the flux of 511-keV photons that passes through the medium without interaction. The parameter μ is the linear attenuation coefficient and is the probability per unit distance that an interaction will occur.

FIGURE 1-8. Relative probability of Compton scattering (normalized per unit of solid angle) versus scattering angle. At 511 keV, small-angle forward scatter is most likely. (Reproduced with permission from Cherry SR, Sorenson JA, Phelps ME. *Physics in Nuclear Medicine*, W.B. Saunders, New York, 2003.)

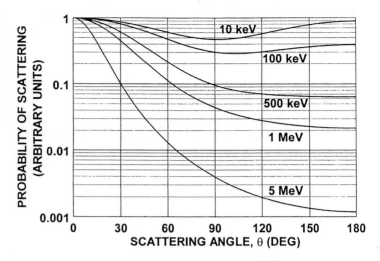

For 511-keV photons, it is largely made up of components due to photoelectric absorption and Compton scattering, such that:

$$\mu \approx \mu_{\text{compton}} + \mu_{\text{photoelectric}} \tag{1-16}$$

For PET imaging, three media are of potential interest: tissue in the body, the detector material, and any material used for shielding or collimation. The attenuation coefficients for soft tissue, bone, for a typical detector material (bismuth germanate or BGO) and for lead and tungsten are shown in Table 1-3. The *half-value thickness*, the thickness of material that is required to cause half of the 511-keV photons to interact, is also given.

The annihilation photons must pass through the body so that they can be detected. The dominant form of interaction for 511-keV photons in tissue (Table 1-3) is Compton scattering. Therefore, photon interactions in the body attenuate the signal by redirecting annihilation photons that would have struck a particular detector pair. The angular correlation between the annihilation photons is randomized by the scattering process, so if the redirected photons still escape the body and are detected in the PET scanner, they will be incorrectly located. This results in a background of scattered events in the images. Unfortunately, even at the high energies of the annihilation photons, substantial numbers are scattered in the body because the Compton scatter cross-section is quite high. Example 1-6 illustrates this point. A number of steps are taken to correct for the

TABLE 1-3. Linear Attenuation Coefficients for Soft Tissue, Bone, Bismuth Germanate (a Detector Material), Lead, and Tungsten at 511 keV.

Material	$\mu_{Compton}$ (cm^{-1})	$\mu_{photoelectric}$ (cm^{-1})	μ (cm^{-1})	Half-value thickness (cm)
Soft tissue	~0.096	~0.00002	~0.096	7.2
Bone	~0.169	~0.001	~0.17	4.1
Bismuth germanate (B60)	0.51	0.40	0.96	0.76
Lead	0.76	0.89	1.78	0.42
Tungsten	1.31	1.09	2.59	0.29

attenuation due to scatter and to minimize and remove the scatter background as explained in Attenuation Correction (p. 56) and Scatter Correction (p. 63). This is, in part, based on the fact that photons that undergo Compton interaction in the body will lose energy (Equation 1-12) and can thus be rejected by a detector if they have sufficient energy discrimination.

EXAMPLE 1-6

Determine the probability that a 511-keV photon emitted 7.5 cm deep inside the brain is Compton scattered. How does this change if the photon is emitted from a point in the liver, 20 cm from the surface of the body?

ANSWER

From Table 1-3, the attenuation coefficient due to Compton scattering for 511-keV photons in tissue is 0.096 cm^{-1}. Using Equation 1-15 we find:

$$I(x)/I(0) = \exp{(-\mu x)}$$

Brain: $x = 7.5$ cm, $I(x)/I(0) = 0.49$ (49% of photons escape unscattered)
Liver: $x = 20$ cm, $I(x)/I(0) = 0.15$ (15% of photons escape unscattered)

This implies that relatively large numbers of photons are scattered. When using PET, we require that both photons are unscattered when they reach the detectors. The probability that neither photon scatters is roughly the square of the probabilities above, assuming both photons pass through equal amounts of tissue.

The function of the PET scanner is to detect those 511-keV photons that escape the body without interacting. The detector material should, therefore, be something that has a high probability of stopping these photons, that is, very dense materials, with large values of μ. An example of such a material is BGO. It is also preferable that the detector has as high a ratio between photoelectric and Compton interactions as possible. Photoelectric interactions are preferred in a detector because they result in all of the energy being deposited locally. Compton scattering can result in multiple interactions within a detector or interactions in adjacent detectors. It can, therefore, be difficult to unambiguously define the location of the interaction.

EXAMPLE 1-7

What thickness of bismuth germanate detector material would be required to cause 90% of the incoming photon flux to interact?

ANSWER

From Table 1-3, the attenuation coefficient for 511-keV photons in bismuth germanate is 0.96 cm^{-1}. Using Equation 1-15 and setting $I(x)/I(0) = 0.1$ (only 10% transmitted, 90% interact) we find:

$$I(x)/I(0) = 0.1 = \exp{(-0.96 \times x)}$$
$$x = \ln{(0.1)} / -0.96 = 2.4 \text{ cm}$$

This demonstrates that detectors will need to be several centimeters thick to be highly efficient at stopping 511-keV photons.

Finally, we may want to shield the detectors from radioactivity that is outside the imaging volume. In addition, some multislice PET scanners use collimators in the axial direction to define the slices of the object that is being imaged. These axial collimators can also be an effective way to decrease the detection of photons that scatter in the body. The idea of collimator or shielding material is to absorb any photons that are incident on them, and so materials with the very highest attenuation values (subject to requirements for ease of machining and cost) are used. Lead and tungsten are two commonly used materials in this regard.

511 keV PHOTON DETECTORS

A PET scanner is comprised of a set of two or more detectors. To obtain the best quality image for a given injected dose of radioactivity, the detectors must have a very high *efficiency* for detecting 511-keV photons that impinge on their surface (the more photon pairs that are detected, the better the signal-to-noise in the image) and must also give precise information on the spatial location of the interaction (this relates directly to the *spatial resolution* of the images). The latter is generally achieved in one of two ways, either by using arrays of small detector elements, in which case the precision of localization is related to the size of the detector elements, or by using a larger area detector that has position-sensing capability built in. It is also important to be able to determine when a photon struck the detectors, so that the time of all detected events can be compared to determine which ones arrived closely enough in time to correspond to an annihilation pair. The ability of a pair of detectors to determine the time difference in arrival of the annihilation photons is known as the *timing resolution* and is typically on the order of 2 to 6 ns. A typical timing window that is used in PET scanners so as not to accidentally reject annihilation photon pairs is typically 2 to 3 times the timing resolution, leading to values in the range of 4 to 18 ns. Finally, the detectors should indicate the energy of the incoming annihilation photon such that those that have scattered in the body (and have thus lost energy as explained in the section on Compton Scattering Interactions (p. 13) can be rejected. The ability of the detector to determine the energy of the photon is known as the *energy resolution*.

    Scintillation detectors are widely used gamma-ray detectors that form the basis for almost all PET scanners in use today. These detectors consist of a dense crystalline *scintillator* material that serves as an interacting medium for gamma-rays and high-energy photons and which emits visible light when energy is deposited inside of them. This light is then subsequently detected by some form of visible light photon detector and converted into an electrical current (Figure 1-9). This section reviews the components of scintillation detectors and shows how they are used as detectors in PET scanners. Other technologies for gamma-ray detection (and therefore annihilation photon detection) are also briefly reviewed.

Scintillators
Scintillators are transparent materials that have the property of emitting light in the visible region of the spectrum when energy from particles or high-energy

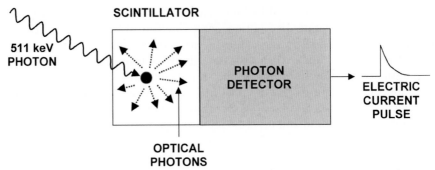

FIGURE 1-9. Basic components of a scintillation detector. The incident annihilation photon interacts in the scintillator (either by photoelectric or Compton interaction). Each annihilation photon that interacts produces a single pulse in the detector, with the amplitude of the pulse being determined by the number of scintillation photons reaching the photon detector and any amplification inherent in the photon detector.

photons are deposited in them. The light is emitted isotropically and the amount of light emitted is proportional to the amount of energy that is deposited in the material. These materials can be organic or inorganic compounds and can come in both solid and liquid forms. An excellent review of scintillators can be found in the textbook by Knoll.[11] Scintillators are characterized by their stopping power, their brightness, the wavelength of the emitted light, and the time over which the light is produced—important considerations in choosing a scintillator for a particular application. For the purposes of PET imaging, the scintillator must be a dense material that can stop a large fraction of the incident 511-keV photons. For this reason, dense, inorganic, solid scintillators are the scintillators of choice. Table 1-4 lists some of the properties of scintillator materials suitable for detecting gamma-rays in the 100 to 1000 keV range. As demonstrated by Example 1-7, a thickness of several centimeters of these scintillators is required to effectively stop a large percentage of incident 511-keV photons. It is also apparent, that even in the most dense available scintillators, Compton interactions are more likely to occur than photoelectric interactions at 511 keV.

While stopping power is a major factor in the choice of a scintillator for PET, other considerations are also important. The brightness of the scintillator (the number of light photons produced per 511 keV interaction) is important because the integrated light signal from the scintillator (converted by the subsequent photon detector from photons into electrons) is used in several different ways. In many detectors, the relative amplitudes of the signals seen by adjacent light sensors viewing a piece of scintillator are used to determine the location of the interaction. The integrated light signal is used as a direct measure of the energy deposited in the scintillator; therefore, by placing a lower threshold on the output, it is possible to reject low-energy photons that have scattered in the body. In both cases, a major source of noise in the measurement (leading to errors in positioning or energy) are statistical fluctuations in the number of scintillation photons detected. These fluctuations are governed by Poisson counting statistics and reduce as $1/\sqrt{N}$ where N is the number of scintillation photons that are detected.

TABLE 1-4. Properties of Scintillator Materials Useful for Gamma-Ray Detection at 511 keV

Scintillator	Density (g/cc)	Light output (photons per 511 keV)	Decay time (ns)	Index of refraction	Linear attenuation at 511 keV (cm^{-1})	Ratio between photoelectric and Compton
Sodium iodide [NaI(Tl)]	3.67	19400	230	1.85	0.34	0.22
Bismuth Germanate (BGO)	7.13	4200	300	2.15	0.96	0.78
Lutetium Oxyorthosilicate (LSO:Ce)	7.40	~13000	~47	1.82	0.88	0.52
Gadolinium Oxyorthosilicate (GSO:Ce)	6.71	~4600	~56	1.85	0.70	0.35
Barium Fluoride (BaF2)	4.89	700, 4900	0.6, 630	1.56	0.45	0.24
Yttrium Aluminum Perovskite (YAP:Ce)	5.37	~9200	~27	1.95	0.46	0.05

Based on data (Table 8.3) from Knoll GF (Radiation Detection and Measurements, 3rd Edition, 2000, Wiley, New York, 2000), light output and decay time data for cerium doped scintillators such as LSO, GSO, and YAP are approximate and can vary by tens of percent depending on cerium concentration, impurities, and growing conditions.

Because PET imaging involves the coincident detection of the two annihilation photons, it will be important to have an accurate assessment of exactly when a photon interacts in a detector. The accuracy of timing is determined in large part both by the decay time of the scintillator and its brightness. A fast, bright scintillator will produce a signal with less timing variation than a slow, dim scintillator. This observation is based on an analysis of the spread of the average arrival times of the first scintillation photons at the photodetector. It is these first photons which trigger the start of a pulse and is the earliest time point that can be detected. Finally, the index of refraction of the scintillator is also important as this determines how efficiently optical photons can be transmitted from the scintillator to the photodetector. Large mismatches in index result in significant internal reflection at the scintillator/photodetector boundary and reduce light transmission to the photodetector.

When discussing PET detectors based on scintillators detectors, it is very important to clearly distinguish between the high-energy annihilation photons (511 keV) that are absorbed by the scintillator and the burst of low-energy optical photons (energy of a few eV) that are subsequently emitted by the scintillator and converted into an electric current. Each interaction of a 511-keV photon in the scintillator ultimately produces a single electrical pulse. The number of visible light photons generated in the scintillator and detected by the photon detector determines the amplitude of that pulse.

Photomultiplier tubes

The vast majority of commercially available PET scanners use *photomultiplier tubes* (PMTs)[12] as the photon detector to convert scintillation light into an elec-

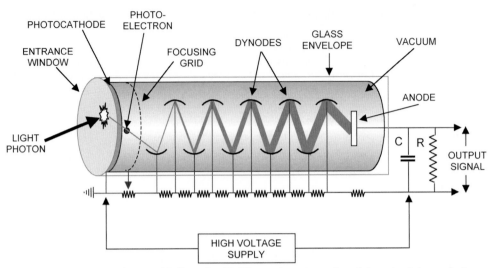

FIGURE 1-10. A photomultiplier tube (PMT) consists of a series of dynodes (electrodes) each of which is held at a greater voltage with a resistor chain. Each dynode is coated with an emissive material in an evacuated glass tube. The inner surface of the entrance window (the photocathode) is also coated with an emissive material. Light photons striking the photocathode can release electrons into the tube, and these electrons are accelerated by a potential difference to the first dynode. Each electron has sufficient energy upon striking the first dynode to release further electrons, which, in turn, are accelerated to the second dynode. After 10 dynode stages, each original electron produced at the photocathode has been amplified into approximately 10^6 electrons, producing a sizeable current at the PMT output (anode). (Reproduced with permission from Cherry SR, Sorenson JA, Phelps ME. *Physics in Nuclear Medicine*, W.B. Saunders, New York, 2003.)

trical current. A cross-section through a typical photomultiplier tube is shown in Figure 1-10. Light from the scintillator is transmitted through the glass entrance window of the PMT and excites the *photocathode*. The photocathode is made from a thin layer of material that can easily liberate electrons as energy is deposited in it. Each light photon from the scintillator has roughly a 15% to 25% chance (depending on wavelength) to liberate an electron. This probability is called the *quantum efficiency* of the PMT. A high potential difference accelerates the electron from the photocathode and directs it to strike a positively charged electrode called the first *dynode*. This dynode is also coated with an emissive material that readily releases electrons, and each impinging electron has acquired sufficient energy to release on the order of 3 to 4 secondary electrons from the dynode. These electrons are in turn accelerated to the second dynode and so forth, ultimately creating an avalanche of photoelectrons. After 10 stages of amplification, each initial electron has created on the order of 10^6 electrons, which, occurring over a period of a few nanoseconds, lead to an easily detectable current in the milliamp range. PMTs come in a wide range of shapes and sizes and also are available as multichannel and position sensitive models. Most PET scanners use round or square single-channel PMTs in the range of 1 to 5 cm in diameter. The advantages of PMTs are their high *gain* (amplification), which leads to high signal-to-noise pulses, their stability and ruggedness, and their fast response (the output pulse from a PMT rises in approximately a nanosecond for a step function input of light into the PMT). The disadvantages are that they are quite bulky and fairly expensive.

Solid state photodetectors

An alternative to PMTs are photon detectors based on the *silicon photodiode.*[13] A simple photodiode consists of a thin piece of silicon (typically a few hundred microns thick), which has been carefully doped with impurities to create a favorable electric field profile in the material (Figure 1-11). A small voltage of 10^2 to 10^3 V is applied across the silicon diode. When a scintillation light photon interacts in the silicon, it often has sufficient energy to liberate an electron from the lattice structure of the silicon. The vacancy it leaves behind, known as a hole, has the properties of a net positive charge. Under the applied electric field, the electron drifts towards the anode (positively charged electrode) and the hole drifts towards the cathode (negatively charged electrode), constituting an electric current that can be measured. The quantum efficiency of photodiodes is approximately 60% to 80%, providing a much more efficient conversion of photons to electrons than is possible with PMTs. However, photodiodes have no internal gain, producing only one detected electron-hole pair per scintillation photon. This leads to a signal that is roughly 10^6 times weaker than a PMT signal, reducing the signal-to-noise of the pulses and degrading the ability to determine the energy deposited in the scintillator. The low signal-to-noise also necessitates the use of long integration times in the electronics, reducing the ability to time the arrival of the pulses (an important aspect for PET). Therefore, photodiodes are generally not suitable for use in PET.

FIGURE 1-11. Schematic cross-section of a typical photodiode. Scintillation photons enter through the entrance window and have sufficient energy to liberate an electron-hole pair in the silicon. The electric field profile in the silicon moves the electrons and holes towards the anode and cathode, respectively, creating a current that can be measured. Each light photon produces at most one electron, so the signal levels are very low. Avalanche photodiodes are very similar in structure, except the applied voltage is much higher, providing electrons with sufficient energy to create further electron-hole pairs in the silicon. Each light photon produces a signal of up to 10^2 to 10^3 electrons through this avalanche mechanism.

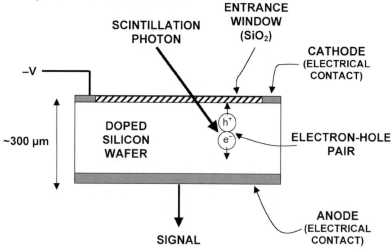

A modification of the photodiode leads to a device known as the *avalanche photodiode* (APD).[14] Here, the voltage applied across the photodiode is much higher and creates a situation where an electron gains enough energy between collisions in the silicon to release further electrons. This leads to an avalanche effect, similar to that seen in the photomultiplier tube. The gain in these devices critically depends on factors such as the applied voltage and temperature. Special care needs to be taken in the fabrication and operation of these devices to obtain stable results. However, gains of 10^2 to 10^3 are typical, yielding improved signal-to-noise over photodiodes. Once again, the quantum efficiency is in the 60% to 80% range. When combined with the relatively high gain, this leads to roughly equivalent performance in terms of energy and timing performance compared with PMT-based detectors. APDs are now available both as single-channel units (ranging in size from 1 mm to over 2 cm in diameter) and as multi-element arrays. APDs allow for a more compact PET scanner design and may in the future replace PMTs as the photon detector of choice.

Block detector

The majority of dedicated PET scanners in use in the early part of the 21st century have detectors based on the block design proposed originally by Casey and Nutt.[15] A schematic of the *block detector* is shown in Figure 1-12. A relatively large block of scintillator material (typically 4×4 cm in area by 3 cm deep) is segmented into an array of smaller detector elements (typically 8×8). The saw cuts are filled with a white reflective material that helps to optically isolate individual elements within the block. The scintillator block is coupled to four single-channel PMTs. The depth of the saw cuts is empirically determined to share scintillation light in a linear fashion between the four PMTs as a function of the position of the annihilation photon interaction within the block. For example, if an annihilation photon interacts in the corner detector element, the deep cuts ensure that virtually all the scintillation light photons that are produced from the interaction end up in the PMT sitting directly underneath that element. Alternatively, an event interacting towards the middle of the block, where the cuts are shallower, results in a roughly equal spread of scintillation light among all four PMTs. By careful design of the depth of the cuts, and with sufficient scintillation light, interactions in each detector element will produce a unique distribution of scintillation light and, therefore, signals on the four PMTs.

In practice, an X and Y coordinate is calculated for each annihilation photon that interacts in the block detector based on:

$$X = (S_A + S_B - S_C - S_D) / (S_A + S_B + S_C + S_D) \qquad (1\text{-}17a)$$

and

$$Y = (S_A + S_C - S_B - S_D) / (S_A + S_B + S_C + S_D) \qquad (1\text{-}17b)$$

where S_A, S_B, S_C and S_D are the four PMT signals shown in Figure 1-12. Figure 1-13 shows the result of an experiment in which the surface of a block detector is uniformly irradiated with 511-keV annihilation photons with the event locations histogrammed into a two-dimensional (2-D) image based on the calculated X, Y locations. This real measurement shows considerable spatial distortions in the array of spots, which is due to the fact that it is not pos-

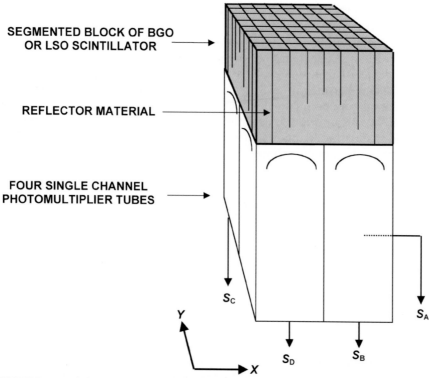

SEGMENTED BLOCK OF BGO OR LSO SCINTILLATOR

REFLECTOR MATERIAL

FOUR SINGLE CHANNEL PHOTOMULTIPLIER TUBES

S_C

S_A

S_D

S_B

Y

X

FIGURE 1-12. Schematic drawing of a typical PET block detector. A block of scintillator is segmented into an 8 × 8 array using a diamond saw. White reflective material is used in the saw cuts to optically isolate elements. Depth of the saw cuts determines the spread of scintillation light onto four single-channel photomultiplier tubes. By looking at the ratio of signals in the four PMTs, the detector element in which an annihilation photon interacted can be determined. (Reproduced with permission from Cherry SR, Sorenson JA, Phelps ME. *Physics in Nuclear Medicine*, W.B. Saunders, New York, 2003.)

FIGURE 1-13. Image resulting from flood irradiating the front surface of a block detector with 511 keV photons, applying Equation 1-17 to the resulting PMT signals and displaying an image of a histogram of the X, Y signals. This measurement is known as a flood histogram. The individual detector elements in this 8 × 8 detector module can be visualized (the edge crystals are hard to see, as they are binned at the extreme edges of the image). Each spot is of a finite size due to the limited number of scintillation light photons contributing to the signal used to calculate X and Y. (Reproduced with permission from Cherry SR, Sorenson JA, Phelps ME. *Physics in Nuclear Medicine*, W.B. Saunders, New York, 2003.)

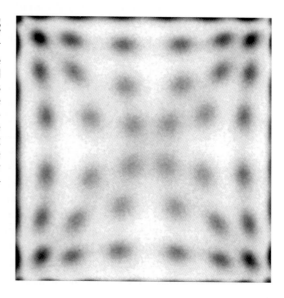

sible to design the cuts such that the response is completely linear across the whole detector face. Therefore, a lookup table is created from these *flood histograms* relating each calculated position *X,Y* to each of the 64 elements in the detector. It is also apparent that the spots are of a finite size and overlap to a certain degree. This is due to statistical fluctuations in the PMT signals used to calculate *X,Y*, which in turn is caused by the limited number of scintillation photons produced and subsequently detected after a 511-keV annihilation photon interacts in the detector. These fluctuations ultimately limit the size and number of detector elements that can be decoded using four PMTs. In the particular example shown in Figure 1-13, the 8 × 8 array of elements are visualized relatively clearly, but had the detector been segmented into a 16 × 16 array of elements, it is highly unlikely that the individual elements could have been resolved from each other.

The block detector is a very cost-effective approach to PET, as it allows on the order of 64 crystals to be decoded from just four PMTs. Because the photodetectors are one of the most expensive components of a PET scanner, this 16:1 multiplexing is the key to developing PET scanners with thousands of detector elements at a reasonable cost. A large number of detector elements implies good solid angle coverage (improving the chances of detecting annihilation photon pairs that are being emitted in all directions). The block design also leads to detector elements that are smaller than the PMTs themselves. Smaller detector elements allow gamma-ray interactions to be better localized leading to improved spatial resolution as well. The spatial resolution of the block detector is primarily determined by the width of the detector elements (assuming scintillation light is sufficient to resolve each of the elements). This width is commonly 3 to 5 mm in current generation block detectors designed for clinical PET scanners.

A further extension of the block detector design leads to the concept of *quadrant sharing*.[16] In this case, larger PMTs are used and each scintillation block is placed on the corner quadrants of four PMTs as shown in Figure 1-14. Four PMTs are still being used to decode each block, but each PMT now actually serves four different scintillator blocks. The block in which the interaction occurs is determined by which four PMTs show a significant signal, and the location of the signal within the block is determined from Equation 1-17. This approach, when extended to large area detector panels, leads to almost another fourfold reduction in the number of PMTs required per detector element, giving a total multiplexing approximately 64:1, and lower overall detector cost. Alternatively, this approach can be used to decode smaller detector elements for the same sized photomultiplier tubes used in the original block detector. One drawback of the quadrant sharing approach is that it requires that blocks be structured into large planar panels and also that there is one half of a PMT width at each end of the panel which is not usable. This unusable space results in relatively large gaps between panels when they are assembled in a hexagonal or octagonal geometry to form a scanner. Because the detector is no longer modular, repair and replacement is also more difficult. However, because of the dramatic cost-saving in this approach, it is being implemented in commercially available PET systems. PET scanners that use block detector and quadrant-sharing approaches are described in more detail in the PET System Design section (p. 107).

STANDARD BLOCK
DETECTOR

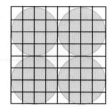

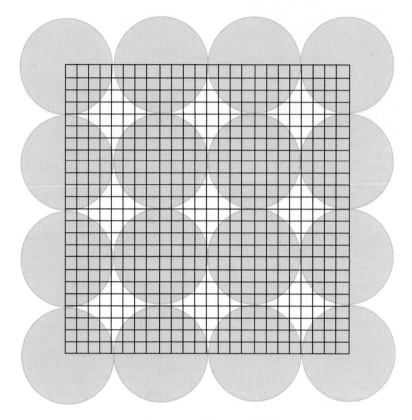

QUADRANT SHARING
DETECTOR

FIGURE 1-14. Concept of quadrant sharing that enables detector elements to be decoded using a smaller number of larger diameter PM tubes. For a given detector element size, this approach can reduce the number of PM tubes by almost a factor of four if large panels are constructed. (Adapted with permission from Cherry SR, Sorenson JA, Phelps ME. *Physics in Nuclear Medicine*, W.B. Saunders, New York, 2003.)

Continuous gamma camera detector

The other major approach to constructing a PET detector is based on a large-area, continuous plate of NaI(Tl) scintillator coupled to a matrix of PMTs as shown in Figure 1-15. This detector is essentially the same that is used in conventional nuclear medicine gamma cameras, although when the detector is designed specifically for PET, a thicker crystal is used to provide sufficient efficiency at 511 keV.[17] The location of an interaction is determined by the

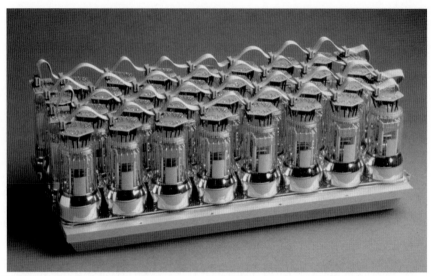

FIGURE 1-15. Photograph of a large-area NaI(Tl) detector designed for PET applications. The scintillator plate is 50 cm long by 15 cm wide by 2.5 cm thick and is read by thirty, 5-cm diameter PM tubes. Six of these detectors have been used in an hexagonal array to form a PET scanner. (Photograph courtesy of Dr. Joel Karp, University of Pennsylvania.)

distribution of scintillation light among the PMTs (Figure 1-16), with the signal from each PMT being digitized and then appropriately weighted such that the position determined from the PMT outputs is linearly related to the position of interaction. The position information provided from these detectors is

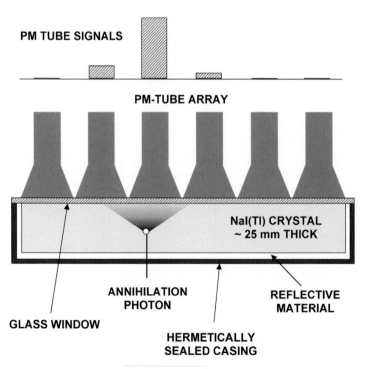

FIGURE 1-16. Schematic cross-section through a continuous gamma camera detector designed for 511-keV annihilation photons. A thick continuous sheet of NaI(Tl) scintillator is viewed by an array of PM tubes. The NaI(Tl) crystal is covered in reflective material on the sides and back to help direct more scintillation light towards the PM tubes and is hermetically sealed in a thin metal case, with a glass front window to allow scintillation light to reach the PM tubes.

continuous. The binning of the position data can be chosen to satisfy sampling criteria for image reconstruction (see Limitations of Filtered Backprojection, p. 80). This differs from the block detector in which position information is determined by which individual detector element produces a signal. The block detector, therefore, produces discrete position information, with a sampling interval equal to the center-to-center spacing of the detector elements.

The performance of continuous detectors critically depends on the number of scintillation photons detected, as this directly impacts the spatial resolution of the detector by determining the signal-to-noise of the PMT signals that are used to calculate the position of interaction on the detector face. Therefore, this approach has only been successfully used with very high light output scintillators such as NaI(Tl). The thickness of the crystal (and, therefore, the efficiency for stopping 511-keV annihilation photons) is limited to approximately 25 mm, as the spatial resolution degrades with increasing crystal thickness. This is due to the fact that the scintillation light will spread over a larger area before reaching the PMTs, producing a lower amplitude signal across a larger number of PMTs. For a constant noise level in the PMTs and electronics, the signal-to-noise of the signals being used to calculate the position is therefore poorer and the positioning accuracy is degraded. With a 10-mm thick NaI(Tl) crystal, it is possible to achieve an intrinsic spatial resolution as high as ~3 mm; at 25 mm thickness this degrades to 4 to 5 mm (Dr. Joel Karp, unpublished observation). Special efforts must also be made with the electronics to allow this large-area detector to handle multiple events occuring in different parts of the detector at the same time. Otherwise, detector *dead time* (the time required to process an event before another event can be properly recorded) becomes a limiting factor in overall performance.

These detectors generally are large flat plates (typically 30–50 cm in size). Significant deadspace occurs at the edges of the detectors due to the need to hermetically encapulsate NaI(Tl) which is highly hydroscopic. Furthermore, the edges of the scintillator plates yield poor spatial resolution due to alteration of the shape of the light distribution by scintillation light that interacts with the edges of the crystal. Curved NaI(Tl) scintillator plates have become available and allow for large-area PET detectors to be constructed as segments of a ring, although regions of poor spatial resolution and gaps in active detector area still remain at the interface between segments. A system for brain imaging has even been made from a single annular NaI(Tl) crystal, eliminating deadspace completely.[18] However, this is a more expensive approach, and crystal failure would result in the loss of the entire system. More details on PET systems based on NaI(Tl) detectors can be found in PET System Design (p. 107).

Other scintillation detectors

Position-sensitive and multi-channel photomultiplier tubes

Several research PET systems have been designed around multi-channel PMTs (MC-PMTs) and position-sensitive PMTs (PS-PMTs). MC-PMTs consist of an array of small, separate PMT channels within a single package. Position-sensitive PMTs have a segmented X and Y readout and are designed such that the output signals are approximately linearly related to the position of the scintillation light that is incident on the photocathode. Both MC-PMTs and PS-PMTs could be used to replace the four single-channel PMTs in a block detector or to decode individual scintillator detector elements arranged into an array. Because of their compact size and the ability to provide positional information, these devices are often used to decode arrays with relatively large numbers of very small scintillator elements for high-resolution PET applications.[19–21] Both MC-PMTs and PS-PMTs often have significant amounts of deadspace around their periphery, and, hence, they have sometimes been used with fiber optic coupling between the scintillator and the PMT to allow tight packing of detectors in a ring configuration.[22] As the cost of PS and MC-PMTs are quite high relative to single-channel PMTs, their use has been largely limited to more specialized applications such as breast and animal imaging where a smaller number of detectors are required.

Depth-encoding detectors

The detectors described so far have all focused on determining the X,Y location of an interaction (the interaction location projected onto the front surface of the detector). This is fine for thin detectors; however, PET detectors typically require a 2- to 3-cm thickness of scintillator to achieve adequate efficiency. The detectors cannot be considered to be thin. The detectors discussed so far do not provide any information on the depth of the interaction of the annihilation photons inside the scintillator. This uncertainty in *depth of interaction* leads to a loss of spatial resolution in PET images as demonstrated in Resolution: Coincidence Response Functions (p. 38). If the PET detector can determine the Z or depth coordinate of the interaction, this resolution degradation would be removed. This is an active area of research and many possible approaches have been proposed. Two methods have emerged that promise a certain degree of success and are now finding their way into PET scanner design (Figure 1-17). The first approach uses two layers of scintillator materials (known as a *phoswich*) to provide a two-level (top half, bottom half) depth encoding capability.[23,24] The scintillator materials are differentiated by their different decay times. The layer in which the interaction occurs can be simply determined by looking at the decay time of the pulses. The second approach places photodetectors at both ends of a scintillator array and uses the ratio of the signals between the two photodetectors to provide a measure of the depth of interaction. The photodetector at the far end must be thin and compact, both from a geometric standpoint, and also to minimize attenuation of the annihilation photons that must pass through this detector before reaching the scintillator. This approach has been studied extensively by Moses and colleagues[25] using a PIN photodiode array at the far end of the scintillator array to identify the crystal of interaction. A single-channel PMT at the back of the scintillator array provides information about the energy of the event and the timing signal. The ratio of the photodiode and PMT signal provides the depth of interaction information. The surface treatment of the scintillator elements and the use of reflectors along the sides of the crystal are critical in determining the distribution of scintillation light to the two ends of the array and hence the success of this approach.[26]

Avalanche photodiodes

Extensive research has been invested in the development and application of APDs (p. 21) for PET. Both single-channel APDs (up to about 15 mm in size) and arrays of smaller APDs are now available. An 8 × 8 array of APD elements

FIGURE 1-17. PET detectors with depth-encoding capability. A: Detector is similar to the standard block detector but is made of two layers of scintillators that have different decay times. An interaction can be assigned to the top or bottom layer, depending on the decay time of the pulse that it generates. This provides one-level (top or bottom) depth of interaction information. (Reproduced from Cherry SR, Sorenson JA, Phelps ME. *Physics in Nuclear Medicine*, 3rd ed, W.B. Saunders, New York, 2003, with permission from Elsevier). B: An array of scintillator elements has photodetectors at both ends. A silicon PIN photodiode is used to determine which crystal the interaction took place in, and the single-channel PMT at the back of the array is used to generate the fast timing signal necessary for PET and a high signal-to-noise measure of the deposited energy. The ratio of the signal in the photodiode and PMT gives an indication of the depth of interaction within the detector element.[25] This provides continuous depth of interaction information but requires careful calibration of the depth information. Abbreviations: LSO, lutetium oxyorthosilicate.

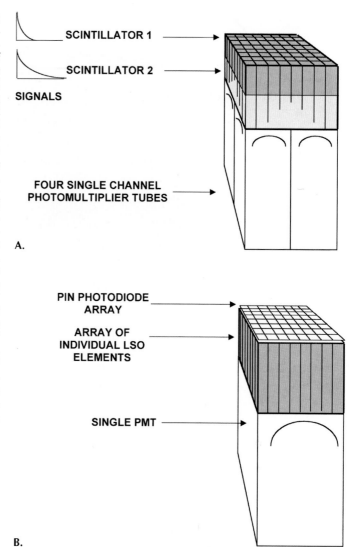

with a 1-mm center-to-center spacing is shown in Figure 1-18. The thin profile of these photodetectors encourages a number of new design possibilities, for example, multiple concentric rings of detectors,[27] or the use of APD arrays on both front and back surfaces of scintillator arrays.[28] Both these designs also provide depth of interaction information, in addition to identifying the detector element in which the interaction occured. APDs have been used successfully on a small scale in PET scanners for animals.[29,30] The stability and longterm reliability of APDs and the need for large numbers of channels of electronics have so far limited their widespread use, although an increasing role is expected in the future.

Other gamma ray detectors

Scintillation detectors have been the dominant detector technology in PET, largely due to their high efficiency, robustness, and reasonable cost, particularly with the block and gamma camera approaches that require a relatively small number of

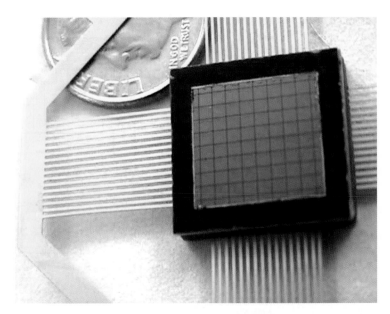

FIGURE 1-18. Photograph of an 8×8 avalanche photodiode photodetector array. Each pixel measures 1×1 mm^2. (Photograph courtesy of Kanai Shah, Radiation Monitoring Devices Inc., Watertown, MA.)

PMTs to read a large surface area of scintillator. However, other technologies have been, and are continuing to be, explored for possible applications in PET.

Multiwire proportional chambers (MWPCs) have long been used in high-energy physics as very cost effective detectors for covering large areas at high spatial resolution. These detectors consist of a chamber of gas with a set of finely spaced anode wires at high positive potential. Above and below the anode wire plane are cathode wires or strips held at ground potential that run in orthogonal directions. When the gas is ionized by a charged particle, the resulting electrons are attracted to the nearest anode wire and, because of the very high electric field close to the wire, an avalanche effect occurs, resulting in further ionization and a large signal. This in turn induces a charge on the nearest cathode strips, which provide information on the x and y position of the event. The fine spacing of the wires and the cathode strips allows very high spatial resolution to be achieved. For applications in PET, the incoming annihilation photons must first be converted into charged particles (electrons). This conversion can be achieved by making the cathode strips from thin layers of lead[31] or by using some form of converter such as a stack of thin lead sheets interlaced with insulating sheets that are then drilled with a fine matrix of holes.[32] Incoming annihilation photons can interact in the lead, ejecting electrons which are then drifted to the anode wires for amplification and detection. Figure 1-19 illustrates the principles of such a detector.

The problem for the application of MWPCs in PET has largely been achieving sufficient efficiency in conjunction with difficulties in matching the counting-rate performance, timing resolution, and energy resolution of scintillation detectors. To improve efficiency, multiple MWPC units have been stacked on top of each other, but even so, the efficiency of these detectors is typically on the order of 1% to 2%, compared to the 30% to 90% efficiency typical of scintillation detectors at 511 keV. Some of this efficiency loss can however be compensated by the good solid angle coverage of these large area detectors when placed in a scanner configuration. A second approach to improving the efficiency of these detectors has been to replace the thin lead convertors with a sheet

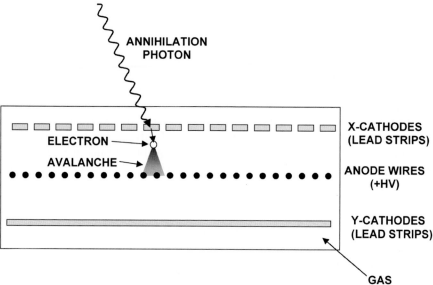

FIGURE 1-19. Diagram showing cross-section through a multiwire proportional chamber (MWPC) detector for PET. The annihilation photon interacts in thin strips of lead, ejecting an electron into the gas which is accelerated by a high potential difference to the anode wires, creating an avalanche of electrons at the wire. This, in turn, induces a signal on the nearby cathode strips that are alternately arranged in the *x* and *y* directions to provide the *x* and *y* coordinates of the event. Multiple units can be stacked on top of each other to improve efficiency and provide depth of interaction information.

or crystals of BaF_2 scintillator material. BaF_2 is one of the few scintillators that produces light as ultraviolet radiation (UV) that has sufficient energy to photoionize the gas tetrakis-dimethylamino-ethylene (TMAE). Incoming annihilation photons interact in the BaF_2, and the subsequent scintillation light ionizes TMAE gas in the MWPC, with the position signal determined by the induced signal on cathode strips or wires as described previously.[33] While this improves efficiency, it still does not match the efficiency of BGO or lutetium oxyorthosilicate (LSO) scintillation detectors; the energy resolution and timing resolution remain poor. Working PET systems based on MWPCs or MWPC/BaF_2 combinations have been developed for clinical studies,[34–36] athough the most successful application to date has probably been in small animal imaging.[32,37]

Direct detection using semiconductor materials

The approach of direct annihilation photon detection using semiconductor materials has been relatively neglected but is likely to gain increasing attention in the future. The concept is to use the semiconductor material itself to directly detect the annihilation photons, thus eliminating the need for a scintillator. The detector would work like a standard silicon photodiode (Figure 1-11); however, in this case the annihilation photons directly create the electron-holes pairs. Silicon, although the most well-developed semiconductor material, has very poor efficiency at 511 keV and would not be the material of choice. Other semiconductor materials such as cadmium telluride (CdTe) or cadmium zinc telluride (CZT) have a stopping power that is similar to NaI(Tl) at 511 keV and might be viable detector materials for PET. These materials are difficult to manufacture in bulk and are costly at this time. Achieving good energy and timing resolution from the relatively thick pieces of material needed to provide reasonable efficiency is a challenge. The approach is attractive in that it eliminates the conversion stage represented by the scintillator. The signal produced is very robust, as each 511-keV photon interaction will produce a large number of charge carriers ($\sim 10^5$). Other, even more dense (and, therefore, better stopping power) semiconductors such as PbI and TlBr exist, but these are in a fairly primitive stage of development and are mainly used as thin films at the present time. Should such materials become available in bulk at a reasonable price, they could be promising alternatives to scintillator-based detectors currently in use for PET.

DATA COLLECTION AND PET SYSTEM CONFIGURATIONS

Coincidence detection

In contrast to other nuclear imaging techniques, PET does not rely on absorptive collimation to determine the direction and location of the emitted photons. Instead, a technique referred to as *coincidence detection* is used. A simple coincidence detection system is illustrated in Figure 1-20, which consists of a pair of radiation detectors with associated electronics (amplifiers, pulse height analyzers, high voltage) and a coincidence circuit. If an annihilation occurs somewhere between two high-efficiency detectors, and the direction of the two 511-keV photons is such that each will have a chance to interact with one of the two detectors, it is very likely that a coincidence event will be recorded. Because all annihilation photons are emitted approximately 180° apart, a recorded coincidence indicates an annihilation occurred somewhere along the line (or more accurately, the volume) connecting the two detectors. This line or volume from which the detector pair can detect coincidences usually is referred to as a *line of response* or LOR. To reconstruct a complete cross-sectional image of the object, data from a large number of these LORs are collected at different angles and radial offsets that cover the field of view of the system (Image Reconstruction, p. 70).

The two detectors and associated circuitry should, under ideal circumstances, simultaneously generate the logic pulses necessary to generate a coincidence. However, due to stochastic processes in the emission of light in the scintillation detectors, a random time delay occurs in exactly when the detectors respond following the absorption of the annihilation photons in the detectors. This uncertainty in response or time resolution depends on the characteristics of the detector, primarily scintillation decay time constant and light output (Scintillators, p. 17). Furthermore, small differences are noted in the arrival times of the two photons depending on the difference in the distance of the annihilation site to each detector (Annihilation, p. 5). To avoid missing coincidence events, the logic pulses must have a certain finite width to ensure that the pulses overlap despite the finite time resolution. Typically, the width of the logic pulses, τ, should be at least as wide as the timing resolution of a pair of detectors (measured in FWHM). A typical timing resolution for a BGO- or NaI(Tl)-based PET detector is approximately 5 to 6 nanoseconds FWHM, while for LSO it is approximately 2 to 3 nanoseconds FWHM. It is important to keep the pulses as narrow

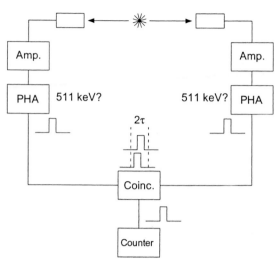

FIGURE 1-20. Diagram of a basic coincidence circuit. The two scintillation detectors with are connected to individual amplifiers (Amp) and pulse height analyzers (PHA). When a photon interacts in either of the detectors, the signals are amplified and analyzed to determine if the energy is above a certain threshold. If the energy criterion is satisfied, a logic pulse is generated by the PHA. These pulses are fed into a coincidence module (Coinc), which determines if there is an overlap of two pulses from the individual channels. An overlap occurs if both pulses occur within a time period of 2τ (e.g., they differ from each other in time by $\leq \tau$), where τ is the width of the pulse. If this is the case, a coincidence has been detected and the coincidence circuit generates a logic pulse that is fed into a counter for registration of the event. In a PET imaging system, the memory location corresponding to the two detectors in which the interaction occurred is incremented by one.

as possible to minimize the detection of events from unrelated decays that happen to strike the detectors within the time window determined by the overlap of the two logic pulses (Types of Events, p. 35).

PET camera: general concepts

The two small detectors shown in Figure 1-20 would not make a very effective PET system. They would only detect annihilation photons from decays occurring in the volume between the detectors and the tiny fraction of those decays in which the annihilation photons are directed towards the detectors. A complete PET system (Figure 1-21) consists of a large number of detectors (e.g., block detectors) placed around the object to be imaged. The most common detector configuration of a PET system is the ring geometry. When referring to directions within the plane of the detector ring, the terms *transverse* or *transaxial* are used. When referring to directions perpendicular to this plane (along the direction of the patient bed), the term *axial* is used. It is also possible to use a smaller number of large-area position sensitive detectors in a polygonal arrangement (e.g., continuous detector panels). Both these geometries allow many different LORs to be measured simultaneously and can sample an entire slice or cross-section of the object that is being imaged with little or no detector motion. This feature is of particular importance if the system is to be used for rapid dynamic imaging of the distribution of radiolabeled tracers.

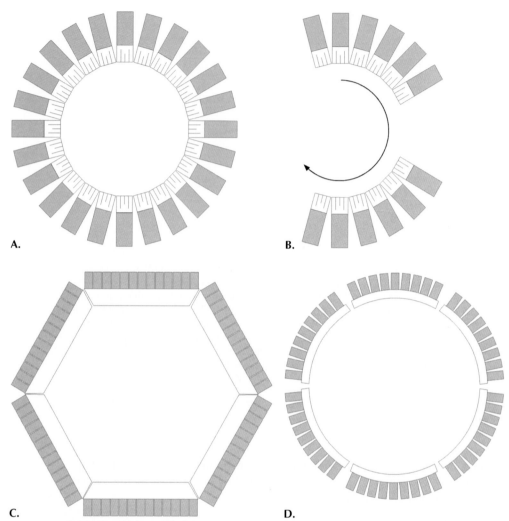

FIGURE 1-21. Schematics of four common PET scanner configurations. A: Stationary block ring system. B: Rotating block ring system. C: Stationary NaI(Tl) system using six flat detectors. D: Stationary NaI(Tl) system using curved continuous panels.

Some lower cost PET systems are comprised of a partial ring of detectors, often two opposing detectors or detector plates. However, to acquire sufficient data to reconstruct a tomographic image, these detectors must be rotated around the object.

To improve the overall detection efficiency in modern PET scanners, the detectors usually extend 15 cm or more in the axial direction. This can be accomplished by stacking several rings of detectors next to each other or by having two-dimensional continuous detectors with large axial dimensions. Many slices of data can then be acquired simultaneously, ultimately producing a set of image slices that can be stacked into a 3-D image volume.

In PET scanners based on large continuous detectors, each detector will be in coincidence with detector heads on the opposing side of the scanner (Figure

1-21). In PET systems constructed from block detectors, the number of possible coincidence combinations is proportional to the square of the number of detector elements. It is, therefore, not practical to have a dedicated coincidence circuit for each possible detector pair. Instead, a large number of detectors are grouped together into detector banks or buckets[38,39] where each detector group will look for coincident events in one or more opposite detector groups. Following the detection of a coincidence event, the electronics will then identify the detector elements (block detector) or detector locations (continuous detector) that produced the coincidence. The electronics will also check that the energy deposited in each detector is in the appropriate range for a 511-keV event. The energy window used is related to the energy resolution of the detector. A typical PET scanner uses an energy window of 350 keV to 650 keV to be sure of including all 511-keV photons, while rejecting photons that have lost a substantial fraction of their initial energy by scattering in the body.

Events that meet both the energy and timing criteria are then conveyed to the sorting hardware that writes the raw data in one of two ways: In *list mode*, each event is individually written to a file, with information about the two locations at which the annihilation photons interacted and the time at which the event occurred. In *histogram mode*, a memory location is assigned to each possible LOR, and each time a valid event is detected in that LOR, that memory location is incremented by 1. This provides the integrated number of events detected in each LOR and is frequently the most efficient manner to store the data, except for short duration acquisitions on cameras with very large numbers of LORs, where the average number of events per LOR < 1. List mode data are advantageous for dynamic studies, as the events can be sorted into time "bins" after the completion of the study. In histogram mode, the events are integrated over a time interval that must be specified prior to data acquisition.

Types of events

Under ideal circumstances, only true coincidences would be recorded, that is, only events where the two detected annihilation photons originate from the same radioactive decay and have not changed direction or lost any energy before being detected. However, due to limitations of the detectors used in PET and the possible interaction of the 511-keV photons in the body before they reach the detector, the coincidences measured are contaminated with undesirable events, which includes *random, scattered* and *multiple* coincidences (Figure 1-22). All these events have a degrading effect on the measurement and need to be corrected to produce an image that represents as closely as possible the true radioactivity concentration. Another point to consider is that the vast majority (typically 90% or more) of photons detected by the PET scanners are *single* events, in which only one of the two annihilation photons is registered. The partner photon may be on a trajectory such that it does not intersect a detector (most PET scanners provide relatively modest solid angle coverage around the object), or the photon may not deposit sufficient energy in a detector to be registered or may not interact at all. These single events are not accepted by the PET scanner, but they are responsible for random and multiple coincidence events (see below). Because they must still be processed by the electronics to see if they form part of a coincidence pair, they are the determining factor in issues related to detector dead time (Dead Time Correction, p. 67).

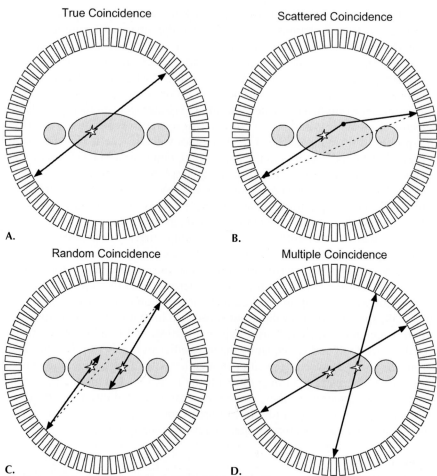

FIGURE 1-22. Illustration of the four main coincidence event types. A: True coincidence. Both annihilation photons escape the body and are recorded by a pair of detectors. B: Scattered coincidence. One or both of the two annihilation photons interacts in the body prior to detection. This results in a mispositioning of the event. C: Random coincidence: A coincidence is generated by two photons originating from two separate annihilations. These events form a background in the data that needs to be subtracted. D: Multiple coincidence: Three or more photons are detected simultaneously. Due to the ambiguity of where to position the events, these normally are discarded. (Reprinted from *Physics in Nuclear Medicine*, 2nd ed, Cherry SR, Sorenson JA, Phelps ME, W.B. Saunders, New York 1986, with permission from Elsevier.)

Accidental coincidences

When positron annihilation occurs, the two 511-keV photons are emitted simultaneously. Therefore, the detectors should ideally respond simultaneously. Because of the finite time resolution of the detectors, as discussed earlier, signals must be accepted if they occur within a certain finite time interval or timing window. Because of the finite width of the timing window, it is possibile that two unrelated single annihilation photons can be detected and registered as a valid coincidence. These unrelated events are referred to as *accidental* or *random* events. Because the random events are produced by photons emitted from unrelated isotope decays, they do not carry any spatial information about the activity distribution and produce an undesired background in the final images. If the individual photon detection rates (counts per second) in a pair of detectors are given by N_1 and N_2, then it can be shown that the rate of random coincidences, N_R (randoms per second) is given by:

$$N_R = 2\tau N_1 N_2 \qquad (1\text{-}18)$$

where τ is the width of the logic pulses produced when a photon is absorbed in the detector. The term 2τ is often referred to as the *coincidence timing window*. Because the individual detection rates N_1 and N_2 are directly proportional to the activity in the field of view of the scanner, the rate of random coincidences is proportional to the square of the activity in the field of view. The randoms rate is directly proportional to the coincidence timing window, which is why it is important not to make this any wider than required by the timing uncertainties in true coincidence events.

EXAMPLE 1-8

Two detectors register a counting rate of 100,000 counts per second each when operating independently. What would the rate of random events be if they were placed in coincidence, and if the logic pulse width generated by each detector had a width of 6 nanoseconds?

ANSWER

From Equation 1-18, the randoms rate would be:

$$N_R = 2 \times (6 \times 10^{-9}) \times (100{,}000)^2 = 120 \text{ random events per second}$$

Scattered coincidences

Scattered coincidences are another type of background event in need of correction. These events are in essence true coincidences, but one or both of the two annihilation photons has undergone a Compton scatter interaction and changed direction before they reach the detector pair. Using the coincidence detection technique, it is assumed that all detected coincidence events originate from an annihilation which, in turn, originates from a position anywhere on a line connecting the detector pairs. Because of the change in direction of the photon(s) in a scattered event, this is not true and the event is assigned to the incorrect LOR. If not corrected, the scattered events produce a low spatial frequency background that reduces contrast. The distribution of scattered events depends on the distribution of the radioactivity and the shape of the scattering medium (i.e., the patient). As will be discussed later, this is probably the most difficult correction to perform in PET. The fraction of scattered events detected can range from 15% to well over 50% in typical PET studies, depending on the size of the object and the geometry and energy resolution of the PET scanner.

Multiple coincidences

Although only two detectors are required to be activated within the coincidence time window to register a valid coincidence, at high count-rates it is possible that three or more detectors are involved. In this case, it becomes ambiguous where the event should be positioned. Because of this ambiguity, these multiple coincidences normally are discarded. However, they can contain information about the quantity and spatial location of positron emissions because these events are often composed of a true coincidence together with a single photon from an unrelated decay. In this situation, up to three possible LORs can intersect the field of view, only one of which will be correct. In some circumstances, it may be better to randomly select one of the possible LORs rather than completely discarding the event.

Prompt coincidences

The total number of events detected by the coincidence circuit in a PET scanner are referred to as *prompt* coincidences. These events consist of true, scattered, and accidental coincidences where the true coincidences are the only ones that carry spatial information regarding the distribution of the radiotracer. It is, therefore, necessary to estimate what fraction of the measured prompt coincidences arise from scattered and accidental coincidences for each of the LORs. The contribution of scattered and accidental coincidences is then subtracted from the prompt coincidences to yield the net true coincidence rate for each measured LOR. Because both the scattered and accidental events are, in general, estimates, the accuracy of these estimates will affect the accuracy of the net calculated true coincidence rate. Any statistical or systematic noise in these estimates will also propagate into the net true coincidence rate.

Resolution: coincidence response functions

As discussed in Positron Range and Noncolinearity (p. 9) an ultimate resolution limit can be achieved in PET due to the physics of the positron decay. In addition to this limit, the design and properties of the detector used in the PET scanner, and the system geometry, will also contribute to the final image resolution. The intrinsic detector resolution can be divided into two main components: geometric and physical. The geometric component can be seen as the best possible resolution that can be attained for a particular design using a scintillation material with ideal detection properties (e.g., 100% detection efficiency). The physical component is caused by nonideal properties of the detectors (e.g., detector scatter, light sharing, cross-talk, and so on).

For a pair of discrete detectors, such as the detector elements in a block detector, the geometric resolution at the mid-point between the detector pair, can be described by a triangular shaped coincidence response function (Figure 1-23A) where the FWHM equals one half the detector width. This response function can be obtained by considering how many coincidence events would be detected as a small source is moved across the detector face. At any position close to either of the two detectors the response function changes and becomes trapezoidal in shape and eventually becomes a square function at the front surface of the detector. The intrinsic resolution in these types of detectors is therefore strongly influenced by the width of the detector elements.

In continuous detector systems, the intrinsic spatial resolution of the detector is largely determined by the number of scintillation photons available for determining the position of the event, not by geometric factors. The same types of physical components listed above, also contribute to the intrinsic spatial resolution. The intrinsic spatial resolution of a continuous detector can typically be approximated by a Gaussian with a particular FWHM. If this is the case, then it can be shown that the coincidence response function at the midpoint between

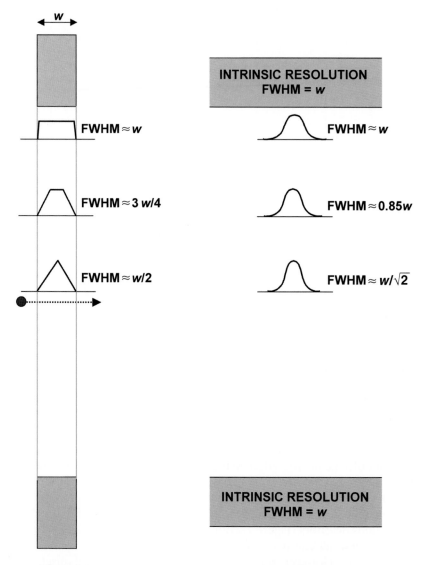

a) DISCRETE
DETECTORS

b) CONTINUOUS
DETECTORS

FIGURE 1-23. A: Geometric spatial resolution as a point source is moved between two discrete detectors. At the center of the field of view, the coincidence response function has a triangular shape with a FWHM equal to half the detector width w. As the source is moved towards one of the detectors, the coincidence response function becomes trapezoidal in shape and the FWHM increases linearly with the distance from the center of the field of view. B: Coincidence response function for a pair of continuous detectors, each with an intrinsic spatial resolution described by a Gaussian with a FWHM = w. The coincidence response function at the center of the field of view is $w/\sqrt{2}$, increasing to w at the detector face. (Reproduced with permission from Cherry SR, Sorenson JA, Phelps ME. Physics in Nuclear Medicine, W.B. Saunders, New York, 2003.)

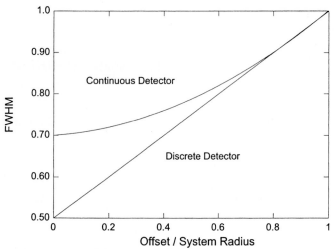

FIGURE 1-24. Comparison of the FWHM of the coincidence response function for discrete and continuous detectors with $w = 1$ (as defined in Figure 1-23) as a function of source position (offset) relative to the two detectors. A source offset of 0 corresponds to a source located exactly halfway between the detectors.

the detector pair is equal to the individual detector resolution FWHM/$\sqrt{2}$. For locations closer to one detector or another, the FWHM resolution will increase and at one detector face will eventually become equal to the intrinsic resolution of the individual detectors (Figure 1-23B). Figure 1-24 shows the change in the FWHM of the coincidence response function for discrete detectors and continuous detectors as a function of the source location.

The thick scintillation detectors used for PET imaging (typically 2–3 cm) lead to another geometric effect that degrades spatial resolution. This effect, which is referred to as *detector parallax* or the *depth of interaction* effect, is caused by the fact that the annihilation photons can interact at any depth in the scintillator material. Consider a ring geometry scanner consisting of either discrete or continuous detectors (Figure 1-21, top left or bottom right). At the center of the field of view, all emitted photons will enter the detectors perpendicular to the detector face. However, when a source is located with a radial offset, the detectors are angled with respect to the line of response and the annihilation photons may penetrate through the first detector they encounter and be detected in an adjacent detector as shown in Figure 1-25. There are two consequences of this effect. The coincidence response function becomes broader (because the detectors are at an angle and present a larger area to the line of response) and the event is also mispositioned towards the center of the scanner with respect to the line joining the two detectors of interaction. The amount of broadening depends on the width and thickness of the scintillator elements, the absorption characteristics of the scintillator material, and the separation of the detectors. It results in a worsening in the radial component of the spatial resolution of PET images as you move away form the center of the field of view. This can be a significant effect in small-diameter PET scanners that use thick scintillation detectors. This effect could be reduced if the depth of the interaction in the detector could be measured, which would allow a correct placement of the event (Other Scintilla-

FIGURE 1-25. In a ring geometry scanner, the point spread function becomes asymmetrical with increasing radial offsets due to detector penetration and the lack of information regarding the depth of interaction within the crystal. The result is a widening of the point spread function (degrading spatial resolution) and mispositioning of events towards the center of the field of view. The severity of these effects depends on detector ring diameter, detector depth, and the detector material.

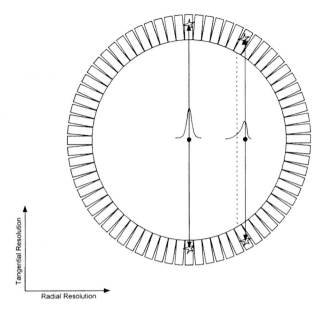

tion Detectors, p. 27). PET scanners based on a polygonal geometry (Figure 1-21, bottom left) also suffer from these detector parallax effects, although the degradation in resolution is spread fairly uniformly across the entire field of view rather than being concentrated towards the peripheral field of view. These effects occur because for all source locations (even at the center of the field of view), annihilation photons enter the detectors with a range of angles with respect to the detector face.

The final system resolution for a particular system design is a convolution of all the resolution response functions, including the positron range, photon noncolinearity, geometric factors, intrinsic spatial resolution (for continuous detectors), and physical factors. In addition, insufficient sampling of lines of response through the object can degrade the resolution in the final reconstructed image (Limitations of Filtered Backprojection, p. 80).

EXAMPLE 1-9

Assuming that detector resolution, positron range, and photon non-colinearity can be approximated by Gaussian functions, calculate the system resolution at the center of the field of view for a clinical PET scanner with an 80-cm diameter and 6-mm discrete detector elements when imaging a ^{18}F-labeled radiopharmaceutical.

ANSWER

From Figure 1-23 the intrinsic detector resolution, R_{int}, at the center of the field of view of the scanner is:

$$R_{int} = 6 \text{ mm}/2 = 3 \text{ mm}$$

From Equation 1-10, the blurring due to photon noncolinearity, Δ_{nc}, is:

$$\Delta_{nc} = 0.0022 \times 800 = 1.76 \text{ mm}$$

From Figure 1-5, the blurring due to the positron range of ^{18}F, Δ_{pos}, has a FWHM of 0.102 mm.

The convolution of multiple Gaussian functions is another Gaussian with a FWHM given by adding the individual component FWHMs in quadrature. The system resolution, R_{sys}, is therefore:

$$R_{sys} \approx \sqrt{R_{int}^2 + \Delta_{nc}^2 + \Delta_{pos}^2} = \sqrt{3^2 + 1.76^2 + 0.102^2} = 3.48 \text{ mm}$$

Sensitivity: detector and geometric efficiencies

One of the most important factors in designing a PET system is to maximize the *system sensitivity*, since this will be a major determinant of final image quality. The more coincidence events that can be detected and used to form the image, the better. The number of events collected is dictated by the amount of radioactivity injected, the fraction of the injected activity that reaches the tissues of interest, the imaging time, and the sensitivity of the PET system. Practical limits are set for the amount of radioactivity that can be administered and on the imaging time. Thus, system sensitivity is a key factor in obtaining high-quality images. The system sensitivity is defined as the number of events (in counts per second) detected per unit of radioactive concentration (cps/Bq/ml) in a specific phantom. It is sometimes also expressed as the fraction of radioactive decays that produce a valid coincidence event (cps/Bq). The system sensitivity is a product of several factors, which include the efficiency of the detectors at 511 keV, the solid angle coverage of the detectors, the location of the radioactivity with respect to the detectors, and the timing and energy windows applied to the data.

The *detection efficiency* ε, of an individual detector is given by the product of the detection probability of the incoming photon in the detector volume and the fraction of these events, Φ, that fall within the selected energy window (typically set at 350–650 keV). The energy window helps to reduce the influence of scattered events by only accepting events that deposit energy close to 511 keV (e.g., photopeak events). The efficiency is:

$$\varepsilon = (1 - e^{-\mu d}) \times \Phi \tag{1-19}$$

where μ is the attenuation coefficient of the detector material (Table 1-4), and d is the thickness of the detector. A valid event requires that both photons be detected in opposing detectors and be within the appropriate energy range. The *coincidence detection efficiency* is, therefore, given by the square of Equation 1-19:

$$\varepsilon^2 = (1 - e^{-\mu d})^2 \times \Phi^2 \tag{1-20}$$

The *geometric efficiency* of the system is determined by the overall solid angle (Ω) coverage of the detectors with respect to the source location and the packing fraction. The solid angle subtended by the detectors of a circular system for a point source placed at the center is given by:

$$\Omega = 4\pi \sin [\tan^{-1} (A/D)] \tag{1-21}$$

where D is the diameter of the detector ring. For a PET scanner consisting of a single ring of detector elements, A is just the height of the detector in the axial direction. For scanners consisting of multiple detector rings (e.g., a ring or rings of block detectors) or continuous detectors, A depends on the maximum acceptance angle over which data will be collected. This is discussed further in the next two sections in this chapter.

In the manufacturing of the detectors in a PET system using discrete detector elements or block detectors, a small gap is always between the detector elements due to the need for reflective material on the detector walls and/or detector encapsulation. This dead space will produce a reduction in the overall efficiency and is referred to as the packing fraction (φ). The packing fraction is the ratio of the detector element area (width of detector element by axial height of detector element) to the total surface area, including the dead space:

$$\varphi = \frac{width \times height}{(width + deadspace) \times (height + deadspace)} \tag{1-22}$$

The overall system sensitivity, η, for a point source placed at the center of a ring scanner is the product of the square of the detection efficiency ε and the geometric efficiency $\varphi \times \Omega$. Expressed as a percentage, it is given by:

$$\eta = 100 \times \frac{\varepsilon^2 \varphi \Omega}{4\pi} \tag{1-23}$$

Notice that ε is squared as a result of the coincidence detection. Because of this, a small reduction in ε, due to either a reduction in the thickness of the scintillator or a tighter energy window, will produce a significant loss in the overall sensitivity. φ appears as a linear term because of the angular correlation of the two photons; however, this is only an approximation and the true contribution of packing fraction losses is position and geometry dependent. For a distributed source, the expression becomes more complex due to variations in both the geometric and detection efficiencies across the field of view (FOV).

EXAMPLE 1-10

Compute the overall system sensitivity for a central point source in a PET scanner consisting of a single ring of BGO crystals if the ring diameter is 80 cm and the detector elements measure 4.9 mm in width (transaxial) by 6 mm in height (axial) by 30 mm deep. Assume the window fraction is 80%. Assume further that the dimensions for each detector element include a 0.25-mm thick layer of reflector all around the crystal, such that the actual size of the BGO elements is 4.4 mm $\times$ 5.5 mm in cross-section.

ANSWER

From Equation 1-19, and using the linear attenuation coefficient for BGO in Table 1-4, the detection efficiency is:

$$\varepsilon = (1 - e^{-(0.96 \times 3)}) \times 0.8 = 0.755$$

From Equation 1-21, the geometric efficiency is:

$$\Omega = 4\pi \sin[\tan^{-1}(0.6/80)] = 0.094$$

The packing fraction is given by Equation 1-22 as:

$$\varphi = (4.4 \times 5.5) \div (4.9 \times 6) = 0.673$$

The overall system sensitivity, from Equation 1-23, is:

$$\eta = 100 \times 0.755^2 \times 0.094 \times 0.673 / 4\pi = 0.287\%$$

This example demonstrates the low sensitivity of a single-slice PET scanner, even when a complete ring of detectors surrounds the patient and high-efficiency detectors are used. In this situation, the geometric efficiency is the limiting factor.

Data representation—the sinogram

Consider a simple PET system consisting of 32 individual detectors in a ring, scanning an object with a 2-D distribution of radioactivity denoted by $a(x,y)$ (Figure 1-26). The raw data, which consists of the detection of annihilation photon pairs, usually is histogrammed into a 2-D matrix, where each element in the matrix corresponds to the number of events recorded by a particular pair of detectors (or along a specific line of response). The matrix is arranged such that each row represents parallel line integrals or a *projection* of the activity at a particular angle ϕ. Each column represents the radial offset from the center of the scanner, r. The relationship that relates which elements in this matrix (r,ϕ) record data from radioactivity in the object at location (x,y) is given by:

$$r = x \cos\phi + y \sin\phi \qquad (1\text{-}24)$$

This 2-D matrix $s(r,\phi)$ is known as a *sinogram* because a point source at a location (x,y) traces a sinusoidal path in the matrix as given by Equation 1-24. The mapping of detector pairs into a sinogram is shown in Figure 1-27. In practice, as Figure 1-27 demonstrates, the data in each row do not come from a single angular view but rather from two adjacent angles that are interleaved together. The samples from the second angle fall exactly half way between those from the first angle. For typical PET scanner geometry, this leads to projection views that

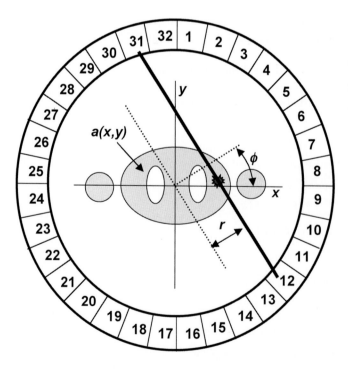

FIGURE 1-26. Imaging geometry for a single-slice PET scanner consisting of 32 detectors. The relationship between the (x,y) coordinate system of the object and the (r,ϕ) coordinate system in which PET data are commonly stored is also shown.

29 20	29 19	30 19	30 18	31 18	31 17	32 17	32 16	1 16	1 15	2 15	2 14	3 14	3 13	4 13
30 21	30 20	31 20	31 19	32 19	32 18	1 18	1 17	2 17	2 16	3 16	3 15	4 15	4 14	5 14
31 22	31 21	32 21	32 20	1 20	1 19	2 19	2 18	3 18	3 17	4 17	4 16	5 16	5 15	6 15
32 23	32 22	1 22	1 21	2 21	2 20	3 20	3 19	4 19	4 18	5 18	5 17	6 17	6 16	7 16
1 24	1 23	2 23	2 22	3 22	3 21	4 21	4 20	5 20	5 19	6 19	6 18	7 18	7 17	8 17
2 25	2 24	3 24	3 23	4 23	4 22	5 22	5 21	6 21	6 20	7 20	7 19	8 19	8 18	9 18
3 26	3 25	4 25	4 24	5 24	5 23	6 23	6 22	7 22	7 21	8 21	8 20	9 20	9 19	10 19
4 27	4 26	5 26	5 25	6 25	6 24	7 24	7 23	8 23	8 22	9 22	9 21	10 21	10 20	11 20
5 28	5 27	6 27	6 26	7 26	7 25	8 25	8 24	9 24	9 23	10 23	10 22	11 22	11 21	12 21
6 29	6 28	7 28	7 27	8 27	8 26	9 26	9 25	10 25	10 24	11 24	11 23	12 23	12 22	13 22
7 30	7 29	8 29	8 28	9 28	9 27	10 27	10 26	11 26	11 25	12 25	12 24	13 24	13 23	14 23
8 31	8 30	9 30	9 29	10 29	10 28	11 28	11 27	12 27	12 26	13 26	13 25	14 25	14 24	15 24
9 32	9 31	10 31	10 30	11 30	11 29	12 29	12 28	13 28	13 27	14 27	14 26	15 26	15 25	16 25
10 1	10 32	11 32	11 31	**12 31**	12 30	13 30	13 29	14 29	14 28	15 28	15 27	16 27	16 26	17 26
11 2	11 1	12 1	12 32	13 32	13 31	14 31	14 30	15 30	15 29	16 29	16 28	17 28	17 27	18 27
12 3	12 2	13 2	13 1	14 1	14 32	15 32	15 31	16 31	16 30	17 30	17 29	18 29	18 28	19 28

ϕ

r

FIGURE 1-27. Formation of a sinogram based on the 32 detector PET system in Figure 1-26. The annihilation event shown in Figure 1-26 would be binned into the highlighted element in the sinogram. Each row in the sinogram corresponds to a projection of the radioactivity within the object at a specific angle ϕ. The angles in a sinogram extend over 180°, the other 180° is redundant as the data are based on pairs of detectors.

closely approximate parallel lines, particularly at the center of the scanner where the patient is located. This small rearrangement of the data from the strict definition results in twice the sampling near the center of the scanner, at the expense of reducing the number of angular samples by a factor of 2. This rearrangement helps produce data that are more appropriately sampled for image reconstruction (Image Reconstruction, p. 70). Figure 1-28 shows the sinogram that would be obtained from a simple cylindrical object containing two smaller

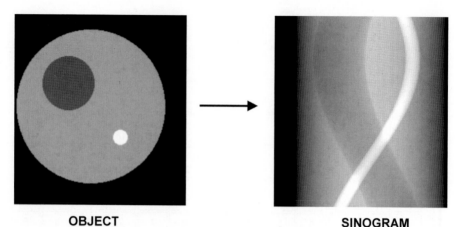

OBJECT   **SINOGRAM**

FIGURE 1-28. A simple object and the sinogram (simulation) that would result from taking projection views over 180° around this object. (Data courtesy of Dr. Andrew Goertzen. Reproduced with permission from Cherry SR, Sorenson JA, Phelps ME. *Physics in Nuclear Medicine*, W.B. Saunders, New York, 2003.)

regions with different radioactivity concentrations. Notice how these regions with different radioactivity uptake trace a sinusoidal path in the sinogram.

EXAMPLE 1-11

What locations in object space will contribute data to a sinogram element at angle 30° and which is offset at a distance 6 cm from the center of the scanner?

ANSWER

From Equation 1-24, we get:

$$6 = x \cos 30° + y \sin 30°$$
$$0.866 \, x + 0.5 \, y = 6$$
$$x = 6.93 - 0.58y$$

This is the equation for a line, and all (x,y) locations that satisfy the equation and lie along the line can contribute data to this particular sinogram element.

Two-dimensional data acquisition

In the first generation of multiring PET systems, coincidences were only recorded in *direct* and *cross planes*, where a direct plane is defined as coincidences between detector elements within the same detector ring and a cross plane are the average of coincidences recorded between detectors in two adjacent detector rings (Figure 1-29A). Collecting coincidences this way allows an improvement in axial sampling because the events collected by the cross planes originate primarily from the volume between the direct planes. Thus, in a system built up of N detector rings, N direct planes and N − 1 cross planes can be defined, resulting in a total of 2N − 1 coincidence planes. Thin tungsten shields, known as *septa*, were used between detector rings to absorb annihilation photons incident at larger angles, thus reducing the overall count rates on the detectors to decrease the

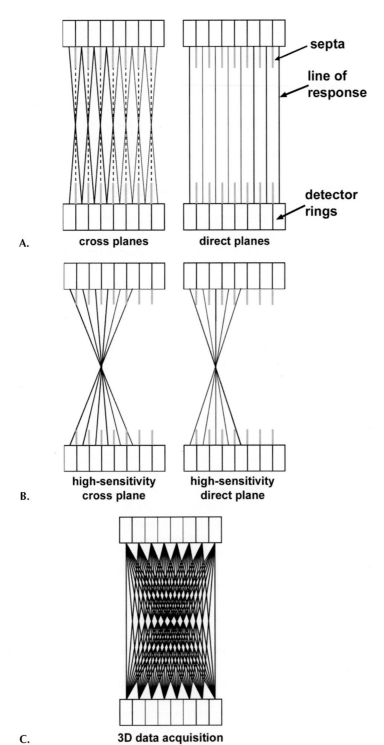

FIGURE 1-29. Axial section through a multiring PET scanner showing 2-D and 3-D sinogram definitions: A) standard 2-D direct and cross-plane definitions, B) high sensitivity 2-D direct and cross-plane definitions used in many scanners, and C) full 3-D data acquisition.

likelihood of random coincidences and also to help absorb photons that had scattered in the body. This mode of operation is commonly referred to as 2-D *data acquisition* because the data collection is restricted to a set of almost parallel 2-D planes.

Newer, higher resolution PET systems are using smaller detector elements. In these scanners, direct and cross-plane definitions are still used, but because of the low sensitivity of each pure direct and cross plane, additional coincidence planes are accepted in which the detector pairs are separated by up to 5 to 6 detector rings (Figure 1-29B). This increases the azimuthal angle over which events will be allowed, also known as the *acceptance angle*. In terms of Equation 1-21, summing these coincidence planes increases the effective value of *A*, leading to higher sensitivity than would be achieved with the original definition of direct and cross planes. The drawback of this method is that the axial resolution at the edge of the FOV is significantly degraded due to the geometric divergence of the lines of response that are contributing to a particular image plane. There are also shadowing effects that come from the septa.[40,41] In addition, the axial sensitivity drops off rapidly at the edge of the axial FOV because no additional cross-plane combinations can be added to the planes at the axial extremes.

In 2-D data acquisition, the data from the selected coincidence planes are averaged to produce a set of 2N − 1 parallel sinograms, each of which can be used to reconstruct a cross-sectional image. Methods for reconstructing these sinograms will be discussed in Image Reconstruction (p. 70).

Three-dimensional data acquisition

The sensitivity of the PET system can be further improved by defining additional coincidence plane combinations, where the ring difference extends well beyond that used in 2-D data acquisition (Figure 1-29C). This requires the removal of the tungsten septa that would otherwise block these oblique lines of repsonse. To avoid unacceptable resolution losses at off-center positions, these oblique coincidence planes are now stored in separate sinograms, with an associated azimuthal angle. This leads to N^2 sinograms for an N-ring PET scanner. Because the coincidence planes are no longer only limited to parallel planes, this acquisition mode is referred to as *3-D data acquisition*. Since the data are acquired in a 3-D manner, an appropriate 3-D algorithm has to be used to reconstruct the images (Three-Dimensional Analytic Reconstruction, p. 82).

The 3-D acquisition mode provides a dramatic improvement in sensitivity (typically a factor of ×5 to ×7) compared to 2-D acquisition,[42,43] as *A* in Equation 1-21 now corresponds to the entire axial length of the scanner. This additional sensitivity can be used to improve signal-to-noise in PET images, reduce imaging time, or to reduce the amount of radioactivity that is injected. The sensitivity increase is not uniform across the field of view. The sensitivity profile for 3-D data acquisition is triangular in shape in the axial direction as shown in Figure 1-30. At the axial extremes of the field of view, the sensitivity is equivalent to that of 2-D data acquisition. The wide-open geometry of 3-D acquisition and lack of interplane septa results in a three- to fourfold increase in the fraction of scattered events detected. Furthermore, noise due to the subtraction of random coincidences becomes a problem at lower activity concentrations than in 2-D because each detector sees more of the radioactivity in the body and, therefore, has a higher singles event rate. This leads to further challenges in accurately cor-

FIGURE 1-30. Measured sensitivity profiles along the axis of a multiring PET scanner in 2-D mode (corresponding to B in Figure 1-29) and 3-D mode (corresponding to C in Figure 1-29). In 3-D mode, sensitivity peaks at the center of the axial field of view. At the extreme edges of the axial field of view, 2-D and 3-D sensitivity are equivalent.

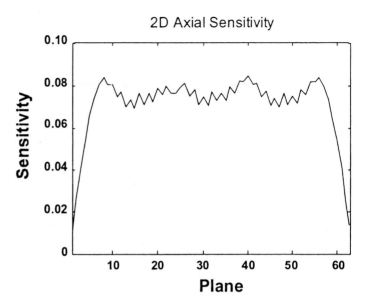

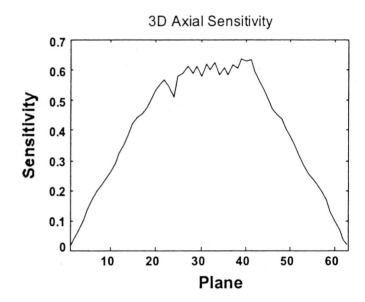

recting data for random and scattered coincidences and can result in relatively poor image quality when large amounts of activity are present in the field of view, for example, when imaging over the bladder region. Many radiotracers are excreted through the kidneys and a significant fraction of the injected activity can end up in the bladder.

As a consequence of the improved sensitivity of the 3-D acquisition mode, the size of the raw data sets also is increased. This presents an additional challenge in handling the data from the initial collection of the data to the final archiving. As an example, the complete, uncompressed, 3-D data set from a high-resolution clinical PET system can be more than 100 Mbytes. With the constant improvement in computing power and data storage, this size may not be a limitation in the near future, but with present technology a data set of this size poses significant challenges. Due to the relatively high-noise levels in the raw data, conventional loss less compression techniques are relatively inefficient in producing significant compression ratios. To produce a more significant reduction in the data sizes, a technique sometimes referred to as angular mashing is used. In the method, adjacent angles (projection angles within each sinogram and/or the oblique azimuthal angle) are simply added together to produce the compression. This is similar to the averaging used in high-sensitivity 2-D data acquisition shown in Figure 1-29B. Using this technique, the 3-D data sets can be reduced to a more managable size of about 20 Mbytes. Because projection angles are added together, this method does produce a loss in both in-plane and axial resolution at off-center positions.

EXAMPLE 1-12
For the same scanner described in Problem 1-10, estimate the system sensitivity at the center of the field of view if there are 16 rings of BGO detectors and the scanner is operated with 3-D data acquisition.

ANSWER
The detector efficiency and packing fraction are the same as in Problem 1-10. The geometric efficiency is now given by Equation 1-21:

$$\Omega = 4\,\pi\,\sin\,(\tan^{-1}\,(A/D)) = 4\,\pi\,\sin\,(\tan^{-1}\,(6 \times 16\,/\,800)) = 1.50$$

The sensitivity Equation 1-23 is therefore:

$$\eta = 100 \times ((0.755)^2 \times 0.673 \times 1.50)\,/\,4\,\pi = 4.57\%$$

The result for 2-D acquisition in Problem 1-10 was 0.29%. This problem shows the dramatic increase in sensitivity at the center of the scanner for 3-D data acquisition compared with 2-D data acquisition.

Data acquisition protocols

The end point in most PET studies is to produce an image, from which diagnostic or quantitative parameters can be derived. These parameters can be as simple as a qualitative comparison of activity concentration in different tissue regions or more complex biologic parameters such as metabolic rate, receptor density, or levels of gene expression. The information that is to be extracted from the image will dictate how the PET data are collected (i.e., static or dynamic sequence).

The most basic data acquisition protocol in PET is the collection of a single data set or static frame over a fixed length of time. The image reconstructed from such a data set represents the average tissue activity concentration during the acquisition. This is the typical acquisition mode used in studies where the tissue activity distribution remains relatively static during the collection of the data. An example where this acquisition mode is commonly used is for 2-deoxy-2-[F-18]fluro-D-glucose (FDG) studies, where the tracer concentration remains fairly stable following an initial uptake period of 30 to 40 minutes. In these types of studies, the biologic parameter of interest (in this case the metabolic rate for glucose) is then assumed to be directly proportional to the measured activity concentration. A detailed discussion on the assumptions inherent in this approach can be found in Chapter 2.

For some radiotracers, it is necessary to follow the dynamic changes in concentration to extract a particular parameter of interest. In these studies, the data are collected as a sequence of dynamic time frames, where the PET images provide information about the changes in activity concentration distribution over time. This information represents the tissue response to the time course of the radiotracer in the plasma following intravenous injection. The tissue time-activity curve can then be processed with a compartmental model to determine the parameters of interest (Chapter 2). These types of studies typically also require additional data such as the plasma radioactivity concentration and the plasma concentration of labeled metabolites, which can be determined from blood samples. An example of a dynamic study is shown in Figure 1-31.

The dynamic acquisition mode also is used in studies where the tissue radiotracer concentration remains constant (e.g., FDG brain scans), but the patient has to remain motionless in the scanner for an extended period of time. By collecting the data in a dynamic sequence (e.g., multiple 5-min frames), it is possible to determine if the subject moved during the acquisition and allow removal, or realignment of frames, when the subject moved.[44]

Most PET systems have a relatively narrow axial field of view that limits the coverage to a single organ (e.g., the brain, heart, kidneys, and so on). To cover a larger extent of the body, the acquisition has to be performed in a series of steps in which the patient is moved through the scanner (Figure 1-32). To minimize the amount of patient motion, these scans are typically limited to 30 to 40 minutes. The main challenge in these whole-body scans is to collect enough counts in both the emission and transmission (see Attenuation Correction, p. 56) scans in this time frame to produce images of diagnostic quality, without excessive noise levels. The problem of noise contamination from the attenuation correction using short transmission scans has been greatly reduced through the development of fast and accurate image segmentation algorithms.[45–47] Also, initial results from clinical PET scanners that are based on fast LSO detectors demonstrate the possibility of acquiring whole-body images in as little as 5 to 10 minutes. In many cases, the relatively high statistical noise originating from the emission data requires that the images be reconstructed using iterative algorithms (see Iterative Reconstruction Methods, p. 86). Although these algorithms tend to be computationally expensive, improvements in both acceleration techniques and a constant improvement in computing hardware, now allow routine reconstruction of high-quality, whole-body PET images in clinically acceptable times.[48,49]

DATA CORRECTION

To produce an image volume in which each voxel value represents the true tissue activity concentration, a number of corrections need to be applied to the raw sinogram data. These corrections are typically applied to the sinograms as a series of multiplicative factors prior to image reconstruction.

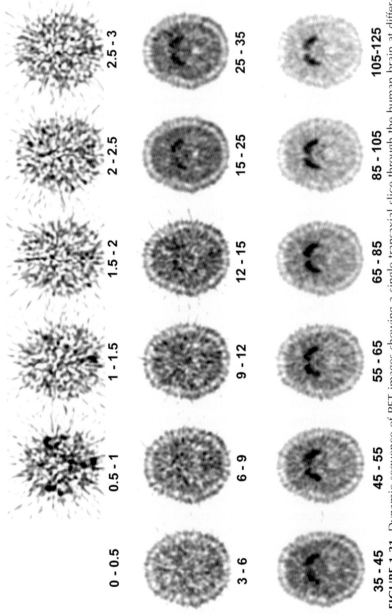

FIGURE 1-31. Dynamic sequence of PET images showing a single transaxial slice through the human brain at different times following the injection of [F18]fluoro-L-DOPA, a radiotracer that reflects dopamine synthesis. Times are in minutes. Notice how the distribution pattern changes over time. The radiotracer is delivered to all brain tissue during the first few minutes. There is a gradual accumulation of the radiotracer in the caudate and putamen (the site to which dopaminergic neurons project) and clearance from other tissues. By 60 minutes, there is clear contrast between the specifically bound radiotracer in the caudate and putamen and the rest of the brain tissues. (Adapted with permission from Cherry SR, Phelps ME. Positron Emission Tomography: Methods and Instrumentation, in *Diagnostic Nuclear Medicine*, 4th Edition, Eds: Sandler MP, Coleman RE, Wackers FJT, Patton JA, Gottschalk A, Hoffer PB. Williams & Wilkins, Baltimore, 2002.)

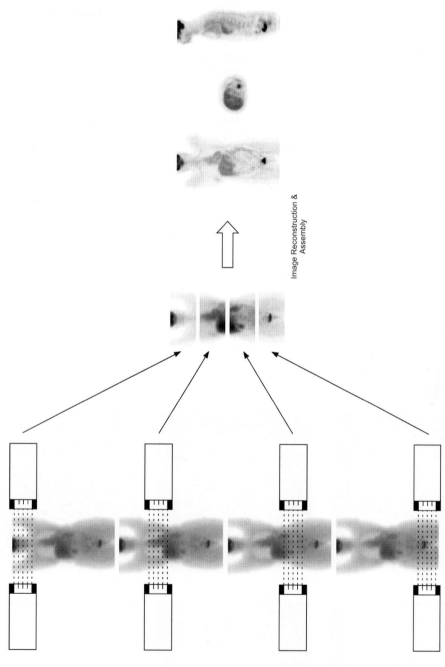

Image Reconstruction & Assembly

FIGURE 1-32. To obtain a whole-body PET image, the body has to be imaged in segments. To achieve this, the patient bed is moved in steps through the scanner. At each discrete bed position, a scan is acquired. The data collected at each bed position are reconstructed and assembled into a whole-body volume which can be reoriented into coronal, sagittal, and transaxial images as shown on the right.

Normalization

Nonuniformities in individual detector efficiencies (physical dimensions), geometrical variations, and detector electronics (e.g., energy thresholds) all contribute to variations in coincidence detection efficiency between different LORs
(i.e., pairs of detector elements) in the system. The normalization corrects each
individual LOR, with a multiplication factor that compensates for these nonuniformities. Figure 1-33 illustrates the effect of normalization on the images from
a scan of a uniform cylinder, acquired in 2-D mode. This figure illustrates that
the normalization is not only a correction on the individual sinogram but is a
volumetric correction that adjusts for any sensitivity variation between the different coincidence planes.

To generate a normalization correction, the individual detector efficiencies
as well as any geometrical efficiency variations are measured. In addition, any
variation in plane-to-plane efficiency is measured. The most straightforward
method to determine the normalization correction factors is to collect data from
a uniform plane source of activity, positioned at 6 to 8 equally spaced projection angles. This method will directly measure the relative variation in coincidence detection efficiencies between all the LORs in the system.[50] To avoid dead
time and pile-up effects, a source of relatively low activity has to be used. Therefore, the main challenge using this method is to acquire enough counts per LOR
(within a reasonable time frame) to provide a good estimate of the efficiencies
with a minimum of statistical noise that would propagate into the final image.

FIGURE 1-33. Effect of normalization on the image of a cylinder containing a uniform
concentration of radionuclide. Row A shows a transaxial cross-section through the reconstructed image of the cylinder, row B an axial cross-section. Without the normalization, the nonuniform axial sensitivity is revealed. The effect of the normalization is
less visible in the transaxial image, but the difference image reveals ring artefacts as
well as a "hole" in the center.

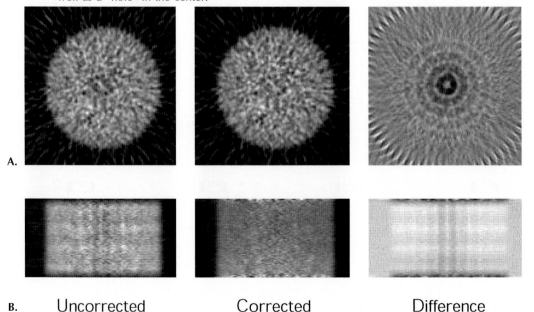

A.

B.   Uncorrected   Corrected   Difference

Furthermore, any nonuniformities in the plane source will propagate into the final image.

EXAMPLE 1-13

Assuming Poisson counting statistics, calculate the number of events that would be needed to normalize a PET scanner with a total of 10^6 lines of response (LORs) if a normalization accuracy of an average of 1% is desired. If the normalization source leads to a coincidence counting rate of 50,000 cps, how long would this normalization scan take?

ANSWER

For Poisson statistics, the standard deviation, σ, is equal to $\sqrt{N}$, where N is the number of events collected. For each LOR, we require that:

$$\sqrt{N}/N = 0.01$$

therefore, $N = 10,000$

For 10^6 LORs, the total number of counts needed in the normalization scan is:

$$10,000 \times 10^6 = 10^{10}$$

For a counting rate of 50,000 cps, the time for the normalization scan would be:

$$10^{10} \div 50,000 = 200,000 \text{ s} = 55.6 \text{ h}$$

This demonstrates the difficulty of making direct measurements of normalization factors for each individual LOR in the system.

An alternative method to determine the normalization matrix is the component-based method, in which the coincidence detection efficiency of a pair of detectors i and j is assumed to be composed of the product of the individual detector efficiencies, ϵ, and geometrical factors, $g_{i,j}$. The normalization correction factors $n_{i,j}$ are therefore given as:

$$n_{i,j} = \frac{1}{\varepsilon_i \times \varepsilon_j \times g_{i,j}} \tag{1-25}$$

These geometrical factors include a correction for the angle of incidence of the annihilation photons, systematic variations in crystal efficiency dependent on the position of the crystal in a detector block modules, and relative plane efficiency. The individual detector efficiencies for all detector elements in the system can be determined from a scan of a uniform cylinder or any circularly symmetric source, centered in the scanner FOV. For each detector element in the system, the sum of the coincidences between the detector of interest and all of its opposing detectors (corrected for random and scattered coincidences) is determined. The assumption is made that by averaging over a large number of opposing detector elements, this sum will be directly proportional to the individual detector efficiency. The geometrical factors are typically determined once for a particular system using very high counting statistical acquisitions at the factory and can be assumed to remain constant. The coincidence detection efficiency for a given LOR in the system is the product of the measured individual detector efficiencies adjusted for any geometrical efficiency variations,[51–53] and the normalization factors that need to be applied to the emission data are the reciprocal of this quantity (Equation 1-25). This method provides an estimate of the normalization factor with virtually no statistical noise because the measurement of detection efficiencies is averaged over a large number of detector elements; however, the method dose depends heavily on a number of measured and empirical geometrical factors that could introduce systematic errors as discussed by Badawi et al.[54] Figure 1-34 shows the projection data before and after correction for detector normalization.

Attenuation correction

At 511 keV, a relatively high probability exists that one or both annihilation photons will interact in the subject, predominantly through Compton interactions.

FIGURE 1-34. A: Unnormalized sinogram. Each detector in the system traces a diagonal line in the sinogram. Detectors that have a high or a low efficiency will lead to bright and dark diagonal lines, respectively. B: Measured normalization factors. C: After multiplying the unnormalized sinogram by the normalization factors, differences in detector efficiencies have been effectively removed. The images on the left show an individual sinogram; the images on the right show normalization effects in the axial direction.

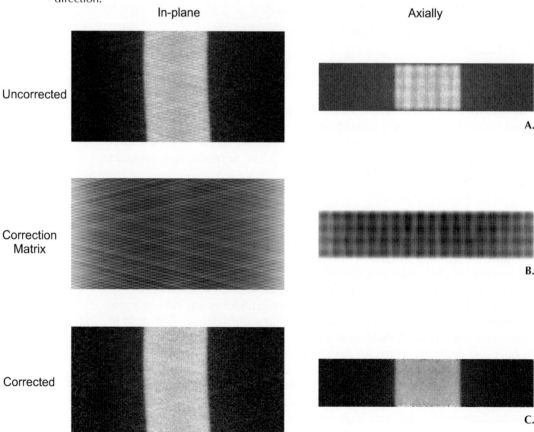

FIGURE 1-35. Effect of attenuation correction on a uniform cylinder.

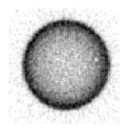
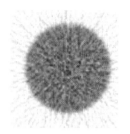

Uncorrected Corrected

As discussed earlier, the results of these interactions are the removal or attenuation of primary photons from a given LOR and the potential detection of scattered photons in a different LOR. Thus, attenuation and scatter are manifestations of the same physical process. Correction involves removing scattered events from the LORs and then subsequently correcting each LOR for the fraction of events that were scattered, or attenuated from, that LOR.

Attenuation of the signal from a given LOR can be corrected either by a direct measurement or using a mathematical model or a combination of the two. Figure 1-35 illustrates the effect of photon attenuation on the image of a cylinder containing a uniform radioactivity concentration. Without the correction, the central portion of the cylinder appears to have lower activity than the outer edge because photons coming from the center of the cylinder, on the average, must pass through more material to reach the detectors than photons at the edge of the cylinder.

Consider a point source located at an unknown depth x in a uniformly attenuating medium with an attenuation coefficient μ. If the thickness of the object is D along the LOR (Figure 1-36), then the probability that annihilation photon 1 will escape the object is the result of Equation 1-15:

$$p_1 = \frac{I(x)}{I(0)} = \exp(-\mu x) \qquad (1\text{-}26)$$

The probability that annihilation photon 2 will escape is:

$$p_2 = \frac{I(D - x)}{I(0)} = \exp(-\mu(D - x)) \qquad (1\text{-}27)$$

FIGURE 1-36. Derivation of the equations for attenuation correction in PET. p_1 and p_2 are the probabilities that each of the two annihilation photons from a source located at an unknown depth x in a uniform attenuator of thickness D will escape the object. The product of p_1 and p_2 is the probability that both annihilation photons will escape the object and be available for detection. The attenuation correction for this line of response is simply $(p_1 \times p_2)^{-1}$, which is independent of the location of the source.

$$p_2 = e^{-\mu(D-x)} \qquad p_1 = e^{-\mu x}$$

$$p_{coinc.} = p_1\, p_2 = e^{-\mu x}\, e^{-\mu(D-x)} = e^{-\mu D}$$

$$\text{Atten. Corr.} = e^{\mu D}$$

The probability that both annihilation photons will escape the object is the product of the individual probabilities:

$$p_1 \times p_2 = \exp(-\mu x) \times \exp(-\mu(D - x)) = \exp(-\mu D) \qquad (1\text{-}28)$$

As can be seen from this equation, the reduction in photon flux is independent of the location of the source and only dependent on the total thickness of the object along the LOR and the attenuation coefficient of the object. This is unique to annihilation coincidence detection and makes attenuation correction straightforward. The attenuation correction factors, $a_{i,j}$, that need to be applied to the emission data for the LOR joining detector i and j, are given simply by the reciprocal of Equation 1-28:

$$a_{i,j} = \exp(\mu D_{i,j}) = I(0)/I(D_{i,j}) \qquad (1\text{-}29)$$

where $D_{i,j}$ is the tissue thickness for the LOR between detector i and detector j. This equation forms the basis for the various methods for correcting photon attenuation in PET.

EXAMPLE 1-14
A line of response passes through 30 cm of soft tissue and 2 cm of bone. Compute the attenuation correction factor that would need to be applied to this line of response.

ANSWER
From Table 1-3, μ(bone) = 0.17 cm^{-1} and μ(tissue) = 0.096 cm^{-1} at 511 keV.

The total attenuation correction factor is the product of the two components:

$$\exp(0.17 \times 2) \times \exp(0.096 \times 30) = 25$$

This demonstrates how to compute attenuation correction factors for a mixture of tissues and the very large correction factors that need to be applied when the annihilation photons have to pass through large amounts of tissue.

Calculated attenuation correction

In its simplest form, the calculated attenuation correction assumes that the outline of the object that being imaged can be approximated with a geometrical shape such as an ellipse. Furthermore, the attenuation coefficient within this object is also assumed to be constant. To generate the attenuation correction, the chord length (representing $D_{i,j}$) is determined for each individual LOR intersecting the ellipse and $a_{i,j}$ is calculated from Equation 1-29.

This method is primarily useful in imaging phantoms where the attenuation coefficient is typically uniform and the shape of the phantom can most of the time be approximated with a geometrical shape such as a circle or ellipse. This method was also used in early PET systems as the attenuation correction in brain studies. To apply this correction, the emission data were initially reconstructed without correction for attenuation. The users then fitted an ellipse to the outline of the skull on each individual cross-sectional slice. From these ellipses, the attenuation correction was calculated and applied to the raw data, which was reconstructed again. This method produces images that are largely free of attenuation artifacts, however, due to the approximations of the shape of the object and the assumption of a uniform attenuation coefficient, the method tends to underestimate the attenuation. This method is also very prone to artifacts, such as asymmetries, depending on the positioning of the ellipse. Furthermore, the method can be very labor-intensive on a system generating a large number of image slices.

An improvement of this method was introduced by Bergström et al[55] and later refined by Siegel and Dahlbom.[56] The outline of the head was determined directly from the sinogram data. This eliminated the need of fitting the ellipse to each individual slice and more accurately models the outline of the head. Furthermore, in this refined method, the attenuation of the skull can be modeled. This method improves the original one but still has a tendency to create quantitative errors and small artifacts, especially at the base of the skull due to the presence of air cavities and thicker bones.

Measured attenuation correction

The most accurate method to determine the attenuation correction is through direct measurements. As was shown in Equation 1-28, the amount of attenuation is independent of the location of the source. This means that if a source is placed outside the object along the LOR of interest, the amount of attenuation would be the same as for a source inside the object. Therefore, by placing a positron-emitting source outside the object, the amount of attenuation can be measured directly. In measured attenuation correction, either a set of ring sources, or a set of rotating rod sources, is placed just inside the detectors, enabling the attenuation factors for all LORs in the scanner to be measured in a single scan. Initially, a reference or a *blank scan* is measured, in which data from these external sources are acquired with no object in the scanner. This corresponds to measurements of $I(0)$ in Equation 1-29 for each LOR. Then the object is placed in the scanner, and a *transmission scan* is acquired. This provides $I(D)$ from Equation 1-29. The attenuation correction factors for each LOR are simply given by taking the ratio between the blank sinograms and the transmission sinograms as shown in Figure 1-37. The normalized emission sinogram is multiplied by these factors to obtain attenuation corrected sinograms. Figure 1-38 shows measured sinogram data before and after applying attenuation correction. The sources used in blank and transmission scans usually are made from ^{68}Ge which has a 273-day half-life. These sources generally need replacing every 12 to 18 months.

The main advantage of this method is that the attenuation is directly measured, and no assumptions are made in regards to the shape of the object nor the distribution of attenuation coefficients. The main difficulty in these transmission scans is to collect an adequate number of counts along each attenuated LOR. It is not unusual to have attenuation correction factors of over 50 in the region of the abdomen, with less than 10 measured transmission counts measured in an LOR. Thus, the statistical quality of the transmission scan is typically very poor and this noise will propagate into the emission data if left unprocessed. The most common method to process the transmission data is to apply a spatial smoothing filter to the blank and transmission scans prior to computing the attenuation correction (i.e., the blank/transmission ratio). This method is typically adequate if the transmission scan is fairly long (> 20 min).

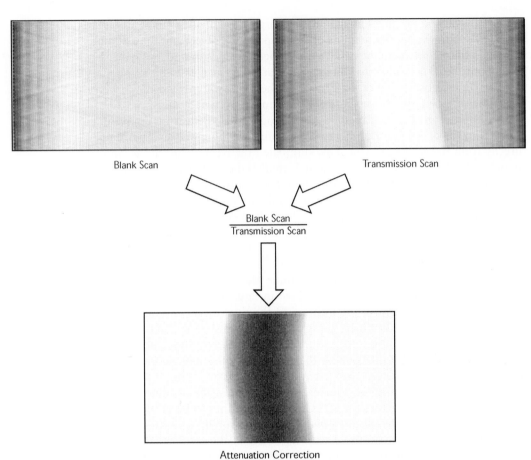

Attenuation Correction

FIGURE 1-37. The measured attenuation correction matrix is created by dividing the blank scan sinogram (acquired without the subject in the scanner) by the transmission scan sinogram (acquired with the subject in scanner). This operation is performed on every element (i.e., line of response) in the sinogram. These blank and transmission scan measurements typically are taken with external ring or rotating rod sources containing positron-emitting radionuclides.

Hybrid techniques of the calculated and measured attenuation correction methods also have been developed, where a virtually noise-free attenuation correction can be created. In these methods, an image of the attenuation coefficients is first reconstructed by taking the natural log of the attenuation correction sinograms and reconstructing these sinograms using computed tomography (CT) techniques. This reconstruction yields a noisy CT-like image, but the information content of these images is typically enough to allow an image segmentation, where the attenuation coefficients in the images are classified or segmented into a fixed number of attenuation coefficients (e.g., soft tissue, lung tissue, and bone). The segmented image can then be traced along each LOR to calculate an almost noiseless estimate of the attenuation correction.[45–47] A drawback of the method is that assumptions about the actual attenuation coefficients must be made and population averages are used.

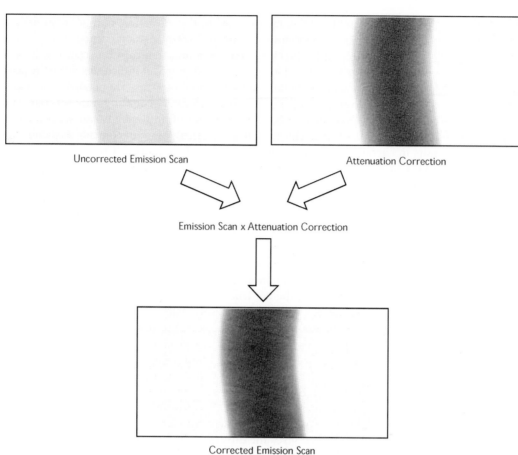

FIGURE 1-38. The attenuation correction is performed by multiplying the normalized emission sinogram with the attenuation correction matrix. This operation is performed on every element in the sinogram.

　　The introduction of rotating rod sources instead of ring sources has allowed a more efficient use of the scanner with the acquisition of transmission scans after the injection of the tracer.[57–59] This approach is known as *post-injection transmission scanning.* In clinical imaging protocols (Data Acquisition Protocols, p. 50), this eliminates the need for the patient to remain in the scanner during the required time for the radiotracer to distribute in the body. Because most transmission sources use a positron emitter, a coincidence originating from the transmission source will be indistinguishable from an emission coincidence. However, when using a rod source, the position of the rod is monitored during the acquisition. If the line of response for a detected event aligns with the location of the rod source, a high likelihood exists that the event originated from an annihilation in the rod source. This assumption can be made if the total activity in the source is much higher than the total emission activity along any given LOR. This is typically the case if the activity in the rod sources is approximately 2 mCi. In areas of high accumulation of radioactivity, such as in the bladder in FDG scans, this assumption may not be true. This can lead to an undercorrection for attenuation in these regions, due to the substantial number of emission coincidences that are erroneously assigned as transmission events.

Using rotating rod sources, the emission and transmission scans can be acquired simultaneously.[60,61] However, several practical difficulties occur in performing simultaneous emission and transmission scans. The relatively high activity in the rod sources produces an elevated counting rate of random coincidences (Types of Events, p. 33), which can, in some instances, exceed the emission counting rate. The subtraction of these random coincidences then results in excessive noise levels in the corrected sinograms (Correction for Random Coincidences, p. 65). To overcome the problems associated with high random counting rates in simultaneous emission/transmission scans, the activity in the rod sources has to be reduced by a factor 4–5. This reduction requires that the transmission data must be corrected for the contamination of emission events. Furthermore, the emission counts also have to be corrected for contamination of transmission events. The main advantage of this method is the perfect spatial registration of emission and transmission data. However, the need for the various cross-contamination factors may introduce systematic errors and noise in the estimation of the net true counting rate for each LOR.

The main reason for the poor statistical quality of many transmission scans is that only a limited amount of activity can be put in the transmission sources. Because the transmission source will be very close to the detector ring, the near detector is always exposed to a very high photon flux. Therefore, the amount of activity in the rod source is primarily dictated by the count rate capabilities of the detector system. One approach to overcome this problem is to only measure the photons that pass through the object instead of requiring coincidence detection.[62] The line connecting the detector element and the position of the transmission source then gives the directional information of the detected photon. This method is generally referred to as *singles transmission scanning* because only one of the two photons is used in the detection process. The main advantage of this method is the improvement in count rate compared to coincidence measurements. A significant drawback of this method is that scattered radiation cannot be rejected by the requirement that the position of the rod source has to align with the coincidence LOR as described above. Therefore, the scatter fraction is typically very high in *singles transmission scans*, which, in turn, results in a significant underestimation of the attenuation correction. The use of rod sources that extend across the entire axial FOV also results in attenuation correction maps with very poor axial resolution that introduce inaccuracies in attenuation coefficients, especially at interfaces of tissues of significantly different attenuation coefficients. To alleviate these problems, single or multiple collimated point sources are typically used instead of a single rod source.[63,64]

Another drawback of using the singles measurement with ^{68}Ge as the transmission source is that postinjection transmission scans cannot be performed because the emission singles cannot be distinguished from the transmission singles. To allow postinjection transmission scans, one can use a transmission source that emits photons of energy different from 511 keV. Several singles transmission systems use ^{137}Cs, which emits 662 keV photons.[63,64] Using a higher photon energy reduces the amount of emission photon cross-contamination of the transmission data. The amount of cross-contamination depends on the energy resolution of the detector system but cannot be entirely eliminated even in systems using NaI(Tl) detectors, where the energy resolution is as good as 10%. The drawback of using ^{137}Cs as the source is that the transmission measurement is performed at a different energy compared to the emission data (i.e., 511 keV). To overcome this problem, transmission images are typically segmented and the appropriate attenuation values are assigned at 511 keV.[63–65]

Scatter correction

Correction for scatter is probably the most difficult correction that is required in PET, mainly because a scattered event is indistinguishable from a true event except on the basis of energy. Unfortunately, there is no simple way to measure the number of scattered events, and it is, therefore, important to minimize the detection of these events, accomplished to a certain degree by energy discrimination, collimation, and geometrical considerations. When an annihilation photon undergoes a Compton interaction in the body and scatters, it will lose some of its energy in the process. The direction of the scattered photon follows the Klein–Nishina probability function (Figure 1-8) and the amount of energy lost in the scattering interaction is given by Equation 1-12. At 511 keV, forward scatter, in which only a small amount of energy is lost in the interaction, is favored. In fact, 50% of all Compton interactions produce photons with a scatter angle of 60° or less. If PET detectors only accepted events with an energy of 511 keV, all scattered events could be eliminated. But this would require a detector with extremely good energy resolution. Most BGO scintillation detectors used in PET have an energy resolution of about 20% to 25%, which makes it very hard to separate small angle, high-energy scattered photons from the primary 511-keV photons. Even PET systems that use high light output NaI(Tl) scintillation detectors have an energy resolution of at best 10%. An additional difficulty in separating scattered events from primary events is caused by the fact that a significant fraction of the primary 511-keV photons will only deposit a portion of the energy within the detector volume. Although these events are "good" events, they are detected in the same energy range as scattered events. Thus, if the system would only accept events within a narrow energy window at approximately 511 keV, the overall detection efficiency of the system would be very poor (see Sensitivity: Detector and Geometric Efficiencies, p. 42). Therefore, to maintain a reasonable detection efficiency, most PET systems operate with a relatively large energy window between 350 keV to 650 keV, which also results in the detection of a certain amount of scattered photons. Energy discrimination is most efficient in rejecting low energy, large angle scatter. The presence of tungsten interplane septa (Figure 1-29) in a PET system helps reduce detected scatter to a relatively low level. For brain imaging, the fraction of the detected events that have undergone Compton scatter is in the range of 0.1 to 0.15 for a 2-D scan with the interplane septa in place. If the septa are removed, and the system is operated in 3-D mode, the scatter fraction for brain imaging increases to approximately 0.3 to 0.4.

Although scattered events are spread across the field of view and have a fairly low spatial frequency distribution, their contribution, particularly in 3-D studies, needs to be corrected to produce images with high contrast and acceptable quantification. Figure 1-39 shows the effects of scatter in images of a phantom. It is important to notice that scatter and attenuation are really one and the same phenomenon. When one of the annihilation photons scatters, the event is removed from its original LOR (attenuation), but because the photon is rarely ac-

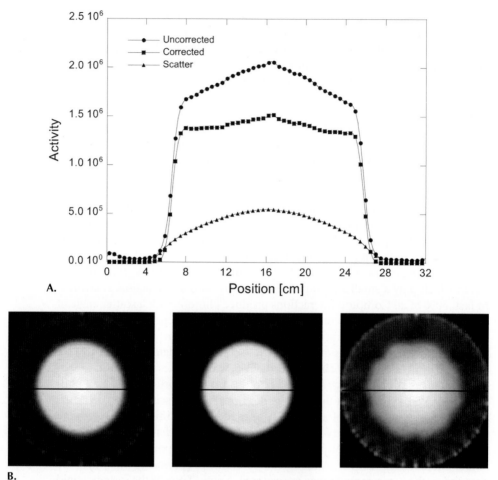

FIGURE 1-39. A: Profiles through the reconstructed images of a cylinder containing a uniform radioactivity concentration showing the contribution of scattered events. The corrected profile is flat, as expected. B: Images corresponding to the profiles; from left to right: Uncorrected image (trues + scatter), corrected image (trues), and scatter image.

tually absorbed in tissue, it may still be detected in a different LOR (scatter). For this reason, the order in which the corrections are applied is important, and scatter correction should be performed prior to attenuation correction. The scatter correction methods can be divided into three main categories: *analytical, dual energy window,* and *simulation methods.*

Analytical methods

In the simplest analytical scatter correction methods, the amount of scatter was estimated by fitting a smoothly varying function to the counts appearing outside the object in the sinograms.[66,67] This method assumes that the scatter distribution varies slowly across the FOV and is relatively independent of both the source distribution and the scattering medium. One of the most widely used analytical methods for scatter correction in 2-D PET is the Bergström et al. method.[68] This method is based on phantom measurements of the scatter distribution from line sources placed at different locations inside scattering media of different dimensions. This information is then used to essentially deconvolve the measured data which is blurred by these scatter distributions. The advantage of this method compared with the fitting method is that it considers the source distribution. However, the shape of the scattering distribution is highly dependent on the shape and size of the scattering medium; thus, the phantom measurements are at best an approximation.

Dual energy method

The dual-energy window technique is based on scatter correction techniques developed originally for SPECT. In this method, coincidences are acquired in two energy windows, for example, 400 keV to 600 keV and 250 keV to 400 keV. The idea is that the upper window contains scattered and unscattered photons and the lower window contains only scattered photons. To correct for scatter, some fraction of the low-energy window counts are subtracted from the high-energy window counts. A difficulty in using this method is that in reality both energy windows contain a mixture of both unscattered and scattered events due to the limited energy resolution of the detectors, and that the low-energy window is more likely to contain multiply scattered photons that in general will have a different spatial distribution than singly scattered photons. This method also requires a set of measured calibration constants to account for efficiency differences in the two windows and to determine what fraction of the low-energy window counts should be subtracted. These constants, in turn, depend on object size. This method is typically only used in studies in which the object geometry is well-defined and remains fairly constant between studies (i.e., brain scans).[69]

Simulation methods

The most accurate scatter correction methods developed to date are probably the simulation-based methods. In these methods, the scatter is estimated by first reconstructing the emission data without scatter correction. Using these images as the initial estimate of the source distribution together with an attenuation map (i.e., reconstruction of the transmission images), the scatter is then simulated, either using a simple single scatter model,[70] an approximate analytical model,[71] or using a Monte Carlo simulation.[72,73] The advantage of this method is that it takes into account the 3-D distribution of radioactivity and attenuation coefficients in the object that is being imaged. The obvious drawback is that it is more time consuming because it involves additional image reconstructions and computationally expensive simulations, especially if a Monte Carlo simulation is performed.

Correction for random coincidences

Random coincidences, like scatter, result in additional events being recorded in LORs.[74] These events, because they contain no spatial information (the two annihilation photons come from separate decays), are distributed quite uniformly across the field of view. Without correction, they lead to a loss in image contrast, adversely affect quantification, and can lead to significant image artifacts. Random correction often is performed in real time in modern PET systems and, therefore, is transparent to the user.

Two main approaches correct random or accidental coincidences in PET. As was shown in Equation 1-18, the random counting rate can be estimated from the singles counting rate for a given detector pair and coincidence time window. In theory, the number of random events for every detector pair in the scanner can be estimated and subtracted. To implement this singles method, one would need a data acquisition system that can, in addition to recording coincidences, also accurately monitor the singles rate for each detector element. In addition, the coincidence time window needs to be accurately known for each detector pair.

A different approach is to directly measure the accidental coincidences, which can be achieved by adding a parallel coincidence circuit to the one measuring the prompt coincidences. In this second coincidence circuit, the logic pulse from one of the two detectors is delayed in time such that the detector pair cannot produce any true coincidences. Therefore, any coincidences seen in this coincidence circuit can only be caused by accidental coincidences, which is also an estimate of the number of accidental coincidences in the prompt circuit.[75]

It should be noted that in both methods, the correction for randoms is not a correction on an event-by-event basis, because a random event is indistinguishable from a true event for the coincidence circuit. Instead, the correction method provides a statistically separate measurement of the number of random events detected by each detector pair which is then subtracted from the prompt (trues + randoms) coincidence measurement. This subtraction of two measurements leads to an increase in the statistical uncertainty of the true coincidence rate. Assuming that Poisson statistics applies, the net number of true counts (N_{true}) after correction are:

$$N_{true} = N_{prompt} - N_{random} \tag{1-30}$$

where N_{prompt} and N_{random} are the number of prompt and random counts, respectively. If the delayed coincidence technique is used for correction, the statistical error in the true counts (ΔN_{true}) is given as:

$$\Delta N_{true} = \sqrt{\Delta N^2_{prompt} + \Delta N^2_{random}}$$
$$= \sqrt{N_{prompt} + N_{random}} = \sqrt{N_{true} + 2 \times N_{random}} \tag{1-31}$$

As can be seen from Equation 1-31, the statistical error in the estimate of N_{true} increases with increasing numbers of random events. If the singles method is used for estimating the accidental rates, then it can be shown using Equation 1-18, and error propagation analysis that the error in the net true coincidence counts is:

$$\Delta N_{true} = \sqrt{N_{true} + N_{random} + 2 \times 4\tau^2 \times N^3_{single}} \tag{1-32}$$

where N_{single} is the number of single events (no coincidence requirement) recorded by the detectors (assumed to be equal in the two detectors). The third term in Equation 1-32 is typically much smaller than N_{random} and can be neglected in terms of its contribution to the statistical error in the estimate of N_{true}. Equation 1-32 does not consider any errors in estimating the coincidence window 2τ, which typically has to be measured.

Comparing Equations 1-31 and 1-32, the singles correction method produces a statistically superior estimate of the number of random events, due to the negligible noise contribution from the term containing N_{single}. On the other hand, there will most likely be systematic, additional measurement errors in the determination of the coincidence time window, which can vary due to differences in cable and trace lengths in the electronics, variations in PMT transit times and other factors that are difficult to measure or account for. Although the delayed coincidence method produces a noisier estimate of the number of random events, this method is virtually free of systematic errors because the delayed coincidences are measured in the same circuitry as the prompt coincidences.

EXAMPLE 1-15

You are performing a 5-minute, whole-body PET study in a patient. The scanner records a prompt coincidence counting rate of 50,000 cps and a randoms rate of 10,000 cps. If there are 10^6 LORs in the scanner, compare the % uncertainty in the number of true coincidences per LOR for the two different randoms correction methods if you assume that the prompt and random coincidences are equally spread among all LORs in the system.

ANSWER

The number of prompt coincidences per LOR is given as:

$$50,000 \text{ cps} \times (5 \times 60) \text{ secs} / 10^6 = 15 \text{ prompts per LOR}$$

The number of random coincidences per LOR is:

$$20,000 \text{ cps} \times (5 \times 60) \text{ secs} / 10^6 = 6 \text{ randoms per LOR}$$

The number of true coincidences per LOR is:

$$15 - 6 = 9 \text{ trues per LOR}$$

From Equation 1-31, the uncertainty in the number of trues for the delayed method is:

$$\Delta N_{true} = \sqrt{N_{true} + 2 \times N_{random}} = \sqrt{9 + 12} = 4.58$$

The % uncertainty in N_{true} is

$$100 \times \frac{\Delta N_{true}}{N_{true}} = \frac{4.58}{9} = 50.9\%$$

From Equation 1-32, the uncertainty in the number of trues for the singles method, assuming that the third term is negligible, is:

$$\Delta N_{true} = \sqrt{N_{true} + N_{random}} = \sqrt{9 + 6} = 3.87$$

The % uncertainty in N_{true} is:

$$100 \times \frac{\Delta N_{true}}{N_{true}} = \frac{3.87}{9} = 43\%$$

This demonstrates the advantage of the singles method, particularly when N_{true} is not much greater than, or even less than, N_{random}.

Dead time correction

In an ideal system, the net true count rate of the system should increase linearly with increasing activity in the field of view. However, there are a number of com-

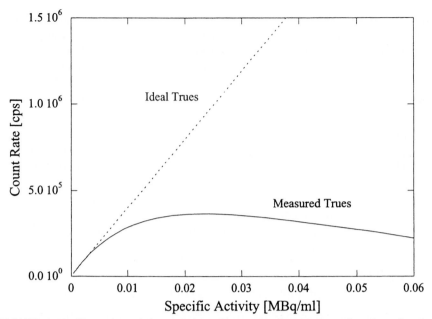

FIGURE 1-40. Illustration of the variation of true counting rate as a function of activity concentration in a uniform cylinder (solid line). The dashed line indicates the ideal linear response of the true counting rate. At low activity concentrations, the measured count rate follows the ideal linear response. As the activity concentration is increased, the deviation from the ideal response increases due to dead time in the processing electronics.

ponents in the detection chain that will experience some level of dead time as the activity increases. This is illustrated in Figure 1-40, where the measured true counting rate is shown as a function of the activity concentration in a 20-cm diameter, 20-cm tall cylinder. The ideal true counting rate is also shown (extrapolated from the measured true counting rate at low activity concentrations). The main source of dead time in most PET systems is the processing of each event in the detector front-end electronics. This dead time is mainly dictated by the extent of signal integration necessary for accurate energy discrimination and event positioning in the detector module. The integration time is, in turn, dictated by the scintillation decay time constant of the crystal material. The integration time is typically set at 3 to 4 times the decay time constant (i.e., 900–1200 ns for BGO and 120–160 ns for LSO). The most common way to characterize dead time is to fit the scanner response using either a paralyzable or nonparalyzable dead time model. Mathematically, these models are described by:

Paralyzable model $R_{Meas} = R_{True} \times \exp\left(-R_{True}\tau\right)$ (1-33)

Nonparalyzable model $R_{Meas} = R_{True} / \left(1 + R_{True}\tau\right)$ (1-34)

where R_{Meas} and R_{True} are the measured (or observed) and true counting rates rates, respectively, and τ is the dead time constant, which in the case of the detector dead time would be the integration time. Thus, if the integration time can be reduced, for instance, by using a faster scintillator, the amount of detector

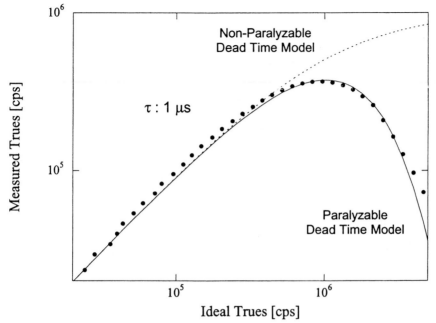

FIGURE 1-41. Measured true counting rate (closed circles) as a function of ideal true counting rate. The solid line shows the fit of the data to a paralyzable dead time model with a dead time constant of 1 μs. The dashed line shows the corresponding fit for a nonparalyzable, dead time model.

dead time can be reduced. Figure 1-41 shows the measured counting rate as a function of true counting rate, using the data from Figure 1-40. Figure 1-41 also shows the best fit of the two dead time models, described by Equations 1-33 and 1-34, to the data. In this particular case, the paralyzable model best characterizes the overall dead time for the system.

Other contributions to dead time in a PET system can come from the coincidence event processing, real-time sorting of data into sinograms, and data transfer.[76] Correction for dead time typically involves a model of the dead time behavior of the system at different count rate levels and will generally be some combination of paralyzable and nonparalyzable dead time factors contributed by the different processing stages in the system. Input to the overall dead time determination is usually the measured average detector singles rates and coincidence rates.[77]

Another problem at high counting rates is pulse pile-up which may result in resolution losses and artifacts. Pulse pileup occurs when two photons are absorbed in the same detector module within the integration time of the electronics. Because of the broad energy windows used in PET and the high likelihood of Compton interactions in the detector, it is quite possible for the total energy deposited by the two photons to fall within the energy window of the system. In this case, the two photons are accepted as a single event and the detector electronics will assign the event to a location between the two interaction positions. This leads to both loss of events (the two events are recorded as one) and mispositioning of the event. At very high counting rates, pile-up can become a limiting factor and may degrade resolution and introduce artifacts.[78]

EXAMPLE 1-16
Determine the true count rate at which 20% of all counts are lost for a BGO ($\tau = 1.2\ \mu s$) and LSO ($\tau = 160$ ns) detector. Assume a paralyzable dead time model.

ANSWER
The 20% count rate loss occurs when:

$$R_{Meas} = 0.8\ R_{True}$$

Using Equation 1-33:

$$0.8\ R_{True} = R_{True} \exp\left(-R_{True}\tau\right)$$
$$R_{True} = -\ln 0.8/\tau$$

For BGO:

$$R_{True} = -ln\ 0.8/1.2\mu s = 186\ kcps$$

For LSO:

$$R_{True} = -ln\ 0.8/160ns = 1.39\ Mcps$$

IMAGE RECONSTRUCTION

The goal of *image reconstruction* is to provide quantitatively accurate *cross-sectional* images of the distribution of positron-emitting radiopharmaceuticals in the object that is being scanned, using the externally detected radiation along with the mathematical algorithms of *computed tomography*. This essentially allows us to see "inside" the body in a completely noninvasive fashion. The reconstruction step is necessary because the raw PET data only defines the location of the emitting atom to within a line across the object (Figure 1-1). To reconstruct tomographic images also requires that data from the object be adequately sampled. For this reason, PET scanners generally consist of rings of detectors that fully encompass the object to be imaged or sets of opposing detectors that can be rotated about the object. Both geometries allow data to be collected from many different angles around the object.

Initially, we will consider a highly simplified PET scanner that consists of a single ring of individual detectors that can localize incident annihilation photons (Figure 1-26). A PET scan consists of the detection of a large number of pairs of annihilation photons (typically 10^6–10^8). During the course of the PET scan, the total number of counts measured by a particular detector pair will be proportional to the integrated radioctivity along the line joining the two detectors. This data are commonly referred to as *line integral* data. The role of image reconstruction is to convert the line integrals measured at many different angles around the object into a 2-D image that quantitatively reflects the distribution of positron-emitting atoms (and, therefore, the molecule to which it is attached) in a slice through the object parallel to the detector plane.

There are two basic approaches to image reconstruction. One approach is analytic in nature and utilizes the mathematics of computed tomography that relates line integral measurements to the activity distribution in the object. These algorithms have a variety of names, including filtered backprojection and Fourier reconstruction. The second approach is to use iterative methods that model the data collection process in a PET scanner and attempt, in a series of successive iterations, to find the image that is most consistent (using appropriate criteria) with the measured data. This section provides a basic introduction to the methods of image reconstruction. A discrete formulation is used, as all real PET data acquired are ultimately sampled in discrete bins rather than on a continuous basis. For more details on the mathematics or details on specific reconstruction algorithms, the reader is referred to the list of further reading at the end of the chapter, as well as the individual references made in the text. An excellent summary review on image reconstruction is given by Leahy and Clackdoyle.[79] Details on analytic reconstructions can be found in the textbook by Kak and Slaney.[80]

Backprojection

A basic algorithm used as part of many reconstruction methods, and an intuitively appealing way to approach image reconstruction, is *linear superposition of backprojections*, often known simply as *backprojection*. First, an image matrix is defined (typically, 128×128 pixels for PET). For a valid line of response (e.g., coincidences between detectors 12 and 31 in Figure 1-26), a line is drawn between the detectors and through the image matrix. The value added to each pixel that is intersected by the line is given by $N \times w$, where N is the number of counts detected by the detector pair (after all corrections described in Data Correction, p. 51, have been applied) and w is a weighting factor proportional to the pathlength of the line through the pixel. The value is therefore larger if the line passes across the center of the pixel and smaller if the line passes through the corner of the pixel. This is illustrated in Figure 1-42. In essence, the counts from a detector pair are being projected back along the line from which they originated. This process is repeated for all valid detector pairs in the PET system, the counts from each subsequent detector pair being added to the counts that have been backprojected for all preceding detector pairs, hence the name linear superposition of backprojections.

There are two different methods to implement simple backprojection on a computer. The first approach, *ray-driven backprojection*, is the method described above. The lines of response, or rays, are traced through the 2-D image matrix, and the pathlength through each pixel is calculated. A more common (and efficient) way to perform backprojection, when the projection data are stored as sinograms (Data Representation: The Sinogram, p. 44) is to use the *pixel-driven backprojection* algorithm. For each image pixel (x,y), and each projection angle ϕ, we calculate the sinogram coordinate r (from Equation 1-24) that will contribute data to that pixel. In general, the calculated value of r will not fall exactly on one of the sinogram elements, and linear interpolation is used between adjacent elements to calculate the contribution to add to pixel (x,y). In this algorithm, each image pixel is handled one at a time, and the calculation proceeds as a loop over all the projection angles ϕ for each image pixel. Mathematically, pixel-driven backprojection can be written as:

$$a'(x,y) = \frac{1}{N}\sum_{n=1}^{N} s(r,\phi_n) = \frac{1}{N} \sum_{n=1}^{N} s(x \cos \phi_n + y \sin \phi_n, \phi_n) \qquad (1\text{-}35)$$

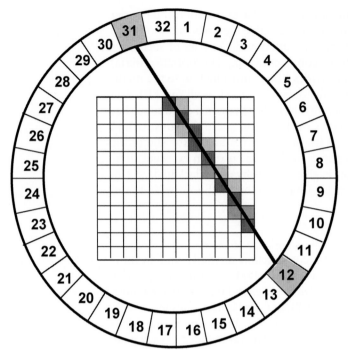

FIGURE 1-42. Illustration of backprojection. An image matrix consisting of an array of square-image pixels is defined. Events detected by a given detector pair (in this case detectors 12 and 31) are placed in pixels intersected by the line joining the two detectors. A weighting factor is applied to account for the pathlength of the line of response through the pixel. This is repeated for all valid detector pairs to build a backprojected image (see Figure 1-43).

where N is the number of different equally spaced projection angles over which data have been obtained, $s(r,\phi_n)$ is the number of counts in the sinogram element at angle ϕ_n and radial offset r, and $a'(x,y)$ is the backprojected image. Both approaches to backprojection are mathematically identical, although results can differ slightly depending on the details of how the weighting factors and interpolations are carried out.

Simple backprojection of the data does result in an image that resembles the true distribution of radioactivity in the object, but it is only an approximation, hence the designation $a'(x,y)$. Backprojection places counts outside the boundaries of the object which is clearly incorrect, and for any complex object, it is readily apparent that backprojection will result in a blurred representation of the object because counts are distributed equally along the line from which they originated. The result of reconstruction of the computer phantom shown in Figure 1-28 by backprojection is shown in Figure 1-43. The blurring in backprojection is proportional to 1/r, where r is the distance from the source. Mathematically, it can be shown that the relationship between the backprojected image $a'(x,y)$ and the true activity distribution $a(x,y)$ is given as:

$$a'(x,y) = a(x,y) \otimes \frac{1}{r} \qquad (1-36)$$

where $\otimes$ denotes the operation of convolution.

Analytic reconstruction: projection slice theorem and direct Fourier reconstruction

To develop a reconstruction algorithm that eliminates the 1/r blurring factor, we turn to an important theorem known as the *Fourier* or *projection slice theo-*

FIGURE 1-43. Simple backprojection reconstruction of the sinogram in Figure 1-28. The reconstructed image bears some resemblance to the object in Figure 1-28 from which the sinogram was measured, but the image is badly blurred. Counts are placed outside of the object where there is no radioactivity. (Data courtesy of Dr. Andrew Goertzen. Reproduced with permission from Cherry SR, Sorenson JA, Phelps ME. Physics in Nuclear Medicine, W.B. Saunders, New York, 2003.)

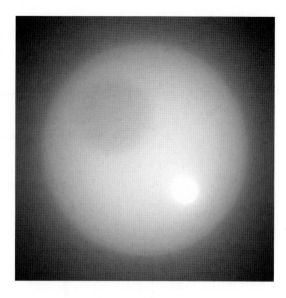

rem (sometimes also known as the *central section* theorem). This theorem states that the measured projection data $s(r,\phi)$ contained within the sinogram can be related to the activity distribution $a(x,y)$ in the object through the use of a widely used mathematical tool known as the *Fourier transform*.

The Fourier transform expresses a function $f(x)$ in terms of its component *spatial frequencies* (expressed as a weighted sum of sine and cosine terms of different frequencies) rather than in terms of its magnitude as a function of position. The component spatial frequencies, v, and the magnitude with which each frequency contributes to the signal, $F(v)$, is determined by the manner with which the signal $f(x)$ changes with position. For example, a signal that is fairly uniform over space can be represented using lower spatial frequencies, while one with sharp discontinuities and regions of rapid change will require higher frequencies for an accurate representation. This is perhaps best illustrated with some simple examples as shown in Figure 1-44. The two extreme cases would be a uniform signal (i.e., $f(x) =$ constant) and a delta function ($f(x) = 0$, except at $x = 0$, where $f(x) = 1$). In the former case, there is no frequency information and the Fourier transform of the function only contains information at the zero frequency. In the latter case, an infinite number of frequencies are required to represent the sharp delta function, and the Fourier transform contains equal contributions at all frequencies. The last function illustrated is a more general and discrete function, such as might be measured as the projection data from a particular angle in a sinogram. Here again, there is a distribution of frequencies, but high-frequency components are limited by the resolution of the detectors that are being used and the spatial sampling of the data. Discrete Fourier transforms of data can be calculated very quickly on computers; many data analysis packages have built-in functions for computing them. In this text, we will not provide details of the exact formulation and calculation of Fourier transforms. This involves the use of complex exponentials and is beyond the scope of this book. The interested reader is referred to the textbook by Bracewell[81] for further details. We will simply denote the Fourier transform $F(v)$ of a function $f(x)$ as:

$$F(v) = FT\ [f(x)] \tag{1-37}$$

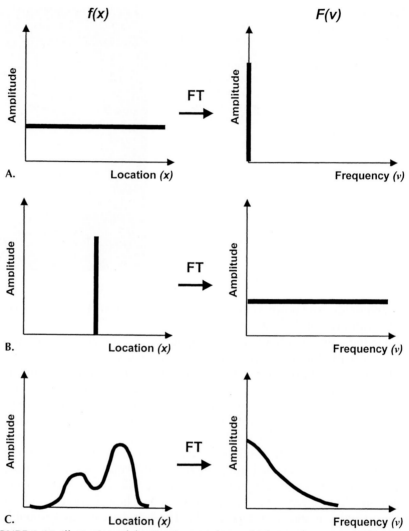

FIGURE 1-44. Illustration of the Fourier transform which expresses a spatially varying signal *f(x)* in terms of its frequency components *F(v)*. Three cases are shown: A (top row): Signal is uniform over space and the only nonzero component of the Fourier transform is at zero frequency. B (middle row): A delta function. All frequencies are required to represent this sharp spike. C (bottom row): A more realistic situation that could represent a profile through the radioactive distribution in a patient. A range of frequencies is required to represent this distribution, with higher amplitudes at lower frequencies. The high-frequency cut-off in real data will be determined by the resolution of the detector and the sampling of the data.

The inverse Fourier transform takes the frequency representation of a function $F(v)$ and computes the spatial representation of the function $f(x)$ and is denoted by:

$$f(x) = \mathrm{FT}^{-1}\left[F(v)\right] \qquad (1\text{-}38)$$

Fourier transforms can also be calculated for 2-D functions $f(x,y)$, where the transform is also a 2-D function $F(v_x, v_y)$ representing spatial frequency components in the x and y directions.

The projection slice theorem states that the one-dimensional (1-D) Fourier transform of a projection at angle ϕ (one row in the sinogram) is equal to the 2-D Fourier transform of the image evaluated along a radial profile at angle ϕ with respect to the x-axis (Figure 1-45), which can be written as:

$$S(v_r, \phi) = A(v_x, v_y)|_{v_x = v_r \cos \phi, \, v_y = v_r \sin \phi} \qquad (1\text{-}39)$$

where $S(v_r, \phi)$ is the 1-D Fourier transform of $s(r, \phi)$ with respect to r, and $A(v_x, v_y)$ is the 2-D Fourier transform of the activity distribution $a(x,y)$ which is the quantity desired to reconstruct in the image. This relationship immediately leads to the direct Fourier reconstruction of a cross-sectional image $a(x,y)$ by the following approach:

1. Take the 1-D Fourier transform of the first row in the sinogram.
2. Interpolate and add onto a 2-D rectangular grid $A(v_x, v_y)$ according to Equation 1-39.
3. Repeat for all subsequent rows in the sinogram.
4. Take the inverse 2-D Fourier transform of $A(v_x, v_y)$ to find the image $a(x,y)$.

The practical difficulty with this approach is that the Fourier-transformed projection data $S(v_r, \phi)$ are sampled along radial lines and must then be interpolated onto a rectangular grid to form $A(v_x, v_y)$ before taking the inverse Fourier transform. Accurate interpolation is computationally intensive, and the resultant image is very sensitive to interpolation errors. However, when properly implemented, this leads to a reconstructed cross-sectional image $a(x,y)$ that will match the distribution of radioactivity in the original object within the limits

FIGURE 1-45. The Projection slice theorem. The object with activity $a(x,y)$ is scanned to produce projection data $s(r,\phi)$ at different angles ϕ (sinogram data). The 1-D Fourier transform (FT) of the projection data at angle ϕ, $S(v_r,\phi)$ is equal to the 2-D Fourier transform of the image $A(v_x, v_y)$ evaluated at angle ϕ. To reconstruct an image, the Fourier transforms of the projection data at each angle are inserted onto a rectangular grid according to this theorem. The reconstructed image can then be obtained by taking the inverse 2-D Fourier transform of $A(v_x, v_y)$ to yield a(x,y).

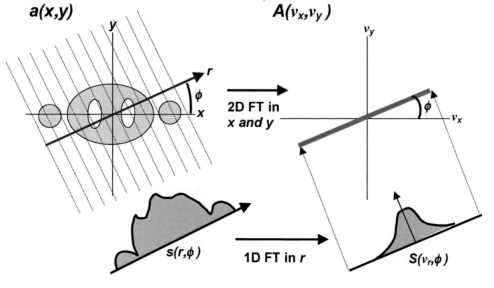

imposed by statistical noise in the measured projection data, errors in quantification of the line integrals (due to any of the factors discussed in Data Correction, p. 51), and resolution and sampling limitations of the data.

Two-dimensional analytic reconstruction: filtered backprojection

A more elegant approach to reconstruction can be achieved by reformulating Equation 1-39 in the spatial rather than frequency domain. The result is:

$$a(x,y) = \frac{1}{N} \sum_{n=1}^{N} s^*(r,\phi_n) \qquad (1\text{-}40)$$

where s^* is the original sinogram data that have been modified by a filter function in the spatial frequency domain with form $H(v) = |v|$:

$$s^*(r,\phi) = \frac{1}{2\pi} FT^{-1}[S(v_r,\phi) \times |v_r|] \qquad (1\text{-}41)$$

$S(v_r,\phi)$ is the 1-D Fourier transform of the original projection data $s(r,\phi)$ with respect to r. Comparing Equation 1-40 with Equation 1-35, it can be seen to be the same equation as for backprojection, the only difference being that the projections have been modified by a filter according to Equation 1-41. Hence, the name *filtered backprojection*.

The reconstruction filter, $H(v)$, is known as the ramp filter because of its shape in the frequency domain (Figure 1-46) which results in a larger weighting factor for higher spatial frequencies. The blurring that occurs in images reconstructed with backprojection can be thought of as suppressing high-spatial frequency information (high-spatial frequencies give "sharpness" to an image). The shape of the ramp filter, therefore, makes sense intuitively, as it amplifies the high-spatial frequencies with respect to the low-spatial frequencies, reversing the effects of the 1/r blurring.

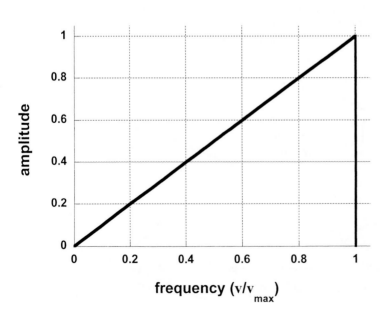

FIGURE 1-46. The reconstruction filter that is applied to the projections in frequency space to achieve accurate reconstructions is a simple ramp function, where the amplitude of the filter is proportional to the frequency, up to a maximum frequency v_{max} which is defined by the sampling of the data.

The implementation of filtered backprojection (FBP) is as follows:

1. Take the 1-D Fourier transform of the first projection angle in the sinogram.
2. Multiply this by the filter function.
3. Take the inverse Fourier transform.
4. Backproject the modified (filtered) projection.
5. Repeat for all angles around the object.

This algorithm is very fast and easy to implement on a computer. It involves only 1-D Fourier transforms and simple linear interpolation (in general, the selection of x, y, and ϕ will result in values of r that do not fall exactly on the line of response defined by a detector pair). It has become the method of choice for analytic reconstruction.

In the discrete formulation of image reconstruction appropriate for PET (the recorded projection data are discrete, not continuous functions), the reconstruction filter $H(v)$ should be cut-off at a maximum frequency v_{max} (Figure 1-46) which is given as:

$$v_{max} = \frac{1}{2 \times \Delta r} \qquad (1\text{-}42)$$

where Δr is the distance between samples in the sinogram and v_{max} represents the highest frequency that can be faithfully recorded in the discrete, sampled data.

The ramp filter often is modified in practice to improve signal-to-noise in reconstructed PET images. A typical projection view contains a range of frequencies, with a tendency for higher amplitudes at low frequencies and lower amplitudes at higher frequencies. Statistical noise (noise related to the finite number of annihilation photon pairs contributing to each element in the profile) has a uniform spectral appearance and contributes equally at all frequencies (Figure 1-47). Thus, if a reconstructed image is too noisy due to limited sta-

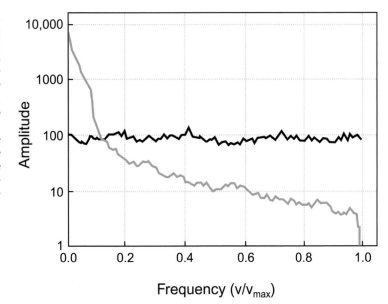

FIGURE 1-47. Fourier transform of the signal (no-noise) (gray line) and the statistical noise (black line) in a projection measurement. Notice how the signal drops off quickly with increasing frequency, while the noise remains quite constant across all frequencies. The individual data points have been smoothed to produce the solid curves to better visualize the trends in the two components. (Data courtesy of Dr. Andrew Goertzen.)

tistics, one option is to attenuate or remove higher frequencies, thus improving signal-to-noise. This improvement, however, is at the expense of degrading image resolution, as the signal contained within these same high frequencies is responsible for the finer detail (rapidly changing activity, sharp edges, and so on) in an image. Thus, by modifying the reconstruction filter, it is possible to trade-off signal-to-noise and spatial resolution in the reconstructed image. A simple way to do this is to cut off the ramp filter at a frequency $v_{cutoff} < v_{max}$. More commonly, apodizing filters are used, which are based on the ramp filter at low frequencies but have a reduced magnitude at high frequencies. These also avoid a sharp change in the filter at the cut-off frequency which reduces the chances of introducing artifacts into the reconstructed images. The functional forms for some of the more common reconstruction filters are:

Ramp: $$H(v) = |v| \tag{1-43A}$$

Hann: $$H(v) = 0.5|v|\left(1 + \cos\frac{\pi v}{v_{cut\text{-}off}}\right) \tag{1-43B}$$

Shepp–Logan: $$H(v) = \frac{2v_{cut\text{-}off}}{\pi}\sin\frac{|v|\pi}{2v_{cut\text{-}off}} \tag{1-43C}$$

In all cases, $H(v)$ is set to zero for $|v| > v_{cut\text{-}off}$; $v_{cut\text{-}off}$ can have a maximum value of v_{max}. These filters are shown in Figure 1-48. Figure 1-49 shows the reconstruction of a dataset using several different reconstruction filters, demonstrating the trade-off between signal-to-noise and resolution as the filter is changed and as $v_{cut\text{-}off}$ is varied. In practice, it is rare that sufficient annihilation photon pairs are collected in a human PET study to reconstruct PET images with a ramp

FIGURE 1-48. Three reconstruction filters that are commonly used in filtered back-projection. The Shepp–Logan and Hann filters reduce the amplitude at high frequencies, improving signal-to-noise but reducing spatial resolution. They also avoid "ringing" artifacts from the very sharp cut-off of the ramp filter at $v = v_{cut\text{-}off}$.

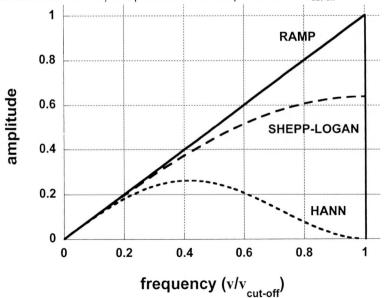

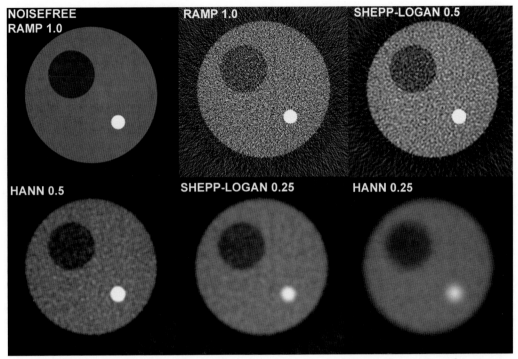

FIGURE 1-49. Effects of filters and cut-off frequencies on the same reconstructed image. Notice trade-off between signal-to-noise and spatial resolution as the filter is changed and its cut-off value is varied. (Data courtesy of Dr. Andrew Goertzen.)

filter cut-off at v_{max}; therefore, these modified filters are almost always used to yield acceptable signal-to-noise images.

So far, this chapter has discussed producing a single 2-D image slice from a single ring of detectors. Most PET scanners, however, consist of multiple rings of detectors or area detectors that can provide information from many different locations along the axis of the patient. These scanners can acquire and reconstruct many parallel and contiguous 2-D image slices simultaneously and can be stacked to form a 3-D volume of image data. The thickness of each slice is determined by the size of the detector elements in the axial direction in the case of block-style detectors—the slice profile is a triangular shape, with the width of the base of the triangle equal to the width of the detector element. For gamma-camera style detectors, the slice thickness is determined by the resolution of the detector in the axial direction. Modern PET cameras produce 3-D image volumes that can be resliced from the transaxial orientation in which they were acquired, into coronal or sagittal views, or any arbitrary orientation that is desired. It is important to notice that even though 3-D image volumes are assembled in this manner, they are produced from a stack of independent 2-D reconstructions. This approach only uses annihilation photons that are emitted parallel, or close to parallel, to the desired image section (see Two-Dimensional Data Acquisition, p. 46). It is also possible to use annihilation photons that are emitted obliquely to the desired image slices, but this requires approximations or a fully 3-D reconstruction algorithm (Three-Dimensional Data Acquisition, p. 48). The reconstruction of 3-D PET data is covered in Three-Dimensional Analytic Reconstruction, p. 82.

Limitations of filtered backprojection

Although 2-D filtered backprojection (FBP) is a fast method for reconstructing cross-sectional images, it has requirements that must be met to successfully reconstruct images. FBP also has assumptions about the data that are approximations in the real world. One major requirement for successful reconstruction using FBP is adequate sampling.[82] Two types of sampling are of concern. The center-to-center spacing between samples in a row in the sinogram (sometimes referred to as linear sampling or projection sampling) and the angular sampling that is defined by the number of rows in the sinogram. Based on the sampling theorem, the data should be sampled with a projection sampling interval Δr that is at least one half the highest anticipated spatial resolution of the reconstructed image. The highest resolution that can be achieved is dictated by the intrinsic resolution of the detectors combined with additional factors such as the blurring effects of positron range and noncolinearity (R_{sys} from Example 1-9). The projection sampling criterion can therefore be expressed approximately as:

$$\Delta r \leq 0.5 \times R_{sys}(FWHM) \qquad (1-44)$$

The required angular sampling depends on the diameter of the object being imaged because the sampling density decreases with distance from the center of the scanner. Reconstructing PET data requires projection data that are acquired over 180°. To achieve a sampling interval equal or better than Δr along the circumference of an object of diameter D over 180° requires that:

$$N \geq \pi D/2\Delta r \geq \pi D/R_{sys}(FWHM) \qquad (1-45)$$

where N is the number of angular samples. Inadequate linear or angular sampling leads to a reduction in spatial resolution and can cause artifacts in the reconstructed images (Figure 1-50).

In PET systems with continuous detectors, the choice of linear and angular sampling intervals is made by the choice of bin size into which the measured interaction coordinates are histogrammed into a sinogram. It is, therefore, quite easy to meet the sampling requirements. In a stationary ring PET system composed of individual detectors, the sampling distance and number of angular samples is fixed by the width of the detector elements and the number of detectors in the ring. In these systems the data are undersampled in the linear direction and, therefore, the projection data usually are rearranged by interleaving adjacent angular views to form a sinogram that has double the linear sampling and half the angular sampling (see Data Representation—The Sinogram, p. 50). This leads to a better balance between linear and angular sampling, although the data are still undersampled based on strict sampling criteria. To address this, some PET systems have a small built-in detector motion (often known as "wobble") that allows Δr and N to be increased so that they meet the sampling criteria.[82] Some PET scanners have inactive or "dead" regions between detector modules or panels, leading to gaps in the sinogram data. In these regions the data are not sampled at all, which can lead to major reconstruction artifacts. This is often solved by rotating the detectors such that these gaps can be filled in or by using extrapolation or other techniques to estimate what the missing data should be.

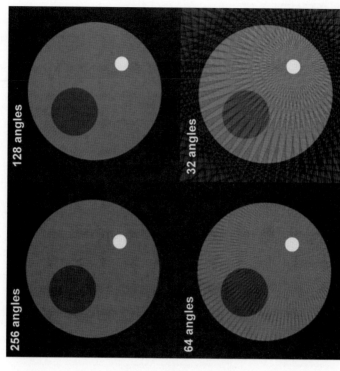

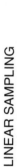

FIGURE 1-50. Effects of linear (A) and angular (B) sampling on reconstructed image quality. Data at top left have sufficient sampling. (Data courtesy of Dr. Andrew Goertzen. Reproduced with permission from Cherry SR, Sorenson JA, Phelps ME. Physics in Nuclear Medicine, W.B. Saunders, New York, 2003.)

EXAMPLE 1-17

A fixed ring PET scanner is made up of 512 detector elements, each 4.9-mm wide, that are tightly packed in a 79.8-cm diameter detector ring. The spatial resolution of each detector is 3.8 mm. Calculate the required projection and angular sampling for this system for imaging an object that is 40 cm in diameter and compare this with the actual sampling intervals.

ANSWER

From Equation 1-44, the required projection sampling for 3.8-mm resolution detectors would be:

$$\Delta r \leq 0.5 \times R_{sys}(FWHM) \leq 1.9 \text{ mm}$$

From Equation 1-45, the required number of angular samples over 180° would be:

$$N \geq \pi D/2\Delta r \geq \pi D/R_{sys}(FWHM) \geq \pi \times 400 \text{ mm} / 3.8 \text{ mm} \geq 330$$

Based on how the sinograms for PET are defined (Figure 1-27), Δr is equal to one half the detector spacing; in this case $\Delta r = 4.90/2 = 2.45$. The number of angles in the sinogram equals half the number of detectors, and so in this case $N = 256$. This demonstrates that PET data are slightly undersampled, although in practice the effects of this level of undersampling on the reconstructed images are relatively small.

The major drawbacks of FBP relate to assumptions that this analytic approach makes about the detection system and the data that are collected. First of all, FBP is based on line integrals and assumes that the PET detectors are point detectors. In practice, PET detectors have finite dimensions, thickness, and resolution; they measure data along a volume joining two detectors. The solid angle subtended by the detectors to points within the volume varies with source position, giving nonuniform sensitivity. Furthermore, FBP cannot model any of the other degrading factors that occur in a PET scanner, such as intercrystal scatter, positron range, and noncolinearity. Lastly, FBP takes no account of the statistical properties of the data. It assumes noise-free data and weights all lines of response equally, independent of signal-to-noise. Because different angular views can never be completely consistent with each other due to the variation of statistical noise from one sinogram element to the next, streak artifacts are common unless very high count data are available for reconstruction. As this is rarely the case in PET, compensation is usually made by using a reconstruction filter that improves signal-to-noise, at the expense of degrading image resolution as explained in Two-Dimensional Analytic Reconstruction: Filtered Backprojection p. 76.

Three-dimensional analytic reconstruction

PET scanners operating in 2-D mode only process data that come from detectors lying in or close to the plane of the desired transverse image. Obliquely angled lines of response are rejected (either physically by the interplane septa or by not enabling these lines of response in the data acquisition system) as discussed in Two-Dimensional Data Acquisition p. 46. This does not make good use of the emitted radiation from a patient, in which annihilation photon pairs are randomly oriented and, therefore, very few of which are aligned parallel to the imaging planes. 3-D PET data acquisition (Figure 1-29C) involves removing the interplane septa and acquiring data between all possible axial locations in the scanner. This makes better use of the emitted radiation, leading typically to the detection of somewhere between ×5 and ×10 more events for a given radiation dose and imaging time.[42,43] 3-D PET data also are usually stored in sinograms, with each sinogram being characterized by an average axial location $\bar{z}$, and an azimuthal angle θ or ring difference δ (Figure 1-51). A scanner where the data are binned into 32 different intervals in the axial direction would, for example, produce 32^2 possible sinograms, with ring differences up to ± 31. To incorporate the oblique lines of response into the reconstructed image requires that the approach described in Two-Dimensional Analytical Reconstruction: Filtered Backprojection (p. 76) be modified.

Several approximate reconstruction methods seek to convert the collected 3-D data into a set of parallel transverse sinograms ($\theta = 0°$) so they can be reconstructed using conventional 2-D filtered backprojection methods. The simplest of these methods, often referred to as *single-slice rebinning*,[83] takes the average axial location, $\bar{z}$, of a detected event and places the event in the sinogram(s) that most closely corresponds to that axial position as illustrated in Figure 1-52. Along the central axis of the scanner, this approximation works perfectly. However, it steadily becomes worse with increasing radial distance. This approach only yields reasonably acceptable images when the object being imaged takes up a small fraction of the field of view and when the axial acceptance angle (the maximum oblique angle accepted) is small. Otherwise, significant blurring of data occurs in the axial direction that becomes apparent when the data are resliced into sagittal or coronal views. It is a very quick way to reconstruct 3-D data, as it only requires that the data are resorted into conventional 2-D sinograms and reconstructed using standard 2-D FBP.

FIGURE 1-51. Definition of sinograms in a 3-D PET system. A sinogram is produced for each possible combination of axial positions in the scanner, which are defined by the azimuthal angle θ (or ring difference δ) and the average location, $\bar{z}$, from which the data come. The sinogram data are therefore denoted as $s(r,\phi,\theta,\bar{z})$ where a separate sinogram is produced for each value of $(\theta,\bar{z})$ viewed by the scanner.

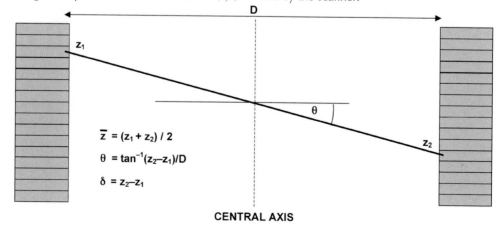

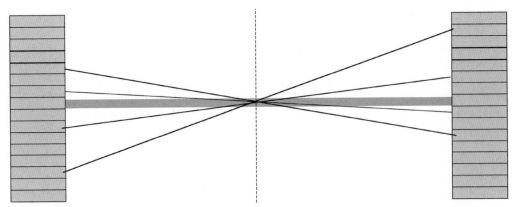

FIGURE 1-52. Illustration of single-slice rebinning in which the 3-D dataset is reduced to a set of parallel 2-D sinograms that can be reconstructed with 2-D FBP. All four lines of response illustrated would be binned into the same sinogram, as they all have the same value for $\bar{z}$. These sinogram data are then assumed to come from radioactivity in the gray slice perpendicular to the scanner axis. At the center of the field of view, data are positioned correctly, but it is clear that the axial resolution will degrade significantly for sources away from the scanner axis, as data are averaged from the divergent lines of response.

More recently, a technique known as *Fourier rebinning* (FORE) has been introduced.[84] The details of FORE are beyond the scope of this text, but it is based on a principle that relates the 2-D Fourier transform of the oblique sinograms ($\theta > 0°$) to the 2-D Fourier transform of the transverse ($\theta = 0°$) sinograms. Although this is still an approximate method, it yields substantially better results than single-slice rebinning, even for large objects and large acceptance angles,[85] while retaining much of the advantage in terms of short reconstruction times. This has become the algorithm of choice for very large 3-D datasets, for example, those from dynamic PET studies involving perhaps 20 to 30 frames of 3-D data.

The gold standard for analytic 3-D image reconstruction is the *3-D reprojection algorithm* (3DRP).[86] It is based on an extension of filtered backprojection methods to 3-D. However, two major differences exist between 2-D and 3-D PET datasets, one of which creates a problem, and the second of which provides a solution to that problem. The first difference is that the 3-D dataset is in some senses incomplete. In 2-D a complete set of angular data is obtained by having a ring of detectors or by rotating detectors around the object. The projection dataset is complete because projections are available for ϕ ranging from 0 to 180°. In 3-D PET, an analogous situation would occur if the scanner had the geometry of a sphere. In this case, projections would be available for both ϕ and θ ranging from 0 to 180°, and all possible projection angles would be measured. However, PET scanners generally have a cylindrical geometry and the limited axial length of the scanner results in projections that are truncated in the axial direction (Figure 1-53). As the azimuthal angle θ is increased, the truncation becomes more severe. An accurate reconstruction requires that this truncation be removed for the azimuthal angles that are to be included in the reconstruction. As it stands, the only angle for which the data are not truncated are the sinograms with $\theta = 0°$ which correspond to the standard 2-D dataset.

The solution for dealing with this comes from the second feature of 3-D PET datasets—data redundancy. We have already discussed how the stack of parallel 2-D sinograms can be reconstructed and stacked into a 3-D image volume. Therefore, sufficient information is contained within the set of transverse sinograms alone to reconstruct the image volume. If the measured 2-D sinogram data were noise-free, there would be no need for 3-D data acquisition and reconstruction. However, statistical noise dominates in PET; hence, there is good reason for wanting to incorporate the data from the oblique sinograms to improve the signal-to-noise of the reconstructed image. Data redundancy provides the solution to the data truncation problem as follows. The conventional 2-D sinograms ($\theta = 0°$) are first extracted from the 3-D dataset. Each is reconstructed with 2-D filtered backprojection and stacked to form a 3-D image volume. This represents a low statistical estimate of the image. This image volume can now be used to estimate the missing data and remove the truncation by adding the activity along oblique lines of response that were not actually measured by the scanner. This process is known as *reprojection* or *forward-projection* and is the inverse process of backprojection. In this way, the missing data are estimated, and the dataset now fulfills the requirements for reconstruction by 3-D filtered backprojection.

Reconstruction then proceeds along the lines of 2-D filtered backprojection, except the dimensionality of the data is increased by one. Each projection, or

FIGURE 1-53. Truncation of projections in the axial direction caused by the limited axial extent of the scanner. For $\theta \neq 0$ A (top), parts of the object (shaded area) are not sampled. These missing lines of response are indicated by the dashed lines. As θ increases, the amount of truncation becomes worse. However, the dashed lines of response can be estimated by reconstructing an initial image volume (B, bottom) using 2-D FBP of parallel sinograms ($\theta = 0$) and then summing the activity along these lines to estimate what would have been measured in the missing sinograms.

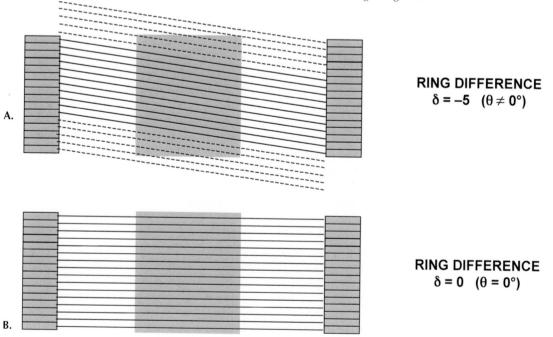

RING DIFFERENCE
$\delta = -5$ $(\theta \neq 0°)$

A.

RING DIFFERENCE
$\delta = 0$ $(\theta = 0°)$

B.

angular view, is now 2-D and represents the projection of activity in (r,z) for a particular value of ϕ and θ. The reconstruction filter is also 2-D and takes on a form dependent on the maximum azimuthal angle, θ_{max}, of the data used in the reconstruction.[87] Finally, the filtered data are backprojected through a 3-D image volume. The steps involved in 3-D filtered backprojection using the 3DRP can be summarized as:

1. Extract 2-D sinograms ($\theta = 0°$).
2. Reconstruct each of these with 2-D FBP and stack to form 3-D image volume.
3. Forward project through 3-D image volume to calculate missing LORs to remove truncation.
4. Extract 2-D projection data for angle ϕ and θ.
5. Take 2-D Fourier transform of the projection.
6. Multiply by 2-D reconstruction filter.
7. Take inverse 2-D Fourier transform.
8. Backproject data through 3-D image matrix.
9. Repeat for all angles $0 \leq \phi < 180°$ and $-\theta_{max} \leq \theta \leq \theta_{max}$.

Because of the need to compute the missing data, and the fact that backprojection occurs through a 3-D volume rather than across a 2-D plane, the computational complexity of 3DRP is approximately an order of magnitude higher than 2-D FBP. Nonetheless, it enables the oblique sinogram data to be accurately incorporated into the reconstructed image leading to significant improvements in signal-to-noise. In many cases, this signal-to-noise improvement allows a higher cut-off frequency to be used in the reconstruction filter, leading to improved spatial resolution if desired. Figure 1-54 shows a comparison of 2-D and 3-D data acquisition and reconstruction demonstrating the signal-to-noise gain in 3-D PET. A detailed review of 3-D reconstruction methods for PET, which also presents a more detailed mathematical treatment, can be found in Bendriem and Townsend.[88]

Iterative reconstruction methods

The analytic techniques described above have historically been the most commonly used reconstruction methods for PET. Another class of reconstruction techniques, known collectively as *iterative reconstruction* methods, offer an alternative approach. These methods are computationally more intensive than FBP; for this reason, they have been found to have less clinical use to date. However, as computer speed continues to improve, and with acceleration techniques, these approaches are beginning to be of more general use.

The basic idea behind iterative reconstruction approaches is summarized in Figure 1-55. An initial guess is made of the image distribution $a^*(x,y)$ (often a blank or uniform grayscale image). The next step is to calculate what projection data would be measured for the radioactivity distribution in the initial guess. The simplest way to do this is to use a process known as *forward-projection*. This is exactly the inverse of backprojection, and involves summing up all the activity in pixels that are intersected by the line of response that corresponds to the measured sinogram element. Once this process is complete, we have a set of estimated projection data based on our initial guess that can be compared with the actual measured projection data. Obviously, they will not agree because it is

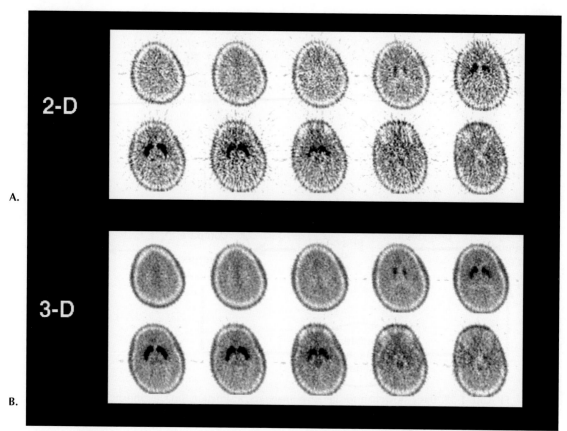

FIGURE 1-54. Comparison of PET images of the brain acquired and reconstructed in A) 2-D (reconstructed with standard 2-D FBP) and B) 3-D (reconstructed with 3DRP). Injected dose and imaging time were the same for both studies. Notice the improvement in signal-to-noise in the 3-D study. (Reproduced from Brain Mapping: The Methods, 2nd ed, Eds: Toga AW, Mazziotta JC, Academic Press, San Diego, 2002, with permission from Elsevier.)

very unlikely that the initial guess of $a^*(x,y)$ is anything like the true radioactivity distribution $a(x,y)$. Based on the differences between observed and measured projections, the initial guess is then adjusted, and the whole process is repeated. If the method by which the image estimate is updated is properly formulated, then with each successive iteration through this process, the image estimate will start to converge towards the true image. After a while, the estimated image should closely match (within the limits imposed by the statistical quality of the data and the resolution and sampling of the detector system) the true distribution of radioactivity in the object.

There are many different types of iterative algorithms each differing in some aspect of their formulation and implementation. One of the factors that distinguish these algorithms is the *cost functions* they use. The cost function is a function that gives a measure of the difference (or similarity) between the estimated and measured projections and is the function that we seek to minimize (maximize) during the reconstruction. The second important component of the algorithm is the search or update function, that is, how the image estimate is up-

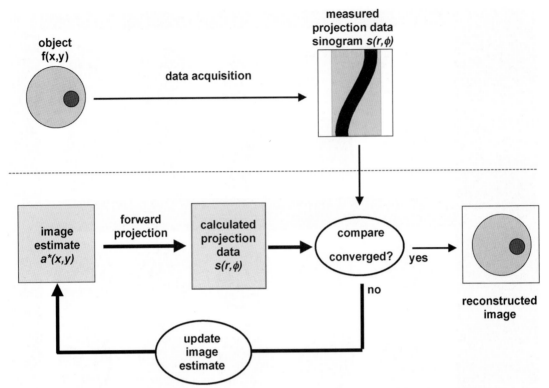

FIGURE 1-55. Basic flowchart for iterative image reconstruction. Image estimate is forward-projected to calculate a sinogram, which is then compared with the measured sinogram. Based on the difference between calculated and measured sinograms, the image is updated. (Reproduced from Cherry SR, Sorenson JA, Phelps ME. Physics in Nuclear Medicine, 3rd ed. W.B. Saunders, New York, 2003, with permission from Elsevier.)

dated at each iteration step. The goal is to use methods that reliably converge to the minimum or maximum of the cost function as quickly as possible. Other differences between algorithms include whether and how the statistical nature of the data is implicitly modeled and whether any other prior information (e.g., the expected smoothness of the image) is considered. Some algorithms also force the reconstructed image to be non-negative. For a concise history and review of different iterative reconstruction methods, refer to the review by Leahy and Clackdoyle.[79]

While simple forward-projection is the most straightforward way of calculating the projection data from an image estimate, most iterative algorithms use a more sophisticated approach that models the probability that a gamma ray pair emitted at point $a(x,y)$ in the object/image space is detected in projection element $s(r,\phi)$. By avoiding the simplistic line integral model that is one of the limitations of filtered backprojection, many of the different factors (e.g., system geometry, object and septa scatter, detector characteristics, positron range, and noncollinearity) that determine whether or not a gamma ray is detected, and where it is detected, can be included in the reconstruction process.[89] The forward-projection step essentially becomes a simulation of the entire imaging system. This can lead to more quantitatively accurate images and improvements in signal-to-noise or spatial resolution.

Two factors make iterative reconstruction approaches much more computationally intensive than their filtered backprojection counterparts. First, each iteration is essentially equivalent in time to a full-filtered backprojection reconstruction. Backprojection is the most time-consuming part of the filtered backprojection algorithm, and backprojection and forward-projection are computationally very similar processes. Most iterative algorithms require multiple iterations (anywhere from 2 up to several hundred, depending on the algorithm and the data) to reach an acceptable image. Second, as soon as the line integral model of simple forward-projection is replaced by a more accurate model of how gamma rays are detected, the time required to compute the projection data increases, as many more image pixels may now contribute to a particular projection element. A number of approximations have been developed to speed up these algorithms. One of the most popular is called *ordered subsets*, also known as OSEM, in which only a subset of the projection angles are used in any one iteration.[90] This speeds up the algorithm, as the time per iteration is directly proportional to the number of angles that need to be forward-projected.

The most widely used iterative reconstruction approaches are based on *maximum likelihood* (ML) methods. *Likelihood*, is a general statistical measure that is maximized when the difference between the measured and estimated projections is minimized. The *expectation-maximization* (EM) algorithm is an iterative algorithm that maximizes likelihood under a Poisson data model. It implicitly treats the projection data as having a Poisson distribution determined by the counting statistics in each projection bin and thus takes into account the statistical noise in the data. The derivation of the form of the algorithm that is used in PET is lengthy and beyond the scope of this book, but the interested reader is referred to articles by Shepp and Vardi[91] and Lange and Carson.[92] It is instructive to examine the implementation of the algorithm and to see how the image is updated on each iteration.

As a starting point, the reconstruction problem can be written as follows:

$$s_j = \sum_i M_{i,j} a_i \qquad (1\text{-}46)$$

where a_i is the activity in an image pixel i and s_j is the number of counts in projection element j. For projection data taken with a PET camera at 128 angles around the object, with each projection measuring 256 elements, the index j would run from 1 to 32768 (128 $\times$ 256). If this is to be reconstructed onto a 128 $\times$ 128 grid, the index i would run from 1 to 16384 (128 $\times$ 128). $M_{i,j}$ is a large matrix (32768 $\times$ 16384 in the example just given) which provides the probability that gamma rays emitted in pixel i will be detected in projection element j. This matrix provides the model of the imaging system and is a much more sophisticated approach than simple forward-projection. This matrix can be determined by calculation, simulations, measurements, or a combination of these approaches. For example, a point source could be placed at a location corresponding to a pixel in the image to determine the counts detected in every projection element for that image location. This would then be repeated for all image pixels. This would be extremely tedious even though symmetry arguments can be used to reduce the number of measurements considerably. In practice, many of the geometric effects can be calculated, and other factors that it may be desirable to include in the matrix (for example detector scatter), can often be simulated.

The ML-EM algorithm for PET can be written as:

$$a_i^{k+1} = \frac{a_i^k}{\sum_j M_{i,j}} \sum_j \frac{M_{i,j}s_j}{\sum_i M_{i,j}a_i^k} \qquad (1\text{-}47)$$

This equation shows how the image pixel intensity a_i at iteration $k + 1$ is calculated based on the estimated image pixel intensity a_i at iteration k and the measured projection counts p_j. Notice that when the estimated projection data exactly equal the measured projection data s_j that (substituting from Equation 1-46):

$$a_i^{k+1} = a_i^k \qquad (1\text{-}48)$$

and the image does not change any more. This never actually occurs in practice because of noise in the data and inevitable errors and approximations in $M_{i,j}$. Figure 1-56A shows the reconstruction of a phantom study as a function of iteration number using the ML-EM algorithm and also shows the reconstructed images obtained using an accelerated OSEM approach.

The iterative reconstruction approach has several key advantages. First, it replaces a simple line integral approximation of what the imaging system is measuring with a model that, if correctly implemented, accurately reflects the probability that a gamma ray emitted at a certain location in the object is detected in a given projection element. This can lead to improved spatial resolution as demonstrated by Figure 1-56B which shows a comparison of FDG brain images reconstructed with filtered backprojection with a maximum a posteriori (MAP) algorithm (155) that contains an accurate model of the PET system used to acquire the data. Second, the sampling criteria are relaxed, in that the effect of missing data tends to produce lower spatial resolution, rather than streak artifacts that would commonly be encountered with FBP. Third, the statistics of each line of response can be taken into account, with more weight being given to measurements that have better statistical quality.

Generally, iterative methods can produce better signal-to-noise at a given spatial resolution than filtered backprojection methods, partly for the reasons above, and partly because they do not directly convolve the data by a filter that amplifies high-spatial frequency components such as noise. In some instances, factors of two improvements in signal-to-noise over FBP have been demonstrated with iterative algorithms, which is equivalent to a fourfold increase in the effective sensitivity of the scanner. Another perspective is that the same quality image could be obtained with iterative methods using just one quarter of the injected activity or in one quarter of the imaging time. The disadvantages of iterative reconstruction relate to the computational issues already discussed and to the fact that these methods are nonlinear, which can make their behavior quite difficult to predict. This un-

FIGURE 1-56. A: Illustration of ML-EM reconstruction of a phantom study as a function of iteration number. Also shown are images reconstructed using an accelerated OSEM algorithm with 4 iterations (using 16 subsets) and 8 iterations (using 16 subsets). The OSEM images are placed under the ML-EM images that are qualitatively of similar quality. In this case, the OSEM required 8 to 16 times fewer iterations compared to the conventional ML-EM algorithm to produce images of similar quality.

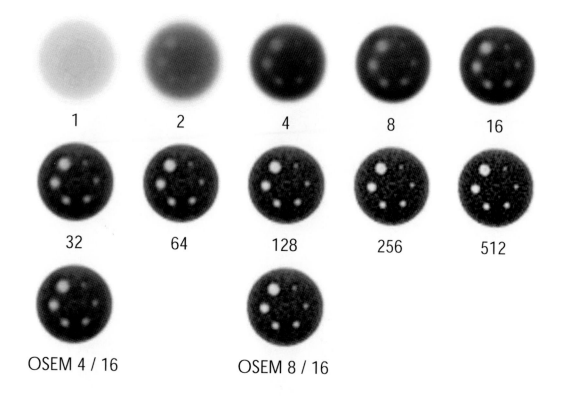

1   2   4   8   16

32   64   128   256   512

OSEM 4 / 16   OSEM 8 / 16

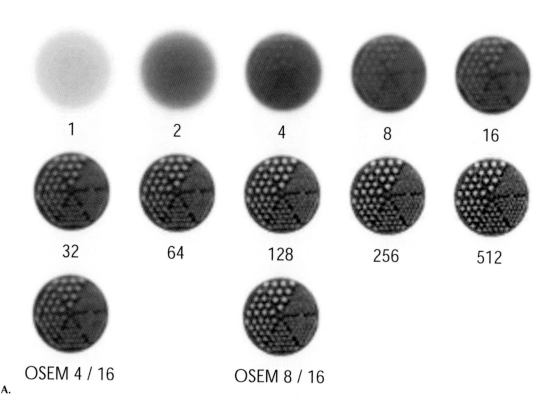

1   2   4   8   16

32   64   128   256   512

OSEM 4 / 16   OSEM 8 / 16

A.

FBP   MAP

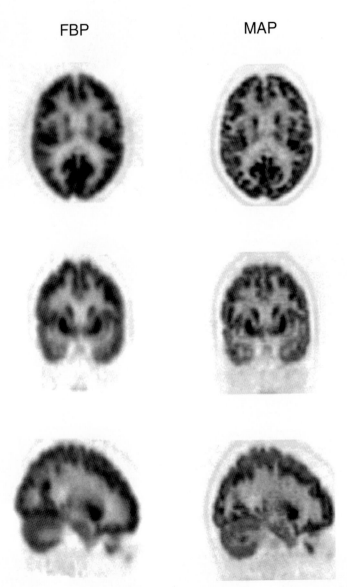

B.
FIGURE 1-56. *Continued.* B: A comparison of filtered backprojection (FBP) and maximum a posteriori (MAP) reconstructions of FDG brain images. Notice the improvement in spatial resolution in the MAP images due in large part to the accurate system model incorporated in this particular algorithm. (Image courtesy of Dr. Richard Leahy, University of Southern California.)

predictability, together with the many different possible implementations of iterative approaches, have caused a certain amount of confusion and concern, which has limited more widespread use. However, the option to use ML-EM algorithms is now found on many commercial PET cameras and powerful multiprocessor desktop computers, and, combined with acceleration techniques such as OSEM, makes reconstruction times acceptable in many instances.

Iterative approaches also can be easily adapted to reconstructing 3-D PET data, although the computational complexity increases dramatically. The matrix $M_{i,j}$ becomes very large because of the added dimensionality of the problem and reconstruction times, even with accelerated approaches or specialized hardware, can take many tens of minutes or longer depending on the specific geometry of the problem.

IMAGE ANALYSIS

Image display

The end result of the PET acquisition and image reconstruction is a 3-D image volume where each individual voxel (volume element) represents the regional tissue radioactivity concentration. The most common way to visualize the data is to display the volume as a series of transaxial cross-sectional images on a gray scale (or pseudo color) display, where each gray level (or color level) represents a particular activity concentration, or if the data are processed through a tracer kinetic model (Chapter 2), a specific biologic parameter. In most modern PET systems, the axial sampling or plane separation is fine enough to allow the re-orientation of the data into coronal planes, sagittal planes, or any other arbitrary orientation. The most common display format for clinical studies is to show coronal sections for whole-body imaging and transaxial sections for brain imaging. It also is common to simultaneously display transaxial, coronal, and sagittal sections in which the cursor is linked between the three image windows, allowing for easy navigation through a large 3-D dataset.

Calibration and region of interest analysis

One of the advantages of PET over some other imaging modalities is that it can accurately determine the activity concentration of the radiotracer within a volume. This can provide information that would allow, for instance, the classification of a lesion in terms of its metabolic rate (see Chapter 2). To do this, it is necessary to accurately calibrate the system such that it is possible to convert the image count density into an activity concentration, which is most commonly done by scanning a uniform cylindrical phantom with a known activity concentration, A (Bq/ml). The phantom data are then corrected for attenuation, scatter, and so on, and reconstructed with the same parameters that are to be used in the clinical studies. From the reconstructed images, the average count density, C (counts per voxel per second), within the central portion of the phantom image is determined. Because the activity concentration in the phantom is known, the calibration factor (CF) between image counts and activity concentration is then:

$$CF = A(Bq/ml) \times B.F. \: / \: C(counts/voxel/sec) \qquad (1\text{-}49)$$

B.F. is the branching fraction, which is the fraction of decays that occur via positron emission for the radionuclide of interest. This term is necessary because the radionuclides used in PET do not necessarily decay by 100% positron emission (Table 1-2). The calibration factor allows the determination of the activity concentration within a region in the reconstructed images. Provided that all corrections have been applied, the accuracy of this activity concentration is typically within 5%.

EXAMPLE 1-18

A region of interest analysis of a noncalibrated ^{18}FDG PET image resulted in an average image count of 3240 counts per voxel/sec. A uniform calibration cylinder (volume 6000 ml) filled with 40 MBq ^{68}Ge/^{68}Ga (branching fraction for ^{68}Ga is 0.89—see Table 1-2) was imaged earlier and resulted in an image count of 72300 counts per voxel/sec. Determine the activity concentration in the region in the ^{18}FDG PET image. The branching fraction for ^{18}F is 0.97.

ANSWER

First determine the calibration factor CF from the ^{68}Ge cylinder data.

$$CF = (40 \text{ MBq} / 6000 \text{ ml}) \times 0.89 / 72300 \text{ (counts per voxel/sec)}$$
$$= 0.082 (\text{Bq} \cdot \text{sec} / \text{ml} \cdot \text{counts per voxel})$$

To determine the activity concentration in the ^{18}FDG PET image, multiply the counts from the image with the CF and correct for the branching fraction for ^{18}F:

$$Act. \text{ Conc.} = 3240 \text{ (counts per voxel/sec)}$$
$$\times 0.082 \text{ (Bq} \cdot \text{sec} / \text{ml} \cdot \text{counts per voxel)} / 0.97$$
$$= 274 \text{ (Bq/ml)}$$

The most common way to determine what the local activity concentration is in a PET image (or volume) is to define a *region of interest* (ROI) on an image, using an image analysis software package. The average voxel value within the region is calculated. Using the calibration factor from Equation 1-49, this value is then converted to an activity concentration in becquerels per milliliter. Because PET data sets usually are made of a stack of images that form a volume, a *volume of interest* (VOI) can be defined by connecting several ROIs defined on multiple contiguous planes into a single VOI. By defining a VOI, the error in the average activity concentration due to counting statistics is reduced.

If a dynamic sequence of images has been acquired, the ROIs or VOI that have been defined can be applied to the same region (or volume) on all images to generate a *time activity curve* (TAC) that shows the radiotracer concentration in a specific region of the body over time. This time dependent data set can then be used with a compartmental model to determine biologically meaningful parameters and to construct parametric images. This is discussed in Chapter 2.

Image segmentation

Image segmentation is an analysis tool used in image processing that classifies pixel elements into regions or classes that are homogenous with respect to one or more characteristics. In the analysis of a CT or MRI study, image segmentation is used to delineate different tissue types, such as the separation of gray and white matter areas in the brain. In the case of a PET study, image segmentation could aid in the determination of the extent of areas of radiotracer uptake. Image segmentation also can be used in combination with image registration techniques (see Image Registration, p. 95) where different tissue types or regions are identified on an image with structural information (such as an MRI or CT image). These regions are then transferred onto a spatially registered PET image to determine the level of activity uptake in these regions.

One of the primary uses of image segmentation in PET is the processing of measured attenuation correction scans as a method to reduce image noise.[45–47] As discussed in Attenuation Correction p. 56, measured attenuation corrections are inherently noisy, and this noise propagates into the final emission image. Image segmentation can be used in the process of the measured attenuation data to reduce the amount of noise that propagates from the measured attenuation correction. Figure 1-57 illustrates the effect of image segmentation on a whole-body transmission scan. Figure 1-57A shows the reconstructed transmission data, in which the gray levels represent the distribution of linear attenuation co-efficients. The relatively high level of noise in this image is due to poor count-ing statistics, which, in turn, are due to the relatively short acquisition time ($\sim$15 minutes). Using image segmentation, where pixel values within specific gray-scale ranges corresponding to air, lung, soft tissue, and bone are replaced with a fixed value or a narrow range of values, the noise in the transmission image is greatly reduced (Figure 1-57B). This image volume is then forward-projected to generate the appropriate attenuation correction factors, which will contain less noise compared to the original attenuation correction.

Image registration

Image registration refers to the process in which image volumes are realigned into a common anatomical coordinate space. The three main applications for image registration in PET are:

1. Correction for patient motion.
2. Correlation of PET images to other imaging modalities (e.g., MRI and CT).
3. Comparison of image data within and between different subjects.

A common complaint about PET imaging is that the entire procedure is lengthy, especially in quantitative research protocols with multiple isotope in-jections. Therefore, patient motion is potentially a problem. Motion during a scan not only introduces a loss in spatial resolution in the final image but may also make regional quantitation impossible in dynamically acquired studies or in studies involving multiple scans. A common clinical protocol for FDG brain imaging is to acquire data for 20 to 40 minutes following the injection and up-take period. For many patients, it is very difficult to remain motionless during the scan time, despite head restraints. Therefore, the data are collected as a se-ries of short frames, which can be viewed, following the acquisition, as a dy-namic sequence to detect patient motion. If the patient moved, then only the frames in which the patient remained stationary are added together, and the frames with motion are discarded. Although the amount of patient motion has been reduced, the drawback is that, by discarding data, the image noise is in-creased due to the lower number of counts that contributes to the final image. This problem could potentially be eliminated if all images are registered, prior to summation; thus, all the acquired information contributes to the final image.

There are many methods for image registration and numerous articles have been published on this subject. An excellent overview of medical image regis-tration techniques is provided by Hill et al.[93] The most successful application of these techniques has been in the registration of brain images, where the regis-tration process for within subject registration is typically limited to rigid trans-lation and rotations of the two image volumes. The challenge in image registra-tion is in determining the transformation that will produce the best possible

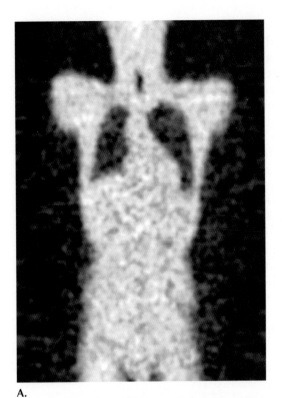
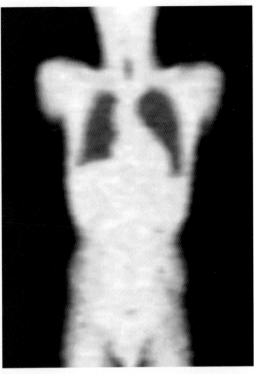

A.   B.

FIGURE 1-57. A (left): Whole-body transmission image. B (right): Segmentation of image on the left in which different gray levels have been segmented out and assigned a narrow range of attenuation values that correspond to the known values for air, soft tissue, and bone.

alignment. One method for aligning two volumes is to view them on a screen and manually identify common features or manually adjust registration parameters until the two volumes appear to match. Using manual alignment methods, a trained user can relatively quickly register two image volumes within a few millimeters, provided the images are free of spatial distortion. Because manual registration can be labor-intensive, several more or less automated algorithms have been developed over the years. One group of these is based on the assumption that the information content in the two images is similar. The main difference between the published implementations is in what criterion is used for determining image correspondence (e.g., stochastic sign difference or the sum of absolute differences).[94,95] This approach is suitable for correction of patient motion within a scan, such as in the example given earlier, or to register two image volumes of the same subject acquired on two different occasions.

   Many times it is desirable to register the image of the same subject obtained using different tracers or, more commonly, to register intramodality images (e.g, PET to CT or PET to MRI). Intramodality registration is of particular interest as it allows the biologically specific PET signal to be mapped onto the high-resolution anatomy provided by MRI or CT. In these situations, the information content in the two data sets are typically dramatically different. Using the similarity criterion generally does not provide a robust solution to the registration problem. Nonetheless, robust registration methods have been developed that seek to maximize the overlap of the volumes or surfaces[96] or minimize the standard deviation of the ratio of the pixel intensities.[97] If the PET radiotracer has very specific uptake in a small fraction of the volume (e.g., [F-18]fluoro-L-DOPA in the human brain) or the images have relatively high noise levels, these methods may fail. In these situations, it might be better to register the PET transmission images rather than the emission images; however, this assumes that the patient remained stationary between the transmission and emission scans.

The most sophisticated type of image registration involves registration of images of different subjects into a standardized atlas (e.g., Talairach space). This application has been extensively used in brain activation studies but also in studies of different types of diseases, such as dementia. Although, at a gross level, the anatomical and functional structure of the human brain is common among individuals, broad deviations are seen in size and shape, and there is significant variation in the appearance of the cortex at the gyral level. To register one person's brain to another, the registration process must involve different nonrigid transformations that deforms or reshapes the brain. The main challenge here is to not only introduce a deformation that makes the two brains similar in shape but also to ensure that functional areas are registered. The process of elastic deformation into a common space is also sometimes referred to as spatial normalization.[98–100] The use of spatial normalization allows the comparison of regions of brain activation across several subjects that are given the same stimulus.[101] Spatial normalization also allows the use of a standardized ROI atlas, from which uptake in specific anatomical or functional areas can rapidly be extracted, thus eliminating the need for manual drawing of regions.[102] Several groups also have assembled databases of the normal uptake of a specific tracer, such as FDG, to which an individual's image is compared to determine areas of abnormal uptakes. This has been applied in the detection of Alzheimer's disease using ^{18}FDG.[103] Figure 1-58 shows an example of intrasubject image registration.

Partial volume effects

One of the main difficulties in the ROI and VOI analysis is to accurately determine the activity concentration in regions or volumes that are small compared with the resolution of the PET scanner. This is of particular importance in the quantitative characterization of small lesions or structures. As discussed earlier, a PET system has limited spatial resolution, such that decays from an infinitely small point source of radiation will be smeared out and appear as a finite-sized blob (equal to the point spread function of the scanner) of lower activity concentration in the reconstructed PET image. This is known as the *partial volume effect*.[104]

The result of the partial volume effect is that small objects appear to have lower activity concentration in comparison to larger objects of equal activity concentration (Figure 1-59). In this figure, a set of spherical sources of equal activity concentration are simulated (A, top row). In Figure 1-59B, a smoothing filter of 10- mm has been applied in all three dimensions to simulate a 10-mm resolution detector system. As can be seen from the profiles (Figure 1-59C) through the images, the activity concentration is accurately measured in the larger objects, although there is smearing at the edge of the sources due to the limited spatial resolution. As the sources become smaller, the plateau of the measured activity concentration in the center of the sources diminishes, and, eventually, a suppression of the peak activity concentration is seen. The degree of

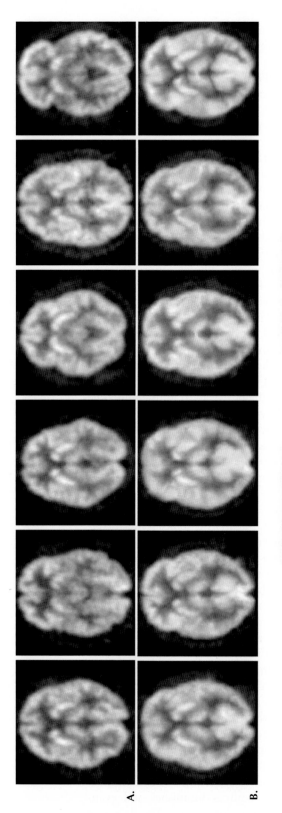

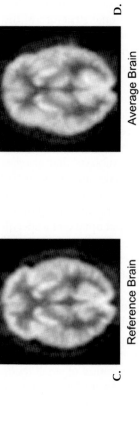

C. Reference Brain

D. Average Brain

FIGURE 1-58. Illustration of intrasubject registration of PET images. A (top row) shows single sections through the midbrain of 6 individuals from their FDG-PET scans prior to any image registration. B (second row) shows the images following a nonlinear registration to a "reference" brain shown in C (bottom left). The sum of the 6 images in B is shown in D (bottom right). Notice the high correlation in location and shape of structures after image registration (B) that allows the scans from these 6 different individuals to be added together while still maintaining resolution of the major brain structures.

A.

B.

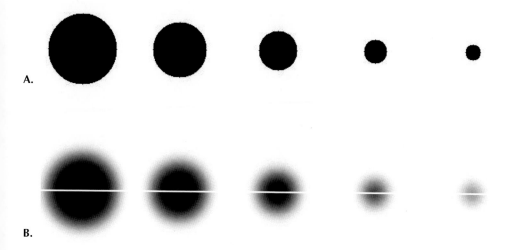

A.

B.

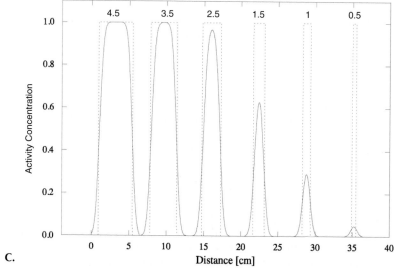

C.

FIGURE 1-59. Simulated data showing the partial volume effect on a set of spherical sources (diameter ranging from 0.5 cm to 4.5 cm) of equal activity concentration (A, top row). Due to the partial volume effect (10-mm Gaussian smearing), the activity concentration in the smaller spheres appears to be lower (B, second row). The sphere diameter in centimeters is given above each profile (C, bottom).

suppression is both a function of object size and the system reconstructed image resolution; it is characterized by the recovery coefficient (RC):

$$RC = \frac{\text{Measured peak activity concentration}}{\text{True activity concentration}} \qquad (1\text{-}50)$$

The recovery coefficient for a spherical object as a function of object diameter, normalized to the image resolution, is shown in Figure 1-60.

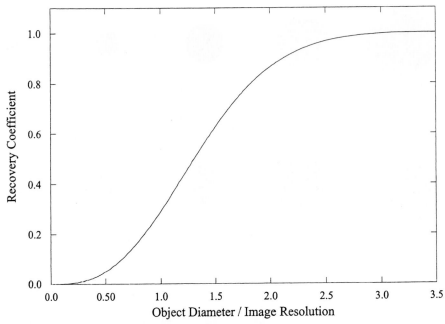

FIGURE 1-60. Calculated recovery coefficient for the system simulated in Figure 1-59. For a sphere with a diameter greater than 3 times the image resolution (FWHM), the activity concentration is accurately preserved.

To accurately estimate the activity concentration using ROI analysis, it is, therefore, important to know the size of the object and the reconstructed image resolution. If the size of the object is approximately three times greater than the image resolution, a small central region of interest placed over the object would accurately represent the activity concentration within the object. The size of the ROI has to be small enough to minimize partial volume effects but also large enough to reduce statistical noise (by averaging across voxels). The curves in Figure 1-61 show the effect of the region of interest size on the measured activity concentration as a function of object size, normalized to the image resolution. As can be seen from this figure, if the size of the region is identical to the object size, underestimation of activity concentration will occur. However, as the ROI size is reduced, the amount of underestimation is reduced.

If the recovery coefficient can be determined, then it is possible to correct for partial volume effects. The recovery coefficient depends on both the physical dimensions of the object and the image resolution. The image resolution of the PET system can be easily determined by measuring its point spread function. However, the dimensions of the structure or lesion of interest are in general much more difficult to measure, with one particular problem being that they cannot easily be determined from the PET images because the extent of the structure or lesion seen in the PET images is distorted by the partial volume effect.[104]

The dimensions of the structure can be estimated if anatomical information from other high-resolution modalities such as either a registered MR or CT is provided with the PET image. Using this information together with the meas-

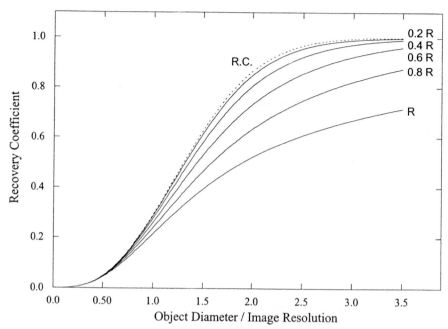

FIGURE 1-61. Effect of the region of interest size (relative to the image resolution R) on the estimated activity concentration for spheres of varying diameter. If the region size is large in comparison to the object size, the estimated activity concentration is underestimated. As the region of interest size approaches zero, the degree of under-estimation approaches the recovery coefficient (RC).

ured PET image resolution, a recovery coefficient can be estimated.[105–107] However, the problem remains a complex one, because not only is it necessary to correct for the apparent suppression of the activity concentration, but if the region of interest is surrounded by tissue with radiotracer uptake, it is also necessary to correct for cross contamination or activity spillover from these surrounding areas into the region of interest due to the limited spatial resolution. An example of this "spillover" effect would be the contribution to the signal in gray matter regions of the brain from activity in the adjacent white matter, or the contribution of signal from radioactivity in the blood to the determination of myocardial activity concentrations due to the large blood pool in the heart. Furthermore, the radiotracer may not be homogeneously distributed in the structure or lesions that are of interest. A more generalized model for partial volume correction that accounts for the cross contamination and heterogeneous tracer uptake has been proposed by Rousset et al.[108] Nonetheless, in most imaging situations, correction for partial volume errors are only estimates at best, as some assumptions are always needed.

PERFORMANCE EVALUATION OF PET SYSTEMS

To objectively compare the performance of different clinical PET systems, the National Electrical Manufacturers Association (NEMA) has developed guidelines on how certain performance parameters, such as spatial resolution and sensitivity, should be evaluated and presented.[109–111] The guidelines allow a user, in the process of selecting a PET system, to obtain a relatively unbiased comparison of system parameters. The ability to make these comparisons is probably of most importance in multicenter clinical trials where a variety of systems may be in use and a certain minimum performance standard is required. The original NEMA standard focused on the system performance using a relatively small phantom (20 cm diameter, 20 cm tall), which is appropriate to use to simulate imaging brain-sized objects. Since the publication of the initial standard,[110] whole-body PET has become the predominant use of PET, at least in routine clinical practice. Therefore, the use of the small phantom does not adequately describe the count rate situation in whole-body PET studies. Furthermore, the short axial extent of the phantom used in the original standard makes comparisons of systems with large axial FOVs to narrow FOV systems difficult. The new NEMA standard, NEMA NU2-2001,[109] takes some of these shortcomings into account and adds an image quality measurement appropriate for whole-body imaging. Approaches for making a number of important performance measurements are outlined below.

Reconstructed spatial resolution

Spatial resolution measurements are made using an ^{18}F-point source (dimensions 1 mm or less). The FWHM and the FWTM are reported for several prescribed source positions in the FOV (Figure 1-62) so that variations in resolution can be determined. At least 100,000 counts are collected for each acquisition and the data are reconstructed with a ramp filter and, if possible, a zoom that results in pixels of dimension of at most 0.1 $\times$ the anticipated FWHM. Three components of resolution are measured by taking orthogonal profiles through the reconstructed image of the point source: the radial and tangential components are in the transaxial plane defined as shown in Figure 1-62, and the axial component is along the axis of the scanner.

Scatter fraction

The *scatter fraction* (SF) is a measure of the contamination of the data from scattered photons, which depends on factors including the geometry of the scanner, the shielding (such as septa), and the energy window. The scatter fraction is defined as the ratio of scattered to total events measured at low counts rate to minimize accidental coincidences and dead time. In the initial NEMA standard from 1994,[110] the scatter fraction is estimated from data acquired with a line source of activity placed at different radial offsets in a cylindrical phantom (20 cm diameter, by 19 cm tall, inner diameter) filled with (nonactive) water. A 24-cm FOV is defined for all scanners. Profiles through the sinogram are used to estimate the number of scattered events within the FOV and the number of true events within a 2-cm radius of the source (Figure 1-63). Scatter within the peak is estimated by assuming a constant background of scatter under the peak. The measurement is repeated at three radial positions: 0, 4.5 and 9 cm. At 4.5 cm and 9 cm, the sinogram profile must be analyzed as a function of angle. The average scatter fraction is calculated by weighting the totals counts and scattered counts measured at each position of the source by the relative area of the annulus at that radius (Figure 1-63):

$$SF = \frac{S(0) + 8 \times S(4.5) + 10.75 \times S(9)}{T_{tot}(0) + 8 \times T_{tot}(4.5) + 10.75 \times T_{tot}(9)} \qquad (1\text{-}51)$$

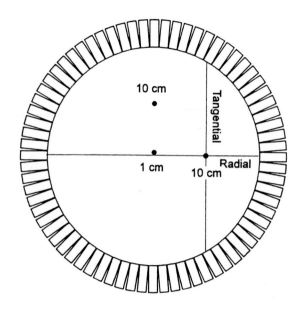

Axial Section

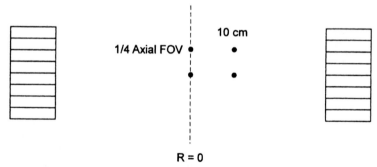

FIGURE 1-62. Illustration of the positioning of the point sources to measure the transaxial and axial resolution in a PET system. Abbreviation: FOV, field of view.

where S is the number of the scattered counts per unit activity and T_{tot} is the total number of counts (true + scattered) per unit activity. This measurement is performed in both 2-D and 3-D. This measurement represents the scatter fraction in brain imaging. In NEMA NU-2 2001,[109] the scatter fraction is defined for whole-body imaging. The scatter fraction is determined in a similar way with the difference that a 20-cm diameter and 70-cm long cylinder is used. Furthermore, the scatter fraction is only determined for a single off-center position (4.5 cm).

Sensitivity

The sensitivity of a PET scanner is defined as the counting efficiency of the system for a known amount and distribution of activity. To measure the absolute sensitivity of the scanner, a 700-mm long, 5-mm diameter tubing is filled with a known amount of activity. The activity in the source should be

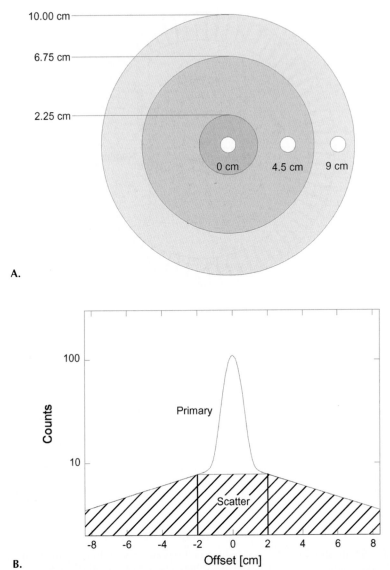

A.

B.

FIGURE 1-63. The scatter fraction is determined from measurements of a line source placed within a 20-cm diameter phantom (A). The sinogram profile (B) is used to estimate the number of scattered events within the FOV and the number of true events within a 2-cm radius of the source. Scatter within the peak is estimated by assuming a constant background of scatter under the peak. The measurement is repeated at three radial positions: 0, 4.5 cm, and 9 cm; at 4.5 cm and 9 cm, the sinogram profile must be analyzed as a function of angle. The average scatter fraction is calculated by weighting the totals and scatter measured at each position of the source by the relative area of the annulus at that radius (Equation 1-51).

low enough to ensure counting losses of less than 1% and a random coincidence fraction of less than 5% of the true coincidence counting rate. To ensure that the emitted positrons annihilate and produce a pair of 511-keV photons, the source has to be surrounded by an attenuating sleeve. Although the sleeve will ensure positron annihilation, it will also attenuate a fraction of the emitted photons, which will prevent a direct measurement of the absolute sensitivity. Instead, by successive measurements of the count rate using different sleeves of known thickness, the attenuation-free sensitivity can be determined by extrapolation.[112] This measurement is performed in the center and at a 10-cm radial offset in the FOV.

Count-rate performance and dead time

Measurements of count rate as a function of activity concentration are performed with a 20-cm diameter, 70-cm long, uniform cylinder phantom initially filled with a high activity concentration (typically 25–50 kBq/ml) and allowed to decay. The recommended radionuclide is ^{11}C because the shorter half-life makes the total measurement time more manageable than with ^{18}F. Data should be acquired until the fraction of random coincidence events and the system dead time are negligible. The rate of prompts (true + scatter + randoms), random (from delayed window) and scattered (using scatter fraction, p. 102) coincidences are recorded at convenient time points (e.g., 4 points per half-life).

The deviation of the trues rate at high activity concentrations from an ideal, linear dependence is due to scanner (detector + electronics) dead time. The percentage dead time, as a function of increasing activity concentration, is defined as: $\%DT = 1 - T/T_{ex}$, where T is the actual trues rate and T_{ex} is the trues rate linearly extrapolated from low count rate data (Figure 1-40). The concentration at which the dead time reaches 50% also is a measure of scanner performance (Figure 1-64). A high sensitivity scanner (e.g., one operated in 3-D) typically saturates at relatively low activity concentration (compared to 2-D), even though the maximum trues rate is higher than that of a less sen-

FIGURE 1-64. Example of a typical dead time curve as a function of activity concentration within a 20-cm diameter cylinder phantom. The concentration at which the dead time is 50% should be reported.

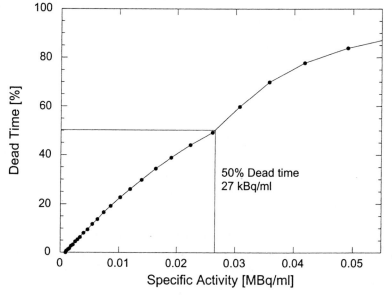

50% Dead time
27 kBq/ml

sitive system which peaks at a higher activity concentration (e.g., the same scanner operated in 2-D).

Noise equivalent count rate

The count rate measurements do not directly indicate image signal-to-noise in the presence of relatively changing trues, randoms and scatter rates. A better measure of signal-to-noise is provided by the *noise equivalent count rate* (NEC),[113] defined by:

$$NEC = \frac{T^2}{T + S + 2\,fR} \qquad (1\text{-}52)$$

where T, S and R are the true, scatter, and random coincidence counting rates, f is the fraction of the sinogram width subtended by the phantom, and the factor 2 comes from on-line randoms subtraction (see Correction for Random Coincidences, p. 65). The NEC provides only a global measure of the signal-to-noise ratio because it is not sensitive to regional variations of the source distribution. Figure 1-65 shows a set of typical count rate curves from a clinical scanner for prompt, true, and random coincidences as well as the resulting NEC count rate.

Image uniformity

Uniformity measures the deviations in the reconstructed image from a uniform response. A 20-cm diameter uniform cylinder is filled with a moderate activity concentration (fraction of random coincidences and dead time < 20%) and imaged when positioned ~2.5 cm off-axis transaxially. An average of 20 million

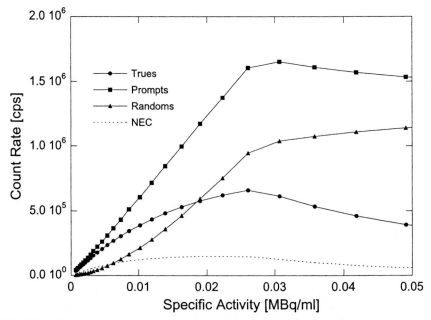

FIGURE 1-65. Example of prompt (squares), random (triangles), and true + scatter (circles) count rate curves. The dashed curve is the resulting NEC curve calculated from the measured count rate curves using Equation 1-52.

counts per slice are acquired and reconstructed with a ramp filter. A grid of 1-cm $\times$ 1-cm regions of interest are inscribed in a circle 18 cm in diameter centered on the image of the cylinder in each slice. Positive and negative nonuniformity (NU) are defined by:

$$NU(+) = +(C_{max} - C_{ave})/ C_{ave} \qquad (1\text{-}53)$$

$$NU(-) = -(C_{ave} - C_{min})/ C_{ave} \qquad (1\text{-}54)$$

where C_{max} is the maximum number of counts in any square ROI within the slice, C_{min} is the minimum number of counts, and C_{ave} is the average number of counts of all regions in the slice. The necessity to collect such high statistics is to minimize the nonuniformity due to statistical effects and focus on those due to scanner imperfections, software corrections, and the reconstruction algorithm.

PET SYSTEM DESIGN

High-performance dedicated clinical PET scanners

Dedicated PET systems have undergone dramatic changes since the first PET systems were designed in the mid 1970s.[112] Although the first systems could produce images at a resolution of 1 cm to 2 cm, these were low-sensitivity, single-slice, small-diameter systems, using heavily collimated NaI(Tl) detectors. State-of-the-art, high-resolution whole-body systems now have an intrinsic resolution of 3 mm to 5 mm, orders of magnitude of higher sensitivity, and an axial coverage of 15 cm or greater, with a minimal amount of collimation.[114–118] The design of the most widely distributed high-end PET systems is fundamentally the same. The detector system in these systems is based on the block detector concept (Block Detector, p. 22). Depending on the manufacturer and the particular model, the size of the individual detector elements vary. For example, they are 4.0 $\times$ 4.4 mm^2 in cross-section on the ECAT HR+ (CTI/Siemens, Knoxville, TN) and 6 $\times$ 8 mm^2 on the Advance (GE Medical Systems, Waukesha, WI). These systems generally cover an axial field of view of 15 cm to 16 cm, producing between 35 to 63 simultaneous cross-sectional image planes. The total number of detector elements in these systems can be as high as 18,000. Table 1-5 summarizes the design and performance of several commercial, dedicated PET systems. A photograph of a typical clinical PET scanner is shown in Figure 1-66 and Figure 1-67 shows a whole-body ^{18}F-FDG PET scan acquired on a similar system.

These systems all have the ability to collect data in both 2-D and 3-D mode, as discussed in Image Reconstruction (p. 86), where the lead septa located between each detector ring can be removed to allow the collection of oblique coincidence lines of response. These systems all have built-in rod sources that can automatically be extended and retracted for the acquisition of transmission data. These high-end dedicated systems provide the user with the maximum flexibility in the type of PET studies that can be acquired. The large number of detector channels allows high count rate studies to be performed with nominal dead time losses (especially in 2-D mode). The full ring geometry allows fast dynamic scans to be acquired.

TABLE 1-5. Comparison of Several Commercially Available Clinical PET Systems

			Scanner			
	ECAT EXACT 47	ECAT EXACT HR+	ECAT ACCEL	Advance NXi	C-PET plus	ALLEGRO
Detector Material	BGO	BGO	LSO	BGO	NaI (Tl)	GSO
Diameter [cm]	82.4	82.4	82.4	92.7	90	90
Detector Dimensions [mm] (Transaxial × Axial × Depth)	6.75 × 6.75 × 20	4.05 × 4.39 × 30	6.75 × 6.75 × 20	3.9 × 8.2 × 30 mm	Curved Panel 500 × 300 × 25 mm	4 × 6 × 20 mm
Detectors per Block or Module	64	64	64	36	1	638
Number of Rings	47	63	47	35	64/128	90
Axial FOV [cm]	16.2	15.5	16.2	15.2	18	25.6
Transverse FOV [cm]	58.5	58.5	58.5	55	57.6	57.6
Septa	Yes	Yes	No	Yes	No	No
Spatial Resolution [mm]						
2-D Transaxial:						
1 cm	6.0	4.6	6.2	4.8	—	—
10 cm	6.7	5.4	6.7	5.4	—	—
2-D Axial:						
1 cm	4.5	4.2	4.3	4.0	—	—
10 cm	5.9	5.0	5.9	5.4	—	—
3-D Transaxial:						
1 cm	6.0	4.6	6.3	4.0	5.0	4.8
10 cm	6.7	5.4	6.8	5.4	6.4	5.9
3-D Axial:						
1 cm	4.6	3.5	4.7	6.0	5.5	5.4
10 cm	6.5	5.3	7.1	6.3	5.9	6.5
Sensitivity [kcps/mCi/cc]						
2D	180	200	200	200	—	—
3D	780	900	925	1100	450	>700
Peak NEC [kCps] NEMA NU-2 (2001)						
2D	44	54	>90	83	—	—
3D	25	38	61	28	16	48

Abbreviations: BGO, bismuth germanate; FOV, field of view; GSO, gadolinium oxyorthosilicate; LSO, lutetium oxyorthosilicate; NaI(Tl), thallium-activated sodium iodide; NEC, noise equivalent counts; NEMA, National Electric Manufacturers Association; PET, positron emission tomography; 3-D, three-dimensional; 2-D, two-dimensional.

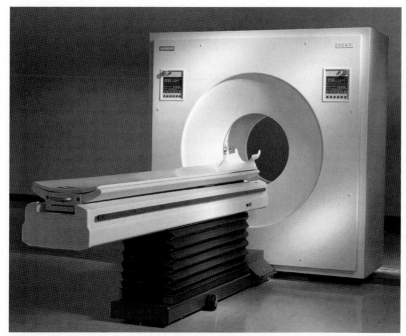

FIGURE 1-66. Photograph of ECAT EXAT clinical PET scanner. (Courtesy of CTI Inc., Knoxville, TN.)

FIGURE 1-67. Whole-body FDG image acquired on the GE Advance clinical PET scanner. (Courtesy of GE Medical Systems, Waukesha, WI.)

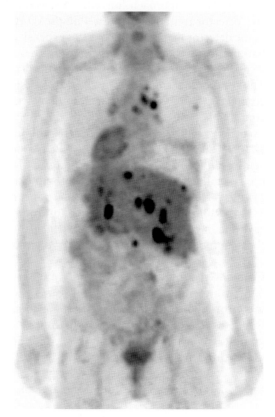

Since the early 1980s, the majority of dedicated PET systems have used BGO as the scintillation material.[119] Although this material has excellent absorption properties, the relatively long scintillation decay time (Table 1-4) limits the count rate performance, especially in the high counting-rate environment of 3-D whole-body scans. Because of this limitation, the injected dose has to be reduced when operating a BGO in this 3-D mode, which tends to offset the sensitivity gain. Recently, the first commercial whole-body system was introduced using LSO as the scintillation material. The speed of LSO allows 3-D scans to be acquired at the full injected dose, which will provide an improvement in image quality and/or improved patient throughput.[120] For example, whole-body scan times can be reduced from about 1 hour to under 10 minutes.

Lower cost clinical PET scanners

The overall cost of a PET scanner is directly proportional to the number of detector modules and the amount of associated electronics. These components account for approximately 50% of the manufacturing cost of a PET system. One approach to reduce the overall cost of the system is to reduce the number of detector channels. This is an approach used in the ECAT ART scanner,[121] which is a partial ring system (Figure 1-21, upper right) in which the detectors rotate to collect a complete data set. To compensate for the lost sensitivity caused by the reduced number of detector channels, this system has no interplane septa and is operated in 3-D mode only. The need for detector motion limits how fast dynamic frames can be acquired.

A different approach for reducing overall system cost is to use less expensive detector technology. In the Philips/ADAC C-PET systems, NaI(Tl) is used as the detector material, which is less expensive in comparison to BGO. This system uses continuous detectors based on curved plates of NaI(Tl) read by a matrix of relatively large PMTs (Continuous Gamma Camera Detector, p. 25).[122] The total number of PMTs used in this design is roughly a factor of 3–4 less compared to PET systems based on the block design. The use of less expensive continuous NaI(Tl) detectors allows the construction of a system with a longer axial FOV, which to a certain degree compensates for the lower efficiency of NaI(Tl). Like the ECAT ART, the C-PET system is also a 3-D-only system. Recently, Philips/ADAC (ADAC Laboratories, Milpitas, CA) introduced the Allegro system, where individual ~4 × 4 mm GSO crystals are mounted on an array of PM tubes. This is similar to the panel detector concept shown in Figure 1-14 (bottom). GSO has both better absorption characteristics and a shorter decay time in comparison to NaI(Tl), which should provide significant improvements in both sensitivity and count rate performance.

Coincidence imaging on gamma cameras

Shortly after the first scintillation camera was invented in the late 1950s, it was proposed to use a pair of these devices, operated in coincidence mode, for detection of annihilation radiation.[123] Since the algorithms for tomographic reconstruction were not yet developed, the device was restricted to planar imaging. With the increased availability of positron-emitting radiopharmaceuticals from distribution centers in the mid 1990s, the idea of using two conventional scintillation cameras in coincidence for tomographic imaging was revived.[124] Because such a system is basically a dual-headed SPECT system, upgraded with coincidence circuitry, this system could then also be used with collimators for conventional nuclear medicine studies using single-photon emitting radionuclides.

One of the difficulties in using standard scintillation cameras for PET imaging is that they are highly optimized for low-energy gamma ray imaging (~140 keV). Because of the high energy of the annihilation radiation (511 keV), the detection efficiency is very poor using standard three-eighths-thick NaI(Tl) detectors. This can be compensated for by increasing the detector thickness; however, this reduces the intrinsic spatial resolution of the detector. The count rate capability of these coincidence systems also is limited, which is caused by the fact that all detected events have to be processed through only two detector channels. Because these coincidence systems are operated with a minimum of collimation and all events have to be processed by only two detector channels, dead-time and pile-up effects become a serious problem at relatively low activity levels. The end result is that the total number of counts that can be collected within a reasonable time frame is limited. This, in turn, requires the use of low-resolution filters in the reconstruction algorithm to keep statistical noise at acceptable levels for diagnostic quality images, which may limit the visualization of small lesions.

To overcome both the detection efficiency and count rate limitation of the coincidence systems, CTI/Siemens (Knoxville, TN) designed a hybrid PET/SPECT, using block detector technology as found in conventional PET systems and the phoswich concept (Figure 1-17, top). Using this technology, several parallel channels process the photon flux. To overcome the efficiency problem, this system uses two layers of scintillators, where a front layer of NaI(Tl) is primarily used for detection of the low-energy gammas from single-photon emitters. A second layer of LSO is used to improve the detection efficiency of the 511-keV photons.[125]

High-performance brain imaging systems

Several companies and universities have developed or are in the process of developing high-performance research PET scanners, with a particular emphasis on high resolution and high sensitivity brain imaging. The *ECAT EX-ACT 3D* (CTI/Siemens, Knoxville, TN) is a 6-ring, 3-D only version of the clinical ECAT EXACT HR+, resulting in an axial field of view of 23.4 cm.[126] This is the highest sensitivity PET scanner built to date, with an absolute sensitivity at the center of the field of view of 10%, and it is largely directed towards low concentration receptor studies in the brain. Another system, the *HRRT (High Resolution Research Tomograph*; CTI/Siemens, Knoxville, TN), introduced a number of new features in the quest for higher spatial resolution in the brain.[127] It combines the quadrant-sharing approach (Figure 1-14) with a LSO/GSO phoswich detector block (Figure 1-17) that provides 1-bit depth of interaction information. This was the first human scanner to use LSO scintillator and the first human PET scanner to have depth of interaction capability. It is also the highest resolution commercial PET system built to date for human imaging, with a reconstructed image resolution as high as 2.5 mm. Figure 1-68 shows one of the first brain studies performed on this

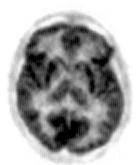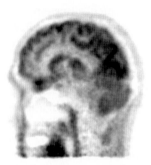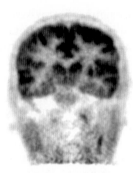

FIGURE 1-68. Brain images showing glucose metabolism acquired on the high-resolution HRRT scanner—the highest resolution commercial human PET scanner currently in existence. (Image courtesy of CTI Inc., Knoxville, TN.)

machine, showing glucose metabolism in the brain that demonstrates the astonishing detail that can now be visualized by PET. Other high performance brain imaging systems based on GSO detectors and depth encoding LSO detectors with photodiode and PMT readout are being developed at the University of Pennsylvania[128] and Lawrence Berkeley National Laboratory,[129] respectively.

Other human PET scanners
A number of other prototype systems based on novel approaches or technologies have been designed and built by research groups across the world. Most notable are scanners based on multiwire proportional chambers with lead or lead glass converters,[35,36] a combination of BaF_2 scintillator with MWPC readout[34] and a variable field of view BGO camera,[130] which also included an early implementation of the quadrant-sharing scheme (Figure 1-14).

There has also been considerable interest in developing dedicated positron imaging systems for breast imaging. FDG-PET has been shown to have high sensitivity and specificity in the detection of breast lesions.[131] By placing detectors around the breast, rather than around the whole cross-section of the patient, sensitivity can be dramatically increased, and it should be possible to achieve higher resolution images at a reasonable noise level. A number of designs have been developed, some of which provide simple projection images through the breast,[132,133] others of which will be capable of some form of tomography. The projection-based systems are designed for incorporation into mammography or biopsy gantries so that coregistered mammograms can be acquired along with the PET data. At the present time, these systems are just entering clinical trials,[134] so the cost-effectiveness and diagnostic utility of these systems for breast imaging have yet to be determined.

Multimodality PET imaging
A major advance in the late 1990s has been the concept of combining molecular imaging by PET with anatomic information obtained from other modalities, using integrated imaging systems rather than software-based approaches.[135] In particular, combined PET and CT scanners have been developed that enable coregistered PET and CT images to be acquired in quick succession.[136] The value

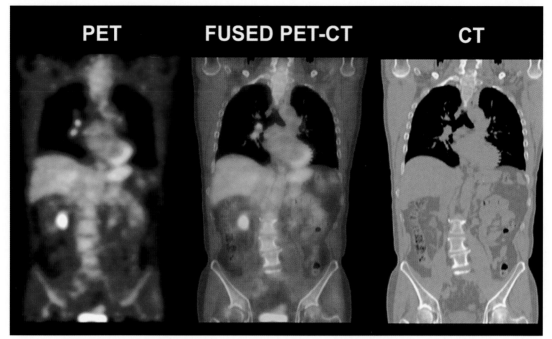

FIGURE 1-69. Fused FDG-PET and anatomical CT images from the Reveal combined PET/CTscanner. (Image courtesy of CTI PET Systems, Knoxville, TN.)

of fused FDG-PET and CT images has become apparent to physicians, particularly in oncology,[137] where the correlation of anatomy (CT) and metabolism (FDG-PET) has become a powerful new diagnostic tool. Furthermore, the CT scan can be used to provide the tissue density information with which to calculate the attenuation correction for the PET images. It is expected that combined PET/CT systems will have important applications in radiation therapy, surgical planning, and guided biopsy procedures.

A number of companies have unveiled products that combine a PET scanner and a CT scanner. One example is the Biograph/Reveal system (CTI/Siemens, Knoxville, TN) which consists of an ECAT HR+ PET scanner (with either BGO or LSO block detectors) integrated with a Siemens Somatom EMOTION spiral CT system. An example of a fused PET/CT image obtained from this system is shown in Figure 1-69. The Hawkeye system (GE Medical Systems, Waukesha, WI) uses a Millenium VG coincidence gamma camera system with a simple CT system based on a linear detector array.[138] A new combined PET/CT system based on the GE ADVANCE PET scanner and a high-end, multi-plane spiral CT has also been released (Figure 1-70). ADAC/Philips (ADAC Laboratories, Milpitas, CA) have a PET/CT system based on their Allegro GSO PET system combined with a spiral CT system. This is a rapidly developing area in clinical PET; systems in which there is more complete integration of the PET and CT systems, in terms of the detector hardware, gantry, and the software, are to be expected.

There have also been some early attempts at producing PET systems that are compatible with MRI scanners so that PET and MRI images can be acquired in

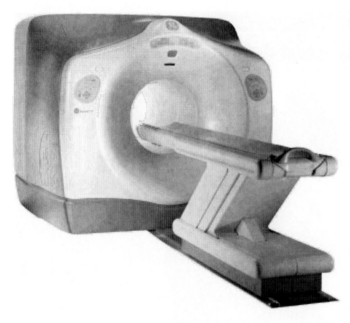

FIGURE 1-70. Photograph of GE Discovery LS combined PET-CT scanner. (Image courtesy of GE Medical Systems, Waukesha, WI.)

the same setting. This research, however, remains at a very preliminary stage and has been limited so far to phantom and animal studies.[139]

Animal scanners

PET has recently increased its impact in basic biological research, leveraged largely by the development of very high-resolution, relatively low-cost PET systems designed specifically for imaging laboratory animals.[140] The ability to measure a range of relevant molecular and biological processes noninvasively in animal models by PET has opened many new possibilities in animal research, both in research laboratories and in the pharmaceutical industry. High-performance PET systems have been developed for brain imaging in nonhuman primates,[141] but perhaps the biggest advances have been in the development of systems for imaging small rodents, particularly mice and rats. An early system based on the same detectors found in clinical scanners provided an initial demonstration of the utility of dedicated animal PET scanners for neuroreceptor studies in the rat brain.[142] Since then, a number of groups have built functional prototype systems using a wide array of PET detector technology including avalanche photodiodes,[28,29] position-sensitive PMTs,[143–145] fiberoptically coupled multichannel PMTs with LSO scintillator,[146] and multiwire proportional chamber technology.[32,37] Figure 1-71 shows the microPET® scanner[146,147] developed for small-animal imaging. This was the first PET scanner to incorporate the new scintillator LSO. When combined with an accurate iterative reconstruction algorithm,[148] this system can produce animal images with a spatial resolution of approximately 1.5 mm. FDG images of the rat brain obtained with this scanner and reconstructed with the MAP algorithm described by Qi et al[148] are also shown in Figure 1-71.

Several companies now offer commercially available animal PET systems. The most widely distributed at the time of writing is the microPET® scanner

FIGURE 1-71. Photograph of microPET® small animal scanner (A, top). Coronal FDG images of the rat brain obtained using this system and reconstructed with an iterative algorithm containing an accurate system model (B, bottom).

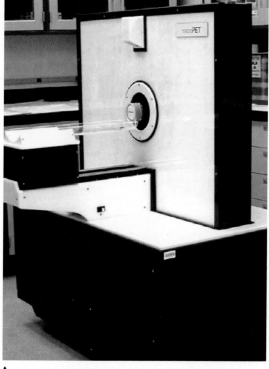

A.

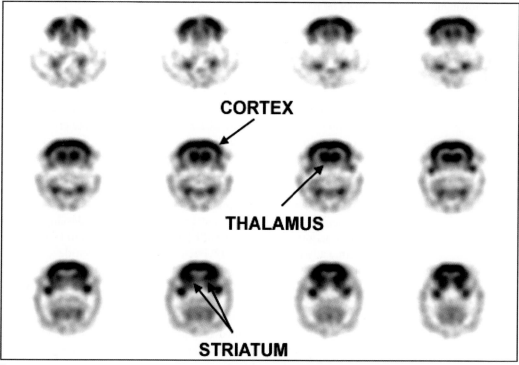

B.

A.

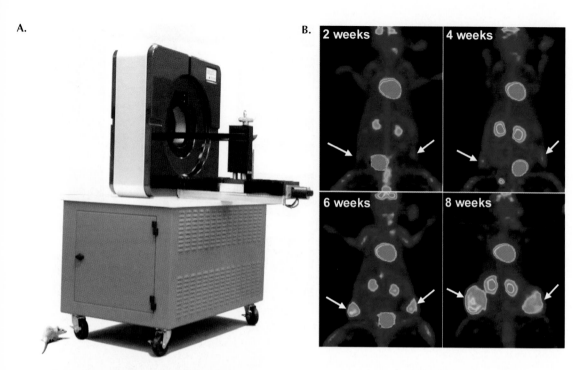

FIGURE 1-72. A: Photograph of the microPET® Focus animal PET scanner with covers removed to reveal ring of detector modules (courtesy of Concorde Microsystems Inc., Knoxville, TN). B: ^{18}F-FDG whole-body imaging in a single mouse showing tumor growth (arrows) in mammary fat pads over a period of eight weeks. (Courtesy of Craig Abbey, UC Davis.)

(Concorde Microsystems Inc., Knoxville, TN). This system is made up from detector modules that consist of an array of 2.2 × 2.2 × 10 mm LSO crystals coupled via a short optical fiber bundle to a position-sensitive PMT.[149] Two different configurations exist, one with a 26 cm diameter bore that can accommodate small non-human primates[149] and a rodent-only version with a 14.8-cm bore.[150] Reconstructed image resolution is approximately 2 mm with filtered backprojection and the sensitivity is 2.2% and 3.4% for the 26 cm and 14.8 cm bore system respectively at the center of the field of view. Images showing the development of tumors in a mouse acquired using a MicroPET® system are shown in Figure 1-72.

A new system, called the MicroPET® Focus, has recently been developed by the same company and uses 1.5 × 1.5 × 10 mm crystals to improve the spatial resolution to around 1.75 mm, with a sensitivity of 3.4%. With MAP reconstruction, this system achieves images with a spatial resolution approaching 1.25 mm. Oxford Positron Systems (Weston-on-the-Green, UK) offers a very high resolution animal PET system[32] called the quad-HIDAC that is based on the multiwire proportional chamber technology. This system achieves 1 mm reconstructed resolution with iterative algorithms and has stacks of detector mod-

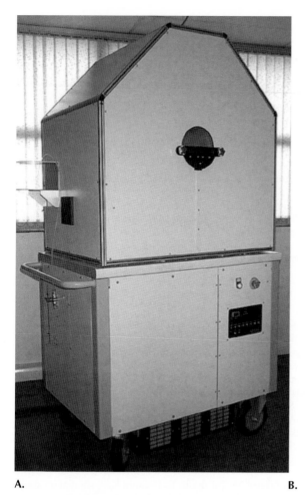

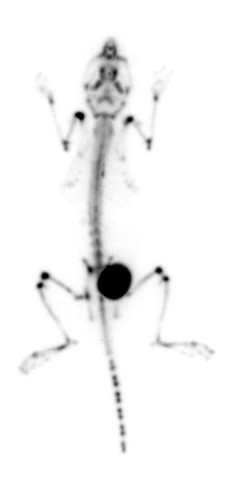

A.

B.

FIGURE 1-73. A: Photograph of the quad-HIDAC small-animal PET scanner. B: ^{18}F-fluoride ion bone scan in a mouse acquired with this system. (Courtesy of Oxford Positron Systems, Weston-on-the-Green, UK.)

ules to provide depth of interaction information, thus minimizing parallax errors. The sensitivity is around 1.8%. An image from this system is shown in Figure 1-73.

It is clearly still possible to make significant improvements in spatial resolution and sensitivity for small-animal imaging. A number of groups are developing detectors and systems that can realize approximately 1-mm reconstructed spatial resolution in all three dimensions, leading to a 1-μl volumetric resolution.[151–153] The combination and integration of small-animal PET with other modalities such as CT[154] and MRI[139] also is being explored. Finally, the development of detector technology for small-animal PET applications has the added benefit of providing a convenient testing ground for technologies that may ultimately also be applicable for clinical PET systems used in humans.

REFERENCES

General references and further reading
Basic Nuclear Physics:
The Atomic Nucleus. R.D. Evans. McGraw-Hill, New York, 1955.
Detectors and Detector Physics:
Radiation Detection and Measurement. G.F. Knoll. 3rd Edition. John Wiley, New York, 2000.
Physics of Nuclear Medicine:
Physics in Nuclear Medicine. S.R. Cherry, J.A. Sorenson, M.E. Phelps. 3rd Edition. W.B. Saunders, New York, 2003.
Image Reconstruction:
Principles of Computerized Tomography. A.C. Kak and M. Slaney. Society for Industrial and Applied Mathematics, 2001.
3-D PET Data Acquisition and Image Reconstruction:
The Theory and Practice of 3D PET. Eds: B. Bendriem and D.W. Townsend. Kluwer Academic Publishers, Dordrecht, The Netherlands, 1998.
Image Processing
Handbook of Medical Imaging: Processing and Analysis. I.N. Bankman. Academic Press, San Diego, 2000.

Cited references

1. Evans RD. *The Atomic Nucleus.* New York: McGraw-Hill; 1955.
2. Phelps ME, Hoffman EJ, Mullani NA, Ter-Pogossian MM. Application of annihilation coincidence detection to transaxial reconstruction tomography. *J Nucl Med.* 1975;16:210–233.
3. Derenzo SE. Precision measurement of annihilation point spread distributions for medically important positron emitters. *Proceedings of the 5th International Conference on Positron Annihilation,* Sendai, Japan, Eds. Hasiguti, RR and Fujiwara, K. The Japan Insitute of Metals, 1979, 819–823.
4. Palmer MR, Brownell GL. Annihilation density distribution calculations for medically important positron emitters. *IEEE Trans Med Imag.* 1992;11:373–378.
5. Levin CS, Hoffman EJ. Calculation of positron range and its effect on the fundamental limit of positron emission tomography system spatial resolution. *Phys Med Biol.* 1999; 44:781–799.
6. Iida H, Kanno I, Miura S, Murakami M, Takahashi K, Uemura K. A simulation study of a method to reduce positron annihilation spread distributions using a strong magnetic field in positron emission tomography. *IEEE Trans Nucl Sci.* 1986;33:597–600.
7. Hammer BE, Christensen NL, Heil BG. Use of a magnetic field to increase the spatial resolution of positron emission tomography. *Med Phy.* 1994;21:1917–1920.
8. Wirrwar A, Vosberg H, Herzog H, Halling H, Weber S, Muller-Gartner HW. 4.5 tesla magnetic field reduces range of high-energy positrons-potential implications for positron emission tomography. *IEEE Trans Nucl Sci.* 1997;44:184–189.
9. Haber SF, Derenzo SE, Uber D. Application of mathematical removal of positron range blurring in positron emission tomography. *IEEE Trans Nucl Sci.* 1990;37:1293–1299.
10. Derenzo SE. Mathematical removal of positron range blurring in high resolution tomography. *IEEE Trans Nucl Sci.* 1986;33:565–569.
11. Knoll GF. *Radiation Detection and Measurement.* 3rd ed. New York: John Wiley & Sons; 2000.
12. Hamamatsu. *Photomultiplier Tube: Principle to Application:* Hamamatsu Photonics K.K.; 1994.
13. Suffert M. Silicon photodiode readout of scintillators and associated electronics. *Nucl Inst Meth.* 1992;A322:523–528.
14. Renker D. Properties of avalanche photodiodes for applications in high energy physics, astrophysics and medical imaging. *Nucl Inst Meth.* 2002;A486:164–169.
15. Casey ME, Nutt R. A multicrystal two dimensional BGO detector system for positron emission tomography. *IEEE Trans Nucl Sci.* 1986;33:460–463.
16. Wong W-H, Uribe J, Hicks K, Hu G. An analog decoding BGO block detector using circular photomultipliers. *IEEE Trans Nucl Sci.* 1995;42:1095–1101.

17. Karp JS, Muehllehner G. Performance of a position-sensitive scintillation detector. *Phys Med Biol* 1985;30:643–655.
18. Freifelder R, Karp JS, Geagan M, Muehllehner G. Design and performance of the HEAD PENN-PET scanner. *IEEE Trans Nucl Sci.* 1994;41:1436–1440.
19. Shao Y, Silverman RW, Cherry SR. Evaluation of Hamamatsu R5900 series PMTs for readout of high-resolution scintillator arrays. *Nucl Inst Meth.* 2000;A454:379–388.
20. Vaquero JJ, Seidel J, Siegel S, Gandler WR, Green MV. Performance characteristics of a compact position-sensitive LSO detector module. *IEEE Trans Med Imag.* 1998;17:967–978.
21. Watanabe M, Omura T, Kyushima H, Hasegawa Y, Yamashita T. A compact position-sensitive detector for PET. *IEEE Trans Nucl Sci.* 1995;42:1090–1094.
22. Cherry SR, Shao Y, Siegel S, et al. Optical fiber readout of scintillator arrays using a multi-channel PMT: a high resolution PET detector for animal imaging. *IEEE Trans Nucl Sci.* 1996;43:1932–1937.
23. Saoudi A, Pepin CM, Dion F, et al. Investigation of depth-of-interaction by pulse shape discrimination in multicrystal detectors read out by avalanche photodiodes. *IEEE Trans Nucl Sci.* 1999;46:462–467.
24. Schmand M, Eriksson L, Casey ME, et al. Performance results of a new DOI detector block for a High Resolution PET-LSO Research Tomograph HRRT. *IEEE Trans Nucl Sci.* 1998;45:3000–3006.
25. Huber JS, Moses WW, Derenzo SE, et al. Characterization of a 64 channel PET detector using photodiodes for crystal identification. *IEEE Trans Nucl Sci.* 1997;44:1197–1201.
26. Huber JS, Moses WW, Andreaco MS, Loope M, Melcher CL, Nutt R. Geometry and surface treatment dependence of the light collection from LSO crystals. *Nucl Inst Meth.* 1999;A437:374–380.
27. Pichler BJ, Boning G, Rafecas M, et al. Feasibility study of a compact high resolution dual layer LSO-APD detector module for positron emission tomography. *Proceedings of the 1998 IEEE Nuclear Science Symposium and Medical Imaging Conference,* 1998; Toronto, ON. IEEE Press, Piscataway NJ, 1998, 1199–1203.
28. Shao Y, Silverman RW, Farrell R, et al. Design studies of a high resolution PET detector using APD arrays. *IEEE Trans Nucl Sci.* 2000;47:1051–1057.
29. Lecomte R, Cadorette J, Rodrigue S, et al. Initial results from the Sherbrooke avalanche photodiode positron tomograph. *IEEE Trans Nucl Sci.* 1996;43:1952–1957.
30. Ziegler SI, Pichler BJ, Boening G, et al. A prototype high-resolution animal positron tomograph with avalanche photodiode arrays and LSO crystals. *Eur J Nucl Med.* 2001;28:136–143.
31. Bateman JE, Connolly JF. A hybrid MWPC gamma ray detecting system for applications in nuclear medicine. *Nucl Inst Meth.* 1978;A156:27–31.
32. Jeavons AP, Chandler RA, Dettmar CAR. A 3D HIDAC-PET camera with sub-millimetre resolution for imaging small animals. *IEEE Trans Nucl Sci.* 1999;46:468–473.
33. Charpak G, Imrie D, Jeanjean J, et al. A new approach to positron emission tomography. *Eur J Nucl Med.* 1989;15:690–693.
34. Duxbury DM, Ott RJ, Flower MA, et al. Preliminary results from the new large-area PETRRA positron camera. *IEEE Trans Nucl Sci.* 1999;46:1050–1054.
35. Marsden PK, Ott RJ, Bateman JE, Cherry SR, Flower MA, Webb S. The performance of a multiwire proportional chamber positron camera for clinical use. *Phys Med Biol.* 1989;34:1043–1062.
36. Townsend D, Frey P, Jeavons A, et al. High density avalanche chamber (HIDAC) positron camera. *J Nucl Med.* 1987;28:1554–1562.
37. Bruyndonckx P, Liu X, Tavernier S, Zhang S. Performance study of a 3D small animal PET scanner based on BaF_2 crystals and a photo sensitive wire chamber. *Nucl Instr Meth.* 1997;A392:407–413.
38. Bohm C, Eriksson L, Bergstrom M, Litton J, Sundman R, Singh M. A computer assisted ring detector positron camera system for reconstruction tomography of the brain. *IEEE Trans Nucl Sci.* 1978;NS-25:624–637.
39. Burgiss SG, Byars LG, Jones WF, Casey ME. High resolution and high speed positron emission tomography data acquisition. *IEEE Trans Nucl Sci.* 1986;33:489–491.
40. Dahlbom M, Reed J, Young J. Implementation of true continuous bed motion in 2-D and 3-D whole-body PET scanning, *IEEE Trans Nucl Sci.* 2001;48:1465–1469.
41. Hoffman EJ, Huang S-C, Plummer D, Phelps ME. Quantitation in positron emission

computed tomography. VI. Effect of nonuniform resolution. *J Comp Assist Tomogr.* 1982;6:987–999.

42. Cherry SR, Dahlbom M, Hoffman EJ. 3D PET using a conventional multislice tomograph without septa. *J Comp Assist Tomogr.* 1991;15:655–668.

43. Townsend DW, Geissbuhler A, Defrise M, et al. Fully 3-dimensional reconstruction for a PET camera with retractable septa. *IEEE Trans Med Imag.* 1991;10:505–512.

44. Andersson JL. A rapid and accurate method to realign PET scans utilizing image edge information. *J Nucl Med.* 1995;36:657–669.

45. Meikle SR, Dahlbom M, Cherry SR. Attenuation correction using count-limited transmission data in positron emission tomography. *J Nucl Med.* 1993;34:143–150.

46. Xu M, Luk WK, Cutler PD, Digby WM. Local threshold for segmented attenuation correction of PET imaging of the thorax. *IEEE Trans Nucl Sci.* 1994;41:1532–1537.

47. Xu M, Cutler PD, Luk WK. Adaptive, segmented attenuation correction for whole-body PET imaging. *IEEE Trans Nucl Sci.* 1996;43:331–336.

48. Meikle SR, Hutton BF, Bailey DL, Hooper PK, Fulham MJ. Accelerated EM reconstruction in total body PET: potential for improving tumor detectability. *Phys Med Biol.* 1994;39:1689–1704.

49. Hudson HM, Larkin RS. Accelerated image reconstruction using ordered subsets of projection data. *IEEE Trans Med Imag.* 1994;13:601–609.

50. Hoffman EJ, Guerrero TM, Germano G, Digby WM, Dahlbom M. PET system calibration and corrections for quantitative and spatially accurate images. *IEEE Trans Nucl Sci.* 1989;36:1108–1112.

51. Defrise M, Townsend DW, Bailey D, Geissbuhler A, Michel C, Jones T. A normalization technique for 3D PET data. *Phys Med Biol.* 1991;36:939–952.

52. Casey ME, Gadagkar H, Newport D. A component based method for normalization in volume PET. *Proceedings of the 1995 International Meeting on Fully Three-Dimensional Image Reconstruction in Radiology and Nuclear Medicine*, Aix-les-Bains, France, 1995, 67–71.

53. Badawi RD, Lodge MA, Marsden PK. Algorithms for calculating detector efficiency normalization coefficients for true coincidences in 3D PET. *Phys Med Biol.* 1998;43:189–205.

54. Badawi RD, Ferreira NC, Kohlmyer SG, Dahlbom M, Marsden PK, Lewellen TK. A comparison of normalization effects on three whole-body cylindrical 3D PET systems. *Phys Med Biol.* 2000;45:3253–3266.

55. Bergstrom M, Litton J, Eriksson L, Bohm C, Blomqvist G. Determination of object contour from projections for attenuation correction in cranial positron emission tomography. *J Comput Assist Tomogr.* 1982;6:365–372.

56. Siegel S, Dahlbom M. Implementation and evaluation of a calculated attenuation correction for PET. *IEEE Trans Nucl Sci.* 1992;39:1117–1121.

57. Huesman R, Derenzo SE, Cahoon JL, et al. Orbiting transmission source for positron tomography. *IEEE Trans Nucl Sci.* 1988;35:735–739.

58. Ranger N, Thompson CJ, Evans AC. The application of a masked orbiting transmission source for attenuation correction in PET. *J Nucl Med.* 1989;30:1056–1058.

59. Carson RE, Daube-Witherspoon ME, Green MV. A method for postinjection PET transmission measurements with a rotating source. *J Nucl Med.* 1988;29:1558–1567.

60. Meikle SR, Bailey DL, Hooper PK, et al. Simultaneous emission and transmission measurements for attenuation correction in whole-body PET. *J Nucl Med.* 1995;36:1680–1688.

61. Thompson CJ, Ranger N, Evans AC, Gjedde A. Validation of simultaneous PET emission and transmission scans. *J Nucl Med.* 1991;32:154–160.

62. deKemp RA, Nahmias C. Attenuation correction in PET using single photon transmission measurement. *Med Phys.* 1994;21:771–778.

63. Karp JS, Muehllehner G, Qu H, Yan XH. Singles transmission in volume-imaging PET with a 137Cs source. *Phys Med Biol.* 1995;40:929–944.

64. Watson CC, Schaefer A, Luk WK, Kirsch CM. Clinical evaluation of single-photon attenuation correction for 3D whole-body PET. *Proceedings of the 1998 IEEE Nuclear Science Symposium and Medical Imaging Conference*, Toronto, ON. IEEE Press, Piscataway NJ, 1998, 1694–1701.

65. Bailey DL, Livieratos L, Jones WF, Jones T. Strategies for accurate attenuation correction with single photon transmission measurements in 3D PET. *Proceedings of the 1997*

IEEE Nuclear Science Symposium and Medical Imaging Conference, Albuquerque, NM. IEEE Press, New York, 1997, 1009–1013.

66. Stearns CW. Scatter correction method for 3D PET using 2D fitted Gaussian functions. *J Nucl Med.* 1995;36:105P.
67. Cherry SR, Huang S-C. Effects of scatter on model parameter estimates in 3D PET studies of the human brain. *IEEE Trans Nucl Sci.* 1995;42:1174–1179.
68. Bergstrom M, Eriksson L, Bohm C, Blomqvist G, Litton J. Correction for scattered radiation in a ring detector positron camera by integral transformation of the projections. *J Comp Assist Tomogr.* 1983;7:42–50.
69. Grootoonk S, Spinks TJ, Sashin D, Spyrou NM, Jones T. Correction for scatter in 3D brain PET using a dual energy window method. *Phys Med Biol.* 1996;41:2757–2774.
70. Watson CC, Newport D, Casey ME, deKemp RA, Beanlands RS, Schmand M. Evaluation of simulation-based scatter correction for 3-D PET cardiac imaging. *IEEE Trans Nucl Sci.* 1997;44:90–97.
71. Ollinger JM. Model-based scatter correction for fully 3D PET. *Phys Med Biol.* 1996; 41:153–176.
72. Holdsworth CH, Levin CS, Farquhar TH, Dahlbom M, Hoffman EJ. Investigation of accelerated Monte Carlo techniques for PET simulation and 3D PET scatter correction. *IEEE Trans Nucl Sci.* 2001;48:74–81.
73. Levin CS, Dahlbom M, Hoffman EJ. A Monte Carlo correction for the effect of Compton scattering in 3-D PET brain imaging. *IEEE Trans Nucl Sci.* 1995;42:1181–1185.
74. Hoffman EJ, Huang S-C, Phelps ME, Kuhl DE. Quantitation in positron emission computed tomography: IV. Effect of accidental coincidences. *J Comput Assist Tomogr.* 1981; 5:391–400.
75. Williams CW, Crabtree MC, Burgiss SG. Design and performance characteristics of a positron emission computed axial tomograph-ECAT-II. *IEEE Trans Nucl Sci.* 1979;26: 619–627.
76. Eriksson L, Wienhard K, Dahlbom M. A simple data loss model for positron camera systems. *IEEE Trans Nucl. Sci* 1994;41:1566–1570.
77. Germano G, Hoffman EJ. Investigation of count rate and dead time characteristics of a high resolution PET system. *J Comp Assist Tomogr.* 1988;12:836–846.
78. Germano G, Hoffman EJ. A study of data loss and mispositioning due to pileup in 2-D detectors in PET. *IEEE Trans Nucl Sci.* 1990;37:671–675.
79. Leahy RM, Clackdoyle R. Computed Tomography. *Handbook of Image and Video Processing.* San Diego: Academic Press; 2000.
80. Kak AC, Slaney M. *Principles of Computerized Tomography.* Society for Industrial and Applied Mathematics; 2001.
81. Bracewell RN. *The Fourier Transform and Its Applications.* 3rd ed. Boston: McGraw-Hill; 2000.
82. Brooks RA, Sank VJ, Talbert AJ, Di Chiro G. Sampling requirements and detector motion for positron emission tomography. *IEEE Trans Nucl Sci.* 1979;26:2760–2763.
83. Daube-Witherspoon ME, Muehllehner G. Treatment of axial data in three-dimensional PET. *J Nucl Med.* 1987;28:1717–1724.
84. Defrise M, Kinahan PE, Townsend DW, Michel C, Sibomana M, Newport DF. Exact and approximate rebinning algorithms for 3-D PET data. *IEEE Trans Med Imag.* 1997;16:145–158.
85. Matej S, Karp JS, Lewitt RM, Becher AJ. Performance of the Fourier rebinning algorithm for PET with large acceptance angles. *Phys Med Biol.* 1998;43:787–795.
86. Kinahan PE, Rogers JG. Analytic 3D image reconstruction using all detected events. *IEEE Trans Nucl Sci.* 1989;36:964–968.
87. Colsher JG. Fully three-dimensional positron emission tomography. *Phys Med Biol.* 1980;25:103–115.
88. Bendriem B, Townsend DW. *The Theory and Practice of 3D PET.* Dordrecht, The Netherlands: Kluwer; 1998.
89. Hutton BF, Hudson HM, Beekman FJ. A clinical perspective of accelerated statistical reconstruction. *Eur J Nucl Med.* 1997;24:797–808.
90. Hudson HM, Larkin RS. Accelerated image reconstruction using ordered subsets of projection data. *IEEE Trans Med Imag.* 1994;13:601–609.

91. Shepp LA, Vardi Y. Maximum likelihood recosntruction for emission tomography. *IEEE Trans Med Imag.* 1982;1:113–122.

92. Lange K, Carson R. EM reconstruction algorithms for emission and transmission tomography. *J Comput Assist Tomogr.* 1984;8:306–316.

93. Hill DLG, Batchelor PG, Holden M, Hawkes DJ. Medical image registration. *Phys Med Biol.* 2001;46:R1–R45.

94. Bacharach SL, Douglas MA, Carson RE, et al. 3-Dimensional registration of cardiac positron emission tomography attenuation scans. *J Nucl Med.* 1993;34:311–321.

95. Hoh CK, Dahlbom M, Harris G, et al. Automated iterative 3-dimensional registration of positron emission tomography images. *J Nucl Med.* 1993;34:2009–2018.

96. Ardekani BA, Braun M, Hutton BF, Kanno I, Iida H. A fully automatic multimodality image registration algorithm. *J Comp Assist Tomogr.* 1995;19:615–623.

97. Woods RP, Mazziotta JC, Cherry SR. MRI-PET registration with automated algorithm. *J Comp Assist Tomogr.* 1993;17:536–546.

98. Minoshima S, Koeppe RA, Frey KA, Kuhl DE. Anatomic standardization—linear scaling and nonlinear warping of functional brain images. *J Nucl Med.* 1994;35:1528–1537.

99. Friston KJ, Frith CD, Liddle PF, Frackowiak RSJ. Plastic Transformation of PET Images. *J Comp Assist Tomogr.* 1991;15:634–639.

100. Andersson JLR, Thurfjell L. Implementation and validation of a fully automatic system for intra- and interindividual registration of PET brain scans. *J Comp Assist Tomogr.* 1997;21:136–144.

101. Friston KJ, Frith CD, Liddle PF, Frackowiak RSJ. Comparing functional (PET) images—the assessment of significant change. *J Cereb Blood Flow Metabol.* 1991;11:690–699.

102. Thurfjell L, Bohm C, Bengtsson E. Surface reconstruction from volume data used for creating an adaptable functional brain atlas. *IEEE Trans Nucl Sci.* 1995;42:1383–1387.

103. Minoshima S, Koeppe RA, Frey KA, Ishihara M, Kuhl DE. Stereotactic PET atlas of the human brain—aid for visual interpretation of functional brain images. *J Nucl Med.* 1994; 35:949–954.

104. Hoffman EJ, Huang S-C, Phelps ME. Quantitation in positron emission computed tomography: I. Effect of object size. *J Comput Assist Tomogr.* 1979;3:299–308.

105. Videen TO, Perlmutter JS, Mintun MA, Raichle ME. Regional correction of positron emission tomography data for the effects of cerebral atrophy. *J Cereb Blood Flow Metab.* 1988;8:662–670.

106. Müller-Gärtner HW, Links JM, Prince JL, et al. Measurement of radiotracer concentration in brain gray matter using positron emission tomography: MRI-based correction for partial volume effects. *J Cereb Blood Flow Metab.* 1992;12:571–583.

107. Meltzer CC, Leal JP, Mayberg HS, Wagner HN, Frost JJ. Correction of PET data for partial volume effects in human cerebral cortex by MR imaging. *J Comp Assist Tomogr.* 1990;14:561–570.

108. Rousset OG, Ma Y, Evans AC. Correction for partial volume effects in PET: principle and validation. *J Nucl Med.* 1998;39:904–911.

109. National Electrical Manufacturers Association. *NEMA Standards Publication NU 2-2001: Performance Measurements of Positron Emission Tomographs.* Rosslyn, VA: National Electrical Manufacturers Association; 2001.

110. National Electrical Manufacturers Association *NEMA Standards Publication NU 2-1994: Performance Measurements of Positron Emission Tomographs.* Washington, DC: National Electrical Manufacturers Association; 1994.

111. Karp JS, Daube-Witherspoon ME, Hoffman EJ, et al. Performance standards in positron emission tomography. *J Nucl Med.* 1991;32:2342–2350.

112. Bailey DL, Jones T, Spinks TJ. A method for measuring the absolute sensitivity of positron emission tomographic scanners. *Eur J Nucl Med.* 1991;18:374–379.

113. Strother SC, Casey ME, Hoffman EJ. Measuring PET scanner sensitivity: relating countrates to image signal-to-noise ratios using noise equivalent counts. *IEEE Trans Nucl Sci.* 1990;37:783–788.

114. Lewellen TK, Kohlmyer SG, Miyaoka RS, Kaplan MS. Investigation of the performance of the General Electric Advance Positron Emission Tomograph in 3D mode. *IEEE Trans Nucl Sci.* 1996;43:2199–2206.

115. Brix G, Zaers J, Adam L-E, et al. Performance evaluation of a whole-body PET scanner using the NEMA protocol. *J Nucl Med.* 1997;38:1614–1623.

116. DeGrado TR, Turkington TG, Williams JJ, Stearns CW, Hoffman JM, Coleman RE. Performance characteristics of a whole-body PET scanner. *J Nucl Med.* 1994;35:1398–1406.

117. Wienhard K, Eriksson L, Grootoonk S, Casey M, Pietrzyk U, Heiss W-D. Performance evaluation of the positron scanner ECAT EXACT. *J Comput Assist Tomogr.* 1992;16: 804–813.

118. Wienhard K, Dahlbom M, Eriksson L, et al. The ECAT EXACT HR: Performance of a new high resolution positron scanner. *J Comp Assist Tomogr.* 1994;18:110–118.

119. Thompson CJ, Yamamoto YL, Meyer E. Positome II: a high efficiency positron imaging system for dynamic brain studies. *IEEE Trans Nucl Sci.* 1979;26:582–586.

120. Knesaurek K. New developments in PET instrumentation: Quo vadis PET? *J Nucl Med.* 2001;42:1831–1832.

121. Townsend DW, Wensveen M, Byars LG, et al. A rotating PET scanner using BGO block detectors—Design, performance and applications. *J Nucl Med.* 1993;34:1367–1376.

122. Smith RJ, Adam LE, Karp JS. Methods to optimize whole body surveys with the C-PET camera. *Proceedings of the 1999 IEEE Nuclear Science Symposium and Medical Imaging Conference*, Seattle, WA. IEEE, Piscataway, NJ, 1999, 1197–1201.

123. Anger HO, Rosenthal DJ. Scintillation camera and positron camera. In: *Medical Radioisotope Scanning.* Vienna, Austria: IAEA, 1959, 163–168.

124. Nellemann P, Hines H, Braymer W, Muehllehner G, Geagan M. Performance characteristics of a dual head SPECT scanner with PET capability. *Proceedings of the 1995 IEEE Nuclear Science Symposium and Medical Imaging Conference*, San Francisco, CA. IEEE, Piscataway, NJ, 1999, 1197–1201.

125. Schmand M, Eriksson L, Casey ME, Wienhard K, Flugge G, Nutt R. Advantages using pulse shape discrimination to assign the depth of interaction information (DOI) from a multi layer phoswich detector. *IEEE Trans Nucl Sci.* 1999;46:985–990.

126. Spinks TJ, Jones T, Bloomfield PM, et al. Physical characteristics of the ECAT EXACT3D positron tomograph. *Phys Med Biol.* 2000;45:2601–2618.

127. Wienhard K, Schmand M, Casey ME, et al. The ECAT HRRT: Performance and first clinical application of the new high resolution research tomograph. *IEEE Trans Nucl Sci.* 2002;49:104–110.

128. Surti S, Karp JS, Freifelder R, Liu F. Optimizing the performance of a PET detector using discrete GSO crystals on a continuous lightguide. *IEEE Trans Nucl Sci.* 2000;47:1030–1036.

129. Moses WW, Virador PRG, Derenzo SE, Huesman RH, Budinger TF. Design of a high-resolution, high-sensitivity PET camera for human brains and small animals. *IEEE Trans Nucl Sci.* 1997;44:1487–1491.

130. Uribe J, Baghaei H, Li HD, et al. Basic imaging performance characteristics of a variable field of view PET camera using quadrant sharing detector design. *IEEE Trans Nucl Sci.* 1999;46:491–497.

131. Flanagan FL, Dehdashti F, Siegel BA. PET in breast cancer. *Semin Nucl Med.* 1998;28: 290–302.

132. Raylman RR, Majewski S, Wojcik R, et al. The potential role of positron emission mammography for detection of breast cancer. A phantom study. *Med Phys.* 2000;27:1943–1954.

133. Thompson CJ, Murthy K, Picard Y, Weinberg IN, Mako R. Positron emission mammography (PEM)—a promising technique for detecting breast cancer. *IEEE Trans Nucl Sci.* 1995;42:1012–1017.

134. Murthy K, Aznar M, Thompson CJ, Loutfi A, Lisbona R, Gagnon JH. Results of preliminary clinical trials of the positron emission mammography system PEM-I: A dedicated breast imaging system producing glucose metabolic images using FDG. *J Nucl Med.* 2000;41:1851–1858.

135. Townsend DW, Cherry SR. Combining anatomy and function: the path to true image fusion. *Eur Radiol.* 2001;11:1968–1974.

136. Beyer T, Townsend DW, Brun T, et al. A combined PET/CT scanner for clinical oncology. *J Nucl Med.* 2000;41:1369–1379.

137. Kluetz PG, Meltzer CC, Villemagne MD, et al. Combined PET/CT imaging in oncology: impact on patient management. *Clin Pos Imag.* 2001;3:223–230.

138. Patton JA, Delbeke D, Sandler MP. Image fusion using an integrated, dual-head coincidence camera with x-ray tube-based attenuation maps. *J Nucl Med.* 2000;41:1364–1368.
139. Shao Y, Cherry SR, Farahani K, et al. Development of a PET detector system compatible with MRI/NMR systems. *IEEE Trans Nucl Sci.* 1997;44:1167–1171.
140. Cherry SR, Gambhir SS. Use of positron emission tomography in animal research. *ILAR J.* 2001;42:219–232.
141. Watanabe M, Okada H, Shimizu K, et al. A high resolution animal PET scanner using compact PS-PMT detectors. *IEEE Trans Nucl Sci.* 1997;47:1277–1282.
142. Bloomfield PM, Rajeswaran S, Spinks TJ, et al. The design and physical characteristics of a small animal positron emission tomograph. *Phys Med Biol.* 1995;40:1105–1126.
143. Seidel J, Vaquero JJ, Barbosa F, Lee IJ, Cuevas C, Green MV. Scintillator identification and performance characteristics of LSO and GSO PSPMT detector modules combined through common X and Y resistive dividers. *IEEE Trans Nucl Sci.* 2000;47:1640–1645.
144. Del Guerra A, Di Domenico G, Scandola M, Zavattini G. YAP-PET: a small animal positron emission tomograph based on YAP:Ce finger crystals. *Proceedings of the 1997 IEEE Nuclear Science Symposium and Medical Imaging Conference*, Albuquerque, NM. IEEE, New York, 1997, 1640–1643.
145. Weber S, Terstegge A, Herzog H, et al. The design of an animal PET: flexible geometry for achieving optimal spatial resolution or high sensitivity. *IEEE Trans Med Imag.* 1997; 16:684–689.
146. Cherry SR, Shao Y, Silverman RW, et al. MicroPET: a high resolution PET scanner for imaging small animals. *IEEE Trans Nucl Sci.* 1997;44:1161–1166.
147. Chatziioannou AF, Cherry SR, Shao Y, et al. Performance evaluation of microPET: a high-resolution lutetium oxyorthosilicate PET scanner for animal imaging. *J Nucl Med.* 1999;40:1164–1175.
148. Qi J, Leahy RM, Cherry SR, Chatziioannou A, Farquhar TH. High-resolution 3D Bayesian image reconstruction using the microPET small-animal scanner. *Phys Med Biol.* 1998;43:1001–1013.
149. Tai Y-C, Chatziioannou A, Siegel S, et al. Performance evaluation of the microPET P4: a PET system dedicated to animal imaging. *Phys Med Biol.* 2001;46:1845–1862.
150. Knoess C, Siegel S, Smith A, et al. Performance evaluation of the microPET R4 PET scanner for rodents. *Eur J Nucl Med.* 2003;30:734–747.
151. Tai YC, Chatziioannou AF, Yang Y et al. MicroPET II: design, development and initial performance of an improved microPET scanner for small-animal imaging. Phys Med Biol. 2003;48:1519–1537.
152. Correia JA, Burnham CA, Kaufman D, Fischman AJ. Development of a small animal PET imaging device with resolution approaching 1 mm. *IEEE Trans Nucl Imag.* 1999;46: 631–635.
153. Miyaoka RS, Kohlmyer SG, Lewellen TK. Performance characteristics of micro crystal element (MiCE) detectors. *IEEE Trans Nucl Sci.* 2001;48:1403–1407.
154. Goertzen AL, Meadors AK, Silverman RW, Cherry SR. Simultaneous molecular and anatomical imaging of the mouse in vivo. *Phys Med Biol.* 2002;47:4315–4328.

CHAPTER 2

Quantitative Assay Development for PET

Sanjiv Sam Gambhir

Positron emission tomography (PET) is a novel imaging tool that permits non-invasive visualization of molecular (biochemical) and biological events in a living subject. Due to its highly unique capabilities, it permits the development of quantitative assays that are currently not possible using most other approaches. *For the purposes of this chapter, the process of developing a PET assay is defined as the collection of approaches for the quantitative estimation of a specific molecular (biochemical) and/or biological process in a living subject.* The approaches are a toolbox of sorts that helps to integrate the data obtained from PET so that quantitative information about the process can be extracted from the data. The process of interest may be the expression of a specific gene, upregulation of a specific cell protein, concentration of receptors on the cell surface, decrease in regional perfusion, increase in glucose utilization, decrease in oxygen consumption, or a whole host of other possible events. The goal of a PET assay is to accurately quantitate one or more of the processes just mentioned through the use of novel positron-labeled probes (tracers) as well as appropriate image acquisition, data analysis, and data modeling methodology.

The individual(s) developing a PET assay must closely interact with all the subdisciplines of PET. In fact, the position taken in this chapter will be that the assay developer must guide staff in all of the other subdisciplines (Figure 2-1). This direct interaction with other PET subspecialists is needed to: 1) understand the biological process to be examined; 2) develop and refine the relevant tracer(s), appropriate utilization of PET equipment, and data acquisition/reconstruction methodology; 3) perform appropriate image analysis, quantitation, modeling, and statistical analysis; and 4) help to interpret the results and their potential limitation(s). In many ways, the assay developer needs to be the most informed about all the issues surrounding the use of PET because development of an assay truly requires integration of all the subdisciplines of PET technology.

In this chapter, the building blocks of assay development are first presented followed by details of quantitation of PET data with a focus on compartmental modeling. Approaches to fit PET data to models are described. Specific assays for measuring molecular and biological processes are also provided. These in-

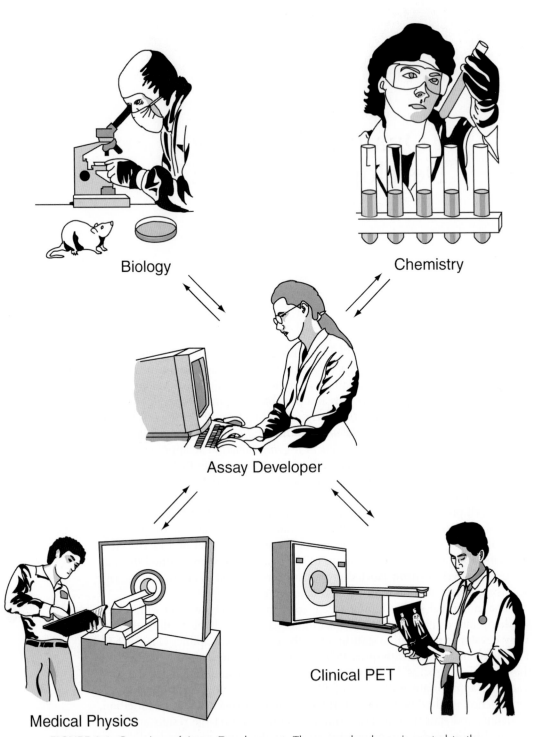

FIGURE 2-1. Overview of Assay Development. The assay developer is central to the process of validating and implementing the use of a tracer for a particular PET application. The assay developer must: (A) work with the biologist to understand the underlying molecular and/or biological process of interest; (B) be able to help utilize the biological information to help the chemists design the proper tracer(s); (C) work with the medical physicists to help properly acquire and quantitate PET data; (D) help clinicians and scientists to properly interpret the PET images and data. This central role for the assay developer helps him or her to refine the development of a specific assay.

clude assays for estimating the following: 1) glucose utilization with 2-deoxy-2-[F-18]fluoro-D-glucose (FDG), 2) regional blood flow with ^{13}N ammonia, and 3) reporter gene expression with various tracers. Key questions with solutions are provided throughout the chapter to help integrate all of the diverse information. The goal is not to provide a comprehensive discussion of all models but rather to teach the principles of modeling biological processes for development of assays appropriate for PET.

PET INSTRUMENTATION AND ASSAY DEVELOPMENT

To develop an assay for any type of experiment, one must have a good understanding of the basic principles and limitations for the instrument(s) used to acquire data for the assay under development. Details of PET instrumentation are provided in Chapter 1, but some specific issues for assay development are briefly reviewed in this section. The PET scanner can be thought of as an instrument that can *estimate* the concentration (C_0) of an administered tracer in a given location as a function of time (Equation 2-1).

$$C_o(i_x i_y i_z i_t) = \int_{i_x \Delta x}^{(i_x+1)\Delta x} \int_{i_y \Delta y}^{(i_y+1)\Delta y} \int_{i_z \Delta z}^{(i_z+1)\Delta z} \int_{t_i}^{t_{i+1}} C(x,y,z,t)dx\,dy\,dz\,dt \quad (2\text{-}1)$$

Note the noise free PET measurement is related to C_0 through a 3-D convolution process that accounts for intrinsic scanner resolution and reconstruction method. Statistical issues usually govern the smallest amount of time ($\Delta t_i = t_{i+1} - t_i$) that can be used to obtain a good image. Typically, at least several seconds to minutes are required. This issue is directly related to the temporal resolution of PET and affects the type of assays that are possible. If the scanner is used to take multiple images of the same object over time (often referred to as dynamic imaging), then one has estimates of C_o for several time intervals (Δt_i) which may or may not be continuous and uniform. It is important to keep in mind that the underlying distribution $C(x,y,z,t)$ is not directly measured; instead, space and time integrals of this distribution are estimated by the scanner.

It should also be made clear that due to the spatial resolution limits of PET (approximately 1–10 mm^3) depending on the exact type of scanner, specific isotope used (each with its own half-life and positron range), counting statistics, and reconstruction algorithm, that C is only obtainable within a finite resolution element (Δx, Δy, Δz). The absolute limit for C depends on the limit of instrument resolution (assuming infinite counting statistics). For example, if the instrument resolution is 1 mm $\times$ 1 mm $\times$ 4 mm (4 mm^3); then, *at best*, C_0 is only obtainable for a 4-mm^3 volume. In fact, if C is spatially heterogeneous within the spatial resolution limit, then there is no way to determine that spatial variance from the reconstructed image. This implies that if many cells (typically millions) are contained within that volume, then there is no way to distinguish potential differences in tracer accumulation between those cells.

Another complicating physical factor for the development of a PET assay is that the resolution limits cause activity within a given region to be underestimated (partial volume effect) and activity from nearby regions to contaminate the area of interest (spillover effect). These issues are discussed in detail in Chapter 1. From an assay development point of view, these two issues must be carefully accounted for to accurately estimate the parameter(s) of interest. It is not that useful information cannot be obtained for small objects but rather that the absolute tracer concentration will be underestimated. If the size of the object of interest is approximately twice the image resolution full-width-at-half-maximum (FWHM), then the partial volume effect is negligible.[1,2] The assay developer must consider the in-plane and axial plane resolution to see if a partial volume effect may apply for each. Several strategies can be used to deal with the partial volume and spillover effects. For a partial volume, if the size of the target object is known (e.g., from anatomical imaging), then a correction factor (called a recovery coefficient) can be used to correct for the amount of underestimation of activity.[1-3] It is also possible in some cases to use the PET images directly to estimate the size of the target object and then to correct using the appropriate recovery coefficient.[4] Care should be taken to validate the recovery coefficients using a phantom with different size objects filled with tracer, then scanned and reconstructed in the same way as data from the target subject of interest. Spillover is much more difficult to directly account for when quantitating PET data. All surrounding objects with activity (both in- and out-of-plane) have the potential to add to the true activity values in the object of interest. One of the most successful methods in dealing with spillover is to treat it as a physical parameter to estimate as part of a tracer kinetic model.[4] Attenuation, scatter, decay correction, and deadtime must also be carefully accounted for and are discussed in Chapter 1.

Regions of interest (ROIs) typically drawn on an image are used to average data from the voxels contained within the ROI—equivalent to integrating $C_0(x,y,z)$ over space. The ROI typically contains spillover information from neighboring tissues and underlying blood vessels. This information becomes important in later sections as data obtained from the ROI is modeled because it potentially represents the tracer in several locations, as well as in different chemical forms (due to metabolism of the tracer). Prior to attempting to quantitate PET data, it is important to visualize the process of tracer movement and modification, described in the next section.

EXAMPLE 2-1

The use of a particular assay will require the injection of two tracers (labeled with two different positron-emitting isotopes) and the concentration of each tracer in tissue regions needs to be estimated. Is this type of assay possible using PET?

ANSWER

This assay is possible as long as both tracers do not need to be injected simultaneously for a given assay. Because both positron emitters will eventually lead to two 511-keV gamma rays (even if two distinct isotopes are used), the PET camera cannot separate the signal from each tracer. However, if the underlying assay allows, one can inject one tracer, estimate its concentration with PET, let it almost completely decay, and then inject the second tracer and estimate its concentration. In some cases, it may also be possible to extract the concentration of the two tracers with simultaneous injection if the half-lives of the two isotopes are sufficiently different and noise levels are not prohibitive to allow mathematical separation.

TRACER THOUGHT EXPERIMENT

For purposes of this chapter, the PET tracer is defined as a molecule labeled with a positron-emitting isotope that is injected or otherwise introduced into a living subject in nonpharmacological (trace) doses. Trace doses are those that usually lead to no more than 10% target occupancy or no more than 10% of the competitive substrate concentration. Further issues surrounding the exact choice of tracer are described in Chapter 4 and in Desirable Properties of Molecular Imaging Probes (p. 158). It is often useful to begin the process of assay development by conducting a virtual experiment in which the investigator pretends to become the tracer. This activity forces one to think about all the regions where a given tracer can distribute and the mechanisms of tracer movement between the various areas. Furthermore, this thought experiment also allows one to better understand what chemical modifications occur to the tracer (if any), what other molecules play a role in that modification, and what other molecules may compete for various processes.

For example, if the assay developer pretends to be molecules of a well-understood tracer such as deoxyglucose labeled with Fluorine-18 (FDG), he or she can experience this tracer thought experiment in detail. FDG, an analog of glucose, has been used extensively to assay for glucose utilization in various tissues. Further details of FDG can be found in FDG Assay (p. 161) and in Chapter 4. The injection route of most tracers such as FDG is intravenous, but some tracers can be delivered through inhalation or other approaches. From the time the assay developer (as labeled molecules) is injected into the intravenous blood pool, he or she has several possibilities: remain in plasma, enter into the circulating blood cells (e.g., white and red blood cells), and/or be bound to plasma proteins. He or she can move between all of these components while flow is occurring within the blood vessel to be pushed through the circulatory system. If in the plasma, he or she can leave the blood vessel by potentially moving into the interstitial space (the space between cells). From the interstitial space, specific cells present in tissues can be entered or return to plasma. In the case of FDG, movement between most blood vessels and the interstitial space and into cells is via facilitated transport. Once inside these cells, he or she can be metabolized by specific enzymes or leave the cell to return to the interstitial space. In the case of FDG, he or she can be phosphorylated (metabolized) by hexokinase type II. When in the phosphorylated form, leaving the cell is not easy (because of being negatively charged). He or she can potentially be dephosphorylated through various intracellular phosphatase enzymes, but this reaction is very slow for FDG-6-P. Thought must be focused on special restrictions. For example, for FDG, as molecules once he or she enters the renal system and is secreted into renal tubules he or she cannot be reabsorbed because FDG (unlike glucose) is not a substrate for active transport (reuptake) in the renal system. FDG will enter the ureters and then the bladder and is then eliminated through urination. Also, for FDG, transport across the blood-brain-barrier is possible because of the presence of glucose transporters, which is not the case for many tracers that have restricted transport across this barrier.

For all of these processes above, we must keep in mind what mechanism(s) transport molecules from one region to another. For example, what carrier(s) if any takes the molecules from the vascular or the interstitial space to the intracellular present space? Please keep in mind that these tracer molecules are not the only molecules present on the journey through the body. For example, when transported or phosphorylated by hexokinase type II, he or she (as FDG) will see that glucose is competing for transporter sites or phosphorylation by hexokinase. Also keep in mind that physiological conditions (e.g., blood flow) can limit the ability to reach certain sites within the body.

This simple thought experiment illustrates the complexity of modeling the journey of a tracer and is very important to perform for each new tracer studied. Often, much is known about the parent molecule (e.g., glucose) of whom the tracer (FDG) is a relative. An assay developer can, therefore, start by doing a thought experiment for the parent molecule. After performing the thought experiment, one can determine what type of quantitation (if any) is needed for a given assay. It may be important to determine the rate of phosphorylation of FDG, or it may be sufficient for a given application for one to know the concentration of FDG and FDG-6-P in a given location. Issues centered on quantitation approaches are discussed in the next section.

QUANTITATION OF PET DATA

A reasonable question to ask in the development of an assay is if *any* quantitation is really needed. Never assume that quantitation and assay development are a necessary part of all PET imaging studies.[5,6] In some applications the PET image alone may be sufficient [e.g., a brain scan with FDG to evaluate for a distinct hypometabolic pattern found in Alzheimer's dementia (see Chapter 7). Ideally, qualitative applications of a tracer should occur after quantitative studies are performed so that the behavior of the tracer is well characterized and used within this knowledge base. Qualitative approaches are often used for practical reasons (e.g., high-throughput routine clinical applications).

Most of this chapter focuses on applications in which some level of quantitation is desired for the development of the assay. In the next section, the chapter begins with semiquantitative approaches and then progresses to more rigorous tracer kinetic modeling approaches.

It is sometimes the case that estimating the concentration of tracer is sufficient, and, therefore, a full kinetic analysis of tracer is not needed. Additionally, sufficient information regarding the tracer may not be present for the proper formulation of a tracer kinetic model. Often assays are initially developed using semiquantitative measures and then eventually refined with full tracer kinetic analysis. The simplest semiquantitation approach is to estimate the concentration of tracer in a given region from the PET images by using an ROI analysis. This approach may be sufficient or one may need to proceed further.

One can calculate the concentration of tracer in a given ROI relative to another ROI (e.g., in the striatum of the brain relative to the cerebellum). This ratio approach is particularly attractive because both the numerator and denominator have calibration factors which cancel out so all one needs to do is draw ROIs.

The percent injected dose per gram of tissue (%ID/g tissue) can also be a useful parameter and is calculated by using Equation 2-2. The %ID/g tissue is the percent of the injected dose of activity that is in a gram of tissue being analyzed:

$$\%ID/g = C_T \cdot \frac{V_T}{W_T} \cdot \frac{1}{D_{Inj}} \cdot 100\% \qquad (2\text{-}2)$$

C_T is the radioactivity in the tissue region with the unit of mCi/cc tissue; it is obtained from the PET images by taking the counts/pixel/time from a PET ROI and converting to mCi/cc tissue using a cylinder calibration factor. W_T and V_T are the weight and volume, respectively, and their ratio produces the density of that region. D_{Inj} is the dose injected with the unit of mCi. The density of tissue is often assumed to be ~1 cc tissue/g tissue. The %ID/g tissue is a way of normalizing the signal imaged at a given location for the amount of tracer injected into the subject. It can range from zero to a value that can exceed 100% if a large fraction of the injected dose accumulates into a site with a mass less than 1 g. The %ID/g tissue can be inaccurate if all of the injected dose is not available to the entire area of the subject (e.g., due to tracer extravasation into tissue at the site of injection). The %ID/g tissue as well as most other approaches just mentioned does not directly account for the mass of the subject or competition of extraction of tracer from various tissue sites relative to the target tissue site. The %ID/g is a relatively crude normalization approach, but it is easy to calculate making it one of the more common approaches used.

The standardized uptake value (SUV) is quite often used as a semiquantitative measure of describing PET data and is given as Equation 2-3. It is related to %ID/g tissue but also normalizes for the mass or surface area of the subject.[7–9] Variations that occur with the use of SUV have been described in the literature.[7,10] The SUV can also be subject to: 1) error if not all of the injected dose is available to the circulation due to extravasation of tracer, or 2) the same variability as %ID/g tissue, except for the mass of the patient. W_s is the weight of the subject in the unit of g:

$$SUV = C_T \cdot \frac{V_T}{W_T} \cdot \frac{1}{D_{Inj}} \cdot W_S \qquad (2\text{-}3)$$

$$= \%ID/g\ tissue \cdot W_S \div 100$$

EXAMPLE 2-2
A patient weighing 70 kg is given 15 mCi of a tracer via a vein in the hand. Approximately 1 hour later, a PET image is obtained to image the liver region. This decay-corrected image shows a 3 cm × 3 cm × 2 cm region of increased radioactivity. A ROI drawn on this area of increased radioactivity shows 0.0005 mCi/cc tissue (after converting counts/pixel/sec to mCi/cc based on a cylinder calibration factor). The image resolution (FWHM) is 8 mm in each dimension. What is the %ID/g tissue and the SUV for this region of increased activity?

ANSWER
Because the size of the area of increased activity is larger than twice the image resolution (0.8 × 2 = 1.6 cm) in each dimension, there is no

need for partial volume correction (e.g., the recovery coefficient (RC) = 1 × 1 × 1 = 1). See Chapter 1 for more details on the recovery coefficient.

%ID/g tissue = ((0.0005 mCi/cc × 1cc/g)/(15 mCi)) × 100
= 0.0033 %ID/g

SUV = (0.0005 mCi/cc × 1cc/g) × (1/(15 mCi)) × (70,000 g)
= 2.33 (a unitless parameter)

TRACER KINETIC MODELING OF PET DATA

All of the previously mentioned approaches are considered semiquantitative because they do not *directly* model and take into account variations from different processes of tracer delivery, uptake, trapping, competition with other molecules, and routes of clearance. Formal tracer kinetic modeling of a PET tracer can be used to develop more theoretically rigorous assays. Tracer kinetic modeling has its roots in pharmacokinetics; therefore, a brief review of pharmacokinetics is provided:

Pharmacokinetics is a relatively old and large field of study that arose out of the need to predict the concentration of drugs in blood and tissues.[11,12] Much of pharmacology has been driven by the need to arrive at optimal drug dosing, frequency of dosing, and drug concentration safety windows. Pharmacologists through sampling the blood concentrations of a drug have therefore developed methods to make predictions based on blood time-activity curves.[11] Fitting of pharmacokinetic data is usually performed with a variety of model assumptions. The goals are not to find a correct model but one that accurately predicts drug concentrations under new exposure conditions or in another experimental subject. These approaches have limited capability to determine the dose of the drug delivered to the target in tissue. PET provides the unique opportunity to make available not only the blood time-activity data but also regional tissue time-activity data. These data allow a dramatic improvement in performing pharmacokinetics. One key difference is that in PET experiments, very low nonpharmacological doses of the tracer are introduced into the subject. Therefore, pharmacokinetic models when used with trace levels of drug or tracer are referred to as tracer kinetic models. Tracer kinetic modeling, however, borrows a lot of tools from pharmacokinetic modeling and is described in detail next. Of course, these two modeling environments merge when the mass of the tracer is intentionally increased to provide kinetic assays under pharmacological conditions.

Tracer kinetic models can be classified as noncompartmental,[13–15] compartmental,[15–17] or distributive.[18,19] The noncompartmental approaches tend to be the simplest, the compartmental models are intermediate in complexity, and the distributive models are the most complex. For most PET analysis, compartmental models have become the model of choice, primarily because they are simpler to implement and often provide adequate parameter estimates. Compartmental models also tend to match how we see the problems to be studied; that is, compartments for blood, tissue, a biochemical reaction, a ligand-receptor interaction, expression of mRNA, and so on, with transport or reactions of tracers between compartments. Before discussing compartmental models further, the other two approaches are briefly reviewed.

Noncompartmental modeling

Noncompartmental approaches do not require the explicit knowledge of the various locations or metabolites of a tracer of interest. These approaches are also referred to as model-independent approaches or statistical moment analysis. The entire body or system of interest is viewed as one large black-box into which tracer is injected and must eventually leave (Figure 2-2). The fundamental principles that govern these approaches are: (1) conservation of matter, (2) assumption of steady state for all parameters of interest (e.g., flux of substrates across membranes, blood flow, concentration of molecular constituents of cells, and so on), (3) linearity with regards to the input. The latter means if two inputs are applied separately and produce two outputs, then if both inputs are simultaneously provided, the output is a linear combination of the two individual outputs. The noncompartmental approaches can be useful as starting tools for predicting general tracer concentrations in tissues or other parameters of interest. Quite often, useful parameters can be extracted from the area under the

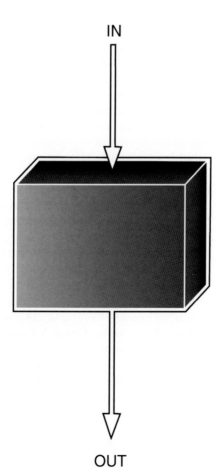

IN

FIGURE 2-2. Noncompartmental Modeling. In this approach, no assumptions are made about the underlying structure of the model. The tracer is introduced into the body (IN) which is treated as a black box, and tracer eventually leaves the body (OUT).

OUT

plasma concentration versus time curve. For example, the clearance of tracer from the body is the ratio of the dose to the area under the plasma concentration versus time curve. Further details of the noncompartmental approaches are covered elsewhere.[15] A specific example of using a noncompartmental approach for radiolabeled anti-cancer drugs has been published by Meikle et al.[20]

The *central volume principle* is a critical noncompartmental concept and helps to relate the mean transit time (τ) to blood flow (F) and the system volume (V). Consider a rigid tube with volume V in which a fluid flows with flow rate F. If a small amount of tracer is introduced at some point A at time zero into the tube, then the tracer will eventually be detected at some point B further along the tube. Not all of the tracer will arrive at point B at the same time. Instead, the arrival time will spread out because of different path lengths and velocities for each individual tracer molecule. If the flow in the rigid tube is reduced, the tracer time-concentration curve at point B will be further spread out. If one defines the mean transit time (τ) as the average time taken by all the tracer molecules to go from point A to B, then it can be shown that $\tau = V/F$.[21] This simple experiment is a good example of a tracer experiment and does not involve formal compartmental modeling. It also illustrates why the term kinetics is often linked with the use of a tracer.

Distributive modeling

Distributed models use capillary beds to model concentration of tracer in the blood and in the extravascular (regions excluding the vasculature) spaces.[18,19] Partial differential equations are used to model the tracer kinetics, and concentration of tracer along a capillary bed are explicitly modeled. This contrasts with compartmental models which do not model concentration gradients within the blood and use simpler differential equations to describe the kinetics of tracers. These models can be useful in various applications, but for PET data, compartmental models are more convenient and more widely used. For examples of PET distributive modeling please see the article by Bassingthwaighte and Holloway.[22]

Compartmental modeling overview

Compartmental models attempt to describe the kinetics of an underlying process through the use of interconnected pools of a tracer in a particular form or space. For example, a pool can represent the location of a tracer in blood or can represent an enzyme-mediated reaction to yield metabolites of the tracer no matter where their physical location is. The reader should not confuse the use of the term pool with a specific location. A pool is a mathematical abstraction which represents a particular form or location of tracer that behaves in a k*inetically equivalent manner*. Compartmental models are usually drawn as boxes that are connected by arrows (Figure 2-3), which represent the movement of tracer between compartments.

The interconnections that govern the movement of tracer between pools can be linear or nonlinear. Linear interconnections are often constant values which can vary from tissue region to region but are not dependent on tracer mass or time. Although most physiological and biochemical processes are nonlinear, as far as tracers are concerned they often behave linearly (or approximately linearly) with regards to transport or chemical reactions.[23] This behavior is primarily due to the fact that the mass of tracer is typically much less than its natural counterpart (see

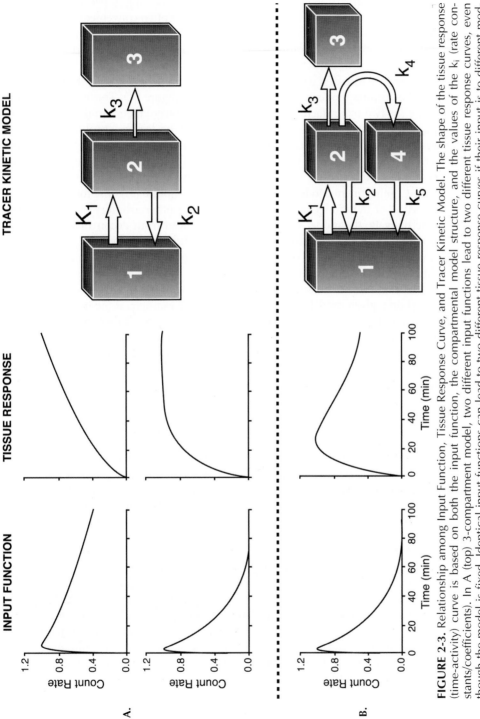

FIGURE 2-3. Relationship among Input Function, Tissue Response Curve, and Tracer Kinetic Model. The shape of the tissue response (time-activity) curve is based on both the input function, the compartmental model structure, and the values of the k_i (rate constants/coefficients). In A (top) 3-compartment model, two different input functions lead to two different tissue response curves, even though the model is fixed. Identical input functions can lead to two different tissue response curves if their input is to different models. This is illustrated by the 4-compartment model (B) compared to the 3-compartment model (A) with the same input function. Given a tissue curve alone, one would not be able to determine the structure of the compartmental model. The input function must also be known. Notice that in A, the tissue response is the sum of compartments 2 and 3, whereas in B (bottom), it is the sum of compartments 2, 3, and 4.

Appendix for this chapter). The fundamental property that governs a complete tracer kinetic model is mass balance, which means that the rate of change of mass for a given compartment must equal the net mass coming in per unit time into a pool minus the net mass leaving per unit time. It is often convenient to write equations that govern a particular compartment in terms of mass balance (instead of concentrations). These complete sets of equations are often referred to as *state equations*.

The structure of a particular compartment model along with the input function determines the tissue response as shown in Figure 2-3. This is important because the two major factors that determine the tracer kinetics in tissue are the input function and model structure. Both must be known to obtain the tissue response. In all cases, the tissue response is obtained by convolving the input function with the solution to the model equations for a unit impulse input function. If a true impulse is used, then the tissue response is just the impulse response (see One-Compartment Model, p. 147). The model impulse response function is characteristic of the model and can be used to scale other arbitrary input functions. Alternatively, the model structure can be deduced from deconvolving the input function from the measured tissue time-activity curve. This may not lead to a unique model, but it can identify the number of compartments under ideal conditions of no noise. As one gains experience in building and fitting tracer kinetic models, it becomes possible to predict the shape of the tissue time-activity curve based on a given model and input function. For example, if the model has effective trapping of the tracer (a compartment exists in which there is tracer moving in but little to no tracer leaving), then the tissue time-activity curve should be increasing as long as the input function remains nonzero. For more complex models [e.g., intermediate compartment(s) between the input and tissue compartment], the tissue activity can decrease for a time and then also increase.

EXAMPLE 2-3

Two patients are given the exact same dose of PET tracer delivered via an infusion pump over 15 seconds into a vein in the hand. The measured arterial input function is different between the two patients. However, the tissue curve is almost identical between the two patients. How is this possible if the same tracer kinetic model can be used for each patient?

ANSWER

The reason that the measured input function can be different between the two patients is that the factors effecting extraction of tracer from the blood (e.g., renal extraction) can be very different even though the same bolus is given. The reason the tissue curve can be the same even though the input function is different is that the underlying model parameters (e.g., rate constants) for the two patients can be quite different, leading to the same tissue response curve even in the presence of distinct input functions.

The process of tracer kinetic modeling is iterative (Figure 2-4) and requires constant revision based on new experimental evidence. The modeling process

FIGURE 2-4. Tracer Kinetic Modeling Overview. The use of compartmental models for developing a PET assay is a step-by-step process that begins with characterizing the goals of the assay. First, goals must be defined (e.g., what underlying biochemical parameter needs to be estimated). Then, a good understanding of the underlying biochemistry and biology involved must be undertaken. After this, potential tracers can be selected that may help to study the underlying process. Next, a comprehensive model is developed using the tracer thought experiment (see Tracer Thought Experiment, p. 129). This comprehensive model must then be reduced to a workable model with a limited number of compartments. As the model is then simulated and used to fit PET data, one must biochemically validate the model itself. Finally, the model is ready to be applied for estimation of parameters of interest. Usually, analysis of real data reveals limitations, and the process can be refined by starting over and selecting a better model and/or a better tracer.

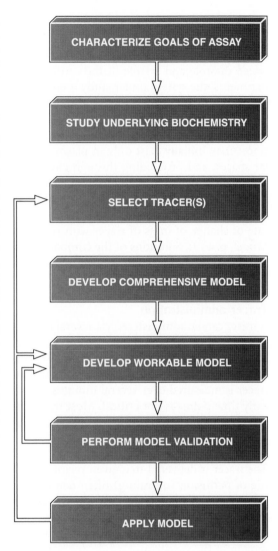

also usually helps to guide future experimentation. Each step in the process involves coordination between different groups of the PET team (Figure 2-1) and should truly be a team effort.

In general, tracer kinetic models cannot be developed from tracer kinetic measurements alone. Biochemical and physiological measurements and a priori knowledge must be utilized to determine the model structure. Kinetic measurements then can determine whether the biochemically and physiological structure of the model is valid. In addition, once an accurate compartment model has been validated, then tracer kinetic measurements can provide very accurate estimates of the biochemical and/or physiological parameters.

Steady state issues

In most tracer experiments, the goal is to study the underlying molecular (biochemical)/physiological process under conditions of approximate steady state.

The definition of approximate steady state is that the rate of change of a specific process with respect to time is negligible or zero. In reality, no biological process is ever under true steady state (e.g., blood flow is not constant but changing between diastole and systole in the cardiac cycle). However, for most tracer experiments, the system under study is effectively in steady state and one attempts not to perturb a steady state. One should also keep in mind that although the process to study is in effective steady state, it is usually important to model the tracer during the time in which the *tracer* is *not* in steady state. For example, a tracer may initially exist only in plasma, moving into the interstitial and cellular spaces, and proceeding through chemical reactions. The changing concentrations within these different regions represent the kinetics by which tracer kinetic assays are performed. The differential equations that govern the mass (or concentration) of tracer in tissue in fact reflect this because they start with the rate of change of mass of tracer with respect to time (see Three-Compartment Model, p. 149). Solutions of the compartmental model at the steady state of the tracer can easily be obtained even if the general time-varying solution is not known.

Tracer administration

A tracer can be administered via several routes (e.g., intravenous, inhalation, and so on), but by far, most PET tracers are introduced intravenously with an administration time of several seconds. The exact rate of administration for a tracer is usually not important because for many models the blood concentration of tracer is measured over several minutes, and the lack of true equilibrium in the early time points is not critical. Most tracers are evenly distributed in the blood pool within a few minutes after intravenous injection.

Perfusion and flow

The tracer is delivered to a given region of tissue as determined by some measure of perfusion (ml/min/g) often denoted by the variable F. Often, this is incorrectly referred to as the flow rate (ml/min): flow and perfusion are different. Blood flow is the rate at which blood flows through vessels in volume/time. Perfusion is blood flow per mass of tissue. Measures of blood flow use tracers that remain in the vasculature, while, for perfusion, tracers that diffuse from vasculature into tissue are utilized. Because diffusion of tracer occurs primarily at the capillary level, perfusion is reflective primarily of capillary perfusion (e.g., at the level where nutrients pass from blood to tissue). Perfusion of tissues becomes important because as one attempts to model biochemical processes, one must keep in mind that there may be a restriction to tracer availability due to delivery. For many PET tracer kinetic models, one does not explicitly see a perfusion term in the model. This is because the perfusion term is modeled as part of a rate coefficient (e.g., K_1 in the FDG model which depends on both blood flow and capillary permeability). In other models, perfusion is explicitly modeled because it is one of the parameters that is to be estimated.

Input function

The term input function usually refers to blood time-activity concentration (TAC) data (Figure 2-5). It is referred to as an input function because the arterial blood delivers the tracer to all tissues of the body. In addition, the blood

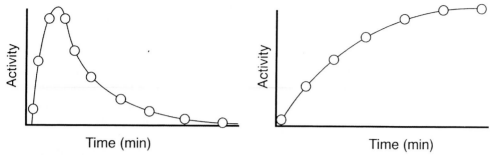

FIGURE 2-5. Blood and Tissue Time-Activity Curves (TACs). The blood TAC (A, left) represents activity in whole-blood or plasma and serves as an input into the tissue compartments. It is also referred to as an input function and tends to peak relatively early in time after intravenous injection of the tracer. It then decreases because tracer is diluted in the total blood pool and extracted from the blood into various tissues. It is also often cleared by the kidneys. The blood TAC can be obtained from direct blood sampling or from PET images of blood pool (e.g., left ventricle). The tissue TAC (B, right) is obtained by placing a region of interest on a set of dynamic PET images and represents the tracer and its potential labeled metabolites. Usually, blood vessels also traverse the ROI so that a portion of the blood TAC can be superimposed on the tissue TAC. In regions where tracer is being trapped, the tissue TAC will increase as shown above. In regions where tracer is not trapped, the tissue TAC can peak and then decrease over time similar to the blood TAC. Each tissue point represents the integrated activity from the PET scanner over a period of time and is often plotted at the *midpoint* of the time acquisition interval.

TAC drives the rest of the tracer kinetic model by serving as an input for the rest of the model. In many experimental processes, it is inconvenient to measure the blood TAC directly; therefore, it is predicted based on injecting a known mass of tracer into blood.[16] It is important to determine the arterial blood concentration as a function of time ($C_a(t)$) of a tracer because this is the concentration that feeds into various tissues. The venous concentration is not in general equal to the arterial concentration and is, therefore, less desirable. It is important to notice that the desired input function is for the original injected tracer. If metabolites are present in the blood, then one must correct for these to obtain the true desired input function. Mathematical approaches for correcting the input function have been studied.[24]

For PET assays, the input function is usually obtained in one of several ways: 1) direct arterial sampling of the blood in order to estimate $C_a(t)$;[25] 2) hand-warmed venous blood in order to estimate $C_a(t)$. Hand-warming dilates the arterial and venous vessels and in effect arterializes the venous blood,[25] allowing one to sample blood from hand veins, which are much easier to sample, and, therefore, estimate the $C_a(t)$; 3) estimation of $C_a(t)$ can also be obtained by dynamic PET imaging of the left ventricle, left atrium, or major arterial blood vessel (e.g., abdominal aorta).[26,27] These image-based approaches have the advantage of being noninvasive but always need to be initially validated for a given tracer by comparing the input function derived from PET images with those derived from direct blood sampling from blood vessels or left ventricle.[28] The imaging approach also samples tracer in whole blood rather than in plasma. It is also important to: 1) remember that if a PET-based approach is used, one is really measuring the input function over a time period (see Equation 2-1) and not at any specific time point, and 2) perform sampling more frequently during early time periods when the concentration is usually changing more rapidly.

In addition, it is important to keep in mind that there can be and generally is a difference between the whole-blood and plasma concentration of a particular tracer because for an image-based approach, one is always obtaining the whole-blood concentration of tracer, whereas for a sampled approach one has the option of spinning down the whole-blood to separate plasma from whole-blood. A tracer kinetic model generally uses the plasma component of the blood TAC to feed into the other compartments of the model. Only tracer in the plasma has the potential to directly leave the intravascular space. Tracer in blood cells would have to first come out of the cells and into the plasma prior to exiting the vascular space (e.g., radioactive oxygen bound to hemoglobin in red blood cells). It is, therefore, important to determine whole-blood and plasma concentrations of tracer as a function of time in each species studied and to use the plasma concentration in the tracer kinetic model. If a relatively fixed ratio exists between whole-blood and plasma (independent of time), then one can use the noninvasive image-based approach to obtain the whole-blood value and correct it to obtain the plasma value (based on hematocrit).

Also, the measured input function is only an approximation of the input function at the site of tissue of interest. For example, if the input function is measured from a *hot* vein in the navel or artery, but one is modeling tissue kinetics in the brain, a difference may exist between the measured input function and the one desired in the brain (due to differences in delay and dispersion from the site of injection to the sampling site in the hand versus the brain). Depending on the exact assay, it may be important to model this delay and dispersion.[29–31] Methods to simplify quantitation by not directly obtaining the input function are also sometimes useful if directly validated against approaches that use the input function to determine what loss in accuracy occurs for estimated model parameters.[32,33] Issues focused on optimal times to sample the input function can also be important and have been studied.[34]

Tissue time-activity curves

One of the most unique features about PET imaging is its ability to provide *regional* tissue time-activity curves (Figure 2-5). These curves would be very difficult to obtain using any other method because of the inability to repetitively sample all tissues of interest. The tissue time-activity curve is actually composed of several curves. Most tissue regions contain blood and extravascular and intracellular spaces. Therefore, the tissue TAC contains a part of the blood TAC. This fraction of the blood curve is sometimes referred to as spillover, not to be confused with the physical spillover due to resolution-related effects (see Chapter 1). In practice, all forms of spillover are often lumped to estimate the combined spillover fraction.[4] Furthermore, the tissue TAC is a measure of total radioactivity and does not separate out tracer from metabolites (if any). The separation of the tracer and its labeled metabolic product(s) must be obtained from the kinetics of the tracer moving through transport and biochemical reaction processes. A vascular compartment can be included in the tracer kinetic model to account for the vascular TAC in tissue. Most investigators use decay-corrected blood and tissue time-activity curves, but for specific models more accurate model parameter estimates may be possible by using nondecay corrected curves and accounting for the decay within the mathematical model.[35] In some cases, it may also be important to account for heterogeneity within an ROI (e.g., FDG uptake in a tumor) so that more accurate model parameter estimates may be obtained.[36] Methods that use factor analysis and related techniques to separate spillover components between time-activity curves have also been extensively studied.[37–41.]

Tracer extraction

Understanding the process whereby tracers leave the blood pool at the capillaries is important in developing a quantitative assay. Tracer concentration entering at one end of the capillary (C_a) will not in general have the same concentration as at the other end (C_v). Some fraction of the tracer is extracted into tissue across the capillary bed while the unextracted fraction remains behind and flows forward. The unidirectional extraction fraction is the fraction of tracer extracted from the blood into tissue. The net extraction fraction is different and refers to the arteriovenous concentration difference divided by the arterial concentration ($C_a - C_v)/C_a$ (Figure 2-6).

When the tracer arrives in the capillaries, some fraction of it is extracted across the capillary walls. The fraction of tracer which is extracted from the capillaries is referred to as the *unidirectional extraction fraction* (E) and is a unitless parameter. The unextracted fraction is washed away in venous blood. It is also important to notice that the *first pass* unidirectional extraction fraction is the extraction fraction during the first *single transit* of a tracer bolus through the capillaries without tracer being extracted back from tissue to blood. Generally, the first pass unidirectional extraction fraction and the unidirectional extraction fraction are used interchangeably. These terms are not to be confused with the *steady state* extraction fraction (E_s) (also referred to as the *net* extraction fraction) which is defined as the ratio of the difference

FIGURE 2-6. A Model of Capillary Extraction of Tracer from Plasma to the Extravascular Space. The blood flow through the capillary is *F*, the arterial concentration of tracer is C_a, and the venous concentration of tracer is C_v.

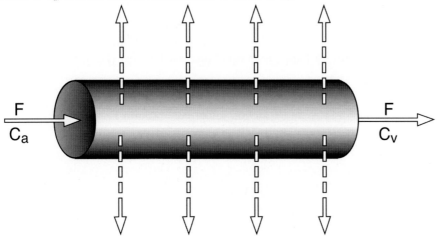

between tracer concentrations in arterial and venous blood over the concentration of tracer in arterial blood at *steady state* conditions (e.g., E_s is approximately constant over time). The steady state extraction fraction takes into account the extraction of tracer out of the capillaries as well as the *backtransport* and/or *backdiffusion* of tracer from the extravascular space back into the capillaries. For most tracers, the value for E is greater than for E_s because of the backtransport of tracer.

The magnitude of the fraction E depends on the total available capillary surface area S, the capillary permeability P for the tracer, and the blood flow F. The unidirectional extraction fraction E will increase if S or P increases. If the blood flow increases, then E tends to decrease because of the decreased time the tracer has to be extracted out of the capillaries. A relationship between E, S, P, and F is given by the Renkin–Crone equation.[42–44]

$$E = 1 - e^{-PS/F} \qquad (2\text{-}4)$$

which is based on considering a rigid cylindrical tube model for the vasculature. Here the units of measure for S, P, and F are cm^2/g, cm/min, and ml/min/g, respectively. As originally derived, P and S are treated as constants, but in experimental applications, it has been found that the PS product increases as flow increases due to either dilation or recruitment of more capillaries at higher blood flows. It is very important to realize that sometimes the extraction fraction as it is used refers to the extraction of tracer into the *cellular* spaces. This extraction occurs because, in some cases (e.g., myocardium), the capillary walls do not pose a significant barrier for tracer transport, but the cellular membranes do. In these cases, the PS value is the permeability surface product of the cellular membranes and capillary walls. This definition of extraction fraction which refers to extraction from capillaries and the interstitial spaces into the cellular spaces is also sometimes known as the *retention fraction* (E_r). Rigorously, the term retention fraction should be reserved for transport into a space from which escape of tracer is not possible or limited over the time of the measurement.

EXAMPLE 2-4

What does the Renkin–Crone equation predict will happen to extraction when the flow is doubled assuming that everything else remains fixed? Assume PS happens to equal the baseline flow ($PS = F_a$).

ANSWER

$$E_a = 1 - e^{-\frac{PS}{F_a}}; \text{ Extraction under condition of Flow} = F_a$$

$$E_b = 1 - e^{-\frac{PS}{F_b}}; \text{ Extraction under condition of Flow} = F_b$$

$$\frac{E_a}{E_b} = \frac{1 - e^{-\frac{PS}{F_a}}}{1 - e^{-\frac{PS}{F_b}}}, \text{ Given that } F_b = 2 \times F_a$$

$$\frac{E_a}{E_b} = \frac{1 - e^{-\frac{PS}{F_a}}}{1 - e^{-\frac{PS}{2F_a}}}, \text{ Now given that } PS = F_a \text{ we obtain}$$

$$\frac{E_a}{E_b} = \frac{1 - e^{-\frac{F_a}{F_a}}}{1 - e^{-\frac{F_a}{2F_a}}} = \frac{1 - e^{-1}}{1 - e^{-\frac{1}{2}}} = 1.61$$

So if flow is doubled, the extraction decreases by a factor of 1.61

If you do the same calculation for decreasing F in half ($F_b = 0.5 \times F_a$), then $\frac{E_a}{E_b} = 0.73$, illustrating the nonlinear response of E to changes in F.

Volume of distribution and partition coefficient

The term *volume of distribution* (V_d) is needed to understand tracer kinetic models and is often highly misunderstood (Figure 2-7). Confusion arises in

A.

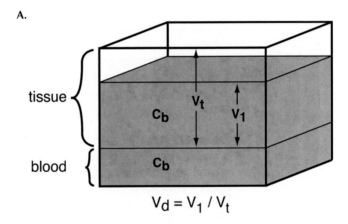

B.

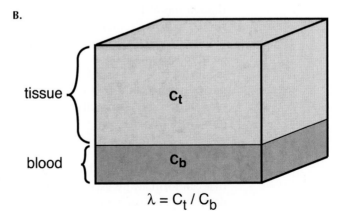

FIGURE 2-7. Volume of Distribution and Partition Coefficient. (A) Volume of distribution (V_d) represents the volume V_1 that tracer would occupy if it had the same concentration in tissue as it does in blood (C_b). (B) Partition coefficient (λ) is the ratio of concentration of tracer in tissue (C_t) to that in blood (C_b) assuming tracer can be distributed over *entire* tissue space with volume V_t.

large part because there is a mistaken tendency to think that the volume must be associated with a physical volume. The term is best understood by doing a tracer thought experiment. If one injects a mass of tracer M intravenously into the blood, and then waits a sufficient period of time Δt and samples the tracer blood concentration C, then one can estimate the volume of distribution $V_d = M/C$ (*units of ml*). Obviously, if the tracer never leaves the blood and is not metabolized, then V_d will equal the blood volume. At the other extreme, if no tracer remains in the blood, then V_d becomes infinitely large. The larger the volume of distribution is for a given tracer, the more this tracer is distributed throughout the body tissues. For a system in which all the tracer leaks out (an open system), one can perform a similar experiment except a continuous infusion of tracer into the blood is used so as to achieve a steady state condition. The volume of distribution can also be defined mathematically as the equilibrium ratio and has units of volume per mass (e.g., milliliters per gram):

$$V_d = (\text{g of tracer/g of tissue})/(\text{g of tracer/ml of blood}) \qquad (2\text{-}5)$$

The *partition coefficient* (λ) arises from thinking about the capillary wall as forming a partition such that the tracer on either side of the wall need not be equal. The ratio of tracer concentration in tissue to that in blood at equilibrium is the partition coefficient and is also given by Equation 2-5. The terms V_d and λ were originally used for inert tracers at equilibrium but have been subsequently used for all tracers, including those that are undergoing transport and/or metabolism. It is likely that most tracers do not distribute uniformly over the entire tissue space nor do they have the same concentration in tissue as they do in blood. Regardless, Equation 2-5 best describes both V_d and λ.

Transport steps in a comprehensive model

A tracer thought experiment can be laid out as a comprehensive compartmental model by formally describing all the locations and forms of a given tracer. The tracer thought experiment done earlier for FDG (see Tracer Thought Experiment, p. 129) can be laid out as a comprehensive model (Figure 2-8). Even such a model is not truly comprehensive and reduces the thought experiment into the major important components. For example, even though blood flow is not fixed, in the comprehensive model it is usually assumed to be fixed. Also, even though tracer moves between plasma and whole blood, the vascular space is often represented as one lumped compartment. A comprehensive model is usually reduced into no more than 3 to 4 compartments because it is usually very difficult to fit data provided from a PET scanner to more than 3 to 4 compartments.[45,46] This is the result of very similar rates of transport between groups of compartments, inadequate temporal sampling, and noise.

Model reduction

It is important to be able to reduce a comprehensive model into a working model that can formally be used to estimate model parameters with PET time-activity data. Two approaches of performing model reduction can be utilized: First, the

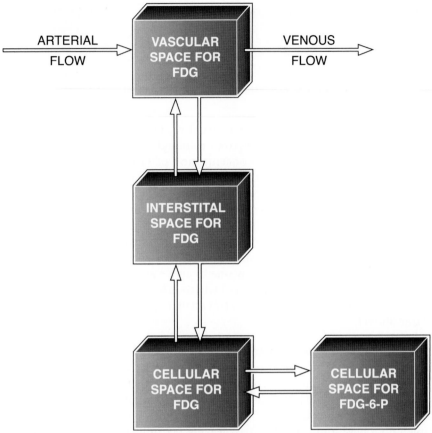

FIGURE 2-8. Comprehensive Model for FDG. The model assumes there is a fixed flow rate in the vascular space. FDG can leave the vascular space and enter the interstitial space. From here, it can be transported into cells and enter the cellular space. Once inside cells, it can be phosphorylated to form FDG-6-P. All the steps are reversible.

relative magnitudes of transport and reaction rates (if available) can be used to decide which compartments to lump together. When two compartments have rate constants that are much faster than other rate constants in the model, then those two compartments can usually be lumped together. In reality, most compartments represent several subcompartments. Fast transport rates between subcompartments cause concentrations of the subcompartments to be approximately in equilibrium at all times and support the subcompartments being lumped into a single compartment. Second, certain rate constants are fixed to specific values based on a priori knowledge (e.g., in vitro data). This in effect reduces the model to be more workable and is commonly referred to as constrained estimates because the model is constrained by setting some of the variables to fixed values. If, however, the fixed values vary significantly, this can cause problems in the working model.[47]

The comprehensive tracer kinetic model for FDG can be simplified to the model shown in Figure 2-9. Several compartments have been lumped together to arrive at this simplified model. The assumptions of this model de-

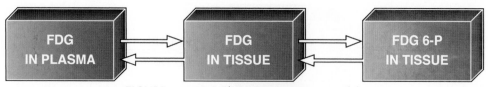

FIGURE 2-9. FDG Three-Compartment Model.

serve detailed description and are instructive. First, if the PS (see Equation 2-4) value is relatively small compared to blood flow, there is relatively low extraction of FDG and plasma concentration of FDG does not vary significantly down the capillary length.[25,48,49] This allows one to eliminate the effects of blood flow and greatly simplifies the model. Furthermore, for FDG the concentration ratio between the interstitial space and cellular space is in near equilibrium at all times allowing one to lump these two compartments together because the rate-limiting steps are movement of tracer out of the capillary wall (facilitated by transporters) and phosphorylation by hexokinase.[50] These simplifications allow one to arrive at the reduced FDG 3-compartment model shown in Figure 2-9 where FDG in tissue (the second compartment) represents FDG in the extravascular space (both extracellular and intracellular).

Differential equations for a compartmental model

The equations that govern a compartmental model are based on the physical principles of mass balance. The equations are usually best written in terms of mass but can often also be written in terms of concentration. The rate of change of mass for a given compartment must equal the net mass coming in per unit time into a pool minus the net mass leaving per unit time. The rate of change is written as the differential d/dt, and the rate of change of mass in a given compartment is often written as $d(M)/dt$. At steady state, when there is no change with respect to time, the differential equals zero. Solving the differential equation at steady state is easy because the time-derivative is eliminated. For each compartment, the differential equation is written separately. The compartment that represents the blood pool does not need an explicit equation because the blood time-activity curve is already available as the input function to the model. Equations from multiple compartments can often be combined into matrix notation to simplify a complicated set of equations.[16] The differential equations are considered linear if all mass terms q_i for compartments are to the power 1 and nonlinear if any one term is of a power greater than 1

(e.g., $\dfrac{dq_1(t)}{dt} = -K_1 q_1(t) + k_2 q_2(t)$ is linear

and $\dfrac{dq_1(t)}{dt} = -K_1 q_1^2(t)$ is nonlinear).

Solutions to the differential equations for linear compartmental models can be derived using a variety of mathematical techniques including Laplace transforms.[51] Nonlinear models often require computational approximations. Specific examples of differential equations and solutions can be found in the following section.

FIGURE 2-10. One-Compartment Model.

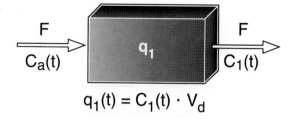

$$q_1(t) = C_1(t) \cdot V_d$$

One-compartment model

Consider the single compartment linear model shown in Figure 2-10. This model might represent the delivery and removal of tracer into tissue as governed by perfusion rate F. The tracer is homogeneously distributed in the compartment with a concentration $C_1(t)$ (g/ml).

Let $q_1(t)$ = mass of tracer in compartment 1 at time t.
F = perfusion of tracer (ml/min/g tissue)
V_d = volume of distribution of tracer (ml/g tissue)
$C_a(t)$ = arterial input function

With mass balance the rate of change in tracer in the compartment is equal to the net mass coming in per unit time minus the net mass leaving per unit time:

$$\frac{dq_1(t)}{dt} = FC_a(t) - \frac{F}{V_d} q_1(t) \qquad (2\text{-}6)$$

This is a system with zero initial state, such that $q_1(0) = 0$. The solution to the above model can be obtained by Laplace transforms[51] and is given as:

$$q_1(t) = e^{-\frac{F}{V_d}t} \otimes FC_a(t) + q_1(0)e^{-\frac{F}{V_d}t} \qquad (2\text{-}7)$$

where $\otimes$ is the convolution operator[51] and the convolution of two functions $f(t)$ an $g(t)$ is given as:

$$f(t) \otimes g(t) = \int_0^t f(s)g(t - s)ds \qquad (2\text{-}8)$$

EXAMPLE 2-5

Show that for the one compartment model depicted in Figure 2-10 the solution shown in Equations 2-7 and 2-8 satisfies the model differential equation shown in Equation 2-6. Use the definition of convolution given in Equation 2-8 to solve.

ANSWER

We are told that the solution to Equation 2-6 $\left[\dfrac{d}{dt} q_1(t) = FC_a(t) - \dfrac{F}{V_d}(q_1(t)) \right]$ is given as:

$$q_1(t) = FC_a(t) \otimes e^{-\frac{F}{V_d}t}$$

If we differentiate the left and right hand sides of the above equation (the given solution), we obtain:

$$\frac{d}{dt}\,q_1(t) = \frac{d}{dt}\left[FC_a(t) \otimes e^{\frac{-F}{V_d}t}\right]$$

$$= \frac{d}{dt}\int_0^t FC_a(\tau)e^{\frac{-F}{V_d}(t-\tau)}\,d\tau$$

$$= F\frac{d}{dt}\left[e^{-\frac{F}{V_d}t}\int_0^t C_a(\tau)e^{\frac{F}{V_d}\tau}\,d\tau\right]$$

$$= F\frac{-F}{V_d}e^{-\frac{F}{V_d}t}\int_0^t C_a(\tau)e^{\frac{F}{V_d}\tau}\,d\tau + Fe^{-\frac{F}{V_d}t}\,e^{\frac{F}{V_d}t}\,C_a(t)$$

$$= -\frac{F}{V_d}\int_0^t FC_a(\tau)e^{-\frac{F}{V_d}(t-\tau)}\,d\tau + Fe^{-\frac{F}{V_d}t}\,e^{\frac{F}{V_d}t}\,C_a(t)$$

$$= -\frac{F}{V_d}(FC_a(t)\otimes e^{\frac{-F}{V_d}t}) + FC_a(t)$$

Such that:

$$\frac{d}{dt}\,q_1(t) = FC_a(t) - \frac{F}{V_d}(q_1(t))$$

The above equation is the original differential equation (Equation 2-6), so we are done. This question illustrates that even if one does not know how to obtain an answer to a tracer kinetic model differential equation(s), one can at least verify that a given solution is correct by differentiating the answer.

Two-compartment model

Consider the 2-compartment model shown in Figure 2-11. This model might represent the movement of tracer between the blood pool (compartment 1) into the tissue pool (compartment 2).

Let: $q_1(t)$ = mass of tracer in compartment 1 at time t.
$q_2(t)$ = mass of tracer in compartment 2 at time t.
K_1 = rate coefficient for transfer from 1 to 2 (ml/min/g).
k_2 = rate constant for transfer from 2 to 1 (1/min).
Here, $q_1(0) = q_2(0) = 0$.

By mass balance one obtains:

$$\frac{dq_1(t)}{dt} = -K_1q_1(t) + k_2q_2(t)$$

$$\frac{dq_2(t)}{dt} = K_1q_1(t) - k_2q_2(t)$$

(2-9)

These two equations can be solved for $q_1(t)$ and $q_2(t)$. However, if $q_1(t)$ is explicitly known (e.g., $q_1(t)$ is the measured blood time-activity curve), then one only need solve for $q_2(t)$ and obtain:

$$q_2(t) = K_1q_1(t) \otimes e^{-k_2t}$$

(2-10)

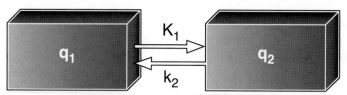

FIGURE 2-11. Two-Compartment Model.

Three-compartment model

Consider the 3-compartment model shown in Figure 2-12. This model might represent tracer in the blood pool (compartment 1), tracer in the extravascular pool (compartment 2), and a metabolite of the tracer in the extravascular pool (compartment 3).

Let $q_1(t)$ = mass in compartment 1 at time t.
$q_2(t)$ = mass in compartment 2 at time t.
$q_3(t)$ = mass in compartment 3 at time t.
K_1 = rate coefficient for transfer from 1 to 2 (ml/min/g).
k_2 = rate constant for transfer from 2 to 1 (1/min).
k_3 = rate constant for transfer from 2 to 3 (1/min).
k_4 = rate constant for transfer from 3 to 2 (1/min).
Here, $q_1(0) = q_2(0) = q_3(0) = 0$.

By mass balance one obtains:

$$\frac{dq_1(t)}{dt} = -K_1 q_1(t) + k_2 q_2(t)$$

$$\frac{dq_2(t)}{dt} = K_1 q_1(t) - k_2 q_2(t) + k_4 q_3(t) - k_3 q_2(t) \qquad (2\text{-}11)$$

$$\frac{dq_3(t)}{dt} = k_3 q_2(t) - k_4 q_3(t)$$

The solution to the above (assuming $q_1(t)$ is explicitly known) is given by:

$$q_2(t) = \frac{K_1}{\alpha_2 - \alpha_1} q_1(t) \otimes \left[(k_4 - \alpha_1)e^{-\alpha_1 t} + (\alpha_2 - k_4)e^{-\alpha_2 t} \right]$$

$$q_3(t) = \frac{K_1 k_3}{\alpha_2 - \alpha_1} q_1(t) \otimes (e^{-\alpha_1 t} - e^{-\alpha_2 t}) \qquad (2\text{-}12)$$

where

$$\alpha_{1,2} = \frac{(k_2 + k_3 + k_4) \mp \sqrt{(k_2 + k_3 + k_4)^2 - 4k_2 k_4}}{2}.$$

FIGURE 2-12. Three-Compartment Model.

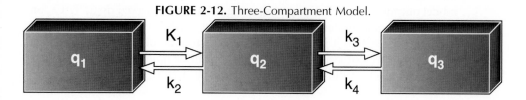

EXAMPLE 2-6

What is the steady state solution for compartment 3 for the three-compartment linear model described previously?

Assume $q_1(\infty) = 0$ and all rate constants are strictly greater than zero.

ANSWER

$$q_3(t) = \frac{K_1 k_3}{\alpha_2 - \alpha_1} \, q_1(t) \otimes (e^{-\alpha_1 t} - e^{-\alpha_2 t})$$

$$q_3(t) = \lim_{t \to \infty} \left[\frac{K_1 k_3}{\alpha_2 - \alpha_1} \, q_1(t) \otimes (e^{-\alpha_1 t} - e^{-\alpha_2 t}) \right]$$

$$= \frac{K_1 k_3}{\alpha_2 - \alpha_1} \lim_{t \to \infty} \left[q_1(t) \otimes (e^{-\alpha_1 t} - e^{-\alpha_2 t}) \right]$$

$$q_3(\infty) = 0$$

Notice that one could reason out the answer (without performing the mathematical steps) because eventually all the tracer would leak out of the last compartment due to a nonzero k_4.

Model validation

Model validation is a critical component for understanding the utility of the model in predicting future experimental results and is generally based on kinetic and biochemical validation. Kinetic validation aims to determine if the model predictions of time-activity curves is consistent with observed data. Biochemical validation compares biochemical data on concentration of tracer and/or metabolites with model predictions for each compartment in the model at specific points in time. It is important to notice that, in either case, one might deal with a true in vivo environment (e.g., a mouse or human subject) or an isolated tissue environment (e.g, isolated heart preparation). Regardless of the exact methods used to perform model validation, it is never the case that a model is proven to be true by the validation process. The validation process simply helps lend support to using the model to estimate the process it was intended to describe under the conditions of the validation.

One can initially determine if the qualitative behavior of the model is consistent with the observed data. The qualitative behavior of the model can be based on studying the equations governing the model and solving them for time-to-peak activity, steady-state mass levels, and so on. These solutions may be based on the blood time-activity curve (input function). It often helps to have an example of a blood time-activity curve for a particular tracer prior to starting model validation. In addition, one can also simulate the model using software tools if one has some estimates of the underlying model parameter(s). By studying the model output and qualitatively comparing this to the observed tissue TACs, one may have a better understanding of the model's validity. The limiting factor in this approach is that it is often the case that estimates of model parameters (F, K_1, k_2, etc.) are not available; model output can be quite dependent on these.

Model kinetic validation is most accurately performed by fitting observed data to a given model and in the process estimating model parameters (Figure 2-13). Through the study of the fitted curve, one can begin to understand model limitations (if any). If the model does not fit the data well, parameter estimates may still be available, but the predicted curve will not fit the data well (Figure 2-13). This process can be made fully statistical by determining if residuals (the difference between model prediction and observation) are randomly distributed about zero (Figure 2-13), which would indicate that model equations provide a good representation of the data. If the residuals are correlated, then the model is not supported by the kinetic data. Once parameters are estimated, and residuals statistically tested for lack of correlation, one can compare the value of the estimated parameter to known physiological and biochemical parameters. If one or more parameters are clearly out of the range of underlying physiology and biochemistry, then the model is suspect.

The standard errors of the parameter estimates can also be important in helping to understand a given model. Large standard errors (e.g., 100%) usually imply that the model has too many parameters unless the data are extremely noisy. When a model has too many parameters, it is usually possible to simplify the model by decreasing the number of parameters. If two models fit the observed data near-equivalently, then usually the model with the fewer number of parameters is the one of choice. Formal statistical methods do exist to test models against each other to determine which one is optimal in terms of the number of parameters and the goodness of each model's fit.[45,46] A careful balance of studying all of the above issues helps to build confidence that one has developed a reasonably good model.

Biochemical validation is necessary to provide the greatest degree of confidence in a particular tracer kinetic model. This approach requires direct estimates of tracer and labeled reaction product(s) concentrations from tissues at various points in time. These estimates can then be directly compared to model predictions from one or more compartments. Biochemical separation of the tracer from labeled reaction product(s) in tissue samples by high performance liquid chromatography (HPLC) or other chemical assay are typically required. The ideal biochemical validation would be achieved by performing dynamic PET scanning and model fitting of blood and tissue time-activity data in order to estimate model parameters. These estimates would then be used to calculate the relative fraction or concentration of tracer in each of the compartments. Tissue samples would be obtained directly after PET scanning and then the concentration of tracer and labeled reaction products in various forms determined. It may be necessary to stop the experiments at various time points in order to test the model during the early and late kinetic phases of the study. It is much more difficult to obtain human tissue samples so that most biochemical validation is done using animal models. Specific examples of biochemical validation can be found elsewhere.[52]

Model parameter estimation

The use of a tracer kinetic model along with measured PET time-activity data allows for the estimation of model parameters. The most robust method for performing this estimation is weighted nonlinear regression.[53,54] The term weighted refers to the fact that different data points can be given more or less weight in the calculation based on how that point may be more or less accurate relative

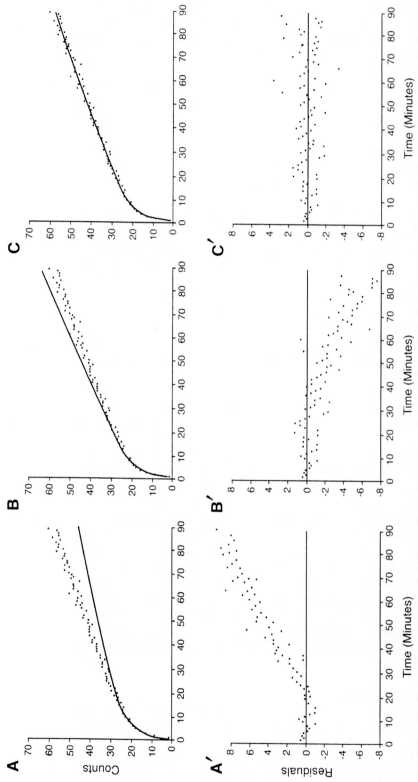

FIGURE 2-13. Fitting Data to a Model with Nonlinear Regression. Panel A shows hypothetical data (individual points) and the model predicted fit during an early iteration. Notice that the solid line does not go through all of the data well especially at late time points. Panel A' shows how well the curve in panel A fits the data as measured by residuals (the difference between fit and observations). Notice that the residuals increase for later time points indicating a poor data fit. As the fitting routine iterates, panels B and C show improved fits as evidenced by the residual plots B' and C'. The residuals should be randomly distributed about zero for a good fit as occurs in C'.

to another point primarily due to statistical accuracy of the data points. Weighted nonlinear regression is an iterative process in which starting estimates of all parameters along with equations that govern a particular model are used to generate a refined estimate of the parameters. This approach is repeated until some criteria are met for achieving convergence. Typically, one wishes to minimize the square of the difference between the observation and model prediction for all observations—often referred to as the weighted residual sum of squares (WRSS) given as:

$$\Theta = WRSS = \sum_{i=1}^{N} w_i(y_i - y_{pi})^2 \tag{2-13}$$

Here N is the number of time points for which there is an observation as well as a model prediction, w_i are the relative weights for each of the $y_i = y(t_i)$ observations taken over time t, and y_{pi} are the model predicted values at each time point $y_p(t_i)$. There is no guarantee in these iterative methods that a global minimum will be achieved, but if multiple distinct initial guesses lead to the same converged final estimates, then it is likely that a global minimum has been reached.[55]

EXAMPLE 2-7

Determine the WRSS if the model being fit to is $y = \exp(-p^*t)$ (a decaying monoexponential curve) for $t = 0, 0.1, 0.2, 0.4, 0.8, 1.0$, with the observed values being $y_i = 0.9, 1.1, 0.93, 0.77, 0.7, 0.55$. Here p is the parameter being estimated. Assume $p = 0.5$ for the value of the parameter for which the WRSS is desired and observations should be weighted equally with a weight $= 1$. If all the weights are equal, WRSS is often referred to as residual sum of squares (RSS).

ANSWER

To calculate the WRSS, we utilize Equation 2-13 and note that $N = 6$, $w_i = 1$ for all i.

i	t_i	y_i	y_{pi}	$w_i (y_i - y_{pi})^2$
1	0	0.9	$\exp(-0.5^*0) = 1.0$	0.01000
2	0.1	1.1	$\exp(-0.5^*0.1) = 0.95$	0.02213
3	0.2	0.93	$\exp(-0.5^*0.2) = 0.90$	0.00063
4	0.4	0.77	$\exp(-0.5^*0.4) = 0.82$	0.00237
5	0.8	0.7	$\exp(-0.5^*0.8) = 0.67$	0.00088
6	1.0	0.55	$\exp(-0.5^*1.0) = 0.61$	0.00319

WRSS = (0.01000 + 0.02213 + 0.00063 + 0.00237 + 0.00088 + 0.00319)
$$= 0.039$$

Shown in Figure 2-14 is an example of a model-predicted surface Θ generated for a model with parameters p_1 and p_2. This surface represents the value of Θ for all possible combinations of the two parameters. The goal of nonlinear regression is to start somewhere on this type of surface (based on the initial guess) and to find the minimum value of Θ. The algorithms developed avoid having to generate the whole surface and, instead, use approaches to find the minimum with only starting guesses.

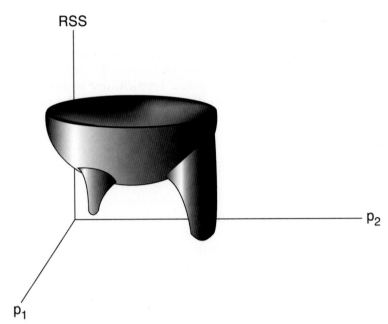

FIGURE 2-14. Residual Sum of Squares Surface for 2 Parameters. Each of the two parameters p_1 and p_2 generates a model predicted estimate of an observed value for each time point. If each of these is used along with Equation 2-13 and the observed data, one can calculate the residual sum of squares (RSS) or WRSS. Every combination of p_1 and p_2 can then be used to obtain a surface for which we wish to find the minimum point. There may be one or several local minima, but the goal is to find the unique global minimum.

Because nonlinear regression is slow and has difficulty in converging when high levels of noise are present, several linearizing methods have been explored to help minimize the computational time required for estimating model parameter(s). These methods also sometimes help deal with noise. If data can be transformed to a linear form, then there is an explicit solution that estimates the slope and y-intercept. One such method is the *Patlak plot*,[56,57] which can be applied to many models in which the tracer is effectively trapped. Effectively trapped refers to a tracer that is nearly totally trapped during the time for which the process is studied. The Patlak equation predicts that after some time $t > t^*$ that a plot of:

$$\frac{C_T^*(t)}{C_P^*(t)} \quad \text{vs.} \quad \frac{\int_0^t C_P^*(s)\,ds}{C_P^*(t)}$$

(where C_T^* is the total tissue activity and C_P^* is the plasma activity) will be essentially linear with a slope of K^* (see Example 2-11 for derivation). In addition to linearizing methods, other methods have been studied including generalized linear least squares (GLLS)[58–60] and neural network approaches[61,62] to speed up the process of parameter estimation. Additional methods are beyond the scope of this chapter. Issues related to models for noise in PET data and how this affects the estimation process are discussed elsewhere.[63–69]

EXAMPLE 2-8

Time-activity data are being fit using nonlinear regression. It is desired to estimate the 4 parameters K_1, k_2, k_3, k_4 of the 3-compartment model shown in Figure 2-12. One individual obtains one set of values for estimates of K_1, k_2, k_3, k_4 and the other individual obtains an entirely different set. Both individuals are using the same software tool and the same model definition. How is this possible?

ANSWER

Nonlinear regression depends on an *initial guess* for *each* parameter to be estimated. Based on these initial guesses, the software algorithms attempt to minimize the RSS. It is possible though that, based on one initial guess, the routine converges into a local minimum, whereas with a different initial guess a true global minimum is reached. The only way to maximize the chance that the converged set of parameter values are the correct ones is to try many different initial guesses to make sure they are all leading to the same set of final parameter estimates. If some initial guesses do not lead to the same parameter estimates, then the converged parameter values that lead to the lowest RSS are likely the correct ones. There is, however, no absolute guarantee with nonlinear regression that the absolute (global) minimum RSS has been found.

It is sometimes desirable to optimize the times at which an underlying kinetic process is sampled to obtain the best estimates of the underlying model parameters. Based on some pilot experiments, it is usually possible to apply specific criteria to maximize the precision of the parameter estimates in an iterative fashion. One such approach, using D-optimal criterion for estimating myocardial beta-adrenergic receptor concentrations[70] and FDG parameter estimation[71], illustrates some of the issues involved.

Physical interpretation of model parameters

In general, the value of rate constants and coefficients in a compartmental model are related to, but different from, the biochemical steps of transport and biochemical reactions or physical parameters such as perfusion. This is because the compartmental model has rate constants that help to determine tracer flux (mass of tracer per unit time leaving or entering a compartment of interest) based on both tracer concentration and volume of distribution of the tracer. A bidirectional transporter does not imply that the rate constants are equal in both directions. The bidirectionality applies to the physical and chemical rate constants which depend on chemical concentrations on either side of the membrane or between reactants and products. Because the rate constant of a compartment model is expressed with respect to the tracer in a compartment, it is related to both concentration and the volume of space represented by the compartment. This change in physical interpretation of the model parameter needs to be taken into account when assigning parameter values as a part of model reduction, model validation, or interpreting model parameters and predictions.

EXAMPLE 2-9

A 2-compartment model as shown in Figure 2-11 has $K_1 = 0.5$ ml/min/g and $k_2 = 0.2$ min^{-1}. At $t = 10$ min, the mass of tracer $q_1(10) = 1.0$ and $q_2(10) = 1.0$, are both in grams. The concentration of tracer $c_1(10) = 0.1$ and $c_2(10) = 0.05$, both in grams per milliliters g/ml.

What is the effective volume for each compartment and what is the mass flux (mass per unit time) out of compartment 1 and 2 at time 10 minutes?

ANSWER

The effective volume of each compartment is:

$$V_{d1} = q_1/c_1 = 1.0 \text{ g}/(0.1 \text{ g/ml}) = 10.0 \text{ ml}$$
$$V_{d2} = q_2/c_2 = 1.0 \text{ g}/(0.05 \text{ g/ml}) = 20.0 \text{ ml}$$

The flux out of a compartment is in units of mass per unit time.

For compartment 1, this would be $q_1(10) \times [c_1(10) \times K_1] = 1.0$ g $\times$ [0.1 g/ml $\times$ 0.5 ml/min/g] = 0.05 g/min.

For compartment 2, this would be $q_2(10) \times k_2 = 1.0$ g $\times$ 0.2 min^{-1} = 0.2 g/min.

Notice that the rate coefficients and rate constants are not equal to the flux. The flux of mass out depends on the current mass in the compartment.

Parametric imaging

Parametric imaging seeks to develop an image of a parameter based on applying a tracer kinetic model to an image set obtained over time. Instead of drawing a specific region of interest (ROI), and then using the input function and tissue time activity curve (TAC) to fit to a model, multiple tissue TACs, each from a voxel, are fit to the model. By applying a tracer kinetic model on a voxel-by-voxel basis, one can estimate a specific parameter of the model, and then display the parameter value on a voxel-by-voxel basis as an image of the parameter. If multiple model parameters exist, then multiple corresponding parametric images can be created. For example, if one takes a set of PET images of the tracer N-13 ammonia as it distributes in myocardial tissues over time and fits those data to a tracer kinetic model, one can develop a parametric image of myocardial perfusion. This allows an image of perfusion in addition to an image of N-13 Ammonia concentration to be studied. An example of such a perfusion parametric image is shown in Figure 2-15A.

Several issues deserve special consideration for parametric imaging. Although in principle the concept of a parametric image is simple, the ability to generate such an image can be quite difficult. Data from each voxel over time can be quite noisy, leading to difficulties in attempting to fit any time-activity curve derived from a single voxel. In addition, the tracer kinetic model may not apply to all areas of the image and artifacts can result. Long computation times can also be involved. Methods to account for partial volume effects on a pixel-by-pixel basis are quite challenging but various approaches that rely on some anatomical information have been studied.[72] Approaches to directly obtain parametric im-

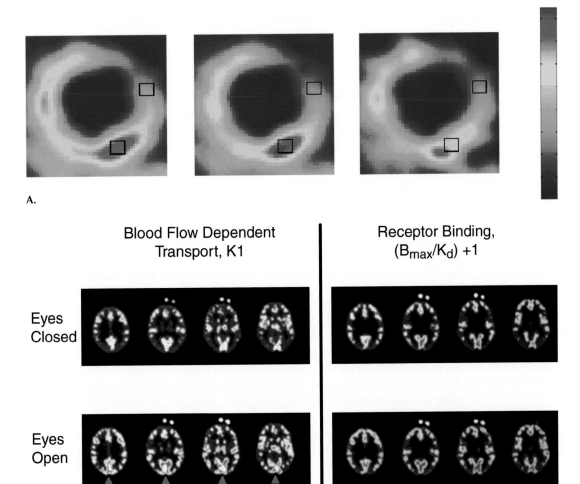

FIGURE 2-15. A: N-13 Ammonia Perfusion Parametric Images of Canine Myocardium. Shown are images of pixel-by-pixel calculated perfusion from time-activity data obtained from dynamic image sets from a canine N-13 Ammonia study done with a 2-compartment model. The input function used was obtained from arterial sampling. The images represent perfusion and not just tracer concentration. The left image was obtained using a neural networks approach, the middle by using weighted nonlinear regression and the right with a Patlak approach. The square ROIs are placed on regions of myocardial tissue and directly yield perfusion values. (Reproduced with permission from reference 62). B: F-18-Flumazenil Brain Parametric Images with Eyes Closed and Open. F-18-Flumazenil human brain tracer kinetic data were fit to a 3-compartment model to estimate the flow-dependent K_1 and receptor binding parameter $(B_{max}/K_d)+1$, under conditions of eyes closed and eyes open. In terms of the tracer thought experiment, "you" would experience your initial blood-flow-dependent forward diffusion to get into the brain (top left) and then subsequently you switch to your longer term existence in tissue being dependent on your association with benzodiazapine receptors (top right). Further, when the brain performs a function like "seeing" that requires increases in glucose delivery through an associated increase in flow, "your" ride into tissue is accelerated (bottom left), but since this increase in visual activity does not change the work of the benzodiazapine receptors, the later part of your journey into the tissue remains unchanged (bottom right). (Images provided courtesy of Dr. Kirk Frey, University of Michigan. Reproduced with permission from 74.)

ages from projection data have also been utilized and are discussed elsewhere.[73] In the latter, the temporal data for each point in the projection data are used to calculate a model parameter (e.g., blood perfusion) and then the image reconstruction algorithm is applied to the projections of the parameters.

Parametric images can also be useful for creating images that reflect different portions of a kinetic process. For example, images can be created that use the early time-points of a diffusible tracer to estimate perfusion followed by use of the later phases to estimate a subsequent reaction. Figure 2-15B illustrates how this can be a powerful method to visualize dynamic PET data.[74]

Modeling software packages

Software packages for PET assay development include tools to help reconstruct images, image analysis, and tracer kinetic modeling.[75] This section focuses on tracer kinetic modeling tools, which can be helpful for simulating what a given model might predict for time-activity curves based on certain fixed parameter values (forward problem) and/or might be used to fit PET time-activity data to a specific model to estimate model parameters (inverse problem). Tools that allow graphical construction of the tracer kinetic model and then interactive adjustment of model parameters are particularly useful when comparing model behavior and exploring different model configurations.[76] For example, one could study how a particular model parameter affects only the late time portions of the tissue time-activity curve while having little effect on the rest of the curve. One could also formally study the sensitivity of the model output with regards to each model parameter. Simulation is particularly useful for students starting to learn tracer kinetic modeling to build confidence with regards to the underlying mathematics.

Developers of PET assays often find difficulty in fitting PET-derived time-activity curves to a given tracer kinetic model. One difficulty is specifying the *explicit* solution of a given tracer kinetic model so that data can be fit to the solution. Most tracer kinetic models have differential equations that are difficult to explicitly solve, especially because the input function is convolved with the solution of the other compartments (see One-Compartment Model, p. 147). Some software packages require that an explicit solution to the tracer kinetic model be already available. In addition, because the input function is usually convolved with other equations, it is important to have tools that support convolution. Software packages that can fit observed time-activity curves directly to the model equations (without requiring the explicit solution) are, therefore, highly desirable. Software tools that show each iteration of fitting a time-activity curve can be quite useful for monitoring the fitting process. Support for batch operations in which many regions of interest can be fit are also useful for working with large data sets. A software package named COMKAT incorporating many of the desirable features for PET assay development has recently been described;[77] details may also be found at www.nuclear.uhrad.com/comkat.

DESIRABLE PROPERTIES OF MOLECULAR IMAGING PROBES

It is important that the development of a PET assay is tightly coupled to the development of positron labeled tracers. In practice, several iterations usually occur to optimize an assay by using a specific tracer, performing the assay, improving the tracer, and so on (see Figure 2-4). Chemical and biochemical criteria for selecting PET tracers are reviewed in detail in Chapter 4, but specific issues warrant discussion here.

Regarding nomenclature, the radioisotope refers to the atom that will decay to produce a positron, and a molecule of interest when coupled to the isotope of choice is referred to as the tracer. It is referred to as a tracer because it will trace out the biochemistry of the parent molecule and because it is administered in trace or low mass amounts. The use of a trace amount allows the underlying system not to be significantly perturbed. The process of administering a tracer is sometimes referred to as the tracer experiment.

The choice of tracer is a complex issue and is in practice an iterative process that leads to one or more tracers that can be used to assay a given process of interest. The two general categories of tracer are: 1) the molecule labeled such that there is a direct isotopic substitution (e.g., ^{12}C replaced with ^{11}C) referred to as the parent molecule and 2) one in which there is a chemical modification to the parent molecule, referred to as a chemical analog. For most applications, it is preferable to use the analog molecule to isolate a few steps in a complex biochemical pathway (see FDG Assay, p. 161). This is often done in basic biochemistry experiments in order to prevent the chemical analog from interacting with more than a limited set of molecules to allow accurate estimates of the process of interest. This approach is also often used by the pharmaceutical industry in order to design drugs to interact with a specific target and minimize any side or subsequent reactions.

Fluorine-18 (^{18}F) is a good substitute for either H or OH because its small size avoids steric hindrance. Furthermore, the C—F bond is relatively strong (~110 Kcal). Of all of the isotopes for PET, ^{18}F is one of the best due to its reasonable half-life, relatively low positron range, and high positron yield. If an analog does not contain a Fluorine atom or if the Fluorine introduced is at a different site on the molecule, it is important to realize that the ^{18}F labeled analog may not behave exactly like the nonlabeled analog. This is because ^{18}F is highly electronegative and may change the properties of the molecule. Fluorine is sometimes found on drugs because of its chemical value in producing drugs where fluorine is used to block unwanted biochemical reactions without significantly altering the desired properties of the drug.

Experimentation *in vitro*, in cell culture, and in living animals to determine the efficacy of a particular tracer is important to perform *early* in the assay development process. Quite often, investigators immediately proceed in labeling a given molecule with a positron emitter without performing fundamental studies that will help to determine if a particular assay will be feasible with a given molecule. For example, if a particular molecule has a slow clearance rate from certain tissues (e.g., blood), it may be desirable to choose a long-lived positron emitter (e.g., ^{124}I, ^{64}Cu, see Table 2-1 for properties of various positron emitting radioisotopes). One can perform initial tests using a beta-emitter (e.g., ^{3}H or ^{14}C) attached to the molecule of interest in order to not be limited by the half-life of short-lived isotopes. In some cases, however, it is relatively easy to label the molecule with a positron emitting isotope, and therefore, it may be more efficient to test the PET tracer directly. After a molecule has been chosen to assay a particular molecular event, a search should be made for ^{3}H or ^{14}C-labeled analog of the molecule. Such molecules are often available from com-

TABLE 2-1. Properties of Drugs versus Imaging Tracers

Property	Drug	Tracer
High affinity for target	Yes	Yes
Efficient transport into tissue	Yes	Yes
Stable in plasma	Yes	Yes
Rapid clearance from tissue	Not necessary	Yes
Limited interaction with nontarget tissue	Yes	Yes
Plasma $T_{1/2}$	Hours to days	Minutes to hours
Target to background	Can be less than 1	Must be greater than 1

panies that routinely provide β-emitter-labeled tracers or from drug companies that have been studying the molecule as a potential drug. Alternatively, it may be possible to rapidly synthesize a ^{3}H or ^{14}C-labeled molecule. The use of these tracers early in the assay development process will aid in the selection of molecules that have the right characteristics to become molecular imaging probes. Good communication between the chemists and the assay developer is needed to carefully discuss these and related issues.

Specific activity issues are highly important for assay development. Specific activity is a measure of the number of molecules capable of producing a radioactive signal at a given time, divided by the total number of available molecules (units in Curies/mmole). It is important to realize that when one uses a certain quantity of a tracer, that not all available molecules can lead to radioactive decay because some molecules will have cold element on them (e.g., some of the FDG contains ^{19}F). In fact, the specific activity is constantly changing because the radioisotope is constantly decaying. The maximum theoretical specific activity of a particular isotope is inversely proportional to the half-life of the isotope[78] (see also Chapter 4). Specific activity may be very important for some assays because an insufficient specific activity may not allow estimation of a desirable parameter because the target site may become saturated by the mass of tracer used. For example, in using a radiolabeled ligand to estimate receptor density, it is generally the case that a relatively high-specific activity is needed (e.g., >1,000 Ci/mmole) in order to determine relatively low levels of receptor concentration (e.g., nanomolar)[79] without occupying a significant percentage of the receptors with unlabelled compound. Specific activity issues also apply when considering ^{3}H and ^{14}C-labeled tracers for use with in vitro, cell culture, and cell or whole-body autoradiography. Further examples of choice of tracer and radiolabel can be found in Assays for Imaging Reporter Gene Expression, p. 175.

Mass perturbation issues are important to keep in perspective for the development of any PET assay. Ideally, one would like to not perturb the underlying biochemistry while performing the assay of it. Typically, in PET assays nanograms of materials are injected resulting in picomoles or femtomoles of tracer per gram of tissue so the potential for perturbation is minimal. One should, however, always attempt to verify this by quantitating the effects of perturbation. For example, what is the fraction of receptors that will be occupied by the PET tracer? In animal experiments, the perturbations may not be minimal because of the relatively small blood volume; potential consequences of this are discussed elsewhere.[80]

SPECIFIC ASSAYS FOR PET

Many different assays have already been developed primarily by the PET research community, covering a wide range of biochemical and physiological processes. Although FDG is the most commonly used assay, there are many other assays available. Some of the more important assays are reviewed next to exemplify different categories of assays.

FDG assay

Deoxyglucose (DG) was originally characterized in terms of its affinity for glucose transporters[81,82] and its affinity for hexokinase.[83,84] The use of DG to block glycolysis in tumors was studied in detail in the 1950s[85] and although it failed as a drug, it opened the door to a new group of imaging agents.

Historically, several tracers for glucose metabolism have been investigated both for the fields of autoradiography as well as PET. Earlier work with autoradiography in rats[49] (the Sokoloff model) and monkeys[86] using [^{14}C]deoxyglucose (DG) was successful in estimating regional glucose utilization in the brain. DG is very useful because it provides a good record of the initial events that a glucose molecule normally undergoes.[83,87] DG competes with glucose for plasma brain barrier and cell facilitated transport carriers and is phosphorylated, but at this stage, it is not further metabolized within typical experimental times used.[88] The phosphorylated DG is essentially trapped in cells because the now charged molecule cannot traverse the cell membrane. It can, however, be slowly hydrolyzed back to DG.[89,90] Early work with DG gave rise to a compartmental model to mathematically describe the behavior of DG in cerebral tissue.[88] With the use of radioactivity concentrations in arterial plasma (DG) and in local tissue (DG and DG-6-PO$_4$), and in conjunction with the mathematical model that contains a proper correction for transport and phosphorylation of glucose versus DG, one can calculate the regional cerebral glucose utilization rates (in units of μmoles/min/g tissue).

DG can be labeled with Carbon-11 (C-11) for use with PET imaging.[91,92] The relatively short half-life of C-11 (20 minutes), however, limits the ability to minimize the background signal from the blood and free DG in tissue. Additionally, one has to rapidly utilize the tracer which cannot be conveniently distributed from commercial radiopharmacies. It does have the advantage of allowing more rapid, repetitive imaging as compared to FDG.

The tracer [C-11] glucose has also been used in conjunction with PET.[93] Short retention times in tissue due to clearance of labeled metabolities (e.g., C-11 labeled CO$_2$ and lactate), along with other problems related to the modeling of the multiple steps of glucose metabolism do not make it the tracer of choice.

In the mid 1970s, Ido, Fowler, and Wolf[94] developed a method to synthesize FDG. FDG is analogous to DG in its competition with glucose for transport and phosphorylation because the hydroxyl in the 2 position of glucose has been substituted by Fluorine. The affinity of FDG for hexokinase has previously been reported.[95] The mathematical model initially developed for DG and autoradiography was later modified[25,48] to mathematically model the hydrolysis of FDG-6-P to FDG that can occur at later times after administration. Therefore, complete trapping of FDG in tissue did not have to be assumed, as was done with the original DG model, although the amount of dephosphorylation that occurred in the 40- to 60-minute time after injection was found to be small.[25,48] The initial validation and use of FDG with PET was for studies of cerebral metabolism[25,48,96] with later extensions for other applications.

Compartmental model

Depicted in Figure 2-16 is the compartmental model used to describe FDG kinetics. The six compartment model is often represented by only showing the top three compartments in the figure. The purpose of showing two sets of three compartments is to emphasize the fact that the transport of FDG and enzyme-mediated reactions are distinct from those for glucose, although FDG does compete for the same carriers and enzymes and occupies the same physical spaces as glucose. This model is a direct extension of the Sokoloff model developed for DG and autoradiography[49] discussed in the previous section, allowing for a nonzero value of k_4^* and k_4.

The three top compartments in Figure 2-16 represent FDG in plasma, FDG in tissue, and FDG-6-P in tissue. The concentrations of FDG or FDG-6-P are C_P^* (mg/ml blood), C_E^* (mg/g tissue), C_M^* (mg/g tissue), respectively. Similarly, the glucose and glucose-6-P concentrations in the three bottom compartments are C_P (mg/ml blood), C_E (mg/g tissue), and C_M (mg/g tissue). All symbols with the asterisk represent quantities associated with the tracer, whereas quantities related to the natural substrate (glucose) are denoted without the asterisk.

The key feature that makes FDG a useful tracer for studying glucose metabolism is that FDG-6-P is not a substrate for further metabolism, as is glucose-6-P, and so it accumulates (due to a small k_4^*) in tissue in proportion to the glucose metabolic rate. This isolates the transport and phosphorylation steps from the rest of glycolysis, making the mathematical modeling of FDG simpler. In addition, tracer assays with accumulation of end products provide a record of the process trapped within the tissue.

The FDG molecules are initially confined to the vascular space when they are injected into the subject. As the tracer distributes through various capillary beds, it diffuses out into the interstitial space, and from there it is transported by the same carriers which would normally transport glucose into the cellular

FIGURE 2-16. Compartmental Model for FDG and Glucose Transport and Metabolism. The three compartments on top represent FDG kinetics between plasma FDG, extravascular FDG, and cellular FDG-6-P. The bottom three compartments represent the analogous compartments for glucose (Glc). The parameters k_2^* through k_4^* and k_2 through k_4 represent first order rate constants for FDG and Glc, respectively, which govern the movement of material between the compartments. The parameters K_1^* and K_1 are rate coefficients for FDG and Glc, respectively. The rate constants and rate coefficients have units of inverse time and volume/time/mass, respectively.

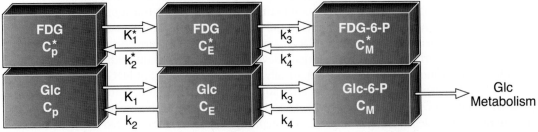

spaces. FDG is phosphorylated within the cell. It can also be slowly dephosphorylated and eventually return to the interstitial space and from there to the vascular space. In the 3-compartment model for FDG tracer kinetics, the extravascular space refers to the interstitial and the intracellular space which are lumped together to form the FDG tissue compartment. This is a simplification based on the assumption that the capillary and cell membrane can be treated as one rate-determining barrier (e.g., capillary transport is much slower than transport across the cell membranes).

The forward transport *rate coefficients* between the first two compartments (see Figure 2-16) are K_1^* and K_1 for FDG and glucose, respectively. The reverse transport rate constants between the first two compartments are k_2^* and k_2 for FDG and glucose, respectively. The rate constants between the second and third compartments denote the hexokinase-mediated phosphorylation and the phosphotase-mediated dephosphorylation reactions, and are k_3^*, k_4^* for FDG and FDG-6-P, and k_3, k_4 for glucose and glucose-6-P. Notice that the rate coefficients K_1^* and K_1 are in milliliters per minutes per gram, whereas the rate constants ($k_2 - k_4$, $k_2^* - k_4^*$) are in units of min^{-1}. The reason that K_1^* and K_1 are in different units than the other parameters is because they take into account blood flow and tracer extraction (see Equations 2-24 and 2-25). A rate constant of 0.1 min^{-1} indicates that an amount of tracer equal to 10% of that in the compartment will be transported out of the compartment every minute.

State equations
The state equations in matrix notation governing the concentration of tracer in the compartments are given as:

$$\begin{bmatrix} \dot{C}_E^* \\ \dot{C}_M^* \end{bmatrix} = \begin{bmatrix} -(k_2^* + k_3^*) & k_4^* \\ k_3^* & -k_4^* \end{bmatrix}\begin{bmatrix} C_E^* \\ C_M^* \end{bmatrix} + \begin{bmatrix} K_1^* \\ 0 \end{bmatrix} C_P^*$$

$$C_T^*(t) = \begin{bmatrix} 1 & 1 \end{bmatrix}\begin{bmatrix} C_E^* \\ C_M^* \end{bmatrix}$$

(2-14)

where a dot over a quantity represents the derivative with respect to time of that quantity. Notice also that the model response $C_T^*(t)$ is activity from both the extravascular FDG and FDG-6-P pools (the component of the measurement due to vasculature in tissue can be accounted for separately). Notice that in Equation 2-14 the plasma measurement is treated as an input into the other compartments, thereby not requiring the plasma compartment to be modeled explicitly. The direct solution of the coupled differential Equations in 2-14 (through the use of Laplace transforms) gives:

$$C_E^*(t) = \frac{K_1^*}{\alpha_2 - \alpha_1}\left[(k_4^* - \alpha_1)e^{-\alpha_1 t} + (\alpha_2 - k_4^*)e^{-\alpha_2 t}\right] \otimes C_P^*(t)$$

$$C_M^*(t) = \frac{K_1^* k_3^*}{\alpha_2 - \alpha_1}(e^{-\alpha_1 t} - e^{-\alpha_2 t}) \otimes C_P^*(t)$$

(2-15)

$$C_T^*(t) = \frac{K_1^*}{\alpha_2 - \alpha_1}\left[(k_3^* + k_4^* - \alpha_1)e^{-\alpha_1 t} + (\alpha_2 - k_3^* - k_4^*)e^{-\alpha_2 t}\right] \otimes C_P^*(t)$$

where

$$\alpha_1 = \frac{(k_2 + k_3 + k_4) - \sqrt{(k_2 + k_3 + k_4)^2 - 4k_2k_4}}{2}$$

$$\alpha_2 = \frac{(k_2 + k_3 + k_4) + \sqrt{(k_2 + k_3 + k_4)^2 - 4k_2k_4}}{2} \quad\quad (2\text{-}16)$$

EXAMPLE 2-10

The $[^{18}\text{F}]$FDG 3-compartment model is shown in Figure 2-16 and the solution to the model is given by Equation 2-15. Calculate the theoretical volume of distribution for free $[^{18}\text{F}]$FDG. Notice that the definition of all terms is provided in FDG Assay (p. 161).

Assume that $k_4^* = 0$.

ANSWER

C_P^* is the concentration of $[^{18}\text{F}]$FDG in plasma, C_E^* is the extravascular (tissue) concentration of FDG (free FDG), and C_M^* is the concentration of $[^{18}\text{F}]$FDG-6-P in tissue. The model equation for this 3 compartment model when $k_4^* = 0$ can be obtained from Equation 2-14:

$$\frac{dC_E^*(t)}{dt} = K_1^* C_P^*(t) - k_2^* C_E^*(t) - k_3^* C_E^*(t)$$

$$\frac{dC_M^*(t)}{dt} = k_3^* C_E^*(t)$$

The units of the variables are:

$$K_1^* = \text{ml blood/min/ml tissue, } C_P^* = \mu\text{Ci/ml blood}$$
$$C_E^*, C_M^* = \mu\text{Ci/ml tissue, } k_2^*, k_3^* = 1/\text{min}$$

If k_3^* is not zero, then C_E^* can never reach an equilibrium state, and the metabolite compartment C_M^* can never reach steady state; the concentration in it will increase monotonously. From the above equations, it is seen that the free compartment can reach steady state when $dC_E^*(t)/dt = 0$, and this leads to $C_E^*/C_P^* = K_1^*/(k_2^*(+ k_3^*)$.

Also, when $k_3^* = 0$, the concentration in the compartment C_E^* can reach an equilibrium state when $K_1^* C_P^*$ equals to $k_2^* C_E^*$. Such that the volume of distribution of $[^{18}\text{F}]$FDG in the free compartment in the situation of steady state is:

$$[V_{d(f)}^*]_{\text{ss}} = K_1^*/(k_2^* + k_3^*)$$
$$[V_{d(f)}^*]_{\text{eq}} = K_1^*/k_2^*$$

The subscript in the expression *f* means the free FDG compartment (C_E^*), *ss* denotes steady state, and *eq* denotes equilibrium. Equilibrium is never reached unless $k_3^* = 0$ and then $[V_{d(f)}^*]_{\text{ss}} = [V_{d(f)}^*]_{\text{eq}}$. This also implies that one can conduct a dynamic FDG PET study, estimate the rate constants, and from this directly estimate the volume of distribution of FDG without ever achieving steady state during the course of the PET study.

State equations for integrated activity

In some cases, it will be necessary to account for the fact that a measurement from a scan from time points t_{i-1} to t_i represents the *integrated* activity (AC) during that time period. This can be accomplished by minor modifications to Equations 2-15 and 2-16. Let

$$AC^\star(t) = \int_0^t \left[C_E^\star(s) + C_M^\star(s) \right] ds$$

$$\frac{d[AC^\star(t)]}{dt} = C_E^\star(t) + C_M^\star(t) \text{ with } AC^\star(0) = 0.$$

Then the system state equations can be modified to give:

$$\frac{d}{dt} \begin{bmatrix} C_E^\star \\ C_M^\star \\ AC^\star \end{bmatrix} = \begin{bmatrix} -(k_2^\star + k_3^\star) & k_4^\star & 0 \\ k_3^\star & -k_4^\star & 0 \\ 1 & 1 & 0 \end{bmatrix} \begin{bmatrix} C_E^\star \\ C_M^\star \\ AC^\star \end{bmatrix} + \begin{bmatrix} K_1^\star \\ 0 \\ 0 \end{bmatrix} C_P^\star \quad (2\text{-}17)$$

$$C_T^\star(t) = \begin{bmatrix} 0 & 0 & 1 \end{bmatrix} \begin{bmatrix} C_E^\star \\ C_M^\star \\ AC^\star \end{bmatrix}$$

Then the quantity $[C_T^\star(t_i) - C_T^\star((t_{i-1}))]$ represents the measurement obtained from a scan over time t_{i-1} to t_i. The state equation forms are important because computer routines are readily available to solve these equations directly without using the explicit solutions. The above equations can easily be modified to include a spillover term to account for that fraction of measured PET activity that is from underlying blood pool and neighboring regions that physically spill into the region of interest.[97]

The estimation of the microparameters $K_1^\star$, $k_2^\star - k_4^\star$ is necessary but not sufficient for estimating regional glucose utilization. To estimate regional glucose utilization, the competitive kinetics between FDG and glucose must be taken into account. If one focuses on the compartment for C_M, by using mass balance one obtains:

$$\frac{dC_M(t)}{dt} = -k_4 C_M(t) + k_3 C_E(t) - MRglc \quad (2\text{-}18)$$

Here, the metabolic rate of glucose utilization (MRglc) is the parameter of interest. At steady state, the above equation can be set equal to zero in order to solve for MRglc. Subsequently, using the principles of competitive kinetics, a lumped constant (*LC*) can be introduced to relate the behavior of the tracer FDG to glucose in order to obtain:[25,48]

$$MRglc = \left(\frac{K_1^\star k_3^\star}{k_2^\star + k_3^\star} \right) \frac{C_P}{LC} = K^\star \frac{C_P}{LC} \quad (2\text{-}19)$$

Here C_P is the plasma concentration of glucose, also assumed to be in steady state, and $K^\star = \dfrac{K_1^\star k_3^\star}{k_2^\star + k_3^\star}$. Further details of this derivation and the lumped constant are provided in the Appendix p. 213. It has been shown that the lumped constant is relatively fixed under various physiological conditions,[98,99] but for applications to extreme conditions, it should be revalidated. Under most conditions, phosphorylation is limited over transport. States can be reached where transport can become rate limiting (e.g., extreme hypoglycemia or low blood flow) and the *LC* will change. This occurs because glucose is preferred over FDG for phosphorylation by hexokinase, but FDG is preferred over glucose by transporters. Thus, when the rate-limiting step shifts from phosphorylation to transport, the lumped constant will change.

Alternative methods for estimating glucose utilization that have been used are also available. These approaches stem from the need to use practical and simplified methods that are conducive to clinical applications. It requires more time to obtain the full FDG kinetics so many approaches have been studied to estimate the glucose utilization rate under specific assumptions. The Patlak plot[56,57] is one approach which does not require direct estimation of the microparameters K_1^*, $k_2^* - k_4^*$ and, instead, only requires the estimation of the macroparameter K^*. Through a transformation of the time-activity data, one can obtain a set of points which can be fit to a linear equation with the slope proportional to K^*. One can, therefore, obtain as little as three time-points (from three dynamic PET images), and estimate K^*.[100]

EXAMPLE 2-11A

The Patlak equation predicts that after some time $t > t^*$ a plot of

$\dfrac{C_T^*(t)}{C_P^*(t)}$ (y-axis) vs. $\dfrac{\displaystyle\int_0^t C_P^*(s)\,ds}{C_P^*(t)}$ (x-axis) (where C_T^* is the total tissue activity and C_P^* is the plasma activity at time t) will be essentially linear with a slope of K^*. Derive that this is the case for the FDG model with $k_4^* \approx 0$.

ANSWER

Because $k_4^* \approx 0$, we can view the C_M^* compartment as irreversible. By this we mean that the tracer is essentially trapped once it enters this compartment. We begin by writing:

$$C_T^*(t) = C_E^*(t) + C_M^*(t) \qquad (1)$$

$$\frac{dC_M^*(t)}{dt} = \text{total input} - k_b^* C_M^*(t) \qquad (2)$$

where the total input is the amount of tracer that enters into the irreversible region per unit of time from both the plasma pool and the interstitial pool. Assuming that k_b^* is sufficiently close to zero, the total input in the above equation is approximately the same as when $k_b^* = 0$. In order to obtain the total input, we proceed by letting $(C_M^*)_0$ represent the amount of tracer present if in fact $k_b^* = 0$ (subscript 0 will be used to designate the case $k_b^* = 0$). Then we may write Equation 2 as

$$\frac{d(C_M^*)_0(t)}{dt} = K^* C_P^*(t) \qquad (3A)$$

so that by integrating the above over all time and solving for K^* we obtain:

$$K^* = \frac{(C_M^*)_0(\infty)}{\int_0^\infty C_P^*(s)\,ds} \left(\frac{\text{mg/g}}{(\text{mg/ml})\text{min}} = \text{ml/g/min} \right) \quad (3B)$$

Now we will also assume that for times greater than time t, the plasma concentration of tracer is zero, then we will have:

$$\int_0^t C_P^*(s)\,ds = \int_0^\infty C_P^*(s)\,ds \quad (4)$$

We also notice that the concentration of tracer in the irreversible compartment at time infinity will equal the amount that is there at time t plus the amount that is in the interstitial pool that does not go back to the plasma pool and out of the system. If we let $G(t)$ represent the fraction of the amount of tracer in the irreversible compartment that *does go back* into the plasma and leaves the system, (notice that this fraction in general is a function of time) we can obtain:

$$(C_M^*)_0(\infty) = (C_M^*)_0(t) + [1 - G(t)]C_E^*(t) \quad (5)$$

Substituting Equations 3 and 4 into the above, we obtain:

$$K^* \int_0^t C_P^*(s)\,ds = (C_M^*)_0(t) + [1 - G(t)]C_E^*(t) \quad (6)$$

Solving Equation 6 for $(C_M^*)_0(t)$ and differentiating, we obtain:

$$\frac{d(C_M^*)_0(t)}{dt} = K^*C_P^*(t) - \frac{d\{[1 - G(t)]C_E^*(t)\}}{dt} \quad (7)$$

By comparing this to Equation 2, we notice that the total input must be equal to the right hand side of Equation 6 (the value of the total input is the same whether or not $k_b^* = 0$). Therefore, by substituting the right hand side of Equation 7 into Equation 2 we obtain:

$$\frac{dC_M^*(t)}{dt} = K^*C_P^*(t) - \frac{d\{[1 - G(t)]C_E^*(t)\}}{dt} - k_b^*C_M^*(t) \quad (8)$$

Solving the above differential equation (Equation 8) and integrating by parts, and using Equation 1 to obtain $C_T^*(t)$ gives:

$$C_T^*(t) = \int_0^t e^{k_b^*(s-1)}\{K^*C_P^*(s) + k_b^*[1 - G(s)]C_E^*(s)\}\,ds + G(t)C_E^*(t) \quad (9)$$

If the change in the plasma concentration eventually becomes small enough, then there will be a t^* such that for all $t > t^*$, $C_E^*(t) = C_P^*(t)$ (an effective steady state is reached), and $G(t)$ will become a constant G. Now since $[1-G(t)] < 1$, $k_b^* \sim 0$, so that *for $t > t^*$* Equation 9 simplifies to:

$$C_T^*(t) = K^* \int_0^t e^{k_b^*(s-1)}C_P^*(s)\,ds + GC_P^*(t) \quad (10)$$

This last equation shows that if one plots:

$$\frac{C_T^*(t)}{C_P^*(t)} \quad \text{vs.} \quad \frac{\int_0^t C_P^*(s)\,ds}{C_P^*(t)}$$

a straight line will result (after $t > t^*$) and that the slope of this line will be K^* and the y-intercept will be G.

EXAMPLE 2-11B

The data table below contains simulated sampling times and the plasma time-activity values (Plasma) in columns 1 and 2, respectively, and sampling times and the tissue time-activity values (Tissue) in columns 3 and 4, respectively.

Graph the plasma and tissue time-activity curves and the Patlak plot. Also estimate the slope of the Patlak plot. *Note the last two columns of the table below will help you to make the Patlak plot.*

Time	Plasma	Time	Tissue	$\dfrac{\int_0^t C_P^*(s)\,ds}{C_P^*(t)}$	$\dfrac{C_T^*(t)}{C_P^*(t)}$
0.28	0.02	0.23	0.00	0.00	0.00
0.73	200.84	1.23	32.85	0.50	0.03
0.98	1149.70	2.23	95.47	2.27	0.13
1.48	1453.60	3.48	124.92	6.25	0.33
1.95	832.43	5.48	145.45	13.08	0.64
2.97	477.88	8.98	155.05	33.75	1.47
3.47	379.32	17.48	158.32	102.60	3.90
4.97	249.13	27.48	163.35	209.56	7.64
7.97	119.83	37.48	168.13	336.42	12.15
11.95	62.38	47.48	171.82	462.43	16.64
19.95	30.93	57.48	174.68	641.48	23.03
29.95	18.24	67.48	176.80	819.18	29.36
39.95	12.39	77.48	178.59	1028.30	36.82
59.97	6.90	87.48	179.92	1367.60	48.92
89.95	3.39	97.48	180.94	1694.40	60.55
119.95	1.79	112.48	182.09	2329.30	83.13

ANSWER

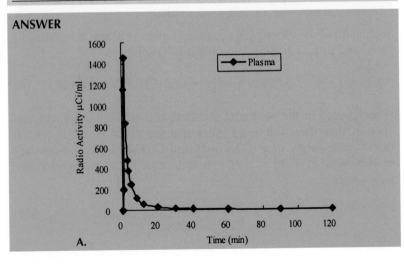

A.

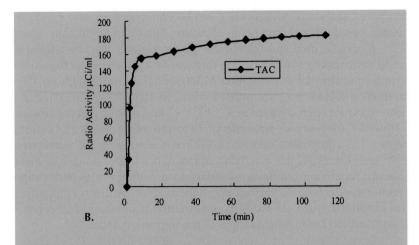

B.

Figures A and B above are the plasma and the tissue time-activity curves (TAC), respectively.

The Patlak plot (Figure C, below) is obtained by plotting:

$$\frac{\int_0^t C_p^*(s)\,ds}{C_p^*(t)} \text{ (x-axis, units of time) vs. } \frac{C_T^*(t)}{C_p^*(t)} \text{ (y-axis, unitless).}$$

The slope of the regressed line is estimated at 0.036 which should equal K^* in Equation 2-19.

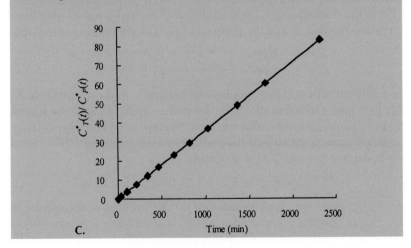

C.

There are also approaches in which a single time point (single PET image) can be obtained at relatively late times after the FDG injection; Equation 2-20 is then used for estimating MRglc:

$$MRglc$$

$$= \frac{\dfrac{C_P}{LC}\left\{ C_T^*(T) - \dfrac{K_1^*}{\alpha_2 - \alpha_1}\left[(k_4^* - \alpha_1)e^{-\alpha_1 t} + (\alpha_2 - k_4^*)e^{-\alpha_2 t}\right]\right\} \otimes C_P^*(t)}{\dfrac{k_2^* + k_3^*}{\alpha_2 - \alpha_1}(e^{-\alpha_1 t} - e^{-\alpha_2 t}) \otimes C_P^*(t)} \quad (2\text{-}20)$$

In the above equation α_1 and α_2 are given by Equation 2-16, and $C_T^*(T)$ is the PET image-based value of tracer concentration. The mean population values for K_1^*, $k_2^* - k_4^*$ can be used and $C_P^*(t)$ must be determined (e.g., by arterial sampling and radioactivity counting). One might at first glance expect that equation 2-20 would not do well in estimating MRglc because mean values for the microparameters K_1^*, $k_2^* - k_4^*$ are utilized when, in fact, changes in rates of metabolism occur through changes in K_1^*, $k_2^* - k_4^*$ and plasma glucose concentration. However, for relatively late times of 40 to 120 minutes after FDG injection, the term $C_T^*(T)$ dominates relative to the term containing the microparameters,[25,48] and, therefore, the exact rate constants for a specific rate of metabolism are not required. Modifications of Equation 2-20 have also been proposed for specific applications to various populations.[101,102] A direct comparison of various simplified approaches to FDG quantitation in oncology studies has been published and further highlights some of the important issues.[103]

^{13}N ammonia perfusion assay

Blood flow is the amount or volume of blood supplied during a time interval to an organ or tissue type of interest. Flow has units of volume per unit of time (ml/min). Perfusion is defined as flow per unit of mass of tissue (ml/min/g tissue). *The term blood flow as used in this section refers to blood perfusion.* To understand the modeling of ^{13}NH$_3$ tracer kinetics, it is important to incorporate the concepts of extraction fraction discussed earlier (see Tracer Extraction, this chapter).

Studies with ^{13}NH$_3$ and canine myocardium[104,105] using residue function measurements have shown the relationship between the first pass extraction fraction E and the perfusion (F). These studies also showed a relationship between the retention fraction E_r and the perfusion (F). The relationships are given as:

$$E = 1 - 0.096e^{-1.09/F} = 1 - e^{-(2.34F+1.08)/F}$$
$$E_r = 1 - 0.607e^{-1.25/F} = 1 - e^{-(F/2+1.25)/F}$$

$$(2\text{-}21)$$

where F is in units of milliliters per minute per gram. In these equations, E represents first pass extraction of ^{13}NH$_3$ from the capillaries into the interstitial space, and E_r represents the extraction from the capillaries and interstitial spaces into a *slowly exchanging* myocardial pool from metabolism of ^{13}NH$_3$. By comparing Equations 2-4 and 2-21 one obtains:

$$PS \text{ (ml/min/g)} = F/2 + 1.25 \text{ for } F \text{ in ml/min/g} \qquad (2\text{-}22)$$

where this PS represents the permeability surface product of the *cellular membranes*. Notice that the PS product is not a constant but a function of flow, as compared to the rigid tube model shown in the Renkin–Crone equation (Equation 2-4).

By defining the retention fraction to be the ratio of tracer extracted by the tissue to the total amount delivered, one can write the concentration of tracer in tissue (C_m) at time T to be

$$C_m(T) = E_r F \int_0^T C_P(t)\,dt \qquad (2\text{-}23)$$

where $C_p(t)$ is the concentration of tracer in the blood. This equation is sometimes useful for quantitating the product of E_r and F but does not account for changes in the retention fraction as a function of flow. It can, however, be solved for F if one can use a known relationship such as Equation 2-21 for the dependence of E_r on F.

$^{13}NH_3$ two-compartment model

Shown in Figure 2-17 is the $^{13}NH_3$ two-compartmental model used for the estimation of regional myocardial blood flow (rMBF). This model was originally proposed by Smith[106] and has previously been validated in canine myocardium by comparing estimates obtained from PET studies and model fitting against the microsphere method. The two compartments represent the mass of tracer in a relatively fast pool (Q_f^*) which has a volume of distribution V_f (ml/g) and mass of tracer in a slower pool (Q_s^*). The units of Q_f^* and Q_s^* are in counts per pixel (equivalently, c/g tissue).

The tracer is brought into the fast pool by blood which arrives at a mean perfusion F (ml/min/g) (F is equivalent to rMBF). The tracer may leave the fast pool through venous outflow at a mean perfusion F, or it may be transported into the slow pool as governed by a parameter K_1^* (F) (ml/min/g), which is not a constant, but depends on the blood flow. Tracer may also slowly be exchanged between the slow pool back to the fast pool as governed by the rate constant k_r^* (min^{-1}).

Many features of this model must be understood before proceeding. The fast and slow pools can be associated with their biochemical and physiological counterparts but this must be done with caution. Isolated rabbit heart septum experiments suggest that $^{13}NH_3$ tracer kinetics have 2 fast and 1 slow exponential components, suggesting that three compartments are necessary, but applications to PET data indicate that only two exponential components are separately identifiable. This is primarily because of the inadequate temporal resolution of PET. Various sources of noise can also make the separation of the two fast components difficult. The two compartments in this model represent a free space, composed of vascular and freely diffusible $^{13}NH_3$, and a second compartment for

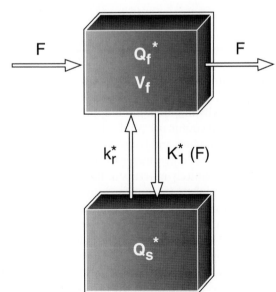

FIGURE 2-17. Two-compartment ^{13}N Ammonia Model. The two compartments represent fast and slow turnover pools for the tracer. Tracer arrives at a flow rate F (or rMBF) into the fast compartment which has a volume of distribution V_f. From the fast compartment, the tracer can move to the slowly exchanging compartment as governed by the parameter K_1^* (F). It can also slowly return to the fast pool as governed by the rate constant k_r^*.

products of $^{13}NH_3$ metabolism. This model essentially lumps the free $^{13}NH_3$ ammonia regardless of whether it is in the vasculature, interstitial space, or even within cells. This freely diffusible pool is the relatively fast pool. The metabolically bound $^{13}NH_3$ (primarily in the form of ^{13}N-glutamate and glutamine) is the slow pool where the tracer is effectively trapped.

The parameter $K_1^* (F)$ can be explicitly written once the compartmental extraction fraction is known. The extraction of tracer from the fast to the slow compartment can be written as (for $k_r^* = 0$):

$$E_r = \frac{K_1^*}{(K_1^* + F)} \tag{2-24}$$

which is an alternate way[107] of describing the *compartmental* extraction fraction as compared to the standard Renkin–Crone equation discussed previously (see Tracer Extraction, p. 141). This equation can also be used with E (as opposed to E_r), depending on the process being modeled. By equating the retention fraction of Equation 2-21 to Equation 2-24 we obtain:

$$K_1^* (F) = F \left[e^{\frac{F/2+1.25}{F}} - 1 \right] \tag{2-25}$$

Equation 2-25 forms the basis for why K_1^* is written as $K_1^* (F)$ in the $^{13}NH_3$ 2-compartment model. E_r is used to obtain $K_1^* (F)$ because E_r represents extraction of tracer from the fast to the slow pool.

State equations

The state equations governing the amount of tracer in the compartments are given as

$$\begin{bmatrix} \dot{Q}_f^* \\ \dot{Q}_s^* \end{bmatrix} = \begin{bmatrix} \dfrac{-(K_1^* + F)}{V_f} & k_r^* \\ \dfrac{K_1^*}{V_f} & -k_r^* \end{bmatrix} \begin{bmatrix} Q_f^* \\ Q_s^* \end{bmatrix} + \begin{bmatrix} F\rho_b \\ 0 \end{bmatrix} C_p^* \tag{2-26}$$

$$C_m^*(t) = \begin{bmatrix} 1 & 1 \end{bmatrix} \begin{bmatrix} Q_f^* \\ Q_s^* \end{bmatrix}$$

where a dot over a quantity represents the derivative with respect to time of that quantity. The parameter ρ_b is the density of blood (~ 1 g/ml). Here C_p^* represents $^{13}NH_3$ activity in blood and is approximated by the LV time-activity curve which is in units of counts per pixel. The model response $C_m^*(t)$ is activity from both the slow and fast pools and is also in units of counts per pixel. In the above state equations, K_1^* is not a parameter to be estimated but is instead given by Equation 2-25 which is entirely in terms of the flow parameter. Although these equations are easily extended to account for scan duration and integrated activity, the midtime scan approximation can be used, so that $C_m^*(t_n)$ will represent the activity measurement at the midtime of scan number n in counts per pixel per second.

This 2-compartment model has successfully been used to estimate rMBF while fixing $V_f = 0.8$ ml/g, fixing $k_r^* = 0$ min^{-1}, and using a dynamic imaging protocol with several short duration (10–15 seconds) scans followed by some longer scans during which the myocardial wall is better imaged. The earlier scans allow for adequate sampling of the blood time-activity curve as approximated by the LV time-activity curve. Strictly speaking, the blood time-activity data must be corrected for metabolites before using the data with this model. The blood time-activity curve must also be corrected for the fraction of blood pool activity that is due to components other than $^{13}NH_3$. For use of data at later times, one must additionally account for metabolites that may be taken up from blood by myocardial tissue.

In human studies, the model fitting can be performed with time-activity data from approximately the first 2 minutes only, during which time the effects of metabolites in blood have been shown to be negligible.[108,109] This removes the need for metabolite determination and blood time-activity curve correction. The model fitting can be accomplished with the same model described above. The primary assumption is that E_r (see Equation 2-24) is still given by the relationship determined for canine myocardium. The use of this relationship in human studies will need further investigation. Applications of the $^{13}NH_3$ assay for measuring myocardial perfusion can be found in Chapter 6.

Other tracer kinetic models and quantitation approaches for perfusion while using ^{13}N Ammonia have also been proposed in the literature and are discussed elsewhere[110,111] and in Chapter 6. Practical simplifications to the ^{13}N ammonia model including a Patlak approximation have also been reported.[112] Other issues related to tracer kinetic modeling specifically for nuclear cardiology studies are discussed elsewhere.[113]

Receptor-ligand assays

Some assays for PET require modeling a process in which the PET tracer is a ligand for one or more tissue receptors. The binding of ligand to receptor may be reversible or irreversible. Important parameters in these assays include B_{max} (concentration of receptors typically in moles of receptor per gram of tissue), k_{off} (disassociation rate constant for an *in vitro* experiment where ligand in a dialysate or supernatant is exposed to a tissue sample which contains receptors), k_{on} (association rate constant *in vitro*), K_d (which equals k_{off}/k_{on}) (Figure 2-18), and finally the rate coefficients and constants in a tracer kinetic model for modeling the *in vivo* behavior of the radiolabeled ligand (Figure 2-19).

In many cases, a three-compartment model is assumed to adequately describe ligand kinetics in areas where there are receptors. The first compartment represents the arterial concentration of tracer, the second represents the free compartment (consisting of several regions including interstitial fluid and intracellular cytoplasm), and the third compartment is the region of specific binding. The nonspecific binding compartment is often lumped with the free compartment because in practice this compartment is in rapid equilibrium with the free compartment. In regions

FIGURE 2-18. Receptor-ligand Model in vitro. *In vitro* compartment model for describing kinetics of receptor ligand assays. A dialysate or supernatant containing ligand can interact with a tissue sample containing receptor. The rate of association (k_{on}) and disassociation (k_{off}) govern ligand-receptor kinetics.

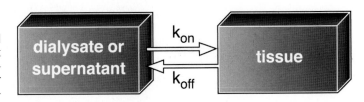

k_{on} = association rate constant
k_{off} = dissociation rate constant

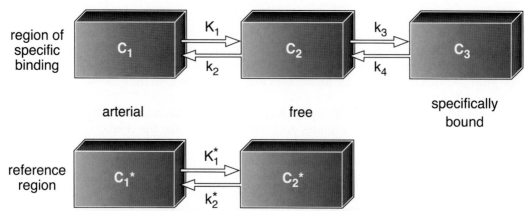

FIGURE 2-19. Receptor-ligand Model *in vivo*. The reference region contains no receptors and, therefore, is represented by a two-compartment model. The specific binding to receptor is represented by compartment 3 and the kinetics are represented by k_3 and k_4.

where there are no receptors, a two-compartment model usually suffices. In contrast to *in vitro* experiments, for a single injection of radioligand, one can only determine variables that are proportional to B_{max}/K_d instead of each individual parameter separately,[114] commonly referred to as the binding potential.

If multiple tracer injections are performed at different specific activities, then it becomes possible to estimate B_{max} directly.[115] Another important distinction between *in vitro* experiments and PET experiments for receptor and ligand interaction is that for PET experiments the ligand does not usually reach equilibrium; however, the time-activity data are fit to derive parameters found at equilibrium. One of the most common errors is to assume that the tracer kinetic model parameters are *equivalent* to parameters in the *in vitro* assay; they are related but not equivalent. If an input function is not available, then approaches have been developed that use reference regions.[114] Further details of various models and approaches to fitting PET receptor and ligand data may be found elsewhere.[114,116,117] For examples of specific PET receptor ligand assays, the reader is referred to Chapter 7 and the following references:[64,70,118–140]

EXAMPLE 2-12

Show $\dfrac{B_{max}}{K_d} = \dfrac{[LR]}{[L]}$ where $[L]$ is ligand concentration in serum, $[LR]$ is the concentration of bound ligand to serum, $[R]$ is the unbound receptor concentration, and $\dfrac{k_{off}}{k_{on}} = K_d$ for models in Figure 2-19.

ANSWER

$$\frac{dC_3(t)}{dt} = k_3 C_2(t) - k_4 C_3(t)$$

$$\frac{dC_2(t)}{dt} = K_1 C_1(t) - k_2 C_2(t) - k_3 C_2(t) + k_4 C_3(t).$$

At equilibrium we have $\dfrac{k_3}{k_4} = \dfrac{C_3}{C_2}$ and $K_1C_1 + k_4C_3 = C_2(k_2 + k_3)$ by setting the above two equations to 0.

By definition at equilibrium, we have $V_3 = \dfrac{C_3}{C_1}$ and $V_2 = \dfrac{C_2}{C_1}$, therefore $\dfrac{k_3}{k_4} = \dfrac{V_3}{V_2}$ $k_{on}[L][R] = k_{off}[LR]$, and rearranging gives

$$\frac{[LR]}{[L]} = \frac{k_{on}[R]}{k_{off}}$$

But $\dfrac{k_{off}}{k_{on}} = K_d$ and $[R] = B_{max}$, so that $\dfrac{B_{max}}{K_d} = [R] \cdot \dfrac{k_{on}}{k_{off}} = \dfrac{[LR]}{[L]}$

Assays for imaging reporter gene expression

For discussion of this assay, a different approach than that used in previous sections will be used. We will discuss this assay so as to integrate some of the concepts discussed throughout this chapter. We will go through each of the steps of model development as shown in Figure 2-4 to reinforce the issues related to assay development. We will first begin with some background information on reporter genes to establish the foundation of the environment to be modeled and then proceed to the development of a PET-based assay.

The process of gene expression involves *transcription* of a gene into messenger RNA (mRNA), and *translation* of mRNA into protein[142] (Figure 2-20). The process of transcription is regulated by regulatory regions (e.g., promoters/enhancers) leading to control over levels of mRNA expressed. These regulatory regions are coded in the DNA and bind various proteins, leading to transcription of a specific gene. The fact that some genes are only transcribed in some cells and not others is due to the presence of cell-type-specific regulatory proteins that interact with the regulatory DNA regions, as well as cell-type-specific DNA methylation and histone modification patterns. Many potential targets of PET tracers are proteins either on the cell surface and/or within the cells. One of the potential limiting issues for PET assay development is the need for new tracers for each and every new cellular target. Approaches to working around this limitation include the use of reporter gene assays described next.

Molecular biologists have long used reporter genes both in cell culture and *in vivo* to monitor gene expression. The term reporter is used because the reporter gene can report back on one or more cellular events. Reporter genes can be used to study promoter/enhancer elements involved in gene expression by *mutating* the regulatory regions to determine what are the critical regions involved in regulation. Inducible promoters (e.g., tetracycline responsive elements) can be used to look at the induction of gene expression by externally controlled inducers (e.g., doxycycline), and endogenous gene expression can be *indirectly* studied through the use of transgenes containing the endogenous gene promoters fused to the reporter gene. In all of these areas of application, the introduction of a transgene into the target tissue(s) has to be first accomplished. Subsequently, expression of the reporter gene can be tracked, and therefore, gene expression can be studied. The key is that regulatory regions (promoter/enhancer) can be fused with reporter genes to study many different processes

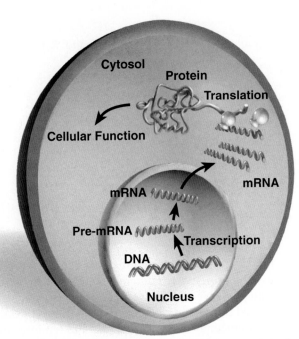

FIGURE 2-20. Cellular Gene Expression. DNA is transcribed into pre-mRNA in the cell nucleus under the control of regulatory regions known as enhancers/promoters. The pre-mRNA is processed into mRNA which is then transported to the cytoplasm and translated by ribosomes into proteins. The proteins are responsible for the structure and various biochemical functions of the cell. These functions include regulation of gene expression itself, metabolism of substrates, cell cytoskeletal structure, cell surface receptors, substrate transporters, and so on. Most PET assays to date are aimed at quantitation of protein levels (e.g., receptor and enzyme assays and reactions mediated by these proteins).

of interest without developing a new probe (tracer) for each process of interest. Although these approaches are *indirect*, they are powerful because they allow the study of many different processes.

Specific examples of conventional reporter genes include the bacterial gene chloramphenicol acetyl transferase (CAT) and the lacZ gene which codes for β-galactosidase. Autoradiography of a chromatogram (when using CAT) or enzyme assay (when using lacZ) can then be used to assay cell extracts for the product of the reporter gene.[141] For tissue specimens, the same reporter genes can also be used, with the use of immunohistochemistry or histochemical staining. A reporter gene (e.g., alkaline phosphatase) which can lead to a protein product secreted into the blood stream can also be used, thereby allowing monitoring in living animals. However, the location(s) of the reporter gene is (are) not determined in this case because only the blood can be sampled easily.

Conventional reporter gene methods are limited by their inability to noninvasively determine the *location(s)* of gene expression in *living* animals and do this repeatedly over time in the same animal. Approaches using fluorescence with green fluorescent protein (GFP)[142–145] and bioluminescence with firefly/renilla luciferase[142–146] have proven to be useful in rodents due to the relatively small amount of tissue that visible light must traverse through for external detection. However, these imaging techniques are limited because of their lack of generalizability (e.g., GFP would not work with most human applications) and detailed tomographic resolution. Further details of optical approaches can be found elsewhere.[147–149]

PET imaging offers the means for monitoring the location(s), magnitude, and time-variation of reporter gene expression (with potentially very high sensitivity) for *in vivo* use in animals and humans. Shown in Figure 2-21 is the general approach in which a PET reporter gene which encodes for either an enzyme or receptor can lead to the *trapping* of a radioactive imaging reporter probe (tracer), thereby allowing imaging of reporter gene expression.

Properties of the ideal reporter genes for PET imaging

The ideal reporter gene/reporter probe assay should have the following characteristics:[150,151]

1. The reporter gene should be present in mammalian cells but not commonly expressed (this will prevent an immune response).
2. When expressed, the reporter protein should produce specific reporter probe accumulation only in those cells in which it is expressed.
3. When the reporter gene is not expressed, there should be no significant accumulation of reporter probe in cells.

FIGURE 2-21. PET Reporter Gene Schematic. Introduction of a PET reporter gene into target cell(s), with subsequent expression of the reporter gene leads to trapping of an imaging PET reporter probe. The reporter gene is driven by a promoter of choice leading to transcriptional control of the reporter gene. The reporter probe can be trapped due to an enzyme or receptor mediated mechanism. The imaging probe does not have to enter the cell if the reporter gene encodes for a receptor located on the surface of the cell. Cells that do not express the reporter gene should not significantly trap the reporter probe leading to specific signal only from those cells in which the reporter gene is expressed.

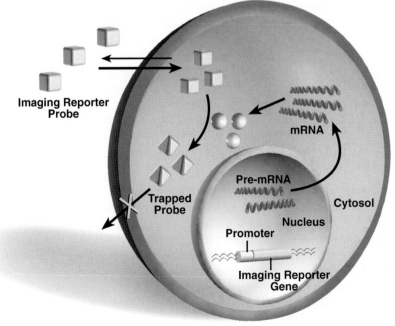

4. There should be no significant immune reaction to the reporter gene product unless one is desired (e.g., cancer therapy).

5. The reporter probe should be stable *in vivo* and not be converted to *peripheral* metabolites that complicate the development of a quantitative assay.

6. The reporter probe should be rapidly cleared from the blood and nonspecific sites in tissues and preferably have an elimination route that does not interfere with the detection of specific signal.

7. The reporter probe should be conveniently radiolabeled with a variety of radionuclides without significant change in its properties and should be labeled with an appropriate specific activity.

8. The reporter probe or its metabolites should not be cytotoxic at the concentrations used. This is likely to be the case for most tracer applications, which are based on very low concentrations of tracer.

9. The size of the reporter gene and the promoter driving it should be small enough to fit in the delivery vehicle (e.g., for a conventional adenoviral vector the upper limit is ~7 Kb). This requirement can be relaxed for animal applications such as transgenics in which a delivery vehicle is usually not needed.

10. The reporter probe must be able to reach the area(s) of interest without transport across membranes being a significant limitation.

11. The reporter probe image signal should correlate well (over the range of concentration relevant to the study paradigm) with levels of reporter gene mRNA and protein in vivo.

12. The reporter gene assay should correlate well with levels of endogenous gene expression, if the reporter gene is being used to indirectly monitor endogenous gene expression.

No single reporter gene/reporter probe system currently meets all these criteria. It is likely that each reporter gene /reporter probe system will only meet some of the above criteria, and therefore, different reporter systems will have to be chosen based on the intended application. The development of multiple reporter gene/reporter probe systems will help to provide a choice, based on their application of interest, for future investigators. Furthermore, by having multiple reporter gene assays, it should be possible to monitor the expression of more than one reporter gene in the same living animal or human. Several reporter gene assays have already been developed or are under active investigation.[149,152] This section we will focus on one of the more extensively studied reporter genes, the herpes simplex virus Type-1 thymidine kinase (HSV1-tk) reporter gene. Notice that *HSV1-tk* denotes the gene and *HSV1-TK* denotes the enzyme.

Assay for HSV1-tk reporter gene expression

In order to develop the HSV1-tk reporter gene assay, this section will strictly follow the approach outlined earlier in Figure 2-4. First, characterize the goals of this assay. It is desired that from the PET time-activity data of a reporter probe (e.g., a tracer such as radiolabeled penciclovir that is phosphorylated by HSV1-TK), that one can estimate the rate of reporter probe phosphorylation and, therefore, the relative concentration of HSV1-TK. Although the assay is referred to as one to measure HSV1-tk reporter gene expression, it is more specifically an assay to measure HSV1-TK enzyme activity. The link between HSV1-TK enzyme activity and levels of HSV1-tk messenger RNA (mRNA) are not directly determinable by using a reporter probe for HSV1-TK alone. Furthermore, the rate of transcription of the HSV1-tk gene is also not directly determinable. However, in some applications it may be the case that levels of active HSV1-TK correlate well with levels of gene transcription and mRNA translation. Furthermore, if the HSV1-tk reporter gene is being used to monitor an endogenous gene of interest (by using an endogenous promoter to drive transcription), then it may also be the case that the assay can indirectly quantitate levels of *endogenous* gene mRNA and/or protein.[153] The motivation for quantitating HSV1-tk reporter gene expression is that it may allow determining the levels of gene expression in target tissue(s), monitoring of specific cell populations that are expressing the reporter gene, as well as a whole host of other applications discussed later. Notice it is *not* the goal of the assay being discussed here to understand the rate of ganciclovir/penciclovir uptake/phosphorylation as in a treatment paradigm while using an imaging tracer to monitor treatment. The assays as derived here do not assume any competition with a pharmaceutical agent.

The next step in assay development is to work with the biologist and chemists to characterize the underlying biochemistry for this reporter system. Two known *mammalian* thymidine kinases are a mitochondrial and a cytosolic enzyme.[154] These kinases are responsible for catalyzing the transfer of the γ-phosphate from ATP to the 5′-terminus of deoxythymidine to form deoxythymidine monophosphate (dTMP). When cells are infected with the Herpes simplex virus, the *viral* thymidine kinase is also expressed. The viral thymidine kinase has relaxed substrate specificity as compared to the mammalian thymidine kinases and is capable of phosphorylating both pyrimidine and purine nucleoside derivatives,[155] as well as deoxythymidine. These compounds, when phosphorylated, are trapped intracellularly (due to their negative charge). Figure 2-22 shows some of the tracers utilized for the HSV1-tk reporter gene assay and their full chemical names and abbreviations. These tracers include 8-[^{18}F]-fluoroacyclovir (FACV), 8-[^{18}F]-fluoroganciclovir (FGCV), 8-[^{18}F]-fluoropenciclovir (FPCV), 9-[(3-[^{18}F]fluoro-1-hydroxy-2-propoxy)methyl]guanine (FHPG), 9-(4-[^{18}F]-fluoro-3-hydroxymethylbutyl)guanine (FHBG), and 5-iodo-2′-fluoro-2′-deoxy-1-β-D-arabinofuranosyluracil (FIAU). Figure 2-23 illustrates some of the biochemical issues for the HSV1-tk reporter gene that must be considered in developing an assay.

The discovery that 9-(2-hydroxyethoxymethyl)guanine (acyclovir) is phosphorylated by the viral thymidine kinase but not significantly by the mammalian TKs resulted in one of the most successful approaches to the treatment of Herpes simplex virus (HSV) infection.[156] Subsequent phosphorylation of acyclovir monophosphate by guanylate kinase to form acyclovir diphosphate, followed by phosphorylation by various cellular enzymes leads to the formation of acyclovir triphosphate. Acyclovir triphosphate leads to DNA chain termination when it is incorporated into DNA and acts as a more potent inhibitor of the viral DNA polymerases than of cellular polymerases (enzymes that are involved in synthesis of DNA/RNA). The DNA polymerases of HSV Type 1 and 2 also use acyclovir triphosphate as a substrate and incorporate it into the DNA primer-template to a much greater extent than do the cellular enzymes. The viral DNA polymerase binds strongly to the acyclovir triphosphate-terminated template and is thereby inactivated.[156] Multiple substrates for HSV1-TK including ganciclovir

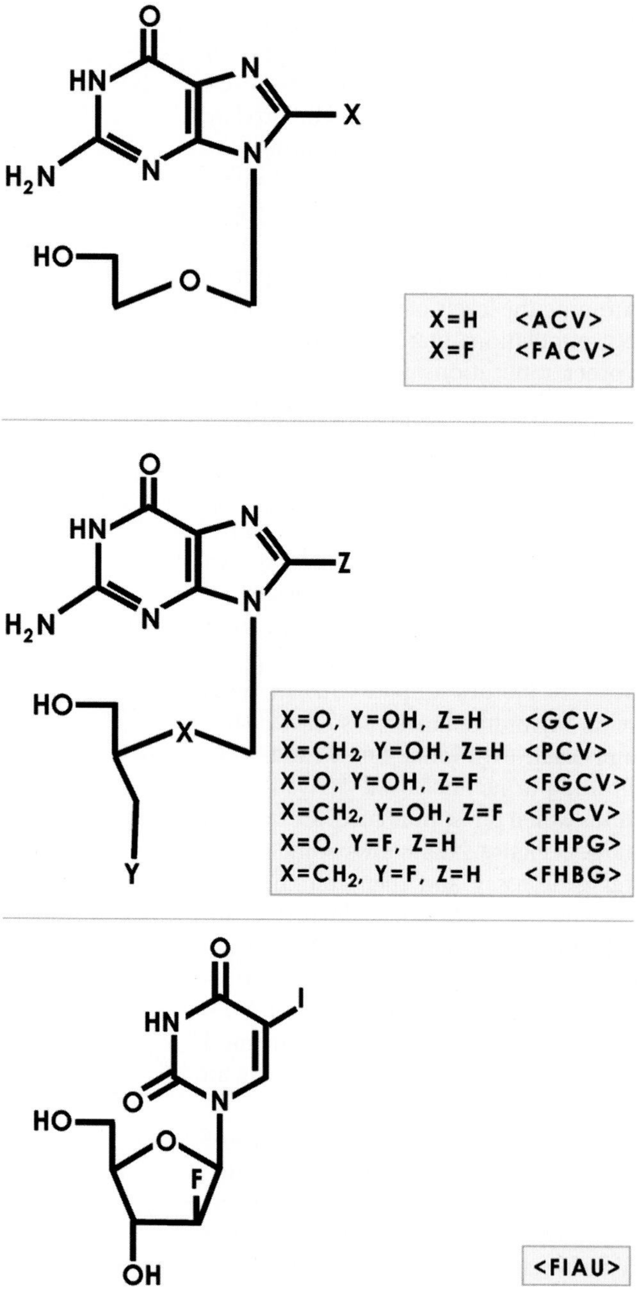

FIGURE 2-22. Chemical Structures of Various Substrates for HSV1-TK and the Corresponding PET Tracers. Acyclovir (ACV), Ganciclovir (GCV), Penciclovir (PCV), and 5-iodo-2'-fluoro-2'-deoxy-1-β-D-arabinofuranosyluracil (FIAU) are all potential substrates for HSV1-TK that have their roots in therapeutics. By labeling with either Fluorine-18 to produce FACV, FGCV, FPCV, FHPG, FHBG, or Iodine [124]I to, in turn, produce FIAU, one has potential PET tracers for monitoring HSV1-tk reporter gene expression. Notice FHPG and FHBG have labeling of Fluorine-18 on the side chain and produce a racemic mixture of two distinct compounds. Although FIAU has a fluorine, it is not easy to replace this with a Fluorine-18, so it has instead been labeled with Iodine-124.

X=H	<ACV>
X=F	<FACV>

X=O, Y=OH, Z=H	<GCV>
X=CH$_2$ Y=OH, Z=H	<PCV>
X=O, Y=OH, Z=F	<FGCV>
X=CH$_2$, Y=OH, Z=F	<FPCV>
X=O, Y=F, Z=H	<FHPG>
X=CH$_2$, Y=F, Z=H	<FHBG>

<FIAU>

(9-[[2-hydroxy-1-(hydroxymethyl)ethoxy]methyl]guanine) and penciclovir (9-(4-hydroxy-3-hydroxymethylbutyl)guanine) have subsequently been synthesized and reported in the literature as antiviral agents.[157] *As is often the case with PET assays, knowledge of existing pharmaceutical agents helps to develop PET tracers for imaging assays.* Please see Chapter 4 for measures of affinity of HSV1-TK for various substrates.

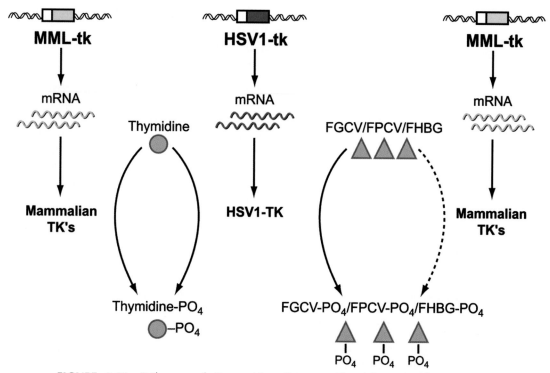

FIGURE 2-23. Pathways of Competition Between Thymidine, Acycloguanosines (FGCV/FPCV/FHBG), and the Mamallian (MML) and HSV1 thymidine kinases (tk). In a cell in which the HSV1-tk gene is being transcribed, there will be mammalian thymidine kinases (MML-TK) as well as HSV1-TK. HSV1-TK can potentially phosphorylate thymidine and various substrates (e.g., fluorinated derivatives of ganciclovir and pencicloivr). However, the MML-TK does not significantly phosphorylate FGCV/FPCV/FHBG.

The use of HSV1-tk as a reporter gene is possible because it can potentially lead to trapping a reporter probe only in those cells in which it is expressed. Several characteristics of HSV1-tk make it an ideal reporter gene:

1. Several substrates (e.g., acyclovir, ganciclovir, penciclovir, thymidine analogs) can be trapped in cells by the HSV1-TK enzyme through phosphorylation.
2. The FGCV, FPCV, and FHBG substrates for HSV1-TK are not significantly phosphorylated by the mamallian thymidine kinases and thymidine analogs only minimally so.
3. Each enzyme molecule can potentially phosphorylate many individual substrate molecules leading to significant signal amplification.
4. Various substrates can potentially be labeled with Carbon-11, Fluorine-18, or Iodine-124 to produce a PET compatible tracer.

In addition to these advantages, some potential disadvantages are:

1. The HSV1-tk gene is a foreign gene and produces a protein (HSV1-TK) that can lead to an immune response.
2. There is the necessity of transport of any potential substrate (tracer) into the cell in order for HSV1-TK to subsequently phosphorylate the tracer.

3. Enodgenous substrates (e.g., thymidine) could potentially compete with the tracer of choice for both transport and phosphorylation.
4. Expression of the reporter gene may interfere with normal cellular processes, although at low levels of expression this should be negligible.

One potential use of HSV1-tk as a reporter gene coupled with a reporter probe (e.g., Fluorine-18 labeled ganciclovir/penciclovir) is illustrated in Figure 2-24. This particular use verifies successful viral infection of target tissue(s).

The next step in assay development is to select tracers for measuring HSV1-TK enzyme activity. Several previously discussed pharmacological agents are known to be useful because of their ability to be phosphorylated by HSV1-TK. As is often the case, tracers for PET imaging have their origins as pharmacological agents that may or may not be therapeutically useful. The structure of some of the potential tracers for HSV1-TK are shown in Figure 2-22. It must be kept in mind that in order to select the best tracer for this assay, many variables come into play. First, even if a substrate has a favorable affinity[17] for HSV1-TK, this

FIGURE 2-24. Herpes-Simplex Virus Type 1 Thymidine Kinase (HSV1-tk) Reporter Gene and FGCV Reporter Probe. Adenoviral mediated delivery of the herpes simplex virus Type 1 thymidine kinase (HSV1-tk) reporter gene driven by the cytomegalovirus (CMV) promoter. Delivery and subsequent expression of the HSV1-tk reporter gene lead to accumulation of a PET reporter probe (e.g., FGCV, FHBG) only in cells that express the HSV1-tk reporter gene. The accumulation of probe is due to phosphorylation of the probe by the HSV1-TK enzyme. Although the adenovirus is depicted as delivering the HSV1-tk reporter gene, many alternative approaches for delivering the reporter gene to target cells could be utilized.

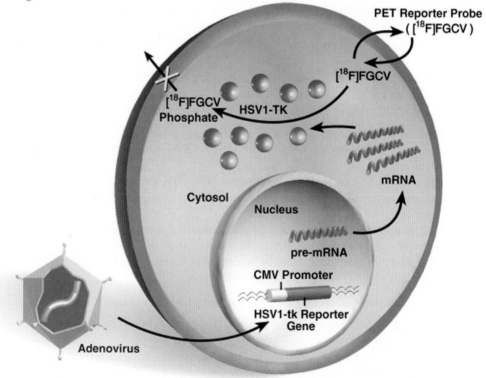

may not be enough. Transport of the substrate into and out of the cell is a key step, and if transport is limited, it may negatively effect the assay. If the substrate does not compete well against endogenous substrates (e.g., thymidine) for phosphorylation by HSV1-TK, then this may be an additional limitation. If the substrate has a favorable affinity for mammalian TKs, then this will lead to undesirable background signal in those cells that do not express HSV1-tk. At the time of this writing, it is not clear which substrate is the best choice based on the above considerations. It is clear, however, that penciclovir is likely a better candidate than ganciclovir and acyclovir.[158] It is not clear if thymidine analogs (e.g., FIAU) are always better than the acycloguanosines, but recent data suggest that, for the HSV1-TK enzyme, they should be superior.[159]

EXAMPLE 2-13

From an assay development perspective, which labeling strategy, a Fluorine-18 labeling of penciclovir in the Carbon-8 position (FPCV) versus the side-chain Fluorine-18 labeling of penciclovir (FHBG), is better and why in choosing a reporter probe for HSV1-TK? Assume that the fluorine chemistry would not limit either labeling approach.

ANSWER

The 8-position labeling is a better strategy because it does not lead to a racemic mixture of probes. The side-chain labeling leads to a chiral carbon and this complicates the assay significantly because of the potential for different uptake, clearance, and phosphorylation rates for the two resulting compounds.

The side-chain, however, is better in practice because of the higher affinity of the tracer and the ease of labeling with F^- rather than F_2. Tracer and assay development are an iterative process as illustrated in Figure 2-4. Notice also that F^--labeling reactions also produce imaging probes with higher specific activity (see Chapters 3 and 4).

Even if there were a clear choice of substrate for HSV1-TK, it should be noted that the ability to radiolabel the substrate with a positron-emitting isotope can significantly effect the final choice. For example, FIAU can theoretically be labeled with F-18, I-124, N-13, O-15, or C-11, but it is difficult to know which might be the best choice without performing some biological studies. In addition, a high-specific activity for the final tracer would be desirable, and this may effect the choice of the isotope and labeling strategy selected. All of these issues for tracer development must carefully be discussed with the chemists (see Chapters 3 and 4).

To be guided when choosing radiolabel for a given substrate, it is often desirable to first use ^3H, ^{14}C, or other beta emitters in cell culture and whole-body autoradiography studies. This allows one to determine the pharmacokinetics of the tracer in cell culture and *in vivo*. If the pharmacokinetics show that the tracer is relatively slow in achieving a high target to background ratio then positron-emitting isotopes with a longer life may have to be used to label the substrate. A further discussion of these issues can be found in Desirable Properties of Molecular Imaging Probes p. 158.

Initial studies in the author's laboratories used $^3H/^{14}C$ ganciclovir in cell culture to examine some of these issues.[160] C6 rat glioma cells were infected with varying titers (e.g., amounts) of an adenovirus carrying the HSV1-tk reporter gene driven by the cytomegalovirus (CMV) constitutive promoter (Ad-CMV-HSV1-tk). This was done to achieve different levels of HSV1-tk reporter gene expression. The adenovirus is replication incompetent so that it can infect cells and deliver the HSV1-tk reporter gene but does not lead to viral replication and cell death. The C6 cells were then exposed to different levels of 3H/14C acyclovir and ganciclovir, and it was determined that 1 to 2 h of exposure to tracer was sufficient to maximize the ratio of accumulated activity to initial activity in the cell medium.[160] Furthermore, it was found that increasing levels of HSV1-TK enzyme activity and HSV1-tk mRNA normalized to GAPDH (a housekeeping protein in the cell) correlated well with levels of 3H-ganciclovir accumulation. This is important because it meets the requirements of the assay that accumulation of tracer correlate with levels of reporter gene expression.

Although the cell culture data support the use of isotopes with a half-life of 1 h or greater, it is important to verify if this is the case *in vivo*. Simple biodistribution studies in which tracer is injected and mice are sacrificed at some time later for counting of organ radioactivity can be quite useful.[160] Mouse models were studied in which varying titers of Ad-CMV-HSV1-tk were injected in a tail vein followed 48 h later by an injection in a tail vein of 14C-ganciclovir.[160] The introduction of the adenovirus via a tail vein leads to the expression of HSV1-tk primarily in the liver due to presence of coxsackie adenoviral receptor on hepatocytes.[161,162] Shown in Figure 2-25 is a digital whole-body autoradiogram (DWBA) of three mice 1 h after an injection of 14C-ganciclovir in a tail vein. The DWBA confirm several issues, including: 1) Sufficient tracer has cleared from the blood and tissues not expressing HSV1-TK at 1 h after injection of the tracer; 2) background routes of clearance include the kidneys and liver; 3) the liver is the primary site of accumulation of tracer and 4) greatest tracer accumulation in liver occurs in the mice injected with the highest viral titer. However, viral titer does not correlate well with DWBA liver signal, as the titer injected does not correlate well with levels of HSV1-tk expression in the liver as measured directly by analysis of liver samples for HSV1-TK activity.

FIGURE 2-25. Digital Whole-body Autoradiography for 14C-Ganciclovir. A1, B1, and C1 and A2, B2, and C2 are anterior and posterior coronal longitudinal sections, respectively. A1 and A2 are of a mouse injected with 1.0×10^9 plaque-forming units (pfu) of control virus. B1, B2 and C1, C2 are of mice injected with 0.5×10^9 and 1.0×10^9 pfu of AdCMV-HSV1-tk virus, respectively. In each case, a mouse coronal-section photograph (left side) and the corresponding digital whole-body autoradiogram (right side) are shown. Each mouse was injected with virus ~48 h prior to the injection of [8-^{14}C]-GCV. Each mouse was sacrificed ~60 minutes after the injection of [8-^{14}C]-GCV. Horizontal scale bar = 10 mm. The DWBA pixels represent the % ID/g tissue as shown in each intensity scale to the right of the DWBA. Notice that each scale is nonlinear and different for each DWBA to enhance the outline of the mouse relative to the various signals seen within a given coronal section. Abbreviations: B, brain; BL, bladder; DWBA, digital whole-body autoradiography; I, intestine; K, kidney; L, liver; M, muscle. (Reproduced with permission from Herz J, Gerard RD. Adenovirus-mediated transfer of low density lipoprotein receptor gene acutely accelerates cholesterol in normal mice. Proc Natl Acad Sci USA 1993;90:2812–2816.)

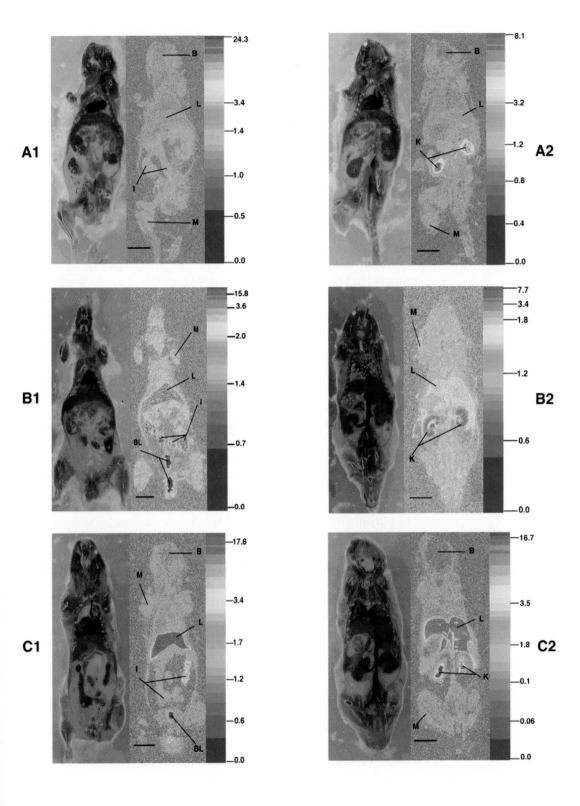

Subsequent to the DWBA mouse studies, it was concluded that the pharmacokinetics supported the use of a Fluorine-18 (half-life = 2 h) ganciclovir reporter probe for microPET imaging of HSV1-tk reporter gene expression. The author and colleagues initially decided to pursue an 8-position labeling of ganciclovir[163] with Fluorine-18 because it does not lead to a racemic mixture as does a side-chain labeling approach to produce FHPG. It was also subsequently discovered that 3H-penciclovir has greater accumulation than 3H-ganciclovir in C6 cells expressing HSV1-tk[158] and therefore decided to label penciclovir in the 8 positions with Fluroine-18 to produce FPCV. Studies with both FGCV and FPCV reveal that they have significantly decreased ability to be phosphorylated by HSV1-TK than do ^{3}H-ganciclovir and ^{3}H-penciclovir.[158] The 8-position labeling with fluorine does interfere with the binding of substrate to enzyme, perhaps due to the significantly higher electronegativity of fluorine relative to hydrogen. Several laboratories have utilized FHPG[164,165] and FHBG[166] and subsequently validated that FHBG is the best PET reporter susbstrate for HSV1-TK as compared to FHPG, FPCV, FGCV, and FACV.[158,167] Current synthesis of FHBG does, however, produce a *racemic mixture.* Research is being conducted to produce methods to synthesize a single isomer so as to make modeling of the tracer simpler and more quantitatively rigorous, as well as to improve the specificity of the probes.

Several groups have also explored Iodine-124 radiolabeling of FIAU[168] as well as its derivatives. These thymidine analogs may have advantages over the acycloguanosines and will require further investigation. Iodine-124 has a long half-life ($t_{1/2}$ = 4 days) which has advantages for certain applications (e.g., for mouse imaging in which one needs to clear bladder and gastrointestinal activity by waiting for many hours after tracer injection) and disadvantages for others (e.g., repetitive imaging of gene expression must wait 10 to 12 days or one must use techniques to subtract activity from previous injections). A recent study demonstrates that ^{124}I-FIAU is superior to FHBG for imaging HSV1-tk reporter gene expression in stably transfected tumors.[159] This same study also lends support to pursuing an ^{18}F labeling of FIAU due to reasonable imaging contrast within 15 to 30 minutes after tracer injection in living rodents. The author and colleagues have demonstrated that ^{14}C-FIAU and FHBG may be comparable in imaging sensitivity in cell culture and in living mice when adenoviral delivery approaches are used to image HSV1-tk reporter gene expression in the liver.[169] Further work will be needed to better clarify advantages of FHBG versus FIAU. Several novel studies have been performed with HSV1-tk and FIAU[170–176] and demonstrate the ability to utilize FIAU for various reporter gene imaging paradigms.

It is likely that no one tracer will meet the needs for all applications and that research into improved substrates will continue to be an iterative process. In fact, the work discussed above was iterative with substrates proceeding from FACV to FGCV to FPCV to FHPG to finally FHBG. It is important to notice that the labeling of a molecule with Fluorine-18 (or any other element or chemical group substitution) can change the characteristics of that molecule (e.g., ^{3}H-penciclovir vs. FPCV), and that it is important to repeat all studies *in vitro* and in cell culture comparing the PET tracer and its analog in a head-to-head fashion. Although much of the process of assay refinement for the HSV1-tk reporter gene assay was and continues to be an iterative process, this section will progress to compartmental modeling for the tracer FHBG, even though developing compartmental models for FGCV and FPCV was initially attempted.

EXAMPLE 2-14

For the HSV1-tk reporter gene assay, is it possible to improve the sensitivity of the assay without developing better reporter probes with a higher affinity for the HSV1-TK enzyme? How can this be done? Improved sensitivity means the ability to detect lower concentrations of HSV1-TK enzyme.

ANSWER

Yes, this is possible. In this assay, a reporter gene has to be introduced into a cell which will encode for an enzyme that will trap the reporter probe. Therefore, one can introduce a gene which encodes for a super enzyme that has improved ability to phosphorylate reporter probe(s). Such an approach has been published using a mutant HSV1-tk reporter gene using random site directed mutagenesis (see below). This approach illustrates the power of merging modern day molecular biology with molecular imaging approaches. One is not necessarily limited to the development of alternate tracers.

The structure of the HSV1-TK enzyme itself can be modified to achieve greater sensitivity for a specific substrate or reporter probe and alleviate some of the limitations with this assay. A mutant HSV1-sr39tk reporter gene has been studied which was selected because of its ability to better phosphorylate acycloguanosines and also a poorer ability to phosphorylate thymidine.[177] The mutant HSV1-sr39TK reporter protein was specifically developed with the substrates acyclovir and ganciclovir in mind but has also worked well with FGCV, penciclovir, FPCV, and more recently FHBG.[177] The mutant was created by random site directed mutagenesis followed by subsequent isolation of mutants that have the improved ability to use acyclovir and ganciclovir as well as decreased ability to use thymidine.[178,179] The HSV1-sr39tk mutant has about a two- to threefold better imaging sensitivity than the wild type tk.[177] The fact that this mutant is less sensitive to changes in endogenous thymidine may particularly be important for various applications because thymidine levels are not controllable. Future mutant reporter protein specifically optimized for FHBG may produce even better results. *For purposes of assay development we will therefore focus on HSV1-sr39tk and FHBG, since together they produce the best level of signal.*

Shown in Figure 2-26 is a dynamic microPET study of a mouse tail vein injected with ~200 μCi of FHBG and the corresponding time-activity curves from various organs. Initial microPET studies can help validate the autoradiography results while utilizing a PET tracer and provide more detailed kinetic results. Clearly, the ability to get kinetic information is critical in building the PET assay and is well facilitated with the microPET. Animal subjects can also be sacrificed immediately after the PET study and organs counted or autoradiography performed with the PET tracer. Measurement of the input function can be performed by direct left ventricular blood sampling or by drawing regions of interest over the heart if the heart does not itself accumulate tracer.[180] After ob-

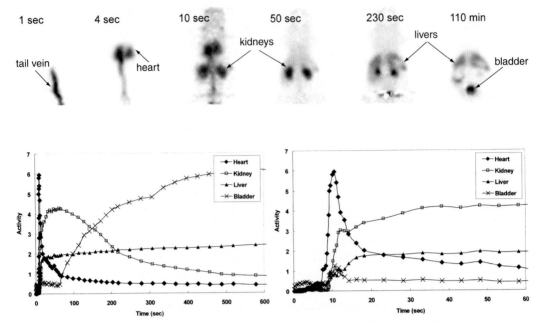

FIGURE 2-26. Dynamic microPET Data for FHBG in Mice. The mouse tail vein was injected with 1×10^9 pfu of Ad-CMV-HSV1-tk and scanned with ~200 μCi of FHBG 48 h later. Clear trapping of radioactivity is visualized in the liver at later times secondary to HSV1-TK-mediated phosphorylation of FHBG. Routes of eliminating FHBG including the renal system (kidneys and bladder) and hepatobiliary system are also seen. High blood pool activity is noted in the early time points (1-, 4-, and 10-second images) and rapidly decreases over time due to elimination of FHBG from the blood. Control mice (not shown) do not show any liver trapping of activity. The time-activity curves obtained by drawing regions of interest over the microPET images are also shown (600-second time scale—bottom left; first 60 seconds—bottom right). The blood ROI (squares) shows an early peak and then rapid decrease for the input function. Rapid accumulation of activity (triangles) in the liver is seen. The kidneys time-activity curve (diamonds) shows an increase followed by a decrease as the activity subsequently clears into the bladder. The bladder (crosses) shows minimal activity for about 50 seconds followed by accumulation of activity into the bladder. (Figure courtesy of Dr. Arion Chatziioanou.)

taining multiple time-activity curves from several animal groups, one can proceed to the next phase of assay development. It is important that issues of partial volume correction, spillover, cylinder calibration factor, and so on, are carefully addressed in conjunction with medical physicists at this stage of assay development (see Chapter 1).

The next assay development step is to build a comprehensive model (Figure 2-27) for the tracer of interest. To perform this step, return to the tracer thought experiment (see Tracer Thought Experiment, this chapter). Assume that there is expression of HSV1-sr39tk in the hepatocytes of the subject and in no other tissues. From the time we as the tracer are injected into the intravenous pool, we have several possibilities. We can remain in plasma, enter into the circulating blood cells (e.g., white and red blood cells), and/or bind to plasma proteins.

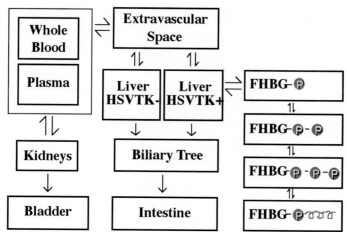

FIGURE 2-27. Comprehensive Model for FHBG and HSV1-sr39tk. Compartmental model showing trapping of FHBG in the hepatocytes of the liver due to HSV1-tk expression. FHBG is phosphorylated by HSV1-TK, and then other cellular enzymes lead to further phosphorylation and eventual incorporation into DNA. Also shown are the routes of clearance via the renal kidneys and hepatobiliary systems.

We can move between all of these components while flow is occurring within the blood vessel to push us through the circulatory system. We can leave the blood vessel by moving into the interstitial space (the space between the blood vessels and cells). From the interstitial space, we can enter into specific cells present in tissues. In the case of FHBG, movement between most blood vessels and the interstitial space and then back to blood is via diffusion, but transport into cells is via one of several transporters. Once inside these cells, we can be phosphorylated by HSV1-sr39TK and by mammalian TKs or leave the cell to go back to the interstitial space. When we are in the phosphorylated form, we cannot easily leave the cell (because we are now negatively charged). We can potentially be dephosphorylated through various intracellular enzymes. In both hepatocytes that do and do not express HSV1-sr39tk, we can also be eliminated via the hepatobiliary system. We must also think about special restrictions placed on us. For example, for FHBG, we cannot cross the blood-brain-barrier. We can also be cleared from the blood via the kidneys.

Taking all of these issues into account, one can develop a comprehensive model for FHBG. This comprehensive model assumes several issues that deserve specific comment. First, it makes the assumption that the two chiral forms of FHBG behave identically in every aspect. It assumes that there is no significant reabsorption from the intestine back into blood. It assumes that the blood/plasma input function is known exactly so that one does not have to worry about modeling FHBG delivery to other tissues. It assumes blood flow does not effect movement of FHBG from blood to the extravascular space.

The next step is to develop a workable model. A three-compartment model has been recently preliminarily validated for FHBG kinetics in mice while using adenoviral-mediated HSV1-sr39tk gene delivery to the liver.[181] For tissues that do not express HSV1-sr39tk, a two-compartment model applies.[181] These tracer

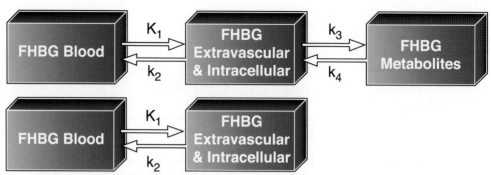

FIGURE 2-28. Workable Tracer Kinetic Models for FHBG. The top model is applicable for tissues in which FHBG can be phosphorylated due to the presence of HSV1-sr39TK. The bottom model is applicable for tissues in which FHBG cannot be significantly trapped. Notice that K_1 is a rate coefficient (ml/min/g) and k_2–k_4 are rate constants (1/min).

kinetic models are depicted in Figure 2-28. Several pools have been lumped together to obtain a usable three-compartment model. The first compartment represents FHBG in plasma/whole blood. A measurable difference is noticed in the ratio between plasma and whole-blood FHBG concentration in mice and humans[181,182] so that this must be properly accounted for. The second compartment can be thought to represent extravascular (interstitial and intracellular FHBG). Finally, the third compartment can be thought to represent all the various intracellular phosphorylated forms of FHBG. The rate constant k_3 is well correlated with direct measurements of HSV1-sr39TK enzyme activity obtained from liver tissue samples.[181] The two-compartment model is identical to the three-compartment model except that there is no compartment representing FHBG metabolites because tissues that do not express HSV1-sr39tk do not have significant metabolites over the course of the 1 to 3 h of the study. These models assume: 1) The racemic mixture of FHBG behaves equivalently with regards to all kinetics (e.g., uptake, phosphorylation, clearance); 2) levels of thymidine do not significantly effect the rate coefficients/constants of the model; 3) the two mammalian thymidine kinases do not significantly phosphorylate FHBG. The two- and three-compartment models have undergone preliminary kinetic validation,[181,183] but further work will be required to confirm their more generalized applicability.

Model validation is the next step in assay development. Initial model validation relies on fitting the two- and three-compartment models to time-activity data. This work shows that for tissues expressing HSV1-sr39tk, the two compartment fits poorly with correlated residuals (see Figure 2-13 for use of analysis of residuals) and the three-compartment model fits very well with low residuals.[181] For tissues that do not express HSV1-sr39tk, the two-compartment model is superior. To further validate the FHBG 3-compartment tracer kinetic model, one has to determine if the rate constant k_3 correlates with active HSV1-sr39TK enzyme activity. This correlation should be high if k_3 is related to active HSV1-sr39TK enzyme activity. Furthermore, no other rate constants should correlate well with levels of active HSV1-sr39TK. To perform this type of validation, mice have been injected with different levels of Ad-CMV-HSV1-tk so as to achieve different levels of HSV1-sr39TK expression in hepatocytes. These mice are then subjected to dynamic microPET scanning so that time-activity data for the liver and blood can be determined.[184] Immediately after scanning, the mice are sacrificed and their livers assayed for HSV1-sr39TK activity.[184] Fitting of time-activity data to the three-compartment tracer kinetic model shows a high correlation of k_3 with relative HSV1-sr39TK activity ($r^2 > 0.8$). Furthermore, all the other model parameters show very poor correlations with HSV1-sr39TK. This lends good biochemical validation that k_3 is the key parameter related to the trapping of FHBG. Additional biochemical support is obtained by performing dynamic microPET studies and comparing model predicted results of relative fraction of tracer in each of the three compartments at various time points as compared to liver extracts from HPLC to separate nonphosphorylated from phosphorylated tracer.

Finally, one is ready for the application of the tracer kinetic model so that the original goals of the assay can be achieved. For example, if one wanted to compare FHBG uptake (K_1) versus phosphorylation (k_3) in different stable transfected tumors *in vivo*, this would now be possible (assuming adenoviral mediated and stable transfected cells behaved identically). One can in fact have large K_1 values and low k_3 values and, therefore, be looking at predominantly unphosphorylated FHBG in tissue. The tracer kinetic model helps to separate transport from phosphorylation so that one can separate that component of the PET signal that represents phosphorylated from unphosphorylated FHBG because the phosphorylated FHBG provides the record of HSV1-tk expression.

Throughout the development of the HSV1-tk reporter gene assay, the assay developer must work with the entire PET team (see Figure 2-1). Specifically, the biologists must provide significant input into the underlying cell biology of gene expression, adenoviral construction and use, and animal models. The chemists are actively involved in the process of choosing and refining substrates, type and positioning of radiolabel (8-position vs. side-chain), specific activity issues, as well as HPLC metabolite analysis. The medical physicists are involved with the autoradiography and microPET instrumentation, acquisition, and image reconstruction/analysis. Finally, as this assay begins to be applied in humans (e.g., clinical human gene therapy trials), clinicians with expertise in medicine and nuclear medicine will play a role. Once the assay is validated and standardized, then it can be used as a routine assay for the study of biology and disease.

The tracer FHBG has been studied in normal human volunteers and, fortunately, its pharmacokinetics and radiation dosimetry profile are quite favorable.[182] It clears readily from the blood via the renal and hepatobiliary systems just as seen in the microPET studies with mice. A recent study has also been published with FIAU PET imaging after liposomal-mediated delivery of HSV1-tk in human gliomas and appears encouraging, with one out of five patients showing some specific FIAU trapping.[185] It is likely that human applications will play a greater role over the next decade.

Other PET reporter gene assays

Several other PET reporter gene assays are under active exploration and are reviewed in detail elsewhere.[149,152] These include the dopamine Type 2 receptor (D2R) reporter gene with 18F-fluorethylspiperone (FESP) reporter probe,[186] and the sodium/iodide symporter[187–191] which can be adapted for PET imaging with

Iodine-124. Reporter gene approaches with SPECT imaging are also under active investigation and are discussed elsewhere.[152,192]

Receptor-based approaches may initially seem as if they would be inferior to an enzyme-based approach due to the fact that one ligand molecule binds to one receptor without any signal amplification as in the enzyme approach. However, because these approaches do not necessarily require intracellular transport of ligand, they offer unique advantages. To date, we have found that the D2R/FESP system is comparable in sensitivity to the HSV1-sr39tk/FHBG reporter gene,[193] but more detailed comparisons are needed. For the D2R reporter gene, the author and colleagues recently studied a mutant that uncouples signal transduction while maintaining ligand affinity,[194] and, therefore, endogenous ligand that may bind to the receptor will not significantly perturb the cell in which the reporter gene is expressed. The D2R reporter gene is also endogenously expressed and should not be immunogenic. It is clear that many more reporter gene assays will be needed in the future and that no single assay will serve the needs of all applications.

Applications of PET reporter genes

The applications of PET reporter genes are numerous. They include: 1) Marking a specific cell population with a reporter gene *ex vivo* and then introducing the cells back into a living subject.[172,195] The reporter gene can be driven by a strong constitutive (e.g., always on) promoter so that high levels of reporter gene expression allow these cells to trap high levels of reporter probe. Cells can then be repetitively followed for their location(s) by readministering reporter probe to the animal. They can also be premarked with reporter probe prior to injection allowing potentially greater sensitivity for tracking them up to two to three half-lives of the isotope used for the reporter probe. Cells can also be marked with two reporter genes (one that is constitutively expressed and one that is expressed based on a specific event such as recognition of a target tissue or a specific molecular event). These trafficking studies will allow an understanding of immune system dynamics, cancer cell trafficking, as well as a whole host of other studies. 2) Imaging the location(s), magnitude, and time-variation of therapeutic gene expression. This can be done by linking the therapeutic gene to the PET reporter gene through one of several methods (see Figure 2-29).[196–198] The linked system can then be delivered by one of many approaches (e.g., liposomal, adenoviral, lentiviral, and so on) that are currently being developed.[199,200] Methods to enhance transcription using molecular amplification techniques have also been studied and will likely prove useful for tissue-specific gene expression with relatively weak promoters driving therapeutic and PET reporter genes.[171,201–203] 3) Indirectly monitoring endogenous gene expression by driving expression of the PET reporter gene using the endogenous gene promoter (see Figure 2-30). This is a particularly powerful approach because it does not require that a tracer exists for the mRNA or protein of a specific gene of interest—the same reporter gene is used and one changes the promoter driving the reporter gene to be the promoter for the endogenous gene of interest. Then the expression of the endogenous gene is followed *indirectly* by quantitating levels of the PET reporter protein. This approach has recently been validated for the albumin gene using the albumin promoter to drive the HSV1-sr39tk PET reporter gene.[153] This indirect approach does have its limitations, however, be-

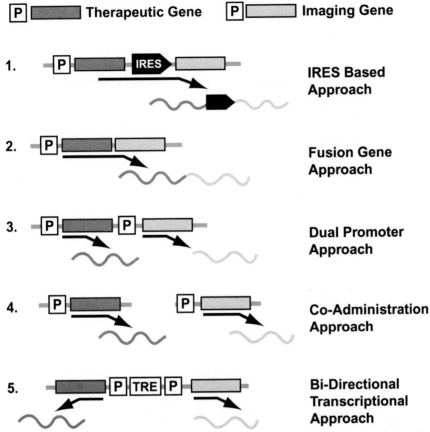

FIGURE 2-29. Approaches to Coupling a Therapeutic Gene with a PET Reporter (imaging) Gene. Several approaches can link the expression of the two genes. Shown is the gene and the corresponding mRNA(s). By monitoring the imaging (reporter) gene, one can indirectly monitor the therapeutic gene. In the internal ribosomal entry site (IRES)-based approach, a single mRNA is transcribed, but two proteins are produced.

cause it may be the case that levels of the reporter protein (as assessed by an assay using the reporter probe) do not correlate well with levels of the endogenous protein. This could occur for many reasons including post-transcriptional regulation of the endogenous gene and inability to mimic upstream and downstream regulatory elements.

Multimodality optical and PET reporter genes offer some unique possibilities that deserve special discussion. Although PET reporter genes offer a powerful approach for applications from animals to humans, they are less useful when considering work which spans from cell culture to small animal models. It is not easy to determine if intact cells are expressing a PET reporter gene. One has to either perform cell uptake assays with radioactive reporter probes or assay cell extracts using radiolabeled probes for the presence of reporter proteins.

For fluorescent optical reporters [e.g., green fluorescent protein (GFP)], it is much easier to determine cell expression by simply looking at the cells under a fluorescent microscope and/or by performing flow cytometry. The bioluminescence optical approaches (e.g., bioluminescence with firefly or renilla lu-

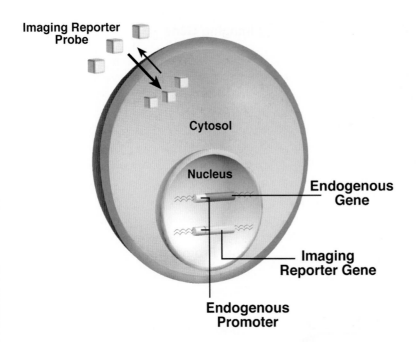

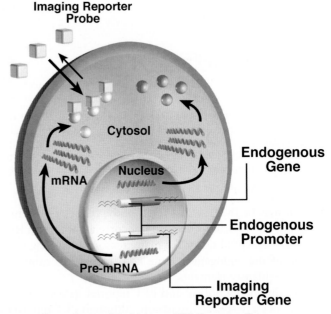

FIGURE 2-30. Monitoring Endogenous Gene Expression Using a PET Reporter Gene. The goal is to use a reporter gene to image expression of an endogenous gene. An imaging reporter gene fused to the promoter of the endogenous gene of interest can be utilized. If the endogenous gene is not expressed, then the reporter gene is also not expressed because of the common promoter, and no reporter probe is trapped (top left). If the endogenous gene is expressed, then the reporter gene is also expressed and leads to the accumulation of reporter probe (bottom right).

ciferase) provide rapid throughput in small animal models without the use of radioactivity but at the expense of tomographic detail and variable response with tissue location.[204] It would be ideal to have a *unique* reporter gene approach that spans the bridge from cell to human applications. One approach is by using fusion reporter genes (e.g., renilla luciferase fused to HSV1-sr39tk) and by utilizing one reporter probe (e.g., colenterazine) to detect the optical protein and a second reporter probe to detect the PET reporter protein (e.g., FHBG).[146,205] Research of various approaches to making it easier to go from cells to humans is ongoing.

Antisense imaging assays

To image transcription directly, tracers need to be developed to interact with pre-mRNA or mRNA. Assays for imaging mRNA levels are currently being investigated through the use of small (12-35 nucleobases long) modified **r**adiolabeled **a**ntisense **o**ligodeoxy**n**ucleotide (RASON) probes targeted toward a specific mRNA (Figure 2-31). This RASON antisense probe is complementary to a small segment of target mRNA. RASON probes have the potential for imaging gene expression specifically at the transcription level. The RASON must be: sta-

FIGURE 2-31. Radioactive Antisense Oligodeoxynucleotide (RASON) Use for Cellular Interrogation of mRNA Levels. The RASON must be able to get into the cell and able to have the rate of binding to target mRNA compete with the rate of efflux and non-specific binding to various cellular proteins and RNA. These competitive kinetics must be such that, at a reasonable imaging time, the concentration of RASON bound to target mRNA exceeds the general RASON concentration in tissue. In those cells that do not express target mRNA, the RASON must rapidly efflux and then be cleared from the blood.

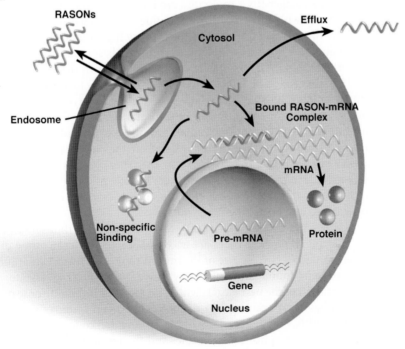

ble against degradation from nucleases, able to enter and efflux from cells, and of sufficient specific activity to detect relatively low levels of mRNA. The antisense method is a general approach because the RASON probe sequence could easily be modified to target many mRNAs of interest (while keeping the radiolabeling chemistry unchanged). RASONs have the distinct advantage of easy modification (by changing the sequence of bases using DNA synthesizer technology) to target a new mRNA.

The pharmaceutical industry has been investigating both DNA and mRNA as targets for antisense drugs for over a decade.[206–208] DNA is an ideal target for a drug because, by binding an antisense drug to a specific gene (via Hoogsteen base pairing in the major groove), one could theoretically prevent the production of mRNA and, therefore, stop protein production. For diseases in which stopping the production of an aberrant protein is beneficial, this approach holds significant promise. Companies that focus specifically on the development and testing of antisense drugs targeted towards various mRNAs are now testing third-generation antisense drugs. However to date, clinical trials using antisense drugs have met with limited success (reviewed by Wagner and Flanagan[209]). Progress towards developing more stable antisense oligodeoxynucleotides with improved uptake, issues of cellular efflux, characterization of biodistribution regarding intracellular access and nonspecific binding, and the understanding of appropriate controls are important for developing RASON probes. Much of what may be possible with imaging applications utilizing RASON probes depends on the significant progress on antisense pharmaceuticals made by the pharmaceutical industry over the last decade.

Of the two choices, DNA and mRNA, only mRNA is a good target for developing an assay for imaging endogenous gene expression. Every cell has the DNA (gene) of interest, but only cells in which the gene has been transcribed have the mRNA of interest. Messenger RNA concentrations are typically in the range of 1 to 1000 pM.[210] Messenger RNA molecules are ideal targets due to their ability to very specifically pair with antisense oligonucleotides through hydrogen bonds. The binding affinity of antisense drugs for mRNA is very high, but a single mismatch (using a base that does not pair with the target mRNA base) can drop the affinity by as much as 300-fold.[207] It has been mathematically shown that a minimum of only 11 to 15 bases need to be targeted to hybridize *uniquely* to any of the mRNA in the human genome.[211] That is, a relatively small oligodeoxynucleotide or RASON is needed to code for any mRNAs in the human genome. This calculation is based on assuming that 0.5% of the human genome is expressed as mRNA. The two numbers correspond to the extreme cases where the oligonucleotide contains only C and G (n = 11) or only A and T (n = 15). Therefore, an antisense probe of relatively short length can be used to target a specific mRNA (Figure 2-32). In addition, changes in the base sequence in these small antisense probes provide the means to switch to any one of the other mRNAs.

Messenger RNA molecules are typically several hundred to thousands of base pairs long, but not all of these bases are accessible to an antisense probe due to the secondary and tertiary structure of the mRNA molecule. Intracellular mRNA is invariably protein bound, and only a few sites are probably available for base pairing. The location of the best targets within an mRNA for the antisense mRNA which to bind has been examined in detail.[212] The main findings are that, in general, the best mRNA locations are the 5′ cap or initiation codon (AUG) regions. There are, however, exceptions to this rule, and the tertiary (folding) structure

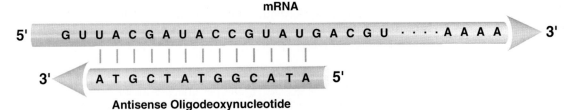

FIGURE 2-32. Hybridization of Antisense Oligodeoxynucleotide to Its Target mRNA. A small 11- to 20-base antisense probe is sufficient to uniquely target any mRNA which can be thousands of bases long.

of the mRNA must be considered to predict potential binding sites. It is important not to generalize mRNA regions that are useful for targeting; instead, for each mRNA, careful studies must be performed to identify good target sites.

Because mRNA-antisense probe interaction is stoichiometric (e.g., for each mRNA there is at most one bound RASON) and, therefore, equivalent to a receptor-ligand interaction, one can attempt to answer questions about the minimal levels of mRNA that can be detected by a given antisense probe. Variables such as the concentration of target mRNA, binding affinities of antisense probe and mRNA, antisense probe specific activity, free intracellular antisense tracer concentration, sensitivity of detection (typically only 0.5% to 2% of annihilation events are detected by PET), and target (specific binding) to background (nonspecific binding) levels all play key roles. Based on these parameters, it has been estimated that mRNA concentrations as low as 1 pM in tissue in establishing the feasibility of the assay can probably be imaged with PET, using RASON probes with the common specific activities of ~1,000 to 10,000 Ci/mmole used in PET radiolabeling.[213]

EXAMPLE 2-15

An assay is desired to measure the levels of messenger RNA (mRNA) in cells using a tracer that can specifically hybridize to a small region of the mRNA through complementary hydrogen bond formation (an antisense tracer). Given the following assumptions and variables, what are the counts in the target versus background?

ASSUMPTIONS

SA = Specific Activity (Ci/mmole) of antisense tracer
    = 1,000 Ci/mmole
n = cell concentration (cell number/ml)
    = 2×10^8 cells/ml
m = mRNA copies per cell = 1,000 copies mRNA/cell
1 Ci = 3.7×10^{10} disintegrations/s
H = percent of mRNA bound by antisense = 10%
C = contrast or target to background ratio = 3
    = (Target + Background) ÷ Background
S = sensitivity of PET instrument = 0.5%
Target volume = 0.5 cm × 0.5 cm × 0.5 cm = 0.125 cm³

Antisense tracer is labeled with Fluorine-18 with a half-life of 110 minutes and scanning has a 15-minute acquisition time at 1-h after injection of antisense tracer.

ANSWER

First, we calculate the density (moles per grams of tissue) of mRNA:

$$2 \times 10^8 \text{ cells/ml} \times 1 \text{ ml/g tissue} \times 1,000 \text{ copies mRNA/cell}$$
$$\times 1 \text{ mole mRNA}/6.02 \times 10^{23} \text{ copies mRNA}$$
$$= 3.32 \times 10^{-13} \text{ moles mRNA/g tissue} = 0.332 \text{ picomoles mRNA/g tissue}$$

Next, we calculate how much mRNA is bound by antisense tracer using H = 10%:

$$= 0.332 \times 10^{-12} \text{ moles mRNA/g tissue} \times (0.10) \times (1 \text{ g/cm}^3)$$
$$\times (0.5 \text{ cm} \times 0.5 \text{ cm} \times 0.5 \text{ cm})$$
$$= 4.15 \times 10^{-15} \text{ moles}$$
$$= 0.00415 \text{ pmol of bound mRNA in a } 0.125\text{-cm}^3 \text{ target volume}$$

Now, if the injected antisense probe has a specific activity = S = 1,000 Ci/mmole, then:

$$1,000 \text{ Ci/mmole} \times 0.00415 \times 10^{-12} \text{ moles} \times (1,000 \text{ mmole/mole})$$
$$= 0.415 \times 10^{-8} \text{ Ci of mRNA bound activity}$$

For a contrast ratio of 3:1, we obtain:

$$(0.415 \times 10^{-8} \text{ Ci} + Y \text{ Ci})/Y \text{ Ci} = 3,$$

so that nonspecific background activity = Y = 0.2075×10^{-8} Ci

So total activity in target is:

$$(0.415 + 0.2075) \times 10^{-8} \text{ Ci} = 0.6225 \times 10^{-8} \text{ Ci}$$

So for a 15-minute scan time, the total nondecay corrected counts one would observe are:

$$\text{Target counts} = 0.6225 \times 10^{-8} \text{ Ci} \times 3.7 \times 10^{10} \text{ decays/second/Ci}$$
$$\times 60 \text{ sec/min} \times 15 \text{ min} = 20.73 \times 10^4 \text{ decays}$$

For a scanner with a sensitivity = 0.5%, and taking into account that the scanning is 1 h after injection:

$$= 20.73 \times 10^4 \text{ decays} \times 0.5\% \times \exp^{(-\ln (2) \times 60 \text{ min}/110 \text{ min})}$$
$$= 10.37 \times 10^2 \times 0.685$$
$$= 710 \text{ decays}$$

The background counts would be = 236 (based on Target/Background = C = 3)

It is likely that 710 versus 236 counts could be statistically distinguished under most conditions. The only way to improve the number of target counts (without significantly longer acquisition times) would be to increase the specific activity to 10,000 Ci/mmole or have a scanner which could operate with 10 times greater sensitivity, S = 5%. It would be difficult to get below 100 copies of mRNA/cell unless both specific activity and sensitivity could be increased to 10,000 Ci/mmole and 5%, respectively. Furthermore, the above calculations assume that one can inject enough mass of tracer at a given specific activity with a reasonable radiation dosimetry profile and still have 10% of mRNA bound, and enough time to allow tracer to clear to achieve the Target ÷ Background = C.

Oligonucleotides are readily hydrolyzed (cleaved) by nucleases *in vivo*.[214] A nonhydrolyzable analogue of an oligonucleotide is, therefore, required so that sufficient amounts can reach the target in effective concentrations. Oligodeoxynucleotides are more stable *in vivo* when compared with oligoribonucleotides,[214] and are, therefore, the probes of choice. Various investigators have used modified oligodeoxynucleotides (e.g., phosporothioates) for greater stability against degradation.[206,215,216] Additional modifications that confer stability are alpha oligodeoxynucleotides, as well as 2′ modified moieties.[208]; 3′ end modifications may be particularly useful because they can prevent exonuclease-based degradation. Polypeptide nucleic acids (PNAs),[217] in which nucleobases are attached to a pseudopeptide, have also been explored as potential drugs to block translation of mRNA, but they may suffer from little to no cellular uptake. PNAs do, however, have improved stability against nucleases and may even have enhanced sequence selectivity for target mRNA.

Uptake of oligonucleotides by cells appears to occur via several mechanisms. The surprising and essential feature is that relatively short oligonucleotides (e.g., fewer than 40 bases) are readily taken up by many different cells. This uptake is critical to insure that a RASON probe can be delivered to the intracellular target mRNA by injection into the venous plasma space. Most oligonucleotides (except methylphosphonates) are polyanionic and do not passively diffuse across cell membranes. Transport mechanisms include receptor mediated endocytosis, adsorptive endocytosis, as well as fluid-phase pinocytosis.[218-221] There is a fast (minutes) as well as a slow component (hours) of uptake. A ~ 80-kD protein associated with the cell membrane has also been isolated from several cell types that seem to be responsible for oligodeoxynucleotide binding and possible internalization.[218,219] The exact transport mechanism seems to be different for various cell types. There have been some preliminary attempts to model oligonucleotide cell transport,[220] but no mathematical model is currently available. It is likely that nondiffusible oligodexoynucleotides end up in cellular endosomes, but it is not clear how they leave the endosomes or what the efflux rate is from endosomes to reach mRNA in the cytoplasm. Several groups have shown that exogenously administered oligonucleotides appear to localize readily in the nucleus, mitochondria, or both within hours.[220]

The oligonucleotide, once inside the cell, must be able to bind to the target mRNA, and excess unhybridized oligonucleotide must also be able to leave cells during the time in which the oligonucleotide and target mRNA complex is stable. Charged oligonucleotides can nonspecifically interact with intracellular proteins. This leads to nonspecific binding, and the potential inhibition of oligonucleotide internalization for transport into cells.[219] To obtain sufficient specificity of the image signal, the rates of exocytosis and mRNA binding must exceed the rate of nonspecific binding. Exocytosis follows a multicompartmental model, with a rapid phase (half-life of 10 minutes) as well as a slower phase (half-life of 30 minutes) in some cases, but varies depending on the cell type and the type of oligodeoxynucleotide. Both truncated fragments as well as chain extension products efflux from cells. Some studies have reported desired pharmacologic effects of a decrease in protein production with *nonantisense* oligodeoxynucleotides; this may be due to interaction of the oligodeoxynucleotide drug with proteins. It is important that a true antisense mechanism is demonstrated by using controls with sequentially increasing numbers of nucleobase mismatches before proceeding with *in vivo* studies. As the number of mismatches in bases increases, the binding to target mRNA should decrease. Without these appropriate controls, it is possible that nonspecific binding of oligodeoxynucleotide to protein(s) leads to a desired therapeutic effect (e.g., reduction in protein production).

Numerous investigators have explored the use of antisense oligonucleotides, both *in vitro* and *in vivo*, as therapeutic agents for decreasing protein production.[222] These include targeting the 35S RNA of the Rous sarcoma virus,[223] various mRNAs for use against HIV,[224] as well as many oncogene mRNAs including c-myc. Most of this work has shown that antisense oligonucleotides can work effectively in suppressing mRNA translation. After binding of oligodeoxynucleotide to target mRNA, the mRNA can be digested by ribonuclease H. Direct translation inhibition can also occur. In either case, the net result is a direct decrease in translation of mRNA to the protein product.

Biodistribution of oligodoexynucleotides in normal animals has been reported.[225] Phosphorothioate oligonucleotides, for example, bind to serum proteins ($\sim$400 μM dissociation constant for albumin). The plasma disappearance is extremely rapid and is well described by a two-compartment model. A relatively large volume of distribution is observed for phosphorothioates demonstrating a very wide-spread distribution to many tissues *in vivo*. The kidneys and liver have the greatest concentrations, with no significant penetration across the blood-brain-barrier. Natural phosphodiester oligonucleotides are very rapidly degraded to monomers *in vivo* and would probably have limited use for targeting gene expression. Animal whole-body autoradiography has also been used to assess the biodistribution of various radiolabeled oligodeoxynucleotides (see, for example, Phillips et al[226]).

Although much can be learned from the development and use of antisense oligodeoxynucleotides as drugs, several distinctions must be kept in mind for using them as imaging probes. First, any isotope labeling modification to the oligodeoxynucleotide must not significantly decrease its stability or its cellular influx, efflux, specific interaction, or hybridization affinity. Second, the relative rate of hybridization to target mRNA must exceed the net effect of the nonspecific interactions and efflux rates. *Also, the efflux and clearance rates must dominate if no target mRNA is expressed, so as to lead to minimal background signal.* The isotope half-life, biological half-life, and specific activity of the RASON are also important parameters to consider when attempting to target a specific mRNA *in vivo*. Potential toxicity also has to be studied.

To our knowledge, the first RASON probe to be developed specifically for nuclear imaging was an Indium-labeled oligodeoxynucleotide targeted against the amplified c-myc oncogene.[227] A 15-mer oligonucleotide sequence was synthesized, aminolinked (sense and antisense phosphodiester and monothioester) and bound with diethylenetriamine pentaacetate (DTPA) containing Indium-111. Subsequently, oligodeoxynucleotides labeled with Technetium-99m[228] and

Iodine-125[229] have been reported. More recently fluorine-labeled oligodeoxynucleotides for use with PET[213,230] have been synthesized. As described earlier, it is essential that high specific-activity probes should be developed for targeting the lowest possible levels of mRNA. Fluorine-18 labeling may achieve high-specific activities of 1,000 to 10,000 Ci/mmole but has the disadvantage of a relatively short isotope half-life of 110 minutes. A recently published report using modified PNAs labeled with Iodine-125 show some promise towards targeting an endogenous mRNA in the brain[231] and will need further validation. Detailed reviews on antisense imaging approaches can be found elsewhere.[232–234]

A potentially interesting approach would be to take advantage of the amplification inherent in an enzyme-based reporter gene with the specificity provided by an antisense sequence to image endogenous mRNA levels. The author and colleagues are currently exploring two such approaches in which amplification may be possible. In the first approach, they are using a decoy reporter mRNA that would trans-splice into the target mRNA based on antisense specificity, which would then lead to a message that encodes simultaneously for the target and reporter proteins.[235–237] In an alternate approach, they are developing split reporter proteins that are inactive until they are brought into close proximity. They have already validated this approach for imaging protein-protein interactions in living subjects[238] and are attempting to link these split reporters to antisense oligodeoxynucleotides so that they may be brought into close proximity only in the presence of the appropriate mRNA. In both the trans-splicing and split reporter approach, delivery of the sequence will still be an issue, but background signal should not be, because the systems are designed to be relatively silent till they interact with target mRNA.

TRANSLATION OF ASSAYS FROM MOUSE TO HUMANS

PET imaging offers the unique ability to rapidly translate preclinical imaging assays directly into the clinical imaging environment.[239] The development of the microPET facilitates rapid testing of new tracer assays in small rodent models and larger animal PET systems allow validation in other larger animals. Tracers that have been validated in animal models can directly be translated into testing in clinical applications after a few key steps. First, it must be demonstrated that there are no acute or chronic toxic effects in the animal model. For filing of an investigational new drug, this typically requires that after giving 100 times the normal tracer dose, no changes in physiological parameters (e.g., body temperature, EKG) or blood chemistries (e.g., cell blood count, serum electrolytes) can be demonstrated. Cold substrate is usually administered to accomplish this testing. It is unlikely that such testing will show any pharmacological effects due to the relatively low dose administered, but it is important to document for safety issues and regulatory agencies. Next, radiation dosimetry predictions can be made based on time-activity data in animals. Residence times of tracers in various organs can be used to extrapolate data to radiation dosimetry to various organs in humans using the MIRD software package.[240,241] Finally, sterility issues must be documented for the tracer prior to its injection into clinical subjects. Initial human testing should document the safety of the tracer by recording acute and chronic toxicity issues and radiation dosimetry estimates.

Typically, the problems that are encountered when one transitions the tracer from animals to humans are related to different behaviors of the tracer in humans compared with animal studies. The stability to the radiolabel can be quite different leading to increased complexity in tracer kinetic models or changes in image signal to background. Defluorination of Fluorine-18 typically leads to a whole body image that in part reflects the skeletal structure due to the affinity of Fluorine ion for bone. Different metabolic rates in humans relative to animals can also lead to different kinetic rates of tracer transport, delivery, metabolism, clearance, and so on. The biodistribution pattern in humans needs to be carefully studied. Tracers that fail in animal experiments can still be effective in humans and vice versa. The relative importance of different routes of clearance can change in humans relative to animals. Tracer kinetic models must be revalidated in humans as there is no guarantee that the models developed for animals will be completely effective. Kinetic validation is relatively easier and biochemical validation is much tougher due to the inability to obtain tissue samples from various sites in humans. However, since the relationship between biochemical and tracer kinetic results have been established in animals, this provides a reasonable foundation to use only tracer kinetic validation in humans.

FIGURE 2-33. Iterative Assay Development through Use of microPET and Clinical PET. Conventional assay development in mice and humans usually has been subdivided into four phases. This approach starts out with a few animals (Phase I) and progresses to more animals (Phase II) and then to a pilot study in humans (Phase III), followed by testing in many more human subjects (Phase IV). This conventional progression from Phase I to Phase IV can be slow and costly. A new iterative model may be more effective. In this new model, investigations progress from Phase I to Phase III (A), then back to Phase II (B), and then finally to Phase IV (C). By quickly transitioning to humans, one can detect problems with the assay much earlier, making the process possibly more cost- and time-efficient. MicroPET and Clinical PET become a team to help in the assay development effort.

A Clinical Trials Demonstration Project

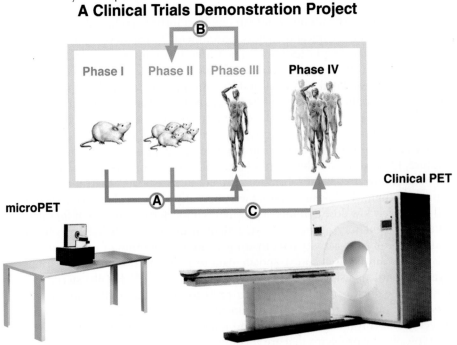

Just as assay development is an iterative process, even if one has no plans to go beyond studying animals (Figure 2-3), it also is iterative when one needs to perform imaging in both animals and humans (Figure 2-33). Ideally, one should develop an assay and rapidly migrate it to human studies and then come back and refine it in more animals prior to going to more humans. This is because often tracer assays that work relatively well in animals may not do so in humans or will have somewhat different characteristics in humans. A tracer that is not working well in an animal can actually work well in humans. The use of microPET and clinical PET can facilitate the early transition of an assay from mouse to humans. Because PET uses trace quantities, the probes are generally safe so these studies can be performed with little risk to humans.

The same principles that guide iterative development of a tracer assay from mouse to humans are also potentially the same for drug development. Pharmaceutical development shares many features with tracer development, and they can be thought of as two sides of the same coin (Table 2-1). Although tracers are administered at nonpharmacological doses and requirements for efflux of tracer out of nontarget sites and the blood are more stringent than that for pharmaceuticals, in most other ways the two tasks are almost identical. Pharmaceuticals that can be radiolabeled with positron emitters early on in the development process can have their biodistribution studied in small animal models and then quickly assessed in humans at tracer levels with low or no risk. It must be noted that the biodistribution of a drug administered at trace levels may not be the same if the drug is administered at mass levels (e.g., due to protein binding of drug in blood), so that care must be taken in interpreting the results of drug imaging studies in humans. Further examples of the use of imaging in drug development can be found elsewhere.[242] This approach has yet to be fully realized by the pharmaceutical and imaging industries but is being established and is likely to play an important role in accelerating drug development in the near future, maybe even producing a paradigm shift in the drug discovery process.

REFERENCES

1. Hoffman E, Phelps M. In: Phelps M, Mazziotta J, Schelbert H, eds. *Positron Emission Tomography and Autoradiography.* New York: Raven Press; 1986:237–286.
2. Hoffman EJ, Huang S-C, Phelps ME. Quantitation in positron emission computed tomography: 1. Effects of object size. *J Comput Assist Tomogr.* 1979;3:299–308.
3. Geworski L, Knoop BO, de Cabrejas ML, Knapp WH, Munz DL. Recovery correction for quantitation in emission tomography: a feasibility study. *Eur J Nucl Med.* 2000;27:161–169.
4. Gambhir SS. Quantitation of the physical factors affecting the tracer kinetic modeling of cardiac positron emission tomography data. PhD dissertation, University of California, Los Angeles; 1990.
5. Coleman RE. Is quantitation necessary for oncological PET studies? *Eur J Nucl Med Mol Imag.* 2002;29:133–135.
6. Graham MM. Is quantitation necessary for oncological PET studies? Against. *Eur J Nucl Med Mol Imag.* 2002;29:135–138.
7. Schomburg A, Bender H, Reichel C, Sommer T, Ruhlman J, Kozak B, Biersack HJ. Standardized uptake values of fluorine-18 fluorodeoxyglucose: the value of different normalization procedures. *Eur J Nucl Med.* 1996;23:571–574.
8. Kim CK, Gupta NC. Dependency of standardized uptake values of fluorine-18 fluorodeoxyglucose on body size: comparison of body surface area correction and lean body mass correction. *Nucl Med Commun.* 1996;17:890–894.
9. Keyes JW Jr. SUV: standard uptake or silly useless value? *J Nucl Med* 1995;36:1836–1839.

10. Sadato N, Tuschida T, Nakamura S, Waki A, Vematsu M, Takahasi N, Myashi N, Yonekura Y, Isii Y. Non-invasive estimation of the net influx constant using the standardized uptake value for quantification of FDG uptake of tumours. *Eur J Nucl Med.* 1998;25:559–564.

11. Sheiner LB, Steimer JL. Pharmacokinetic/pharmacodynamic modeling in drug development. *Annu Rev Pharmacol Toxicol.* 2000;40:67–95.

12. Boxenbaum H. Pharmacokinetics: philosophy of modeling. *Drug Metab Rev.* 1992;24(1): 89–120.

13. Mari A. Circulatory models of intact-body kinetics and their relationship with compartmental and non-compartmental analysis. *J Theor Biol.* 1993;160:509–531.

14. Cobelli C, Saccomani MP. Accessible pool and system parameters: assumptions and models. *J Parenter Enteral Nutr.* 1991;15:45S–50S.

15. Riviere JE. Basic principles and techniques of pharmacokinetic modeling. *J Zoo Wildl Med.* 1997;28:3–19.

16. Jacquez J. *Compartmental Analysis in Biololgy & Medicine.* Ann Arbor: University of Michigan; 1985.

17. Godfrey K. *Compartmental Models and Their Applications.* London: Academic Press; 1983.

18. Luxon BA, Forker EL. Simulation and analysis of hepatic indicator dilution curves. *Am J Physiol.* 1982;243:G76–89.

19. Forker EL, Luxon BA. Lumpers vs. distributers. *Hepatology.* 1985;5:1236–1237.

20. Meikle SR, Matthews JC, Brock CS, Wells P, Marte RJ, Cunningham VJ, Jones T, Price P. Pharmacokinetic assessment of novel anti-cancer drugs using spectral analysis and positron emission tomography: a feasibility study. *Cancer Chemother Pharmacol.* 1998;42:183–193.

21. Zierler KL. Circulation times and the theory of indicator-dilution methods for determining blood flow and volume. In: *Handbook of Physiology, Section 2: Circulation.* Baltimore: American Physiological Society, Waverly Press; 1962:585–615.

22. Bassingthwaighte JB, Holloway GA Jr. Estimation of blood flow with radioactive tracers. *Semin Nucl Med.* 1976;6:141–161.

23. Carson ER, Cobelli C, Finkelstein L. Modeling and identification of metabolic systems. *Am J Physiol.* 1981;240:R120–129.

24. Burger C, Buck A. Tracer kinetic modelling of receptor data with mathematical metabolite correction. *Eur J Nucl Med.* 1996;23:539–545.

25. Phelps ME, Huang SC, Hoffman EJ, Selin CE, Kuhl DE. Tomographic measurement of local cerebral glucose metabolic rate in humans with (F-18)2-fluoro-2-deoxy-D-glucose: validation of method. *Ann Neurol.* 1979;6:371–388.

26. Ohtake T, Kosaka N, Watanabe T, Yokoyama I, Moritan T, Masuo M, Iizuka M, Kozeni K, Momose T, Oku S. Noninvasive method to obtain input function for measuring tissue glucose utilization of thoracic and abdominal organs. *J Nucl Med.* 1991;32:1432–1438.

27. Germano G, Cher BC, Huang SC, Gambhir SS, Hoffman EJ, Phelps ME. Use of the abdominal aorta for arterial input function determination in hepatic and renal PET studies. *J Nucl Med.* 1992;33:613–620.

28. Weinberg IN, Huang SC, Hoffman EJ, Araujo L, Nienaber C, Grover-McKay M, Dahlbom M, Schelbert H. Validation of PET-acquired input functions for cardiac studies. *J Nucl Med.* 1988;29:241–247.

29. Hove JD, et al. Dual spillover problem in the myocardial septum with nitrogen-13-ammonia flow quantitation. *J Nucl Med.* 1998;39:591–598.

30. Markham J, Schuster DP. Effects of nonideal input functions on PET measurements of pulmonary blood flow. *J Appl Physiol.* 1992;72:2495–2500.

31. van den Hoff J, Burchert W, Muller-Schauenburg W, Meyer GJ, Hundeshagen H. Accurate local blood flow measurements with dynamic PET: fast determination of input function delay and dispersion by multilinear minimization. *J Nucl Med.* 1993;34:1770–1777.

32. Herholz K, Lercher M, Wierhard K, Bauer B, Lenz O, Meiss WD. PET measurement of cerebral acetylcholine esterase activity without blood sampling. *Eur J Nucl Med.* 201;28: 472–477.

33. Di Bella EV, Clackdoyle R, Gullberg GT. Blind estimation of compartmental model parameters. *Phys Med Biol.* 1999;44:765–780.

34. Feng D, Wang X, Yan H. A computer simulation study on the input function sampling schedules in tracer kinetic modeling with positron emission tomography (PET). *Comput Meth Progr Biomed.* 1994;45:175–186.

35. Glatting G, Reske SN. Treatment of radioactive decay in pharmacokinetic modeling: influence on parameter estimation in cardiac 13N-PET. *Med Phys.* 1999;26:616–621.

36. Wu HM, Huang SC, Choi Y, Hoh CK, Hawkins RA. A modeling method to improve quantitation of fluorodeoxyglucose uptake in heterogeneous tumor tissue. *J Nucl Med.* 1995;36:297–306.

37. Wu HM, Hoh CK, Choi Y, Schelbert HR, Hawkins RA, Phelps ME, Huang SC. Factor analysis for extraction of blood time-activity curves in dynamic FDG-PET studies. *J Nucl Med.* 1995;36:1714–1722.

38. Wu HM, Hoh CK, Buxton DB, Kuhle WG, Schelbert HR, Choi Y, Hawkins RA, Phelps ME, Huang SC. Quantification of myocardial blood flow using dynamic nitrogen-13-ammonia PET studies and factor analysis of dynamic structures. *J Nucl Med.* 1995;36: 2087–2093.

39. Hermansen F, Bloomfield PM, Ashburner J, Camici PG, Lammertsma AA. Linear dimension reduction of sequences of medical images: II. Direct sum decomposition. *Phys Med Biol.* 1995;40:1921–1941.

40. Hermansen F, Lammertsma AA. Linear dimension reduction of sequences of medical images: III. Factor analysis in signal space. *Phys Med Biol.* 1996;41:1469–1481.

41. Ahn JY, Lee DS, Lee JS, Kim SK, Cheon GJ, Yeo JS, Shin SA, Chung JK, Lee MC. Quantification of regional myocardial blood flow using dynamic H2(15)O PET and factor analysis. *J Nucl Med.* 2001;42:782–787.

42. Kety SS. The theory and applications of the exchange of inert gas at the lungs and tissues. *Pharmacol Rev.* 1951;3:1–41.

43. Renkin EM. Transport of potassium-42 from blood to tissue in isolated mammalian skeletal muscles. *Am J Physiol.* 1959;197:1205–1210.

44. Crone C. Permeability of capillaries in various organs as determined by use of the indicator diffusion method. *Acta Physiol Scand.* 1964;58:292–305.

45. DiStefano JJ 3rd, Landaw EM. Multiexponential, multicompartmental, and noncompartmental modeling. I. Methodological limitations and physiological interpretations. *Am J Physiol.* 1984;246:R651–664.

46. Landaw EM, DiStefano JJ 3rd. Multiexponential, multicompartmental, and noncompartmental modeling. II. Data analysis and statistical considerations. *Am J Physiol.* 1984; 246:R665–677.

47. Hawkins RA, Phelps ME, Huang SC, Kuhl DE. Effect of ischemia on quantification of local cerebral glucose metabolic rate in man. *J Cereb Blood Flow Metab.* 1981;1:37–51.

48. Huang SC, Phelps ME, Hoffman EJ, Sideris K, Selin CJ, Kuhl DE. Noninvasive determination of local cerebral metabolic rate of glucose in man. *Am J Physiol.* 1980;238: E69–82.

49. Sokoloff L, Reivich M, Kennedy C, Des Rosiers MH, Patlak CS, Pettigrew KD, Sakurada O, Shinohara M. The [14C]-deoxyglucose method for the measurement of local cerebral glucose utilization: Theory, procedure and normal values in the conscious and anesthetized albino rat. *J Neurochem.* 1977;28:897–916.

50. Lund-Andersen H. Transport of glucose from blood to brain. *Physiol Rev* 1979;59:305–352.

51. Spiegel MR. *Theory and Problems of Laplace Transforms.* Schaum Publishing Co: New York; 1965.

52. Krivokapich J, Huang SC, Phelps ME, MacDonald NS, Shine KI. Dependence of 13NH3 myocardial extraction and clearance on flow and metabolism. *Am J Physiol.* 1982;242: H536–542.

53. Bates DM, Watt GW. *Nonlinear Regression Analysis and its Applications.* New York: John Wiley & Sons; 1988.

54. Motulsky HJ, Ransnas LA. Fitting curves to data using nonlinear regression: a practical and nonmathematical review. *FASEB J.* 1987;1:365–374.

55. Bard Y. *Nonlinear Parameter Estimation.* New York: Academic Press; 1974.

56. Patlak CS, Blasberg RG, Fenstermacher JD. Graphical evaluation of blood-to-brain transfer constants from multiple-time uptake data. *J Cereb Blood Flow Metab.* 1983;3:1–7.

57. Patlak CS, Blasberg RG. Graphical evaluation of blood-to-brain transfer constants from multiple-time uptake data. Generalizations. *J Cereb Blood Flow Metab.* 1985;5:584–590.

58. Chen K, et al. Generalized linear least squares method for fast generation of myocardial blood flow parametric images with N-13 ammonia PET. *IEEE Trans Med Imaging.* 17: 236–243.

59. Feng D, Ho D, Lau KK, Siu WC. GLLS for optimally sampled continuous dynamic system modeling: theory and algorithm. *Comput Meth Progr Biomed.* 1999;59:31–43.

60. Cai W, Feng D, Fulton R, Siu WC. Generalized linear least squares algorithms for modeling glucose metabolism in the human brain with corrections for vascular effects. *Comput Meth Progr Biomed.* 2002;68:1–14.

61. Gambhir SS, Keppenne CL, Banerjee PK, Phelps ME. A new method to estimate parameters of linear compartmental models using artificial neural networks. *Phys Med Biol.* 1998;43:1659–1678.

62. Golish SR, Hove JD, Schelbert HR, Gambhir SS. A fast nonlinear method for parametric imaging of myocardial perfusion by dynamic (13)N-ammonia PET. *J Nucl Med.* 2001;42:924–931.

63. Carson R. Parameter estimation in positron emission tomography. In: Phelps M, Mazziotta J, Schelbert H, eds. *Positron Emission Tomography and Autoradiography: Principles and Applications for the Brain & Heart.* New York: Raven Press; 1986.

64. Cunningham VJ, Jones T. Spectral analysis of dynamic PET studies. *J Cereb Blood Flow. Metab.* 1993;13:15–23.

65. Levy AV, Laska E, Brodie JD, Volkow ND, Wolf AP. The spectral signature method for the analysis of PET brain images. *J Cereb Blood Flow Metab.* 1991;11:103–113.

66. Turkheimer F, Moresco RM, Lucignani G, Sokoloff L, Fazio F, Schmidt K. The use of spectral analysis to determine regional cerebral glucose utilization with positron emission tomography and [18F]fluorodeoxyglucose: theory, implementation, and optimization procedures. *J Cereb Blood Flow Metab.* 1994;14:406–422.

67. Meikle SR, Matthews JC, Cunningham VJ, Bailey DL, Livieratos L, Jones Price P. Parametric image reconstruction using spectral analysis of PET projection data. *Phys Med. Biol.* 1998;43:651–666.

68. Turkheimer F, et al. Estimation of component and parameter distributions in spectral analysis. *J Cereb Blood Flow Metab.* 1998;18:1211–1222.

69. Turkheimer F, Sokoloff L, Bertoldo A, Lucignani G, Reivich M, Jaggi JL, Schmidt K. Evaluation of compartmental and spectral analysis models of [18F]FDG kinetics for heart and brain studies with PET. *IEEE Trans Biomed Eng.* 1998;45:1429–1448.

70. Muzic RF Jr, Saidel GM, Zhu N, Nelson AD, Zheng L, Berridge MS. Iterative optimal design of PET experiments for estimating beta-adrenergic receptor concentration. *Med Biol Eng Comput.* 2000;38:593–602.

71. Li X, Feng D, Chen K. Optimal image sampling schedule for both image-derived input and output functions in PET cardiac studies. *IEEE Trans Med Imag.* 2000;19:233–242.

72. Strul D, Bendriem B. Robustness of anatomically guided pixel-by-pixel algorithms for partial volume effect correction in positron emission tomography. *J Cereb Blood Flow Metab.* 1999;19:547–559.

73. Huang SC, Carson RE, Phelps ME. Measurement of local blood flow and distribution volume with short-lived isotopes: a general input technique. *J Cereb Blood Flow Metab.* 1982;2:99–108.

74. Holthoff VA, Koeppe RA, Frey KA, Paradise AH, Kuhl DE. Differentiation of radioligand delivery and binding in the brain: validation of a two-compartment model for [11C]flumazenil. *J Cereb Blood Flow Metab.* 1991;11:745–752.

75. Barrett PH, Bell BM, Cobelli C, Golde H, Schumitzky A, Vicini P, Foster DM. SAAM II: Simulation, analysis, and modeling software for tracer and pharmacokinetic studies. *Metabolism.* 1998;47:484–492.

76. Gambhir SS, Mahoney DK, Huang SC, Phelps ME. Symbolic interactive modeling package and learning environment (SIMPLE), a new easy method for compartmental modeling. *Proceed Soc Comput Simul.* 1996:173–186.

77. Muzic RF Jr, Cornelius S. COMKAT: compartment model kinetic analysis tool. *J Nucl Med.* 2001;42:636–645.

78. Dannals R, Ravert H, Wilson A. Chemistry of tracers for positron emission tomography. In *Nuclear Imaging in Drug Discovery, Development, and Approval.* Boston: Birkhauser; 1993:56–74.

79. Frost JJ. *Receptor-Binding Radio Tracers.* Boca Raton, FL: CRC Press; 1982.

80. Hume SP, Gunn RN, Jones T. Pharmacological constraints associated with positron emission tomographic scanning of small laboratory animals. *Eur J Nucl Med.* 1998;25:173–176.

81. Bachelard HS. Specificity and kinetic properties of monosaccharide uptake into guinea pig cerebral cortex in vitro. *J Neurochem.* 1971;18:213–222.
82. Binder T. Hexose translocation across the blood barrier interface: configurational aspects. *J Neurochem.* 1968;15:867–874.
83. Horton RW, Meldrum BS, Bachelard HS. Enzymic and cerebral metabolic effects of 2-deoxy-D-glucose. *J Neurochem.* 1973;21:507–520.
84. Sols A, Crane RK. Substrate specificity of brain hexokinase. *J Biol Chem.* 1954;210:581–595.
85. Woodward G, Hudson M. The effect of 2-deoxy-D-glucose in glycolysis and respiration of tumor and normal tissues. *Cancer Res.* 1954;14:599–605.
86. Kennedy C, Sakurada O, Shinohara M, Jehle J, Sokoloff L. Local cerebral glucose utilization in the normal conscious macaque monkey. *Ann Neurol.* 1978;4:293–301.
87. Oldendorf WH. Brain uptake of radiolabeled amino acids, amines, and hexoses after arterial injection. *Am J Physiol.* 1971;221:1629–1639.
88. Sokoloff L, Reivich M, Kennedy C, Des Rosiers MH, Patlak CS, Pettigrew KD, Sakurada O, Shinohara M. The [14C]deoxyglucose method for the measurement of local cerebral glucose utilization: theory, procedure, and normal values in the conscious and anesthetized albino rat. *J Neurochem.* 1977;28:897–916.
89. Gallagher BM, Fowler JS, Gutterson NI, MacGregor RR, Wan CN, Wolf AP. Metabolic trapping as a principle of oradiopharmaceutical design: some factors resposible for the biodistribution of [18F]2-deoxy-2-fluoro-D-glucose. *J Nucl Med.* 1978;19:1154–1161.
90. Bidder T. Hexose translocation across the blood brain interface: configurational aspects. *J Neurochem.* 1968;15:867–874.
91. MacGregor RR, Fowler JS, Wolf AP, Shine CY, Lade RE, Wan CN. A synthesis of 2-deoxy-D-[1–11C]glucose for regional metabolic studies: concise communication. *J Nucl Med.* 1981;22:800–803.
92. Padgett HC, Barrio JR, MacDonald NS, Phelps ME. The unit operations approach applied to the synthesis of [1(-11)C]2-deoxy-D-glucose for routine clinical applications. *J Nucl Med.* 1982;23:739–744.
93. Raichle M, Welch M, Grubb R, Higgins C, Larson K. Measurement of regional substrate utilization rates by emission tomography. *Science.* 1978;199:986–987.
94. Ido T, Wan CN, Fowler J, Wolf A. Fluorination with F2:a conveninent synthesis of 2-deoxy-2-fluoro-D-glucose. *J Organ Chem.* 1978;42:2341–2342.
95. Bessel EM, Foster AB, Westwood JH. The use of deoxyfluoror-D-glucopyranoses and related compounds in a study of yeast hexokinase specificity. *Biochem J.* 1972;128:199–204.
96. Reivich M, Kuhl D, Wolf A, Greenberg J, Phelps M, Ido T, Caselia V, Fowler J, Hoffman E, Alavi A, Som P, Sokoloff L. The [18F]fluorodeoxyglucose method for the measurement of local cerebral glucose utilization in man. *Circ Res.* 1979;44:127–137.
97. Gambhir SS. Quantitation of the physical factors affecting the tracer kinetic modeling of cardiac positron emission tomography data. Ph.D. Dissertation, University of California Los Angeles; 1990.
98. Gjedde A, Kuwabara H, Evans AC. Metabolic brain imaging. Direct regional measurement of transfer coefficients and lumped constant. *Acta Radiol Suppl.* 1990;374:117–121.
99. Botker HE, Bottcher M, Schmitz O, Gee A, Hansen SB, Cold GE, Nielsen TT, Gjedde A. Glucose uptake and lumped constant variability in normal human hearts determined with [18F]fluorodeoxyglucose. *J Nucl Cardiol.* 1997;4:125–132.
100. Gambhir SS, Schwaiger M, Huang SC, Krivokapich J, Schelbert HR, Nienaber CA, Phelps ME. Simple noninvasive quantification method for measuring myocardial glucose utilization in humans employing positron emission tomography and fluorine-18 deoxyglucose. *J Nucl Med.* 1989;30:359–366.
101. Brooks RA. Alternative formula for glucose utilization using labeled deoxyglucose. *J Nucl Med.* 1982;23:538–539.
102. Hutchins GD, Holden JE, Koeppe RA, Halama JR, Gatley SJ, Nickles RJ. Alternative approach to single-scan estimation of cerebral glucose metabolic rate using glucose analogs, with particular application to ischemia. *J Cereb Blood Flow Metab.* 1984;4:35–40.
103. Graham MM, Peterson LM, Hayward RM. Comparison of simplified quantitative analyses of FDG uptake. *Nucl Med Biol.* 2000;27:647–655.
104. Schelbert HR, Phelps ME, Hoffman EJ, Huang SC, Selin CE, Kuhl DE. Regional myocardial perfusion assessed with N-13 labeled ammonia and positron emission computerized axial tomography. *Am J Cardiol.* 1979;43:209–218.

105. Schelbert HR, Phelps ME, Huang SC, MacDonald NS, Hansen H, Selin C, Kuhl DE. N-13 ammonia as an indicator of myocardial blood flow. *Circulation*. 1981;63:1259–1272.

106. Smith GT. Quantification of myocardial blood flow. *J Nucl Med*. 1992;33:172.

107. Huang S, Phelps M. In: Phelps M, Mazziotta J, Schelbert H, eds. *Positron Emission Tomography and Autoradiograpy: Principles and Applications for the Brain & Heart*. New York: Raven Press; 1986:287–346.

108. Cooper AJ, Nieves E, Coleman AE, Filc-DeRicco S, Gelbard AS. Short-term metabolic fate of [13N]ammonia in rat liver in vivo. *J Biol Chem*. 1987;262:1073–1080.

109. Rosenspire KC, Gelbard AS, Cooper AJ, Schmid FA, Roberts J. [13N]Ammonia and L-[amide-13N]glutamine metabolism in glutaminase-sensitive and glutaminase-resistant murine tumors. *Biochim Biophys Acta*. 1985;843:37–48.

110. Hutchins GD. Quantitative evaluation of myocardial blood flow with [13N]ammonia. *Cardiology*. 1997;88:106–115.

111. Choi Y, Huang SC, Hawkins RA, Kim JY, Kim BT, Hoh CK, Chen K, Phelps ME, Schelbert HR. Quantification of myocardial blood flow using 13N-ammonia and PET: comparison of tracer models. *J Nucl Med*. 1999;40:1045–1055.

112. Choi Y, Huang SC, Hawkins RA, Kuhle WG, Dahlbom M, Hoh CK, Czernin J, Phelps ME. A simplified method for quantification of myocardial blood flow using nitrogen-13-ammonia and dynamic PET. *J Nucl Med*. 1993;34:488–497.

113. DeGrado TR, Bergmann SR, Ng CK, Raffel DM. Tracer kinetic modeling in nuclear cardiology. *J Nucl Cardiol*. 2000;7:686–700.

114. Meyer JH, Ichise M. Modeling of receptor ligand data in PET and SPECT imaging: a review of major approaches. *J Neuroimaging*. 2001;11:30–39.

115. Morris ED, Alpert NM, Fischman AJ. Comparison of two compartmental models for describing receptor ligand kinetics and receptor availability in multiple injection PET studies. *J Cereb Blood Flow Metab*. 1996;16:841–853.

116. Ichise M, Meyer JH, Yonekura Y. An introduction to PET and SPECT neuroreceptor quantification models. *J Nucl Med*. 2001;42:755–763.

117. Slifstein M, Laruelle M. Models and methods for derivation of in vivo neuroreceptor parameters with PET and SPECT reversible radiotracers. *Nucl Med Biol*. 2001;28:595–608.

118. Arnett CD, Fowler JS, Wolf AP, Shiue C-Y, McPherson DW. [18F]-N-methylspiperone: the radioligand choice for PET studies of the dopamine receptor in human brain. *Life Sci*. 1985;36:1359–1366.

119. Coenen HH, Laufer P, Stocklin G, Wienhard K, Pawlik G, Bocher-Schwarz HG, Heiss WD. 3-N-(2-[18F]fluoroethyl)spiperone: a novel ligand for cerebral dopamine receptor studies with PET. *Life Sci*. 1985;40:81–88.

120. Burns HD, Dannals RF, Langstrom B, Ravert HT, Zemyan SE, Duelfer T, Wong DF, Frost JJ, Kuhar MJ, Wagner HN. (3-N-[11Cmethyl)spiperone, a ligand binding to dopamine receptors: radiochemical synthesis and biodistribution studies in mice. *J Nucl Med*. 1984;25:1222–1227.

121. Hall H, Kohler C, Gawell L, Farde L, Sedvall G. Raclopride, a new selective ligand for the dopamine-D2 receptors. *Progr Neurophychopharm Biol Psychiatr*. 1988;12:559–568.

122. Kessler RM, Ansari MS, Schmidt DE, de Paulis T, Clanton JA, Innis R, al-Tikriti M, Manning RG, Gillespie D. High affinity dopamine D2 receptor radioligands. 1. Regional rat brain distribution of iodinated benzamines. *J Nucl Med*. 1991;32:1593–1600.

123. Laduron PM, Janssen PFM, Leysen JE. Spiperone: a ligand of choice for neuroleptic receptors. 2. Regional distribution and in vivo displacement of neuroleptic drugs. *Biochem Pharmacol*. 1978;27:317–321.

124. Leysen JE, Gommeren W, Laduron PM. Spiperone: a ligand of choice for neuroleptic receptors. 1. Kinetics and characteristics of in vitro binding. *Biochem Pharmacol*. 1978;27:307–316.

125. Mintun MA, Raichle ME, Kilbourn MR, Wooten GF, Welch MJ. A quantitative model for the in vivo assessment of drug binding sites with positron emission tomography. *Ann Neurol*. 1984;15:217–227.

126. Persson A, Ehrin E, Eriksson L, Farde L, Hedstrom CG, Litton JE, Mindus P, Sedvall G. Imaging of [11C]-labelled Ro 15–1788 binding to benzodiazepine receptors in the human brain by positron emission tomography. *J Psychiatr Res*. 1985;19:609–622.

127. Tewson TJ, Raichle ME, Welch MJ. Preliminary studies with [18F]haloperidol: a radi-oligand for in vivo studies of the dopamine receptors. *Brain Res.* 1980;192:291–295.
128. Wagner HN Jr, Burns HD, Dannals RF, Wong DF, Langstrom B, Duelfer T, Frost JJ, Ravert HT, Links JM, Rosenbloom SB. Assessment of dopamine receptor densities in the human brain with carbon-11–labeled N-methylspiperone. *Ann Neurol.* 1984;15:S79–84.
129. Wang WF, Ishiwata R, Nonaka M, Ishii S, Kiyosawa M, Shimada J, Suzuki F, Serda M. Carbon-11-labeled KF21213: a highly selective ligand for mapping CNS adenosine A(2A) receptors with positron emission tomography. *Nucl Med Biol.* 2000;27:541–546.
130. Doudet DJ, Holden JE, Jivan S, McGeer E, Wyatt RJ. In vivo PET studies of the dopamine D2 receptors in rhesus monkeys with long-term MPTP-induced parkinsonism. *Synapse.* 2000;38:105–113.
131. Andree B, Halldin C, Thorberg SO, Sandell J, Farde L. Use of PET and the radioligand [carbonyl-(11)C]WAY-100635 in psychotropic drug development. *Nucl Med Biol.* 2000; 27:515–521.
132. Gunn RN, Lammertsma AA, Grasby PM. Quantitative analysis of [carbonyl-(11)C]WAY-100635 PET studies. *Nucl Med Biol.* 2000;27:477–482.
133. Shiue C, Shiue GG, Benard F, Visonneau S, Santoli D, Alavi AA. N-(n-Benzylpiperidin-4-yl)-2-[18F]fluorobenzamide: a potential ligand for PET imaging of breast cancer. *Nucl Med Biol.* 2000;27:763–767.
134. Zubieta JK, Koeppe RA, Frey KA, Kilbourn MR, Mangner TJ, Foster NL, Kuhl DE. Assessment of muscarinic receptor concentrations in aging and Alzheimer disease with [11C]NMPB and PET. *Synapse.* 2001;39:275–287.
135. Wilson AA, Ginovart N, Schmidt M, Meyer JH, Threlkeld PG, Houle S. Novel radio-tracers for imaging the serotonin transporter by positron emission tomography: synthesis, radiosynthesis, and in vitro and ex vivo evaluation of (11)C-labeled 2-(phenylthio)araalkylamines. *J Med Chem.* 2000;43:3103–3110.
136. Aston JA, Gunn RN, Worsley KJ, Ma Y, Evans AC, Dagher A.
140. Costes N, Merlet I, Zimmer L, Lavenne F, Cinotti L, Delforge J, Luxen A, Pujol JF, Le Bars D. A statistical method for the analysis of positron emission tomography neurore-ceptor ligand data. *Neuroimage.* 2000;12:245–256.
137. Christian BT, Narayanan TK, Shi B, Mukherjee J. Quantitation of striatal and extrastri-atal D-2 dopamine receptors using PET imaging of [(18)F]fallypride in nonhuman primates. *Synapse.* 2000;38:71–79.
138. Watabe H, et al. Kinetic analysis of the 5–HT2A ligand [11C]MDL 100,907. *J Cereb Blood Flow Metab.* 2000;20:899–909.
139. Passchier J, van Waarde A. Visualisation of serotonin-1A (5-HT1A) receptors in the central nervous system. *Eur J Nucl Med.* 2001;28:113–129.
140. Costes N, et al. Modeling [18 F]MPPF positron emission tomography kinetics for the determination of 5-hydroxytryptamine(1A) receptor concentration with multiinjection. *J Cereb Blood Flow Metab.* 2002;22:753–765.
141. Lewin B. *Genes VII.* Oxford: Oxford Press; 2000.
142. Chalfie M, Tu Y, Euskirchen W, Ward W, Prasher DC. Green fluorescent protein as a marker for gene expression. *Science.* 1994;263:802–805.
143. Chalfie M. Green fluorescent protein. *Photochem Photobiol.* 1995;62:651–656.
144. Yang M, et al. Widespread skeletal metastatic potential of human lung cancer revealed by green fluorescent protein expression. *Cancer Res.* 1998;58:4217–4221.
145. Chishima T, et al. Metastatic patterns of lung cancer visualized live and in process by green fluorescence protein expression. *Clin Exper Met.* 1997;15:547–552.
146. Bhaumik S, Gambhir SS. Optical imaging of Renilla luciferase reporter gene expression in living mice. *Proc Natl Acad Sci.* 2001.
147. Contag CH, Jenkins D, Contag PR, Negrin RS. Use of reporter genes for optical measurements of neoplastic disease in vivo. *Neoplasia.* 2000;2:41–52.
148. Weissleder R. Scaling down imaging: molecular mapping of cancer in mice. *Nat Rev Cancer.* 2002;2:11–18.
149. Massoud T, Gambhir S. Molecular imaging in living subjects: Seeing fundamental biological processes in a new light. *Genes Devel.* 2003;17:545–580.
150. Gambhir SS, Barrio JR, Herschman HR, Phelps ME. Imaging gene expression: principles and assays. *J Nucl Cardiol.* 1999;6:219–233.
151. Sundaresan G, Gambhir S. Radionuclide imaging of reporter gene expression. In: Toga

WA, Mazziota JC, eds. *Brain Mapping: The Methods*. Amsterdam: Academic Press; 2002: 799–818.

152. Ray P, Bauer E, Iyer M, Barrio JR, Satyamurthy N, Phelps ME, Herschman HR, Gambhir SS. Monitoring gene therapy with reporter gene imaging. *Semin Nucl Med*. 2001.

153. Green LA, Yap CS, Nguyen K, Barrio JR, Namavari M, Satyamurthy N, Phelps ME, Sandgren EP, Herschman HR, Gambhir SS. Indirect monitoring of endogenous gene expression by Positron Emission Tomography (PET) imaging of reporter gene expression in transgenic mice. *Molec Imag Biol*. 2001;4:71–81.

154. Arner ES, Eriksson S. Mammalian deoxyribonucleoside kinases. *Pharmacol Therapeut*. 1995;67:155–186.

155. De Clercq E. Antivirals for the treatment of herpes virus infections. *J Antimicrob Chemother*. 1993;32:121–132.

156. Elion GB. Acyclovir: discovery, mechanism of action, and selectivity. *J Med Virol*. 1993:2–6.

157. Alrabiah FA, Sacks SL. New antiherpesvirus agents: their targets and therapeutic potential. *Drugs*. 1996;52:17–32.

158. Iyer M, Barrio JR, Namavari M, Bauer E, Satyamurthy N, Nguyen K, Toyokuni T, Phelps ME, Herschman HR, Gambhir SS8-[18F]-Fluoropenciclovir: An improved reporter probe for imaging HSV1-tk reporter gene expression in vivo using positron emission tomography. *J Nucl Med*. 2001;42:96–105.

159. Tjuvajev JG, Doubrovin M, Akhurst T, Cai S, Balatoni J, Alauddin MM, Finn R, Bornmann W, Thaler H, Conti PS, Blasberg RG. Comparison of radiolabeled nucleoside probes (FIAU, FHBG, and FHPG) for PET imaging of HSV1-tk gene expression. *J Nucl Med*. 2002;43:1072–1083.

160. Gambhir SS, Barrio JR, Wu L, Iyer M, Namavari M, Satyamurthy N, Bauer E, Parrish C, MacLaren DC, Borghei AR, Green LA, Sharfstein S, Berk AJ, Cherry SR, Phelps ME, Herschman HR. Imaging of adenoviral directed herpes simplex virus type 1 thymidine kinase gene expression in mice with ganciclovir. *J Nucl Med*. 1998;39:2003–2011.

161. Herz J, Gerard RD. Adenovirus-mediated transfer of low density lipoprotein receptor gene acutely accelerates cholesterol in normal mice. *Proc Natl Acad Sci USA*. 1993;90: 2812–2816.

162. Stratford-Perricaudet LD, Levrero M, Chasse J-F, Perricaudet M, Briand P. Evaluation of the transfer and expression in mice of an enzyme-encoding gene using a human adenovirus vector. *Hum Gene Ther*. 1990;1:241–256.

163. Barrio BR, Namavari M, Phelps ME, Satyamurthy N. Elemental fluorine to 8-fluorpurines in one step. *J Am Chem Soc*. 1996;118:10408–10411.

164. Alauddin MM, Conti PS, Mazza SM, Hamzeh FM, Lever JR. Synthesis of 9-[(3-[18F]fluoro-1-hydroxy-2-propoxy)methyl]guanine ([18F]FHPG): A potential imaging agent of viral infection and gene therapy using PET. *Nucl Med Biol*. 1996;23:787–792.

165. Bading JR, et al. Pharmacokinetics of F-18 fluorohydroxy-propoxymethylguanine (FHPG). *J Nucl Med*. 1997;38:43P.

166. Alauddin MM, Conti PS. Synthesis and preliminary evaluation of 9-(4-[18F]-fluoro-3-hydroxymethylbutyl)guanine ([18F]FHBG): a new potential imaging agent for viral infection and gene therapy using PET. *Nucl Med Biol*. 1998;25:175–180.

167. Iyer M, et al. Comparison of FPCV, FHBG, and FIAU as reporter probes for imaging herpes simplex virus type 1 thymidine kinase reporter gene expression. *J Nucl Med*. 2000;41:80P.

168. Tjuvajev JG, et al. Quantitative PET imaging of HSV1-TK gene expression with [I-124]FIAU. *J Nucl Med*. 1997;38:239P.

169. Min J, Iyer M, Gambhir S. Comparison of FHBG and FIAU for Imaging HSV1-tk reporter gene expression: Adenoviral infection vs. stable transfection. *J Nucl Med*. 2002;43:275P.

170. Blasberg R. Imaging gene expression and endogenous molecular processes: molecular imaging. *J Cereb Blood Flow Metab*. 2002;22:1157–1164.

171. Qiao J, Doubrovin M, Sauter BV, Huang Y, Guo ZS, Balatoni J, Akhurst T, Blasberg RG, Tjuvajev JG, Chen SH, Woo SL. Tumor-specific transcriptional targeting of suicide gene therapy. *Gene Ther*. 2002;9:168–175.

172. Ponomarev V, Doubrovin M, Lyddane C, Beresten T, Balatoni J, Bornman W, Finn R, Akhurst T, Larson S, Blasberg R, Sadelain M, Tjuvajev JG. Imaging TCR-dependent NFAT-mediated T-cell activation with positron emission tomography in vivo. *Neoplasia*. 2001;3:480–488.

173. Tjuvajev J, Blasberg R, Luo X, Zheng LM, King I, Bermudes D.Salmonella-based tumor-

targeted cancer therapy: tumor amplified protein expression therapy (TAPET) for diagnostic imaging. *J Contr Release.* 2001;74:313–315.

174. Doubrovin M, Ponomarev V, Beresten T, Balatoni J, Bornmann W, Finn R, Humm J, Larson S, Sadelain M, Blasberg R, Gelovani Tjuvajev J. Imaging transcriptional regulation of p53-dependent genes with positron emission tomography in vivo. *Proc Natl Acad Sci USA.* 2001;98:9300–9305.

175. Bennett JJ, Tjuvajev J, Johnson P, Doubrovin M, Akhurst T, Malholtra S, Hackman T, Balatoni J, Finn R, Larson SM, Federoff H, Blasberg R, Fong Y. Positron emission tomography imaging for herpes virus infection: Implications for oncolytic viral treatments of cancer. *Natl Med.* 2001;7:859–863.

176. Jacobs A, Tjuvajev JG, Dubrovin M, Akhurst T, Balatoni J, Beattie B, Joshi R, Finn R, Larson SM, Herrlinger U, Pechan PA, Chiocca EA, Breakefield XO, Blasberg RG. Positron emission tomography-based imaging of transgene expression mediated by replication-conditional, oncolytic herpes simplex virus type 1 mutant vectors in vivo. *Cancer Res.* 2001;61:2983–2995.

177. Gambhir SS, Bauer E, Black ME, Liang Q, Kokoris MS, Barrio JR, Iyer M, Namavari M, Phelps ME, Herschman HR. A mutant herpes simplex virus type 1 thymidine kinase reporter gene shows improved sensitivity for imaging reporter gene expression with positron emission tomography. *Proc Natl Acad Sci USA.* 2000;97:2785–2790.

178. Black ME, Newcomb TG, Wilson H-MP, Loeb LA. Creation of drug-specific hepes simplex virus type 1 thymidine kinase mutant for gene therapy. *Proc Natl Acad Sci USA.* 1996;93:3525–3529.

179. Black ME, Kokoris SK, Sabo P. Herpes implex virus-1 thymidine kinase mutants created by semi-random sequence mutagenesis improve pro-drug mediated tumor cell killing. *Cancer Res.* 2001;61:3022–3026.

180. Green LA, Gambhir SS, Srinivasan A, Banerjee PK, Hoh CK, Cherry SR, Sharfstein S, Barrio JR, Herschman HR, Phelps ME. Non-invasive methods for quantitating blood time-activity curves from FDG PET mice images. *J Nucl Med.* 1998;39:729–734.

181. Green L, et al. Tracer kinetic modeling of FHBG in mice imaged with MicroPET for quantitation of reporter gene expression. *J Nucl Med.* 2000;41:58P.

182. Yaghoubi S, Barrio JR, Dahlbom M, Iyer M, Namavari M, Satyamurthy N, Goldman R, Herschman HR, Phelps ME, Gambhir SSHuman pharmacokinetic and dosimetry studies of [18F]-FHBG: A reporter probe for imaging herpes simplex virus type I thymidine kinase (HSV1-tk) reporter gene expression. *J Nucl Med.* 2001;42(8):1225–1234.

183. Green L, Berenji B, Kuo J, Gambhir S. Simulation studies of assumptions of a three-compartment FHBG model for imaging reporter gene expression. *J Nucl Med.* 2001;42:100P.

184. Gambhir SS, Barrio JR, Phelps ME, Iyer M, Namavari M, Satyamurthy N, Wu L, Green LA, Bauer E, MacLaren DC, Nguyen K, Berk AJ, Cherry SR, Herschman HR. Imaging adenoviral-directed reporter gene expression in living animals with Positron Emission Tomography. *Proc Natl Acad Sci USA.* 1999;96:2333–2338.

185. Jacobs A, Voges J, Reszka R, Lercher M, Gossmann A, Kracht L, Kaestle C, Wagner R, Wienhard K, Heiss WD. Positron-emission tomography of vector-mediated gene expression in gene therapy for gliomas. *Lancet.* 2001;358:727–729.

186. MacLaren DC, Gambhir SS, Satyamurthy N, Barrio JR, Sharfstein S, Toyokuni T, Wu L, Berk AJ, Cherry SR, Phelps ME, Herschman HR. Repetitive, non-invasive imaging of the dopamine D_2 receptor as a reporter gene in living animals. *Gene Ther.* 1999;6:785–791.

187. Haberkorn U. Gene therapy with sodium/iodide symporter in hepatocarcinoma. *Exp Clin Endocrinol Diabetes.* 2001;109:60–62.

188. Haberkorn U, Henze M, Altmann A, Jiang S, Morr I, Mahmut M, Peschke P, Kubler W, Debus J, Eisenhut M. Transfer of the human NaI symporter gene enhances iodide uptake in hepatoma cells. *J Nucl Med.* 2001;42:317–325.

189. Chung JK. Sodium iodide symporter: its role in nuclear medicine. *J Nucl Med.* 2002;43:1188–1200.

190. Cho JY, Shen DH, Yang W, Williams B, Buckwalter TL, La Perle KM, Hinkle G, Pozderac R, Kloos R, Nagaraja HN, Barth RF, Jhiang SM. In vivo imaging and radioiodine therapy following sodium iodide symporter gene transfer in animal model of intracerebral gliomas. *Gene Ther.* 2002;9:1139–1145.

191. Petrich T, Helmeke HJ, Meyer GJ, Knapp WH, Potter E. Establishment of radioactive astatine and iodine uptake in cancer cell lines expressing the human sodium/iodide symporter. *Eur J Nucl Med Mol Imag.* 2002;29:842–854.

192. Rogers BE, Zinn KR, Buchsbaum DJ. Gene transfer strategies for improving radiolabeled peptide imaging and therapy. *Q J Nucl Med.* 2000;44:208–223.

193. Liang Q, et al. Noninvasive, repetitive, quantitative measurement of gene expression from a bicistronic message by positron emission tomography, following gene transfer with adenovirus. *Mol Ther.* 2002;6:73–82.

194. Liang Q, et al. Noninvasive, quantitative imaging in living animals of a mutant dopamine D2 receptor reporter gene in which ligand binding is uncoupled from signal transduction. *Gene Ther.* 2001;8:1490–1498.

195. Le LQ, Kabarowski JH, Wong S, Nguyen K, Gambhir SS, Witte ON. Positron emission tomography imaging analysis of G2A as a negative modifier of lymphoid leukemogenesis initiated by the BCR-ABL oncogene. *Cancer Cell.* 2002;1:381–391.

196. Yu Y, Annala AJ, Barrio JR, Toyokuni T, Satyamurthy N, Namavari M, Cherry SR, Phelps ME, Herschman HR, Gambhir SS. Quantification of target gene expression by imaging reporter gene expression in living animals. *Nature Med.* 2000;6:933–937.

197. Yaghoubi SS, Wu L, Liang Q, Toyokuni T, Barrio JR, Namavari M, Satyamurthy N, Phelps ME, Herschman HR, Gambhir SS. Direct correlation between positron emission tomographic images of two reporter genes delivered by two distinct adenoviral vectors. *Gene Ther.* 2001;8:1072–1080.

198. Sun X, Annala AJ, Yaghoubi SS, Barrio JR, Nguyen KN, Toyokuni T, Satyamurthy N, Namavari M, Phelps ME, Herschman HR, Gambhir SS. Quantitative imaging of gene induction in living animals. *Gene Ther.* 2001;8:1572–1579.

199. Iyer M, Berenji M, Templeton NS, Gambhir S. Noninvasive imaging of cationic lipid mediated delivery of optical and PET reporter genes in living mice. *Mol Ther.* 2002;6:555–562.

200. Hildebrandt I, Iyer M, Wagner E, Gambhir S. Optical imaging of transferrin targeted PEI/DNA complexes in living subjects. *Gene Ther.* 2003;10:758–764.

201. Adams JY, Johnson M, Sato M, Berger F, Gambhir SS, Carey M, Iruela-Arispe ML, Wu L. Visualization of advanced human prostate cancer lesions in living mice by a targeted gene transfer vector and optical imaging. *Nat Med.* 2002;8:891–897.

202. Iyer M, Wu L, Carey M, Wang Y, Smallwood A, Gambhir SS. Two-step transcriptional amplification as a method for imaging reporter gene expression using weak promoters. *Proc Natl Acad Sci USA.* 2001;98:14595–14600.

203. Zhang L, Adams JY, Billick E, Ilagan R, Iyer M, Le K, Smallwood A, Gambhir SS, Carey M, Wu L. Molecular engineering of a two-step transcription amplification (TSTA) system for transgene delivery in prostate cancer. *Mol Ther.* 2002;5:223–232.

204. Ray P, Bauer E, Iyer M, Barrio JR, Satyamurthy N, Phelps ME, Herschman HR, Gambhir SS. Monitoring gene therapy with reporter gene imaging. *Semin Nucl Med.* 2001;31:312–320.

205. Ray P, Wu A, Gambhir SS. Optical bioluminescence and positron emission tomography imaging of a novel fusion reporter gene in tumor xenografts of living mice. *Cancer Res.* 2003;63:1160–1165.

206. Agrawal S, Iyer RP. Perspectives in antisense therapeutics. *Pharmacol Therapeut.* 1997;76:151–160.

207. Crooke ST, Lebleu B. *Antisense Research and Applications.* Boca Raton, FL: CRC Press; 1993.

208. Crooke S. Progress in antisense therapeutics discovery and development. *Ciba Found Sympos* 1997;209:158–168.

209. Wagner RW, Flanagan WM. Antisense technology and prospects for therapy of viral infections and cancer. *Molec Med Today.* 1997;3:31–38.

210. Hargrove JL, Hulsey MG, Schmidt FH, Beale EG. A computer program for modeling kinetics of gene expression. *BioTechniques.* 1990;8:654–660.

211. Helene C, Toulme JJ. Control of gene expression by oligodeoxynucleotides covalently linked to intercalating agents and nucleic acid-cleaving reagents. In: Cohen JS, ed. *Oligodeoxynucleotides.* London: MacMillan; 1990:137–166.

212. Goodchild J. Inhibition of gene expression by oligonucleotides. In: Cohen JS, ed. *Oligonucleotides: Antisense Inhibitors for Gene Expression.* London: MacMillan; 1990:53–71.

213. Pan D, Gambhir SS, Toyokuni T, Iyer MR, Acharya N, Phelps ME, Barrio JR. Rapid synthesis of a 5'-fluorinated oligodeoxy-nucleotoide: A model antisense probe for use in imaging with Positron Emission Tomography (PET). *Bioorg Med Chem Ltr.* 1998;8:1317–1320.

214. Wickstrom E. Oligodeoxynucleotide stability in subcellular extracts and culture media. *J Biochem Biophys Meth.* 1986;13:97–102.

215. Matsukura M, Shinozuka K, Zon G. Phosphorothioate analogs of oligodeoxynucleotides: novel inhibitors of replication and cytopathic effects of human immunodeficiency virus (HIV). *Proc Natl Acad Sci USA*. 1978;84:7706–7710.

216. Murakami A, Blake K, Miller PS. Characterization of sequence-specific oligodeoxynucleoside methylphosphonates and their interaction with rabbit globin mRNA. *Biochemistry*. 1985;24:4041–4046.

217. Good L, Nielsen PE. Progress in developing PNA as a gene-targeted drug. *Antisense Nucl Acid Drug Devel*. 1997;7:431–437.

218. Cotten M, Wagner E, Birnstiel M. Receptor-mediated transport of DNA into eukaryotic cells. *Meth Enzymol*. 1993;217:618–644.

219. Loke SL, Stein CA, Zhang XH, Mori K, Nakanishi M, Subasinghe C, Cohen JS, Neckers LM. Characterization of oligonucleotide transport into living cells. *Proc Natl Acad Sci USA*. 1989;86:7595–7599.

220. Wu-Pong S, Weiss TL, Hunt AC. Antisense c-myc oligodeoxyribonucleotide cellular uptake. *Pharm Res*. 1992;9:1010–1017.

221. Wu-Pong S, Weiss TL, Hunt AC. Antisense c-myc oligonucleotide cellular uptake and activity. *Antisense Res Devel*. 1994;4:155–163.

222. Stein CA, Cheng YC. Antisense oligonucleotides as therapeutic agents-Is the bullet really magical. *Science*. 1993;261:1004–1011.

223. Zamecnik PC, Stephenson M. Inhibition of Rous sarcoma virus replication and cell transformation by a specific oligodeoxynucleotide. *Proc Natl Acad Sci USA*. 1978;75:280–284.

224. Zamecnik PC, Goodchild J, Yaguchi Y, Sarin P. Inhibition of replication of expression of human T-cell lymphotropic virus type III in cultured cells by exogenous synthetic oligonucleotides complementary to viral RNA. *Proc Natl Acad Sci USA*. 1986;83:4143–4146.

225. Crooke ST. Progress in antisense therapeutics. *Hematol Pathol*. 1995;9:59–72.

226. Phillips JA, Craig SJ, Bayley D, Christian RA, Geary R, Nicklin PL. Pharmacokinetics, metabolism, and elimination of a 20-mer phosphorothioate oligodeoxynucleotide (CGP 69846A) after intravenous and subcutaneous administration. *Biochem Pharm*. 1997;54:657–668.

227. Dewanjee MK, Ghafouripour AK, Kapadvanjwala M, Dewanjee S, Serafini AN, Lopez DM, Sfakianakis GN. Noninvasive imaging of c-myc oncogene messenger RNA with indium-111-antisense probes in a mammary tumor-bearing mouse model. *J Nucl Med*. 1994;35:1054–1063.

228. Hnatowich DJ, Winnard P Jr, Virzi F, Fogarasi M, Sano T, Smith CL, Cantor CR, Rusckowski M. Technetium-99m labeling of DNA oligonucleotides. *J Nucl Med*. 1995;36:2306–2314.

229. Cammilleri S, Sangrajrang S, Perdereau B, Brixy F, Calvo F, Bazin H, Magdelenat H. Biodistribution of iodine-125 dyramine transforming growth factor alpha antisense oligonucleotide in athymic mice with a human mammary tumor xenograft following intratumoral injection. *Euro J Nucl Med*. 1996;23:448–452.

230. Tavitian B, Terrazzino S, Kuhnast B, Marzabal S, Stettler O, Dolle F, Deverre JR, Jobert A, Hinnen F, Bendriem B, Crouzel C, Di Giamberardino L. *In vivo* imaging of oligonucleotides with positron emission tomography. *Nat Med*. 1998;4:467–471.

231. Lee HJ, Boado RJ, Braasch DA, Corey DR, Pardridge WM. Imaging gene expression in the brain in vivo in a transgenic mouse model of Huntington's disease with an antisense radiopharmaceutical and drug-targeting technology. *J Nucl Med*. 2002;43:948–956.

232. Tavitian B. In vivo antisense imaging. *Q J Nucl Med*. 2000;44:236–255.

233. Hnatowich DJ. Antisense imaging: where are we now? *Cancer Biother Radiopharm*. 2000; 15:447–457.

234. Hnatowich DJ. Antisense and nuclear medicine. *J Nucl Med*. 1999;40:693–703.

235. Puttaraju M, DiPasquale J, Baker CC, Mitchell LG, Garcia-Blanco MA. Messenger RNA repair and restoration of protein function by spliceosome-mediated RNA trans-splicing. *Mol Ther*. 2001;4:105–114.

236. Mansfield SG, Kole J, Puttaraju M, Yang CC, Garcia-Blanco MA, Cohn JA, Mitchell LG. Repair of CFTR mRNA by spliceosome-mediated RNA trans-splicing. *Gene Ther*. 2000; 7:1885–1895.

237. Bhaumik S, Lewis X, Puttaraju M, Mitchell L, Gambhir S. Imaging mRNA levels in living animals through a novel RNA trans-splicing signal amplification approach. *Molec Imag Biol*. 2002;4:517.

238. Paulmurugan R, Umezawa Y, Gambhir SS. Noninvasive imaging of protein-protein interactions in living subjects using reporter protein complementation and reconstitution strategies. *Proc Natl Acad Sci. USA.* 2002;99:15608–15613.

239. Gambhir SS. Molecular imaging of cancer with positron emission tomography. *Nat Rev Cancer.* 2002;2:683–693.

240. Siegel JA, Thomas SR, Stubbs JB, Stabin MG, Hays MT, Koral KF, Robertson JS, Howell RW, Wessels BW, Fisher DR, Weber DA, Brill AB. MIRD pamphlet no. 16: Techniques for quantitative radiopharmaceutical biodistribution data acquisition and analysis for use in human radiation dose estimates. *J Nucl Med.* 1999;40:37S–61S.

241. Bolch WE, Bouchet LG, Robertson JS, Wessels BW, Siegel JA, Howell RW, Erdi AK, Aydogan B, Costes S, Watson EE, Brill AB, Charkes ND, Fisher DR, Hays MT, Thomas SR. MIRD pamphlet No. 17: the dosimetry of nonuniform activity distributions—radionuclide S values at the voxel level. Medical Internal Radiation Dose Committee. *J Nucl Med.* 1999;40:11S–36S.

242. Burns HD, Gibson RE, Dannals R, Siegl P. *Nuclear Imaging in Drug Discovery, Development, and Approval.* Boston: Birkhauser; 1993.

243. Cho A, et al. A pharmacokinetic study of phenylcyclohexyldiethylamine. An analog of phencyclidine. *Drug Metab Dispos.* 1993;21:125–132.

APPENDIX

1. Derivation of Competitive Reaction Kinetics

Suppose A and B are two chemical substances that compete for enzyme E.
Claim: If B is present in trace amounts, then the rate of reaction of B with enzyme E is approximately linear regardless of the concentration of A.

Proof: The rate, r (mol/min), of reaction of B with enzyme E is derived from the principles of competitive chemical or enzyme kinetics to yield (see reference 243 for details):

$$r = \frac{V_{max}^B \cdot B}{K_M^B \cdot V_B \left[\dfrac{B/V_B}{K_M^B} + 1 + \dfrac{A/V_A}{K_M^A} \right]} \tag{A1-1}$$

where:

V_{max}^B = maximal velocity of reaction B with enzyme E (mol/min)
K_M^B = Michaelis-Menten constant for B with E (mol/L)
K_M^A = Michaelis-Menten constant for A with E (mol/L)
V_B = volume of distribution of B (L)
V_A = volume of distribution of A (L)
B = mass of B (mol)
A = mass of A (mol)

If the enzymatic reaction being performed is in a test tube, then $V_A = V_B$; therefore, concentrations of A and B can be used directly. Because the processes described in the text take place in a cell, it is potentially possible that A and B have different volumes of distribution, which is why they are included here.

By assumption that B is in trace amounts, $B/V_B \ll K_M^B$.

Therefore, $\dfrac{B/V_B}{K_M^B} \ll 1$

which implies $\dfrac{B/V_B}{K_M^B} + 1 + \dfrac{A/V_A}{K_M^A} \approx 1 + \dfrac{A/V_A}{K_M^A}$ which is independent of B.

Therefore, $r \approx hB$ where $h = \dfrac{V_{\max}^B}{K_M^B \cdot V_B \left[1 + \dfrac{A/V_A}{K_M^A}\right]}$. Therefore, r is linear in B.

Here h is analogous to the linear parameters k described in the models above.

QED

Corollary 1: If B is present in trace amounts, then the rate of reaction of B with enzyme E is approximately linear even when A is present at saturating conditions.

Corollary 2: If B is present in trace amounts, then the rate of reaction of B with enzyme E is approximately linear when A is absent, i.e., when there is no competitor.

2. Derivation that the lumped constant (*LC*) in equation 2-19 for the FDG
   model shown in Figure 2-16 is given by, $LC = \dfrac{\lambda f}{\Theta'}$,

where, $\Theta' = 1 - \dfrac{k_4 C_M}{k_3 C_E}, f = \dfrac{k_3^*}{k_3} = \dfrac{V_m^* K_m}{V_m K_m^*}, \lambda = \dfrac{K_1^*/(k_2^* + k_3^*)}{K_1/(k_2 + k_3 \Theta')}.$

Proof: Because the system is assumed to be in steady state, MRglc is equal to the net phosphorylation rate of glucose. Therefore, we have (see Figure 2-16):

$$MRglc + k_4 C_M = k_3 C_E$$

$$MRglc = k_3 C_E - k_4 C_M = \left(1 - \dfrac{k_4 C_M}{k_3 C_E}\right) k_3 C_E \qquad (A2\text{-}1)$$

and if we make the substitution:

$$\Theta' = 1 - \dfrac{k_4 C_M}{k_3 C_E} \qquad (A2\text{-}2)$$

we obtain by substituting Equation A2-2 into Equation A2-1:

$$MRglc = \Theta' k_3 C_E \qquad (A2\text{-}3)$$

Here Θ' is the fraction of glucose that is metabolized after it is phosphorylated. At steady state, one can also obtain (by setting the time derivative of $C_E = 0$)

$$-(k_2 + k_3)C_E + k_4 C_M + K_1 C_P = 0 \qquad (A2\text{-}4)$$

Therefore, by substituting for $k_4 C_M$ from Equation A2-2 into Equation A2-4 we obtain:

$$C_E = \dfrac{K_1 C_p}{(k_2 + k_3 \Theta')} \qquad (A2\text{-}5)$$

and by using the result for C_E in Equation A2-4 and substituting into Equation A2-3 we obtain:

$$MRglc = \frac{K_1 k_3 \Theta' \; C_P}{(k_2 + k_3 \Theta')} \qquad \text{(A2-6)}$$

Now by multiplying both the numerator and the denominator by $\dfrac{K_1^* k_3^*}{k_2^* + k_3^*}$, we obtain:

$$MRglc = \frac{K_1^* k_3^*}{k_2^* + k_3^*} \cdot \frac{k_3}{k_3^*} \cdot \frac{K_1/(k_2 + k_3\Theta)' \cdot C_P \Theta'}{K_1^*/(k_2^* + k_3^*)} \qquad \text{(A2-7)}$$

In order to further simplify the above we note that:

$$k_3^* = \frac{V_m^*/K_m^*}{1 + C_E/K_m + C_E^*/K_m^*} \qquad \text{(A2-8)}$$

$$k_3 = \frac{V_m/K_m}{1 + C_E/K_m + C_E^*/K_m^*}$$

where V_m, V_m^* are maximal velocities and K_m, K_m^* are apparent Michaelis-Menten constants for glucose and FDG, respectively. The above equations are workable since FDG and glucose are competitive substrates for the enzyme hexokinase, and, therefore, their rates follow Michaelis-Menten kinetics. Then, let:

$$f = \frac{k_3^*}{k_3} = \frac{V_m^* K_m}{V_m K_m^*} \qquad \text{(A2-9)}$$

$$\lambda = \frac{K_1^*/(k_2^* + k_3^*)}{K_1/(k_2 + k_3\Theta')} \qquad \text{(A2-10)}$$

So that we obtain:

$$MRglc = \frac{K_1^* k_3^*}{k_2^* + k_3^*} \cdot \frac{\Theta'}{\lambda f} \cdot C_P \qquad \text{(A2-11)}$$

Then we may write:

$$MRglc = \frac{K_1^* k_3^*}{k_2^* + k_3^*} \cdot \frac{C_P}{LC} \qquad \text{(A2-12)}$$

where

$$LC = \frac{\lambda f}{\Theta'}.$$

To better understand what Equation A2-12 means, notice that $K_1^*/(k_2^* + k_3^*)$ is a concentration gradient for FDG, multiplication of this by $k_3^* C_P$ converts this into the flux of the reaction, and multiplication by the $1/LC$ converts the measured kinetics with FDG into those for glucose.

The LC is an example of using the principles of competitive reaction kinetics to convert a reaction measured with a tracer that is an analog (FDG) to that of a natural substrate (glucose).

CHAPTER 3

Electronic Generators

Nagichettiar Satyamurthy

In the mid 1970s, when positron emission tomography (PET) was developed as a technology for the noninvasive assessment of various biochemical processes in living humans,[1–8] PET radiopharmaceuticals were synthesized manually in relatively low yields and with significant radiation exposure to the personnel.[9] Moreover, cyclotron technology appropriate to satisfy the particular demands of this new imaging procedure was not fully developed.[10] For widespread use of this technique in research and clinical care, an important technological development was necessary in the areas of cyclotrons, target bodies, and radiosynthesis modules for the production of positron-emitting radiopharmaceuticals.[10]

The acceptance of PET as a clinical diagnostic tool is a result of a joint effort between academia and industry to revolutionize the whole technology.[11] An exciting outcome of this joint endeavor is the initiation of the development of versatile and fully automated radiosynthesis units controlled by a personal computer (PC) that is also integrated with a small and low energy, self-shielded (vide infra) cyclotron. The union of these two segments led to the dawn of a PET technology that is oriented to clinical service and capable of producing multiple doses of a variety of radiopharmaceuticals and completely operated by a technician.[11] Although the ultimate success of PET will be determined by the clinical and biological research values it provides, a necessary part of that success to assure that PET is a reliable and cost-effective clinical technology depends upon continued innovation in the field. One of the key technological advances required in this regard is the miniaturization of the radioisotope production unit and successful engineering of small volume targets and automated synthesizers all integrated into a single-system concept. Integration of a self-shielded small cyclotron and automated synthesizers under a personal computer control is the cornerstone for the concept of an accelerator-based electronic radiopharmaceutical generator or, simply, an electronic generator for the routine production of radiopharmaceuticals for PET.[11]

Discussed in this chapter are the principles behind the basic components of the electronic generators, namely, cyclotron, target systems, and nuclear reactions, radiolabeled precursors for radiopharmaceutical syntheses and automated synthesis modules. Representative examples of commercially available low-energy accelerators, target systems, and automated synthesis units are also discussed from the standpoint of the beginning, evolution, current status, and future prospects for an electronic generator.

ACCELERATORS

An accelerator is a device that produces a well-defined, high-energy beam of charged particles with a high-beam intensity.[12] Production of radioisotopes involves a collision between a positively charged particle and the nucleus of an atom. A high-energy beam is required to overcome the repulsive force a positively charged particle would experience approaching a target nucleus.[13] A high-intensity beam simply increases the probability of collision between the charged particle and the atomic nucleus. Accelerators are broadly classified into two types—linear accelerators, in which the charged particles move in a straight line path, and cyclic accelerators, in which the charged particles move in a circular path. An example of a linear accelerator is a drift-tube accelerator and an example of a cyclic accelerator is a cyclotron.[14] Cyclotrons can accelerate either positively or negatively charged particles, and accordingly, they are classified as positive ion and negative ion cyclotrons. All these devices can accelerate charged particles to several million electron volts of energies. A number of excellent books,[15–22] review articles,[23,24] and book chapters[25,26] describe various aspects of cyclotrons.

Principles of positive ion cyclotrons

The cyclotron is the most widely used particle accelerator for the production of PET radioisotopes.[27] It consists of four major components: 1) magnet system, 2) radiofrequency resonant structure comprising a pair of semicircular hollow copper electrodes (called dees), 3) ion source, and 4) beam extraction system.[28] The entire structure of the cyclotron is kept under high vacuum (10^{-5} to 10^{-7} torr).

A schematic representation of a positive ion cyclotron is provided in Figure 3-1. Positive ions (e.g., protons, deuterons, $^3He^{2+}$, or $^4He^{2+}$) produced by ionization of a gas (e.g., hydrogen) in an arc ion source are injected at the center of the gap between the dee electrodes. A 20 MHz to 30 MHz radiofrequency alternating potential of 30 kV, generated with an oscillator, is applied to the dee structure which is located between the pole faces of an electromagnet with a field strength of 15 kG to 20 kG (1.5–2.0 tesla). A positive ion injected from the ion source will accelerate toward the dee that is at a negative potential at that instant. As the ion travels inside the hollow dee electrode, its velocity remains constant because it does not experience any electric potential. However, the ion will encounter the magnetic field acting at a right angle to the plane of its motion. Elementary electromagnetism dictates that the ion under these conditions will trace a circular path.[29] The magnetic force operating on the ion is the centripetal force and is given by the term $Be\nu$ where B is the magnetic field strength, e is the charge of the ion, and ν its velocity. This centripetal force is exactly balanced by the centrifugal effect $m\nu^2/r$ where m is the mass of the ion and r is the radius of the circular path of the ion. Thus, we have:

$$Be\nu = \frac{m\nu^2}{r}$$

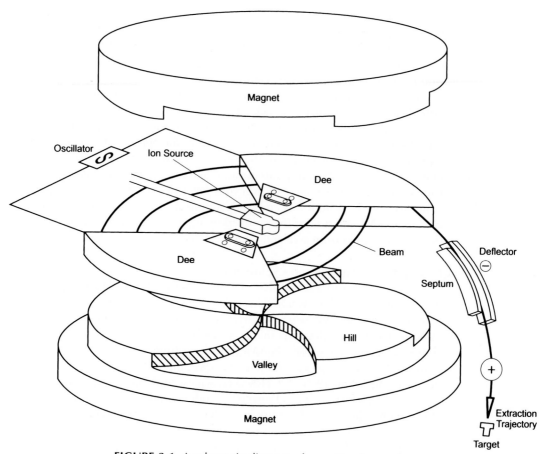

FIGURE 3-1. A schematic diagram of a positive ion cyclotron.

or

$$r = \frac{m\nu}{Be} \qquad (3\text{-}1)$$

This simple equation governs the cyclotron principle.

If the radiofrequency oscillator precisely reverses the polarity of the alternating potential of the dee electrodes exactly at the time the ion emerges from a dee electrode, the ion will be repelled by that dee and will be attracted by the opposite dee. Thus, the velocity ν of the ion will increase as it crosses the gap between the dees. Hence, the radius r of its circular path will also increase so that the relationship described in Equation 3-1 is maintained. The time t taken by the ion to traverse a semicircular path in a dee electrode can be represented by:

$$t = \frac{\pi r}{\nu} \qquad (3\text{-}2)$$

From Equations 3-1 and 3-2, it is evident that:

$$t = \frac{\pi m}{Be} \qquad (3\text{-}3)$$

It is thus apparent that the time required for the ion to traverse a semicircular path in a dee is independent of its velocity and the radius. Equation 3-3 more importantly signifies that if the frequency of the oscillator is tuned to the mass and charge of the ion and the magnetic field strength, the ion will constantly stay in phase with the change in polarity between the dee electrodes. That is, the frequency of oscillation of the accelerating potential will be equal to the frequency of revolution of the ion in the magnetic field. Thus, each time the ion travels the gap between the dees, its velocity (and, hence, the radius) increases due to the repulsive force from one dee and the attractive force from the opposite dee. This results in a steady increase of the energy of the ion with a simultaneous increase in the radius of its orbits. As the ion spirals outward and reaches the periphery of the dees, with an energy in the million electron volts (MeV) range, it is extracted by means of an electrostatic deflector assembly, operating at -30 kV to -60 kV and 0.1 A current to 0.5 A current, for the production of radioisotopes. The radius at which the ion is removed from acceleration is called the extraction radius.

Principles of negative ion cyclotrons

The Equations 3-1 to 3-3 that describe the cyclotron principle are applicable to both positive as well as negative ions of any given mass. Thus, it is possible to accelerate negative ions (e.g., negatively charged hydrogen ion—H^-, a proton associated with two electrons in the K shell) in a cyclotron. Negative ion cyclotron technology has been known for a long time, especially in the research domain. The first negative ion cyclotron was built at the University of California, Los Angeles, in 1966.[30–32] However, widespread and routine utilization of negative ion cyclotrons for radioisotope production did not occur until the mid 1980s mainly due to the difficulty in the high-intensity (volume) production of H^- and the relatively high vacuum required to prevent the neutralization of H^- (called stripping loss) during acceleration.[33,34]

A schematic diagram of a negative ion cyclotron is given in Figure 3-2. Negative ions (e.g., H^-), generated in a specially designed ion source (Penning ion gauge) optimized for negative ion production,[35] are injected at the center of the gap between the dees. The negative ion is accelerated by being attracted by the positive charge and repelled from the negative one at the edges of the dees as it passes through the gap between the dees as described earlier. The interaction of the magnetic field with the negative ion causes it to circulate in a direction opposite to that of the positive ion in a positive ion cyclotron. As the accelerated negative ion reaches the periphery of the dees, it is intercepted with a thin carbon foil (5 μm) which strips the loosely bound electrons from the H^- ion converting it to H^+ ion. This polarity change from H^- to H^+ under the influence of the magnetic field causes the proton to curve outward and thus is extracted from the cyclotron for the production of radioisotopes.

General characteristics of positive and negative ion cyclotrons

The preceding descriptions of the positive and negative ion cyclotrons have considered only the acceleration and extraction of a single ion for the sake of explanation. The ion source obviously provides a continuous stream of charged (positive or negative) ions that are accelerated in pulses in accordance with the radiofrequency of the dee electrodes. The frequency of these pulses are extremely high, approximately 10^7 cycles per second. That is, the time interval between two successive pulses of accelerated particles extracted from the cyclotron is 10^{-7}

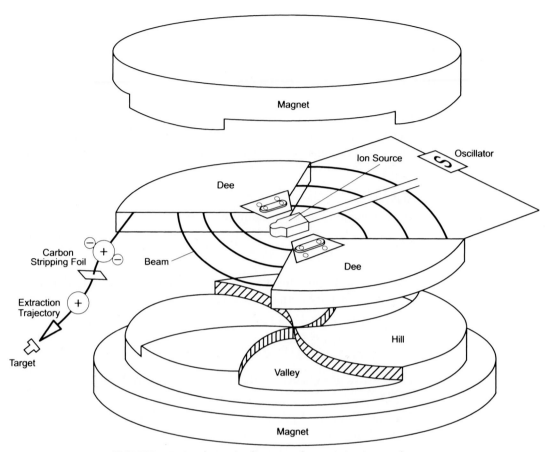

FIGURE 3-2. A schematic diagram of a negative ion cyclotron.

sec. Thus, the cyclotron appears, for all practical purposes, to be producing a continuous stream of ions. This stream of high-energy ions produced by the cyclotron is commonly called the beam.

Maximum kinetic energy

The maximum kinetic energy (E) that an ion can attain in a cyclotron is calculated using the following known relationship:

$$\text{Kinetic energy} = 1/2 \ m \ v^2$$

From Equation 3-1

$$v = \frac{Ber}{m}$$

Thus,

$$E = 1/2 \ m \left(\frac{Ber}{m} \right)^2$$

$$= \frac{B^2 r^2}{2} \left(\frac{e^2}{m} \right) \tag{3-4}$$

For a given cyclotron, the radius of extraction r is generally kept constant and the strength of the magnetic field B is maintained constant. Hence, the kinetic energy that an ion can gain is directly proportional to the square of its charge and inversely proportional to its mass. For protons, the values of e in terms of the electronic charge, and the atomic mass, in terms of atomic mass units, are unity. Hence, protons will gain the same energy as $^4He^{2+}$ ions having the values 2 and 4 for e and m, respectively.

EXAMPLE 3-1

Calculate the maximum kinetic energy of protons, deuterons, $^3He^{2+}$ and $^4He^{2+}$ particles that can be obtained from a cyclotron with an average magnetic field strength of 1.6 tesla and an extraction radius of 42 cm.

ANSWER

Using Equation 3-4, the maximum kinetic energy,

$$E = \frac{B^2 r^2}{2} \left(\frac{e^2}{m} \right)$$

The numerical values for the parameters in the above equation in SI units (Le Système International d'Unites) are as follows:

B = 1.6 tesla = 1.6 kg/A s^2 (A = ampere and s = second)
r = 42 cm = 0.42 m
e = 1.602 × 10^{-19} A s

The mass for proton, deuteron, $^3He^{2+}$ and $^4He^{2+}$ can be obtained from Tables.[36]

m (for proton) = 1.673 × 10^{-27} kg
m (for deuteron) = 2.014 amu (amu = atomic mass unit)
             = 3.344 × 10^{-27} kg
        (1 amu = 1.6604 × 10^{-27} kg)
m (for $^3He^{2+}$) = 3.016 amu = 5.008 × 10^{-27} kg
m (for $^4He^{2+}$) = 4.002 amu = 6.646 × 10^{-27} kg

A) Maximum energy for protons,

$$E_p = \frac{(1.6)^2 (0.42)^2}{2} \times \frac{(1.602 \times 10^{-19})^2}{1.673 \times 10^{-27}}$$

$$= 3.464 \times 10^{-12} \text{ kg m}^2/\text{s}^2$$
$$= 3.464 \times 10^{-12} \text{ J (J = joule and 1J = 1 kg m}^2/\text{s}^2)$$

Since 1.602 × 10^{-19} J = 1 eV (10^{-6} MeV)

$$E_p = \frac{10^{-6} \times 3.464 \times 10^{-12}}{1.602 \times 10^{-19}} = 21.62 \text{ MeV}$$

B) Maximum energy for deuteron,

$$E_d = \frac{(1.6)^2 (0.42)^2}{2} \times \frac{(1.602 \times 10^{-19})^2}{3.344 \times 10^{-27}}$$

$$= 1.733 \times 10^{-12} \text{ J}$$
$$= 10.82 \text{ MeV}$$

C) Maximum energy for $^3He^{2+}$,

$$E_{3_{He}} = \frac{(1.6)^2(0.42)^2}{2} \times \frac{(2 \times 1.602 \times 10^{-19})^2}{5.008 \times 10^{-27}}$$

$$= 4.628 \times 10^{-12} \text{ J}$$
$$= 28.89 \text{ MeV}$$

D) Maximum energy for $^4He^{2+}$,

$$E_{4_{He}} = \frac{(1.6)^2(0.42)^2}{2} \times \frac{(2 \times 1.602 \times 10^{-19})^2}{6.646 \times 10^{-27}}$$

$$= 3.488 \times 10^{-12} \text{ J}$$
$$= 21.77 \text{ MeV}$$

Oscillator frequency

Equation 3-1 can be rearranged and written as:

$$\frac{v}{r} = \frac{Be}{m}$$

The term v/r is the angular velocity ω, for the circular orbits of the ion in a cyclotron. The radiofrequency f of the oscillator required to maintaining the ion in phase with the changes of the electric potential between the dees is given by:

$$f = \frac{\omega}{2\pi}$$

Since

$$\omega = \frac{v}{r}$$

$$f = \frac{v}{2\pi r} \qquad (3\text{-}5)$$

Substituting the value of v from Equation 3-1 we get:

$$f = \frac{Be}{2\pi m} \qquad (3\text{-}6)$$

EXAMPLE 3-2

Calculate the radiofrequency of the oscillator required for the acceleration of protons and deuterons in the cyclotron described in Example 3-1.

ANSWER

The frequency of the oscillator, $f = \dfrac{Be}{2\pi m}$ (Equation 3-6)

$$B = 1.6 \text{ tesla} = 1.6 \text{ kg/A s}^2$$
$$e = 1.602 \times 10^{-19} \text{A s}$$
$$m \text{ (for proton)} = 1.673 \times 10^{-27} \text{ kg}$$
$$m \text{ (for deuteron)} = 3.344 \times 10^{-27} \text{ kg}$$

A) Frequency of the oscillator for proton,

$$f_p = \frac{1.6 \times 1.602 \times 10^{-19}}{2 \times 3.143 \times 1.673 \times 10^{-27}}$$

$$= 24.37 \times 10^6 \text{ cycles/s}$$
$$= 24.37 \text{ MHz (since 1 cycle/s = 1 Hz)}$$

B) Frequency of the oscillator for deuterons,

$$f_d = \frac{1.6 \times 1.602 \times 10^{-19}}{2 \times 3.143 \times 3.344 \times 10^{-27}}$$

$$= 12.19 \text{ MHz}$$

EXAMPLE 3-3

Calculate the magnetic field required to accelerate protons in a cyclotron having a 27 MHz oscillator.

ANSWER

Rearranging Equation 3-6 we can write:

$$\text{the magnetic field, B} = \frac{f2\,\pi m}{e}$$

$$f = 27 \text{ MHz} = 27 \times 10^6 \text{ cycle/s}$$
$$m = 1.673 \times 10^{-27} \text{ kg}$$
$$e = 1.602 \times 10^{-19}\text{A s}$$

Hence,

$$B = \frac{27 \times 10^6 \times 2 \times 3.143 \times 1.673 \times 10^{-27}}{1.602 \times 10^{-19}} = 1.77 \text{ kg/A s}^2$$

Since

$$1 \text{ tesla} = 1 \text{ kg/A s}^2$$
$$B = 1.77 \text{ tesla}$$

In a cyclotron capable of accelerating multiple particles (e.g., protons, deuterons, $^3He^{2+}$, and $^4He^{2+}$), it is rather convenient to maintain the magnetic field strength B constant and to adjust the radiofrequency oscillator in accordance with Equation 3-5.

The beam extracted from a cyclotron is not monoenergetic and has an energy spread of about 1% of the nominal value. However, for isotope production, it is generally not necessary that the cyclotron beam be monoenergetic.

Dee voltage

It is interesting to notice that the maximum energy gained by an ion in a cyclotron as given by Equation 3-4 is independent of the alternating voltage applied to the dees. This can be explained by the number of turns the ion goes through in the dees to reach the extraction radius. When the dee voltage is small, the ion makes a larger number of turns than when the voltage is large. However, in modern cyclotrons, a large dee voltage (30–100 kV) is generally used. In any event, the final energy attained by the ions is the sum of the individual energies gained at each crossing of the gap between the dees. At a dee voltage of 35 kV, the energy gained by a proton in each revolution, in a cyclotron with a magnetic field of 1.8 tesla, is approximately 0.1 MeV. Thus, to reach a maximum energy of 11 MeV, the proton will have to go through 11 MeV/0.1 MeV or 110 revolutions.

Axial focusing and azimuthally varying field (AVF) cyclotron

In a cyclotron, the charged particles generally orbit in a plane between the poles of the magnet (see Figure 3-1). This plane is called the median plane. Accelerating charged particles that deviate from the median plane experience a restraining force from the magnetic field in a direction perpendicular to their motion. This force, known as axial focusing, restores the ions, when necessary, to the median plane.[15–19] For this force to prevail, the magnetic field must decrease at the larger radius. A decrease of the magnetic field with increasing radius has a component of magnetic force that directs any orbiting ions above or below the median plane back toward the median plane. Axial focusing of orbiting charged particles is mandatory for proper functioning of the cyclotron.[16]

An important characteristic of the acceleration of ions in a cyclotron is the manifestation of the relativistic mass increase of the charged particles as they attain higher velocities as defined by Einstein's general relativity equation:

$$\text{m} = \text{m}_o \left[1 - \frac{\nu^2}{\text{c}^2} \right]^{-1/2} \tag{3-7}$$

where m is the mass of the particle in motion, m_o is the mass at rest, ν is the velocity of the particle and c is the velocity of light.[29] For example, a 10-MeV proton has a mass increase of about 1% of its rest mass because it is traveling at 15% of the velocity of light. To maintain the phase relationship stipulated by Equation 3-2, any mass increase of ions due to acceleration would require an appropriate increase in the magnetic field strength, B. Thus, the relativistic mass increase and the axial focusing impose mutually contradicting requirements on the magnetic field B.

A practical compromise for this problem is reached by sinusoidal contouring of the pole faces of the magnet with four spiral sector-shaped pieces of iron (Figures 3-1 and 3-2) so that the space between the poles becomes alternately larger and smaller. This results in alternating strong and weak magnetic fields known as hill and valley regions (Figures 3-1 and 3-2), respectively. An orbiting ion in such a magnetic field experiences alternating strong and weak magnetic fields in the azimuthal direction (around the circular path); this phenomenon is termed azimuthally varying field (AVF).[16] A particle moving in an azimuthally varying field follows a rather distorted circular orbit because the radius r of the ion is inversely related to the strength of the magnetic field B as given by Equation 3-1.

The result of the interaction of the noncircular path of the ion with the azimuthally varying field is a restoring axial focusing force that directs the particle back toward the median plane. The axial focusing thus accomplished permits the increase of the magnetic field strength to compensate for the relativistic mass increase of the ions due to acceleration. This is achieved by decreasing the space between the pole faces of the magnet with increasing radius along with supplemental tuning coils attached to the outer edge of the magnet. Thus, azimuthal variation of the magnetic field in cyclotron results in axial focusing while at the same time maintaining an average magnetic field strength that increases with radius to compensate for the relativistic mass increase. All modern cyclotrons have such magnetic field strength configurations and are often called azimuthally varying field cyclotrons, spiral-ridge cyclotrons, or isochronous cyclotrons.[28]

EXAMPLE 3-4

Calculate (A) the maximum velocity that protons can attain in an azimuthally varying field cyclotron having an extraction radius of 26.37 cm and a magnetic field strength of 1.8 tesla, (B) compare the value obtained for (A) with the velocity of light, (C) what is the relativistic mass increase of the proton at its maximum velocity with reference to its rest mass, and (D) if a proton gains 100 keV energy per orbit, how long would it take for the proton to exit the cyclotron?

ANSWER

A) Equation 3-1 can be rearranged to give:

the velocity of the proton, $v = \dfrac{Ber}{m}$

$$B = 1.8 \text{ tesla} = 1.8 \text{ kg/A s}^2$$
$$e = 1.602 \times 10^{-19} \text{A s}$$
$$r = 26.37 \text{ cm} = 0.2637 \text{ m}$$
$$m = 1.673 \times 10^{-27} \text{ kg}$$

So,

$$v = \frac{1.8 \times 1.602 \times 10^{-19} \times 0.2637}{1.673 \times 10^{-27}} = 4.545 \times 10^7 \text{ m/s}$$

B) Velocity of light, $c = 2.998 \times 10^8$ m/s (from Tables[36])
Therefore, the velocity with reference to that of light is:

$$\frac{4.545 \times 10^7}{2.998 \times 10^8} \times 100 = 15.16\% \text{ of the velocity of light}$$

C) Equation 3-7 provides:

$$\text{the mass, m} = m_o \left[1 - \frac{v^2}{c^2} \right]^{-1/2}$$

$$= m_o \left[1 - \frac{(4.545 \times 10^7)^2}{(2.998 \times 10^8)^2} \right]^{-1/2}$$

$$= 1.01 \, m_o$$

Thus, the relativistic mass is about 1% greater than the rest mass of a proton at this velocity.

D) At exit, the proton has the maximum kinetic energy, given by:

$$E = 1/2 \, mv^2$$
$$= 1/2 \times 1.673 \times 10^{-27} \times (4.545 \times 10^7)^2$$
$$= 1.728 \times 10^{-12} \text{ kg m}^2/\text{s}^2$$

Knowing $1 \text{ kg m}^2/\text{s}^2 = 1\text{J}$ and

$$1.602 \times 10^{-19} \text{ J} = 1 \text{ eV} (10^{-6} \text{ MeV})$$

$$E = \frac{10^{-6} \times 1.728 \times 10^{-12}}{1.602 \times 10^{-19}} = 10.8 \text{ MeV}$$

Thus, to gain 10.8 MeV energy, the proton will go through:

$$\frac{10.8 \text{ MeV}}{100 \text{ keV (or 0.1 MeV)}} \text{ orbits} = 108 \text{ orbits}$$

Time taken by an ion to traverse half an orbit is given by Equation 3-3 as:

$$t = \frac{\pi m}{Be}$$

Thus, the time taken by the proton to traverse one complete orbit is:

$$= \frac{2 \times 3.143 \times 1.673 \times 10^{-27}}{1.8 \times 1.602 \times 10^{-19}} = 3.647 \times 10^{-8} \text{ s}$$

Hence to complete 108 orbits, the proton will take:

$$108 \times 3.647 \times 10^{-8} \text{ s} = 3.94 \times 10^{-6} \text{ s}$$

Advantages of a negative ion cyclotron over a positive ion cyclotron

From the standpoint of performance characteristics, radiation shielding and simplicity of operation, a negative ion cyclotron has several advantages over a positive ion cyclotron. The extraction of the accelerated negative ion (e.g., H^-) beam is very simple. A thin (5 μm) carbon foil, held in a small carousel with a diameter of less than 4 cm, strips the electrons to produce a positive ion (H^+) beam with an efficiency of nearly 100% (Figure 3-3). This electron stripping process does not produce any radiation or induce radioactivity. Thus, the internal parts of a negative ion cyclotron are relatively free from induced radioactivity, lowering the shielding requirements. Beam extraction in a positive ion cyclotron is complex and utilizes a curved and narrow (4 mm) electrostatic channel of 40 cm in length through which the high-energy, accelerated beam is carefully steered (Figure 3-1). The beam extraction efficiency with such an electrostatic deflector assembly is less than 75%. The ~25% of the high-energy beam that is unextracted produces nuclear reactions in the internal parts of the cyclotron making them highly radioactive.[37]

The small size of the carbon foil/carousel extractor assembly permits deployment of multiple extractor systems inside the cyclotron. In the case of the RDS-112 cyclotron (manufactured by CTI, Inc., Knoxville, TN), four extraction carousels are assigned for four different beam delivery lines as shown in Figure 3-3. This avoids the necessity of long-beam transport and steering external to the cyclotron vacuum tank. Overall, a negative ion cyclotron is compact and thus reduces the size and weight of the shielding requirements.

The large size of the electrostatic deflector system restricts a positive ion cyclotron to have only a single-beam delivery line. The beam extracted from the cyclotron is bent by an external steering magnet to divert it to different beam

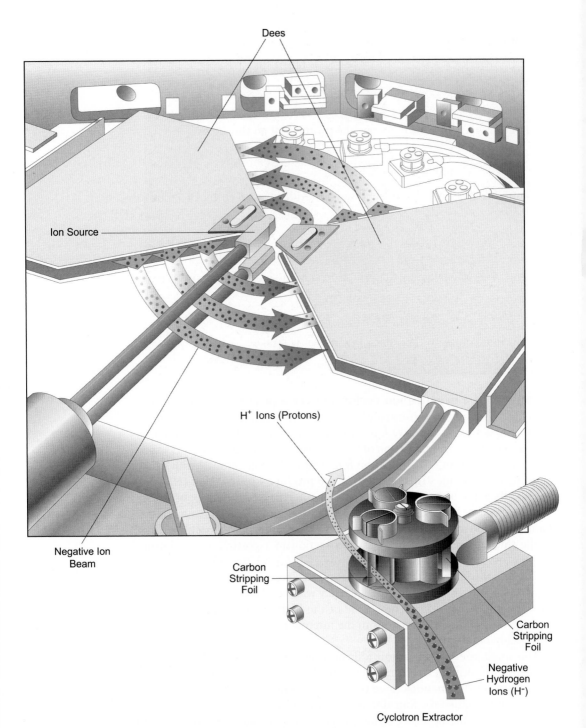

FIGURE 3-3. A schematic representation of the extraction of negative ions using a carbon stripping foil. Shown in the foreground is the carousel that holds three carbon foils for redundancy. The carousel is rotated under computer control to maximize the extraction efficiency of the proton beam. The top of the figure shows four such carousels, each of which can intercept the negative ion beam and deliver the proton beam to different beam lines for different isotope production. (Courtesy of CTI Inc., Knoxville, TN.).

delivery lines. All these make the shielding more extensive for a positive ion cyclotron.

Another major advantage with a negative ion cyclotron is the ability to simultaneously irradiate two targets. This process is illustrated in Figure 3-4. The thin carbon extractor foil is placed partway in the path of the beam. A portion of the beam passes through the foil, electrons are stripped off, and the H^+ ion thus produced is directed to the beam line leading to target A. The remainder of the beam continues for another orbit and is then intercepted by a second extractor foil to generate a second H^+ beam which is steered to target B. Such beam splitting is not practical with positive ion cyclotrons.

The steering of the beam is also simple with a negative ion cyclotron and is accomplished by the position at which the extractor carbon foil intercepts the H^- beam. The carousel holding the foil is rotated under computer control to maximize the amount of the beam extracted.

Finally, the proton beam extracted from a negative ion cyclotron has better beam optics than a H^+ beam derived from a positive ion cyclotron. Beam extraction by the stripping process in a negative ion cyclotron avoids the radial (horizontal) defocusing observed in positive ion cyclotrons and yields roughly circular beam shape. Further, the multiple scattering of the beam in the stripping foil also tends to eliminate inhomogenities (hot spots) in the beam. It is always desirable to have good beam optics for isotope production. Overall, it is advantageous to have a negative ion cyclotron for the production of radioisotopes.

Deep valley cyclotron

The most modern negative ion cyclotrons have a special magnet design, termed deep valley. Deep valley refers to gaps between the hills and valleys of the magnetic system (see Figure 3-2). For example, the RDS-111 (CTI, Inc., Figure 3-5A), an 11 MeV cyclotron with deep valley magnet design, has a ratio of 27:1 for the valley to hill gap (an analogous ratio for a nondeep valley cyclotron is roughly 2:1). This produces a magnetic field strength in the hills that is much stronger than the field strength in the valleys. As the accelerating negative ion passes through the hill region, its trajectory is sharply bent due to the strong magnetic field. On the other hand, the ion experiences only a weak magnetic field in the valley, and its path is nearly a straight line leading to the next strong field hill region. As described earlier, this azimuthally varying magnetic field provides a strong axial focusing effect directing straying particles back toward the median plane. Deep valley magnet design provides excellent efficiency of beam transmission and low activation of the internal structures of the cyclotron, resulting in reduced shielding requirements. The extraction of the beam from a deep valley cyclotron is the same as the negative ion cyclotron beam extraction already described.

Role of cylcotrons in the production of PET radioisotopes

The most popular positron emitting isotopes[35] are ^{15}O, ^{13}N, ^{11}C, and ^{18}F (Table 3-1). Table 3-2 summarizes other important but less common positron emitting isotopes. To date, the cyclotron remains the accelerator of choice for the production of these isotopes. The cyclotrons developed during the 1960s and 1970s are huge, complex, and labor-intensive devices designed generally to support nuclear physics research.[23,38] Occasionally, they are also found useful in a few nu-

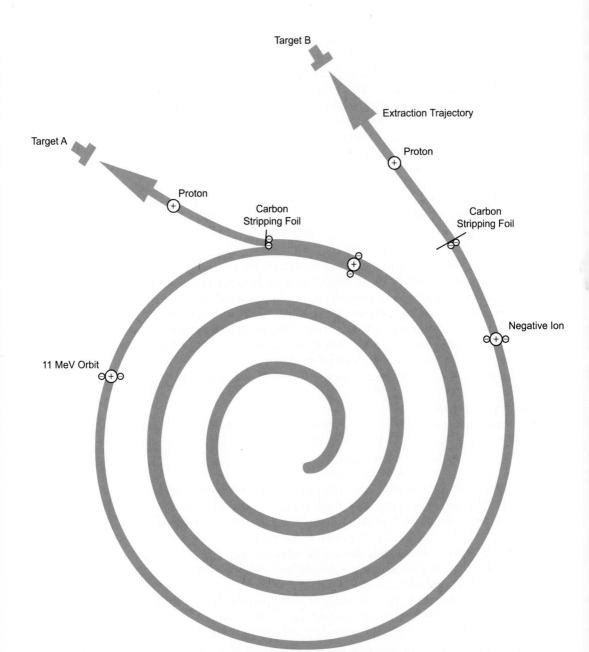

FIGURE 3-4. Schematic illustration of splitting an accelerating negative ion beam into two separate proton beams for dual bombardment. Dual beam extraction permits the production of two different isotopes simultaneously. For example, during the production of a longer lived ^{18}F isotope, it is possible to produce several doses of a shorter lived isotope like ^{13}N or ^{15}O. To enhance the yield of a high demand isotope (e.g., [^{18}F]fluoride ion), two identical targets can be irradiated simultaneously. Such a process is a daily practice in PET radiopharmaceutical distribution companies.

A.
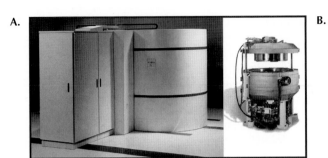

B.
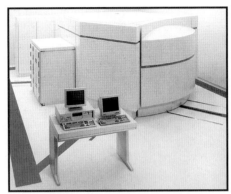

C.
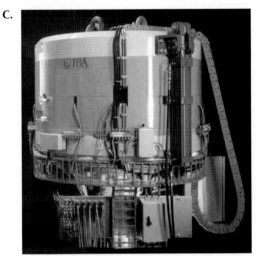

D.
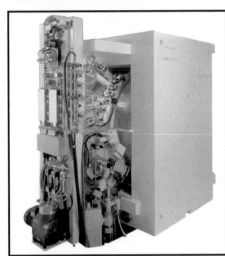

FIGURE 3-5. A: Radioisotope Delivery System—RDS-111 cyclotron (CTI, Inc., Knoxville, TN) with the shield doors in the closed position (left) and the cyclotron inside the shields (right). (Courtesy of CTI.) B: CTI Radioisotope Delivery System—RDS-112 cyclotron with the shield doors in the closed position. The cabinet to the left contains the automated chemistry modules (Courtesy of CTI.) C: IBA Cyclone 10/5 cyclotron without the radiation shield. (Courtesy of IBA Technology Group, Louvain-la-Neuve, Belgium). D: GE PET trace 2000 cyclotron without the radiation shield. (Courtesy of GE Medical Systems.)

TABLE 3-1. Physical Characteristics of Important Positron Emitting Isotopes

Radioisotope	Half-life (min)	Mode of decay[a] (%)	E_{max} for β^+ (MeV)	Theoretical maximum specific activity (Ci/mmol)
^{15}O	2.07	β^+ (99.9) EC (0.1)	1.72	9.08×10^7
^{13}N	9.96	β^+ (100)	1.19	1.89×10^7
^{11}C	20.4	β^+ (99.8) EC (0.2)	0.96	9.22×10^6
^{18}F	109.7	β^+ (97) EC (3)	0.635	1.71×10^6

[a]β^+, positron emission; EC, electron capture.

TABLE 3-2. Physical Characteristics of Less Common Positron Emitting Radioisotopes[66,132,133]

Radioisotope	Half-life	Mode of decay[a] (%)	E_{max} for β^+ (MeV)	Production mode
^{38}K	7.6 m	β^+ (100)	2.68	^{38}Ar (p, n)
^{64}Cu	12.7 h	β^+ (18)	0.66	^{64}Ni (p, n)
		β^- (37)		
		EC (45)		
^{68}Ge (parent)	271 d	EC (100)		^{69}Ga (p, 2n)
↓ generator				
^{68}Ga (daughter)	68.3 m	β^+ (90)	1.90	
		EC (10)		
^{73}Se	7.1 h	β^+ (65)	1.32	^{75}As (p, 3n)
		EC (35)		
^{75}Br	1.6 h	β^+ (75)	1.74	^{76}Se (p, 2n)
		EC (25)		
^{76}Br	16.1 h	β^+ (57)	3.90	^{77}Se (p, 2n)
		EC (43)		
^{82}Sr (parent)	25 d	EC (100)		^{80}Kr (α, 2n)
↓ generator				
^{82}Rb (daughter)	1.3 m	β^+ (96)	3.35	
		EC (4)		
^{124}I	4.2 d	β^+ (25)	2.13	^{125}Te (p, 2n)
		EC (75)		

[a]β^+, positron emission; β^-, electron emission; EC, electron capture.

clear medicine programs of university-based hospitals or the commercial production of medically useful radioisotopes.[40] These cyclotrons provide positive ions (protons, deuterons, ^{3}He^{2+}, and α-particles) with 10 MeV to 50 MeV energies for the production of radioisotopes. These accelerators are installed in specially designed vaults having 6- to 8-ft thick concrete walls for the purpose of radiation protection. The maintenance and operation of these machines require highly trained personnel, often with advanced degrees.

In the mid 1970s, these large, complex cyclotrons were utilized for the production of positron-emitting isotopes in support of emerging PET programs.[23] Chemists, frequently with advanced degrees, utilized these radioisotopes in the preparation of radiopharmaceuticals with remote manual synthesis units.[9,41] Thus, in the 1970s, this combination of a huge, multiparticle positive ion cyclotron for the production of positron emitters and manual synthesis units for the preparation of radiopharmaceuticals served mainly to validate PET as a potential research tool.[39]

In the early 1980s, pragmatic concerns of physical size, complexity, and cost of cyclotrons and the associated facilities led to the introduction of a new generation of small, mini or baby cyclotrons with an expectation of a larger audience participating in PET.[23,42] Unfortunately, the design of these machines closely followed those of the previous generation positive ion cyclotrons and similarly accelerated multiple particles (protons and deuterons and, occasionally, ^{3}He^{2+} and α-particles). These cyclotrons were also installed in huge concrete vaults and operated by interactive manual controls.

The dawn of the personal computer era in the early 1980s was fortuitous for the development of a newer generation of cyclotrons for PET. Thus, in 1984 a fully PC-controlled, low-energy (11 MeV), single particle (proton only), self-shielded cyclotron that did not require the traditional concrete vault was introduced by CTI, Inc. under the trade name RDS-112 (Figure 3-5B). In a self-shielded cyclotron, the cyclotron steel frame or yoke serves as the primary radiation shield. Hydraulically driven movable blocks made of specially formulated concrete surround the accelerator for complete radiation protection. The user-friendly, PC-controlled RDS-112 is based on negative ion acceleration technology.

The RDS-112, the first self-shielded cyclotron designed specifically for the routine production of large quantities of the four important positron-emitting isotopes (^{15}O, ^{13}N, ^{11}C, and ^{18}F) in clinical and research settings, proved to be a trend setter. Other manufacturers developed similar accelerators. Table 3-3 summarizes some of the currently available low-energy cyclotrons appropriately designed for the production of PET radioisotopes.

As PET became a clinical reality in the 1990s, the manufacturers of cyclotrons introduced their latest generation of accelerators for the production of positron emitters specifically developed for installation in hospitals.[11] Common features among these cyclotrons are: 1) negative ion acceleration technology, 2) dual-beam capability for simultaneous production of two different isotopes, 3) self-shielding, 4) complete automation and control by a PC with graphical user interface (GUI) for ease of operation, and 5) low maintenance requirements. Because the self-shielded cyclotrons do not require large and expensive concrete vaults, these devices could be placed in rooms that only require appropriate temperature, humidity, and airflow. Similarly, the personnel costs are also modest as technicians generally operate these automated cyclotrons.

The manufacturers have also concentrated on certain characteristics of the cyclotrons to improve the beam transmission, space requirements, and operating power consumption. For example, IBA's Cyclone 10/5 (IBA Technology Group, Louvain-la-Neuve, Belgium; Figure 3-5C) and CTI's RDS-111 (Figure 3-5A) cyclotrons have a deep valley design for the magnet which reduces the size of the system, enables a better beam transmission, and considerably decreases

TABLE 3-3. Low-Energy Negative Ion Cyclotrons[a] for the Production of Positron-Emitting Radioisotopes

Company	Model	Proton energy (MeV)	Number of targets
CTI	RDS-112	11	4
CTI	RDS-111	11	2×8[b]
IBA	Cyclone 10/5[c]	10	8
GE	PET trace[d]	16.5	6
Ebco	TR 13	13	2×4[e]
NKK-Oxford	—	12	1×7[f]

[a]Self-shielding for CTI cyclotrons is standard. For other companies, it is optional.

[b]Two beam ports each having an eight-target rotating carousel.

[c]Optional 5 MeV deuteron capability available.

[d]Standard 8.4 MeV deuteron capability.

[e]Two beam ports each supporting a four-target rotating carousel.

[f]Single-beam port supporting a seven-target rotating carousel.

the electrical power consumption. On the other hand, NKK-Oxford Instruments have designed a 12-MeV negative ion cyclotron based on a liquid helium-cooled superconducting magnet for stability of the magnetic field, lower weight, and low electrical power consumption. Interestingly, to minimize floor space, GE (GE Medical Systems, Milwaukee, WI; Figure 3-5D) and Ebco (Ebco Technologies, Inc., Richmond, British Columbia, Canada) have developed cyclotrons that accelerate negative ions in a vertical plane.

The choice of low energy (10–16 MeV) cyclotrons (Table 3-3) for the production of sufficient quantities of the four important positron emitters is largely based on the simplicity of design and operation, self-shielding capabilities, and relatively small space and low cost requirements. Overall, these cyclotrons, suitable for a hospital-based production of positron emitters, are fully automated, controlled by a PC, and routinely operated by minimally trained technicians.

Linear accelerators

Recently, considerable interest has focused on the development of a new generation of linear accelerators, as alternatives to cyclotrons, for the production of positron-emitting radioisotopes.[43] They include tandem cascade accelerator (Science Research Laboratory, Somerville, MA),[44] radiofrequency quadrupole (RFQ) accelerators,[45,46] proton linacs,[47,48] Nested High Voltage Generator (North Star Research Corporation, Albuquerque, NM),[49] and Pelletron tandem accelerator (National Electrostatics Corporation, Middleton, WI).[50] In general, these accelerators are capable of providing charged particles (protons, deuterons, or $^3He^{2+}$) in the energy range of 3 MeV to 12 MeV at high milliampere beam currents (as opposed to microampere currents with cyclotrons) for PET radioisotope production. The perceived advantages of these linear accelerators are: 1) lower cost to build, 2) low operating costs due to lower power requirements, 3) reduced radiation shielding, 4) easy to operate and maintain, and 5) better reliability. At this time, many of these characteristics are yet to be realized in practice. Development of suitable target systems for the routine production of positron-emitting radioisotopes with these relatively high-beam current accelerators has so far been a formidable task.[43] The full potential of this newer generation of linear accelerators for the routine production of PET radioisotopes is, however, yet to be established.

NUCLEAR REACTIONS FOR THE PRODUCTION OF POSITRON-EMITTING RADIOISOTOPES

The four most important positron emitting radioisotopes used in positron emission tomography, namely, ^{18}F, ^{11}C, ^{13}N, and ^{15}O, are generally produced by the charged particle irradiation of stable nuclides in a cyclotron. Under a given set of irradiation conditions, the yield of the radioisotope produced depends upon various parameters that govern the nuclear reaction. Selected basic parameters that are relevant in this regard are discussed below.

Nuclear reaction energy, Q

The nuclear reaction energy, customarily called the Q value, represents the release or absorption of energy during a nuclear reaction and is conventionally added to the product side of the nuclear reaction equation.[51] The value of Q can be positive or negative. Nuclear reactions having positive Q value (exoergic) release energy while negative Q value (endoergic) requires a net input of energy. Since the conservation of mass and momentum govern nuclear reactions, the Q value is numerically equal to the difference in rest mass between the reactants and the products, illustrated with the nuclear reaction of stable ^{18}O nuclide with a proton to produce ^{18}F radioisotope and a neutron:

$$^{18}O + p \rightarrow {}^{18}F + n + Q$$

which can also be expressed as:

$$^{18}O(p, n)^{18}F$$

Thus, Q = rest mass of $(^{18}O + p)$ − rest mass of $(^{18}F + n)$

The value Q is more conveniently evaluated using the mass excess Δ (the difference between the mass of an atom and its mass number) readily available from the Table of Radioactive Isotopes.[52] The tabulated values of Δ for the $^{18}O(p,n)^{18}F$ reaction expressed in units of energy are as follows:

^{18} O:−0.7823 MeV	^{18}F : 0.8733 MeV
p : 7.2890	n : 8.0714
6.5067	8.9447

Thus,

$$Q = 6.5067 - 8.9447$$
$$= -2.438 \text{ MeV}$$

Threshold energy, E_t

The threshold energy, E_t, for an endoergic reaction is the minimum kinetic energy that the bombarding charged particle should possess for the nuclear reaction to be energetically possible.[51] The threshold energy would always be greater than the Q value since a fraction of the energy of the bombarding particle must be used to impart momentum to the whole system during the nuclear reaction (conservation of momentum). Calculations show that:

$$E_t = -Q \left(\frac{A_1 + A_2}{A_1} \right) \tag{3-8}$$

where A_1 = mass number of target nucleus and A_2 = mass number of the bombarding particle.

EXAMPLE 3-5
Calculate the threshold energy for the $^{18}O(p,n)^{18}F$ reaction.

ANSWER
The Q value for this nuclear reaction is −2.438 MeV. (see above)

Using Equation 3-8, the value for the threshold energy,

$$E_t = -(-2.438)\frac{(18 + 1)}{18}$$

$$= 2.57 \text{ MeV}$$

Coulomb barrier and starting energy, E_s

For a nuclear reaction to occur, a positively charged particle must overcome the repulsive electrostatic force as it approaches a target nucleus. The minimum energy that the particle should possess to surmount the repulsive force is known as the Coulomb barrier.[52] The starting energy,[53] E_s, required to overcome the Coulomb barrier and the energy of the bombarding particle needed to transmit momentum to the reaction system during collision (conservation of momentum) can be calculated approximately as follows:

$$E_S = \left(\frac{0.96 Z_1 Z_2}{A_1^{1/3} + A_2^{1/3}} \right) \left(\frac{A_1 + A_2}{A_1} \right) \text{MeV} \tag{3-9}$$

where Z_1 and Z_2 are the atomic numbers of the target and the particle, respectively, and A_1 and A_2 are the mass numbers of the target and the particle, respectively.[25] The first term on the right hand side of Equation 3-9 provides the value for the Coulomb barrier alone while the second term represents the fraction of the energy of the particle needed for the conservation of momentum.

EXAMPLE 3-6

Calculate the proton starting energy for the $^{18}O(p,n)^{18}F$ reaction.

ANSWER

Using Equation 3-9, the value for the starting energy,

$$E_S = \left(\frac{0.96 \times 8 \times 1}{18^{1/3} + 1^{1/3}} \right) \left(\frac{18 + 1}{18} \right)$$

$$= 2.24 \text{ MeV}$$

For an endoergic reaction to occur, the minimum energy that the particle should have is given by the larger of the threshold energy E_t or the starting energy E_s.[54] Thus, for the nuclear reaction $^{18}O(p,n)^{18}F$, the minimum proton energy required is given by E_t, which is 2.57 MeV.

An example for an exoergic reaction is $^{20}Ne(d,\alpha)^{18}F$, which has a Q value of +2.80 MeV. The threshold energy for such a nuclear reaction is zero. However, for the nuclear reaction to occur, the deuteron must possess enough starting energy (E_s) to overcome the Coulomb barrier as well as energy to conserve momentum. An approximate value for E_s in this case is given by:

$$E_S = \left(\frac{0.96 \times 10 \times 1}{20^{1/3} + 2^{1/3}} \right) \left(\frac{20 + 2}{20} \right)$$

$$= 2.66 \text{ MeV}$$

Thus, the approximate energy of deuterons needed for the $^{20}Ne(d,\alpha)^{18}F$ reaction is 2.7 MeV, even though the threshold for the reaction is zero.

It is important to note that the calculations involving Coulomb barrier as given above are only approximate. An accurate estimation will require a rigorous quantum mechanical calculation.[51]

Cross section

For a nuclear reaction, the laws of conservation of energy and momentum indicate whether the reaction is possible; the cross-sectional data provide the probability of the reaction to occur. The cross section, σ, is expressed as the effective area (it has nothing to do with the geometrical cross-sectional area, πr^2, of the target nucleus) in a contrived disc for a given nuclei such that when a charged particle passes through it, a nuclear reaction would occur. A mathematical relationship has been derived for the estimation of the cross section for a nuclear reaction wherein a beam of charged particles bombarding a thin target (which does not attenuate the beam) is given by:[51]

$$R = In x \sigma \tag{3-10}$$

where R is the radioactivity expressed in disintegrations/second (dps) for the product nuclei; I is the intensity of the charged particles expressed as the number of particles/second; n is the number of target nuclei/cm^3; x is the thickness of the target in centimeters; and σ is the cross section, expressed in cm^2/nucleus.

The unit of cross section is called a barn, denoted by b, and defined as:

$$1b = 10^{-24} \text{ cm}^2$$

The term barn was humorously proposed as a code word for nuclear cross section during the World War II. The geometrical cross section of a typical nucleus is 10^{-24} cm^2. Thus, a nuclear reaction cross section of 10^{-24} cm^2 is relatively large, and, hence, hitting the nucleus to cause a nuclear reaction is considered as easy as hitting a barn.

A common subunit of barn is millibarn, mb; therefore:

$$1 \text{ mb} = 10^{-3} \text{ b}$$

Assuming the product of a nuclear reaction is radioactive, there will be decay of the product during an irradiation of time t. Equation 3-10 then can be written as:

$$R = In x \sigma (1 - e^{-\lambda t}) \tag{3-11}$$

where t is the time of irradiation in seconds and λ the decay constant for the product radioisotope is given by $\dfrac{0.693}{t_{1/2}}$ where $t_{1/2}$ is the half-life of the radioisotope produced.

The value of R corresponds to the number of product nuclei formed at the end of the bombardment time of t. The value of σ is evaluated by irradiating a thin foil of a material of known mass thickness with a known charged particle flux and measuring the activity after an irradiation time of t using Equation 3-11.

The thickness of the target can be expressed in terms of weight per unit area (occasionally called area density) and is equal to the product of the number of target nuclei per cm^3, n, and the thickness of the target in cm, x. The cyclotron beam current is generally expressed in units of microampere (μA). One μA of current is equal to 6.25×10^{12} electronic charges per second. A proton carries an unit electronic charge. Thus, for a proton beam:

$$1 \ \mu A = 6.25 \times 10^{12} \text{ protons/s}$$

The helium ions ^{3}He^{2+} and ^{4}He^{2+} carry two charges and hence 1 μA of them corresponds to 3.125×10^{12} particles/s.

EXAMPLE 3-7

A 0.1 mg/cm^2-thick foil of ^{11}B (80.2% enrichment) was irradiated for 30 min with a 10-μA beam of 9-MeV protons. The cross section for the ^{11}B(p,n,)^{11}C nuclear reaction is 300 mb. Neglecting the energy degradation of the proton beam in traversing this thin target, calculate the amount of ^{11}C isotope produced.

ANSWER

Applying Equation 3-11 with:

$$I = 10 \times 6.25 \times 10^{12} \text{ particles/s}$$
$$nx = 0.1 \text{ mg/cm}^2$$

Because ^{11}B isotope enrichment is 80.2%, the number of target nuclei in 0.1 mg/ cm^2 is

$$\frac{0.0001 \text{ g/cm}^2}{11 \text{ g/mol}} \times \frac{80.2}{100} \times 6.023 \times 10^{23} \text{ atoms/mol}$$

$$= 4.39 \times 10^{18} \text{ atoms/cm}^2$$

$$\sigma = 300 \times 10^{-27} \text{ cm}^2/\text{nucleus}$$

$$\lambda = \frac{0.693}{20 \text{ min}}$$

$$t = 30 \text{ min}$$

$$R = 10 \times 6.25 \times 10^{12} \times 4.39 \times 10^{18} \times 300 \times 10^{-27} \times \left(1 - e^{\frac{-0.693}{20} \times 30}\right)$$

$$= 5.321 \times 10^7 \text{ dps}$$

Because there are 3.7×10^7 dps/mCi:

$$R = \frac{5.321 \times 10^7}{3.7 \times 10^7} \text{ mCi}$$

$$= 1.44 \text{ mCi}$$

Excitation function

The cross section, σ, depends on the energy, E, of the incident particle beam. A graphical relationship between σ and E is known as the excitation function.[54] Figure 3-6 provides the excitation functions for the production of ^{11}C, ^{13}N, ^{15}O, and ^{18}F isotopes for various nuclear reactions.[55] A knowledge of the excitation function can help in designing a gas target.[56] Excitation function measurements are frequently made to experimentally verify theoretical calculations as well as to elucidate nuclear reaction mechanisms.

Saturation yield

The amount of radioactivity produced in nuclear reactions is generally corrected to the end of bombardment (EOB) to enable a valid comparison between different experiments. For comparison of experiments of different beam currents and irradiation times, a parameter known as saturation yield is used. The saturation yield is the theoretical maximum rate of production

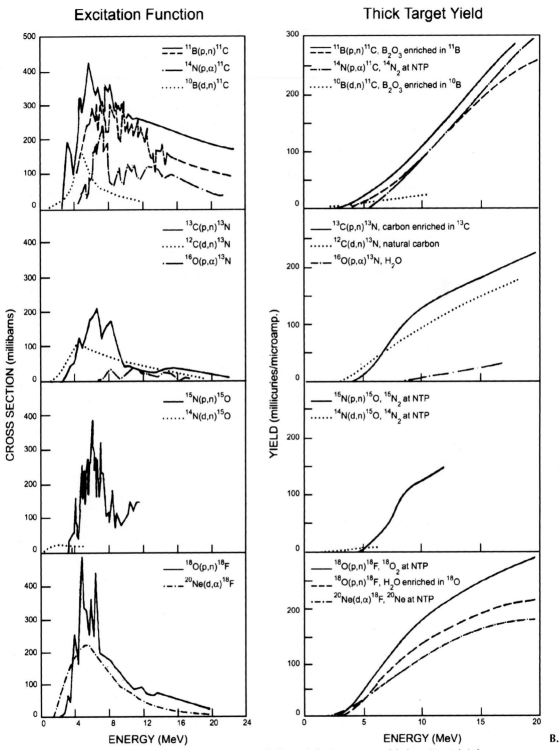

FIGURE 3-6. The excitation function (A, left) and thick target yield data (B, right) for ^{11}C, ^{13}N, ^{15}O, and ^{18}F radioisotopes. (Reprinted with permission from Wieland et al.[55], © 1997 IEEE.)

of a radioisotope for given beam energy conditions.[51] Saturation yield has a unit of mCi/μA and it is calculated using the following equation:

$$\text{Saturation yield} = \frac{A_o}{1(1 - e^{-\lambda t})} \tag{3-12}$$

where A_o is the activity of the product in mCi at EOB; I is the beam current in μA; λ is the decay constant; and t is the time of irradiation in minutes.

Saturation yield data are useful in calculating the radioisotope yield for a given reaction at a given reaction energy.

The term $(1 - e^{-\lambda t})$ in Equations 3-11 and 3-12 is called the saturation factor.[51] It represents the exponential growth of a product radioisotope during an irradiation of a target for time t. The rate of growth of a radioisotope with various irradiation times in terms of its half-life is shown in Figure 3-7. The saturation factor approaches unity as the irradiation time t reaches about 7 half-lives of the product radioisotope. At that point, the rate of production of the isotope will be equal to the rate of decay. Hence, the duration of bombardment of a given target strongly depends upon the half-life of the product nuclide. In the case of PET radioisotopes, the ^{15}O production normally utilizes an irradiation time of 5 half-lives (10 min) while the ^{18}F production bombardment rarely goes beyond 1 half-life (110 min).

Thick target yield

Equations 3-10 and 3-11 are valid only for a beam of charged particles striking a thin target such that the beam is not attenuated or attenuated only infinitesimally. However, charged particles traversing a thick target gradually lose energy due to interactions with electrons; hence, the target nuclei encounter a distribution of energies of the bombarding particles. Because the cross section of a

FIGURE 3-7. Radioactivity buildup with irradiation time. The value 100 represents the saturation when the rate of production and decay are equal.

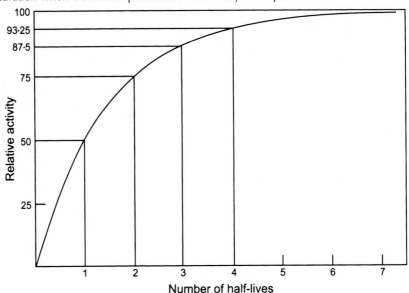

nuclear reaction depends upon the energy of the incident beam, the rate of the nuclear reaction R given by Equations 3-10 and 3-11 should account for this energy loss and its effect on σ, the cross section. Accordingly, an expression for the thick target yield, Y has been derived and shown to be:[53,54]

$$Y = \frac{1.03 \times 10^5}{Z \times A} \int_{E_{in}}^{E_{out}} \frac{\sigma(E)}{dE/dx} \, dE \qquad \text{for } t \gg t_{1/2} \qquad (3\text{-}13)$$

where Y = thick target yield in $\mu Ci/\mu A$;
 Z = atomic number of the bombarding charged particle;
 A = mass number of the target nuclei;
 dE/dx = stopping power or specific energy loss in MeV cm^2/g of the charged particle;
 $\sigma(E)$ = cross section in mb at energy E;
 t = time of irradiation;
 $t_{1/2}$ = half-life of the product radioisotope;
 E_{in} = incident energy of the particle; and
 E_{out} = exiting energy of the particle.

A target is called a thick target if the energy of the particle beam is completely stopped within the target ($E_{out} = 0$) or degraded to an energy less than the threshold for the nuclear reaction. The stopping power, dE/dx values are generally obtainable from range-energy tables.[57,58] Calculations using Equation 3-13 are carried out by considering a thick target as a large number of thin slices stacked together such that the change in σ (due to loss of energy of the beam) in each of those slices is negligibly small.

Thus, the thick target yield can be defined as the radioactive disintegration rate (in mCi or μCi), at saturation, divided by the beam current (in μA). The thick target yield data are generally obtained by the integration of the corresponding excitation function. Typical thick target yield functions for ^{11}C, ^{13}N, ^{15}O, and ^{18}F isotopes are illustrated in Figure 3-6.

EXAMPLE 3-8

Calculate the amount of ^{18}F isotope that would be produced by an irradiation of a thick $H_2^{18}O$ target with 10-MeV protons with a beam current of 20 μA for 60 min, given that the saturation yield for $^{18}O(p,n)^{18}F$ nuclear reaction at 10 MeV is 137 mCi/μA and $t_{1/2}$ for ^{18}F is 110 min.

ANSWER

Equation 3-12 can be rearranged as:

$$A_o = \text{saturation yield} \times 1(1 - e^{-\lambda t})$$

saturation yield = 137 mCi/μA

$$I = 20 \ \mu A$$

$$\lambda = \left(\frac{\ln 2}{t_{1/2}}\right) = \frac{0.693}{110} \ \text{min}^{-1}$$

$$t = 60 \ \text{min}$$

Therefore, activity of ^{18}F isotope produced at EOB:

$$= 137 \times 20 \times \left(1 - e^{\frac{-0.693}{110} \times 60}\right)$$

$$= 862.6 \text{ mCi}$$

EXAMPLE 3-9

A thick target of $^{15}N_2$ was irradiated with 30 μA of 10-MeV proton beam for 10 min to produce 749 mCi of ^{15}O-labeled oxygen gas 3 min after the end of bombardment. Calculate the saturation yield for the $^{15}N(p,n)^{15}O$ nuclear reaction.

ANSWER

The activity of ^{15}O isotope produced at EOB can be calculated using the formula:

$$A_t = A_o e^{-\lambda t}$$

A_t, activity of ^{15}O 3 min after EOB = 749 mCi and $t_{1/2}$ for ^{15}O = 2 min. Therefore, A_o, the activity at EOB

$$= \frac{A_t}{e^{-\lambda t}} = \frac{749}{e^{\frac{-0.693}{2} \times 3}} = 2118.0 \text{ mCi}$$

Applying Equation 3-12 with $t_{1/2}$ = 2 min and I = 30 μA

$$\text{the saturation yield} = \frac{2118.0}{30\left(1 - e^{\frac{-0.693}{2} \times 10}\right)}$$

$$= 72.9 \text{ mCi}/\mu\text{A}$$

TARGETS

A target system is an ancillary unit or part of a cyclotron wherein irradiation of target materials takes place to generate positron-emitting isotopes. The following generic terminology is used for the description of various target systems:

1. Target material—the liquid or gaseous material that undergoes nuclear transformation;
2. Target body—that which holds the target material during the irradiation;
3. Target—the combination of target material and the target body.

Target design

A generic gas target body for the cyclotron production of PET isotopes consists of a cylindrical aluminum tube (10 cm long and 1 cm in diameter) sealed at one end and provided with a thin (usually, 0.0025-cm thick) metal foil at the other end where the beam enters (Figure 3-8). The target body is surrounded by a cooling water jacket which removes the heat generated during the irradiation process. An inlet allows for loading of gaseous target material at ~200 psi, and an outlet permits removal of the irradiated product. Proton beam from the cy-

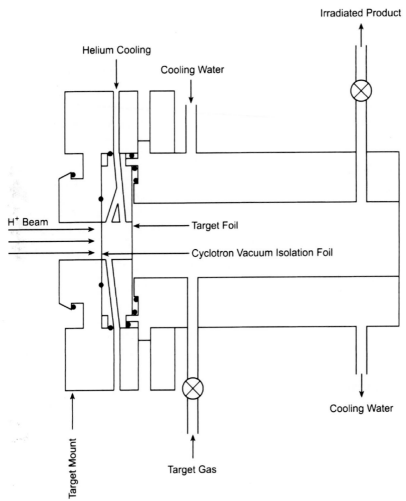

FIGURE 3-8. Generic cyclotron gas target.

clotron travels through a thin vacuum isolation foil, and then the target foil into the target for the nuclear reaction. Cold helium gas is circulated in the annular space between the foils to dissipate the heat generated by the beam in the foils. It is a common practice to use a thick target for the production of radioisotopes. A target is considered thick if the impinging beam is degraded to thermal energy levels. Using range-energy tables,[57,58] the conditions for a thick target are calculated.

Cyclotron target bodies are generally designed to have a feature called low dead volume. The volume of the target material outside the beam path is termed as dead volume. The solenoid valves, fittings, and the associated plumbing of a target system usually provide the dead volume. The heat generated during the irradiation process causes thinning of the target material, known as density reduction, which leads to low radioisotope yield. In low dead volume targets, the reduction of radioisotope yields due to density reduction is minimized.

In general, only 1 in 1,000 charged particles induce a nuclear reaction and the rest interact with atomic electrons and produce heat. The power deposited by the beam in the target is calculated using the formula:

$$\text{Power (in watts)} = \text{beam energy (in MeV)} \times \text{beam current (in } \mu A) \quad (3\text{-}14)$$

EXAMPLE 3-10
Calculate the power in cal/s deposited by a 40-μA proton beam of 10.5 MeV energy on a thick $^{14}N_2$ gas target.

ANSWER
Using Equation 3-14,

$$\text{power (in watts)} = 10.5 \text{ MeV} \times 40 \text{ } \mu A$$
$$= 420 \text{ watts}$$

Since 1 watt = 0.24 cal/s
$$\text{power} = 0.24 \times 420$$
$$= 100.8 \text{ cal/s}$$

Power deposition of this magnitude leads to large pressure rises in gas targets. Failure to cool the target body efficiently would lead to low yields of the product radioisotopes, to target foil rupture or all the way to a target melt down.

Small volume targets for the production of important positron-emitting radioisotopes

Selected nuclear reactions[59–61] with high cross section that are commonly used for the production of ^{15}O, ^{13}N, ^{11}C, and ^{18}F are summarized in Table 3-4. In-

TABLE 3-4. Important Nuclear Reactions for the Production of ^{11}C, ^{13}N, ^{15}O, and ^{18}F Radioisotopes[59–61]

Reaction	Q value (MeV)	Threshold energy (MeV)	Cross section E $(\sigma_{max})^a$ (MeV)	σ_{max} (mb)
^{15}O-isotope				
$^{15}N(p,n)^{15}O$	−3.54	3.7	6.6	230
$^{14}N(d,n)^{15}O$	5.07	0	4.0	227
^{13}N-isotope				
^{13}C $(p,n)^{13}N$	−3.00	3.2	6.7	275
^{16}O $(p,\alpha)^{13}N$	−5.22	5.5	8.0	139
^{12}C $(d,n)^{13}N$	−0.28	0.4	2.3	200
^{11}C-isotope				
$^{11}B(p,n)^{11}C$	−2.76	3.0	9.0	300
$^{14}N(p,\alpha)^{11}C$	−2.92	3.1	7.6	253
$^{10}B(d,n)^{11}C$	6.47	0	2.3	270
^{18}F-isotope				
$^{18}O(p,n)^{18}F$	−2.44	2.6	5.2	630
$^{20}Ne(d,\alpha)^{18}F$	2.80	0	12.3	24
$^{16}O(^3He,p)^{18}F$	2.03	0	6.3	436
$^{16}O(\alpha,pn)^{18}F$	−18.55	23.2	40	250

^{a}Energy of the particle at which the cross-section has the highest value (σ_{max}).

terestingly, the target systems for the production of these isotopes have paralleled the evolution of cyclotron technology as described in Role of Cyclotrons in the Production of PET Isotopes (this chapter). In the 1960s and 1970s, large volume (>100 mL) target bodies containing nonenriched stable isotopes were commonly utilized as target materials for the production of the positron emitters.[62] With the introduction of smaller and self-shielded cyclotrons (Table 3-3) with lower beam energies in the 1980s, a dramatic improvement in target design took place. Overall, the target volumes were reduced substantially (1 mL–3 mL for liquid targets to < 15 mL for gas targets depending upon the radioisotope).[63–65] Based on the thick target yield data (Figure 3-6) proton-induced nuclear reactions for the production of large quantities of ^{15}O, ^{13}N, ^{11}C, and ^{18}F were implemented, and radioisotope yields were optimized based on target shape and volume, beam energy, beam optics, and other related parameters.[66] Utilization of enriched isotopes as target materials for the production of Curie quantities of ^{15}O and ^{18}F is a common practice these days.[63–65] Table 3-5 summarizes the proton nuclear reactions involved in the formation of ^{15}O, ^{13}N, ^{11}C, and ^{18}F isotopes; target volumes and pressures; and the chemical form of the isolated product. Generally, the operation of these target systems are fully automated and controlled by a PC.

In the last decade, a number of advancements in cyclotron target technology have taken place. For example, the RDS-111 cyclotron (CTI, Inc.; Figure 3-5A) has two beam ports, each of which supports a fully automated eight-target rotating carousel for greater flexibility in the production of PET isotopes.[67] The volume of the gas target bodies have been reduced to just 7 mL for an efficient utilization of the expensive enriched target material (e.g., $^{15}N_2$ for $[^{15}O]O_2$ production). This miniaturization of the ^{15}O target has enabled the production of unit doses (20–25 mCi) of ^{15}O-labeled water at a cost of only \$4/dose. In Table 3-6, the routine yields of ^{15}O, ^{13}N, ^{11}C, and ^{18}F radioisotopes obtained (and their chemical form) with 11-MeV protons using the latest generation of target bodies is summarized.

TABLE 3-5. Proton Nuclear Reaction for the Routine Production of Positron-emitting Isotopes

Radioisotope	Nuclear reaction	Target material	Target volume (mL)	Chemical form of product radioisotope
^{15}O	$^{15}N(p,n)^{15}O$	$^{15}N_2 + {}^{16}O_2$ (2.5%)	15[a]	$[^{15}O]O_2$
^{13}N	$^{16}O(p,\alpha)^{13}N$	5 mM ethanol in sterile water	3[b]	$[^{13}N]NH_4^+$
^{11}C	$^{14}N(p,\alpha)^{11}C$	$^{14}N_2 + {}^{16}O_2$ (1%)	15[a]	$[^{11}C]CO_2$
^{18}F	$^{18}O(p,n)^{18}F$	$H_2^{18}O^c$	0.3–3.0[d]	$[^{18}F]F^-$
^{18}F	$^{18}O(p,n)^{18}F$	$^{18}O_2$	15[a]	$[^{18}F]F_2^e$

[a]Target operational pressure: 210 psi.   [b]Target operational pressure: 150 psi.

[c]Using an anion exchange resin column, the target material is separated from the product isotope after irradiation and recycled.[51]

[d]Target operational pressure: 15 psi to 500 psi.

[e]Obtained in a two-step process. After irradiation of $^{18}O_2$, the target gas is cryorecovered leaving ^{18}F isotope on the walls of the target body which is released subsequently by a second irradiation in the presence of small amounts of nonradioactive $^{19}F_2$ (~100 μmol) in argon.

TABLE 3-6. Typical Yields of Positron-Emitting Precursors Obtained with 11-MeV Protons using RDS-111 Cyclotron

	Irradiation			
Radioisotope	Beam current (μA)	Time min	Chemical form	Yield (mCi)
^{15}O	40	10	O_2	2000[a]
	40	10	CO_2	800[b]
	40	10	CO	600[b]
	40	10	H_2O	750[b,c]
^{13}N	40	10	$NH_4{}^+$	100[a]
^{11}C	40	50	CO_2	1500[a]
	40	50	CO_2	3000[a,d]
	40	50	CO	1000[b]
^{18}F	30	60	F^-	1000[a,e]
	100	120	F^-	6900[a,e]
	40	60	F_2	500[a,f]

[a]End of bombardment.   [b]End of synthesis.

[c]Routine production of 20 mCi to 25 mCi doses by computer control would cost less than $4/dose.

[d]Two targets irradiated simultaneously.   [e]$H_2{}^{18}O$ target.   [f]$^{18}O_2$ gas target.

Recycling of enriched target materials

Fluorine-18 and oxygen-15 are the two important positron-emitting radioisotopes that currently utilize enriched stable isotopes as target materials. For example, production of [^{18}F]fluoride ion involves proton irradiation of ^{18}O-enriched water while $^{15}N_2$ is used for the production of ^{15}O isotope.[66] Similarly, the production of ^{18}F-labeled molecular fluorine requires [^{18}O]O_2 as the target material. Typically, only 1 in 1 million of the atoms of the target material undergoes a nuclear reaction during a standard irradiation condition. Thus, it is desirable to recover the untransformed expensive target material, if possible. Scarcity and expense of [^{18}O]water (95% enrichment: $150/g in the year 2003), [^{18}O]O_2 (95% enrichment: $500/L) and $^{15}N_2$ (99% enrichment: $350/L) have led to the development of methods to recover and recycle 2 of these 3 precious target materials.

An excellent method for the recovery (> 90%) of [^{18}O]water after irradiation is commonly used in a number of PET centers. Proton-irradiated [^{18}O]water is passed through a commercially available short column of anion exchange resin (e.g., Waters Accell plus QMA cartridge, Waters Corporation, Milford, MA). The [^{18}F]fluoride ion is efficiently trapped in the resin column and the valuable [^{18}O]water that passes through is collected for recycling.[68] The [^{18}F]fluoride ion is near quantitatively recovered from the resin column by elution with an aqueous base (e.g., K_2CO_3). The recovered [^{18}O]water is purified by distillation before reuse. Alternatively, the used [^{18}O]water could be returned to the manufacturer for purification purposes.

A cryogenic method[69] for recovery and recycling of [^{18}O]O_2 has been known for nearly two decades in the production of [^{18}F]F_2. In this method, [^{18}O]O_2, after proton irradiation, is cryorecovered from the target in a stainless steel cylinder dipped in liquid nitrogen. Essentially 100% of the [^{18}O]oxygen gas is trapped in the cylinder leaving behind the ^{18}F activity produced inside the target surface. The ^{18}F activity is then commonly recovered as [^{18}F]F_2 by adding small quantities of nonradioactive fluorine gas ($\sim$100 μmol) and reirradiating the target. The $[^{18}O]O_2$ thus recovered can be reused without any further purification.

The method of production of ^{15}O isotope by the irradiation of $^{15}N_2$ with protons unfortunately does not lend to recovering the target material. However, using small volume targets as described in Small Volume Targets for the Production of Important Positron-emitting Radioisotopes (this chapter), it is still possible to produce ^{15}O isotope economically.

In any event, the cyclotron manufacturers provide automated target systems for the production of ^{15}O, ^{13}N, ^{11}C, and ^{18}F isotopes. These systems are easy to operate and provide Curie levels of activities for most of these isotopes reliably and reproducibly.

IMPORTANT PRECURSORS FOR PET RADIOPHARMACEUTICALS

Positron emitter-labeled precursors refer to chemically distinct radioactive reagents that are used in the preparation of PET radiotracers. These radiolabeled precursors are invariably simple reactive products that are obtained directly from the target system or produced by certain rapid post-target chemical transformations.[70] These positron-emitting precursors are utilized to incorporate the radiolabel into the PET tracer probes.

Concept of specific activity (SA)

When dealing with the production of radioisotopes, it is extremely important to minimize the isotopic dilution (contamination from stable isotopes of the same element). For example, the production of ^{11}C isotope involves the $^{14}N(p,\alpha)^{11}C$ nuclear reaction, and the target material is 99% $^{14}N_2$ containing 1% $^{16}O_2$ (chemical purity of these gases is 99.9995%). Even a gas mixture of this purity would contain stable isotope of carbon (^{12}C) impurities that would act as an isotopic diluent for the ^{11}C radioactive isotope produced. Carbon-12 contamination could also arise from the surface of the target body, valves, and the associated plumbing of the target. The extent of isotopic dilution is determined by the measurement of the specific activity of the radioactive precursor or the tracer synthesized from it. Specific activity is generally defined as the amount of radioactivity per unit mass of a labeled compound. The mass of the labeled compound includes the mass of the radioactive product as well as the mass of its non-radioactive counterpart. For instance, in the calculation of the specific activity of $^{11}CO_2$ produced with a cyclotron, the investigator should not only account for the mass of $^{11}CO_2$ but also the non-radioactive $^{12}CO_2$ isotopic diluent that would invariably be present in the product. The combined masses of the radioisotope and its corresponding diluent can generally be determined by sensitive spectroscopic or electrochemical methods. The unit for specific activity is mCi/mg, Ci/mmol or Ci/μmol; the latter two are generally preferred.

From the standpoint of specific activity, two distinct methods, namely, carrier-added and no-carrier-added, are used for the production of PET radioisotopes. The term carrier-added preparation of a PET radioisotope refers to a radioactive production during which a known amount of the corresponding stable isotope (generally termed as carrier) has been added. A no-carrier-added preparation involves no intentional or otherwise addition of the stable isotopic carrier during the production of the radioisotope. Thus, the specific activity of an isotope produced via a no-carrier-added method is always higher than the corresponding nuclide made by the carrier-added technique. The specific activity of a carrier-added isotope, of course, depends upon the amount of carrier added during the production. The maximum specific activity that a radioisotope can attain results when every atom of the element is identically radioactive (i.e., entirely free from isotopic dilution) and is called the theoretical maximum specific activity. It can be calculated using the following equation:

$$\text{theoretical maximum SA} = \frac{1.128 \times 10^{13}}{t_{1/2}} \text{ Ci/mol} \qquad (3\text{-}15)$$

when $t_{1/2}$ is expressed in seconds. The theoretical maximum specific activity (Table 3-1) is seldom achieved in practice for any of the PET radioisotopes. Also, it is preferable to report the specific activity of a radiopharmaceutical rather than the SA of its radioactive precursor.

EXAMPLE 3-11
A 10-mCi sample of 2-[F-18]fluoro-2-deoxy-D-glucose (FDG) prepared by no-carrier-added nucleophilic synthesis was found to contain a mass of 0.70 μg of FDG as determined by a pulsed amperometric detector. Calculate the specific activity of the FDG sample.

ANSWER
Number of moles of FDG in 10 mCi sample

$$= \frac{7 \times 10^{-7} \text{ g}}{182 \text{ g/mol}}$$
$$= 3.85 \times 10^{-9} \text{ mol}$$

[In the calculation of the number of moles of FDG in 0.7 μg, the molecular weight (182) of nonradioactive FDG is used since its concentration is $\gg$ that of the ^{18}F counterpart.]

$$\text{The specific activity of FDG} = \frac{\text{activity of FDG}}{\text{mass of FDG}}$$

$$= \frac{10 \text{ mCi}}{3.85 \times 10^{-9} \text{ mol}}$$

$$= 2600 \text{ Ci/mmol}$$

---

^{15}O-labeled precursor
The two common nuclear reactions used for the production of ^{15}O isotope are given in Table 3-4. In both cases, the target material is spiked with 1% stable ^{16}O$_2$ before irradiation to yield ^{15}O in the form of O$_2$. The [^{15}O]O$_2$ can be used directly or as a precursor material for an on-line production of [^{15}O]CO, [^{15}O]CO$_2$, and [^{15}O]H$_2$O[60,62,66,71,72] (Table 3-6). Oxygen-15-labeled butanol has also been synthesized from [^{15}O]O$_2$.[70]

^{13}N-labeled precursor

Among the nuclear reactions used for the production of ^{13}N isotope (Table 3-4), the ^{16}O(p,α)^{13}N reaction is the most popular one.[27,60,62,66,71] Irradiation of 5 mM ethanol in water provides [^{13}N]ammonia[73] which is also the most widely used precursor for ^{13}N-labeled compounds. Nitrogen-13, like ^{15}O radioisotope, finds only limited use in the preparation of more complex radiopharmaceuticals due to its short half-life. The principal utilization of this precursor is in the production of ^{13}N-labeled amino acids using rapid enzyme catalyzed reactions.[74,75]

^{11}C-labeled precursors

When a mixture of oxygen (1%) in pure ^{14}N$_2$ is irradiated with protons, [^{11}C]CO$_2$ is produced.[27,60,62,66,71] This is the principal precursor material for the preparation of a host of secondary ^{11}C precursors as shown in Figure 3-9. With the ^{11}C half-life of 20 min and the ease of production of [^{11}C]CO$_2$ in the Curie levels (Table 3-6), it is quite possible to prepare these secondary precursors not only by simple on-line techniques but also by other rapid synthetic methods. For example, ^{11}C-labeled methane and hydrogen cyanide can be produced by on-line processes while ^{11}CH$_3$I is produced by the reaction of [^{11}C]CO$_2$ with LiAlH$_4$ followed by treatment with HI.[60] The ^{11}CH$_3$I is perhaps the most important precursor for ^{11}C labeling and is used as a methylating agent for a vari-

FIGURE 3-9. ^{11}C-labeled precursors for the synthesis of various classes of radiopharmaceuticals.

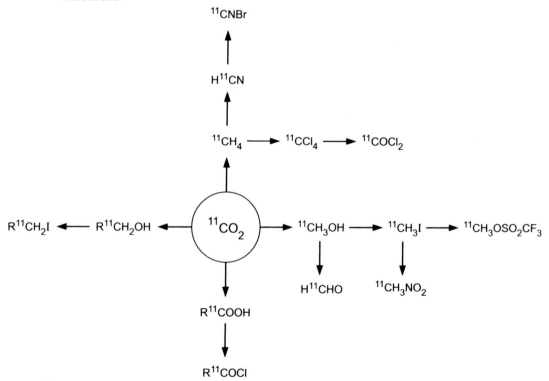

ety of N, O, and S centers in complex pharmaceuticals.[76] A well-designed module for the production of [^{11}C]CH$_3$I has recently been developed by GE Medical Systems.[77] Unlike the [^{11}C]CH$_3$I modules based on gas-liquid phase reactions, the GE module converts [^{11}C]CO$_2$ into [^{11}C]CH$_3$I through an entirely gas-solid phase on-line reaction sequence.[77,78] This automated versatile module can produce very high specific activity (~20,000 Ci/mmol) [^{11}C]CH$_3$I on demand. ^{11}C-labeled methyl triflate has also been prepared from ^{11}CH$_3$I using an on-line technique. The reactivity of [^{11}C]methyl triflate (^{11}CH$_3$OSO$_2$CF$_3$) is several orders of magnitude higher than that of ^{11}CH$_3$I, and hence, it is the more preferred ^{11}C methylating agent.[79]

A number of other precursors such as ^{11}C-labeled nitromethane, phosgene, cyanogen bromide, higher alkyl iodides, acid chlorides, and so on (Figure 3-9), along with ^{11}CH$_3$I, have been found useful in the preparation of amino acids, enzyme inhibitors, and receptor-binding ligands.[27,60,76] Carbon-11-labeled radiopharmaceuticals generally have a specific activity of 2,000 to 20,000 Ci/mmol depending upon the method of production of the ^{11}C precursors. Table 3-7 provides some important ^{11}C-labeled radiopharmaceuticals synthesized by ^{11}C methylation reactions.[76]

^{18}F-labeled precursors

Fluorine-18 labeled precursors are produced in no-carrier-added (high specific activity) and carrier-added (low specific activity) states depending upon the nuclear reaction and the target material used for the irradiation.[66] The relatively long half-life, low positron range (Chapter 1), strong C-F bond (110 kcal) and the ease of cyclotron production in multi-Curie levels make ^{18}F isotope the most useful among the common PET radioisotopes. Fluorine is an important element in its own right for modifying the properties of molecules. In terms of size, replacement of a hydrogen for fluorine in pharmaceuticals produces minimum steric perturbations. However, the strong electron-withdrawing properties of fluorine result in compounds with altered biochemistry and interesting biological properties.[80] Stimulated by this combination, and the increased stability of the carbon-fluorine bond relative to the carbon-hydrogen bond, a variety of fluorinated[81] and radio-fluorinated[82] pharmaceuticals have been synthesized. The im-

TABLE 3-7. Selected ^{11}C-labeled Radiopharmaceuticals and Their Use in PET Studies[76]

^{11}C radiopharmaceutical	Process or target
L-Methionine	Protein synthesis
Thymidine	DNA synthesis
L-Deprenyl	MAO-B enzyme
Nicotine	Nicotinic receptors
Nomifensine	Dopamine reuptake
N-Methylspiperone	Dopamine D-2 receptors
Raclopride	Dopamine D-2 receptors
WIN 35, 428	Dopamine transporter
SCH 23390	Dopamine D-1 receptor
Ro 15-1788	Benzodiazepine receptor
Carfentanil	Opiate receptors
Acetate	Oxidative metabolism and lipid synthesis in tumors

portant routes for the cyclotron production of ^{18}F isotope are summarized in Table 3-4.

The primary carrier-added ^{18}F-labeled precursor is [^{18}F] elemental fluorine. The original production of this isotope utilized ^{20}Ne(d,α)^{18}F nuclear reaction in a nickel target body.[27,61,66] The target gas (a mixture of ^{20}Ne and 0.1% of carrier ^{19}F$_2$) is irradiated with deuterons to produce [^{18}F]F$_2$. Fluorine is the most reactive element known and because of its very high electronegativity (4.0 in Pauling scale), it efficiently undergoes electrophilic addition and substitution reactions. The reactivity of F$_2$ can be tamed to some extent and its propensity for indiscriminate radical reactions can be curtailed by diluting it with inert gases such as nitrogen or noble gases. Thus, the dilute [^{18}F]F$_2$ recovered from the neon gas target found an immediate use in the synthesis of FDG in the late 1970s.[83]

Introduction of low-energy-proton-only negative-ion cyclotrons in the 1980s required a different approach for the production of [^{18}F]F$_2$. Presently, [^{18}F]F$_2$ is produced via ^{18}O(p,n)^{18}F nuclear reaction using [^{18}O]O$_2$ as the target material in an aluminum target body.[84] The expensive target material is cryorecovered as described earlier in Recycling of Enriched Target Materials (p. 246). Secondary precursors that could be produced from [^{18}F]F$_2$ are depicted in Figure 3-10. The main rationale for the preparation of these reagents is to control the reactivity of fluorine. The ^{18}F-labeled reagents OF$_2$, ClF, and NOF are produced in the target itself while ClO$_3$F and CH$_3$COOF (acetyl hypofluorite) are generated on-line.[27,66,85] The fluorosulfonamides,[86] trifluoromethyl hypofluorite, and xenon difluoride-labeled with ^{18}F are prepared with rapid synthetic methods. [85] Among all these carrier-added ^{18}F-labeled precursors, only [^{18}F]F$_2$ and [^{18}F]CH$_3$COOF have found consistent use. Both these reagents are widely used in the synthesis of ^{18}F-labeled aromatic amino acids.[82] Being carrier-added precursors, they produce only low specific activity (1–10 Ci/mmol) radiopharmaceuticals. Selected examples of products synthesized with carrier-added ^{18}F-fluorinating agents are provided in Table 3-8.[87–93]

The primary no-carrier-added ^{18}F-labeled precursor is [^{18}F]fluoride ion, and it is readily obtained in multi-Curie levels by proton irradiation of enriched [^{18}O]water.[66] Secondary ^{18}F-labeled precursors (Figure 3-11) such as the metal

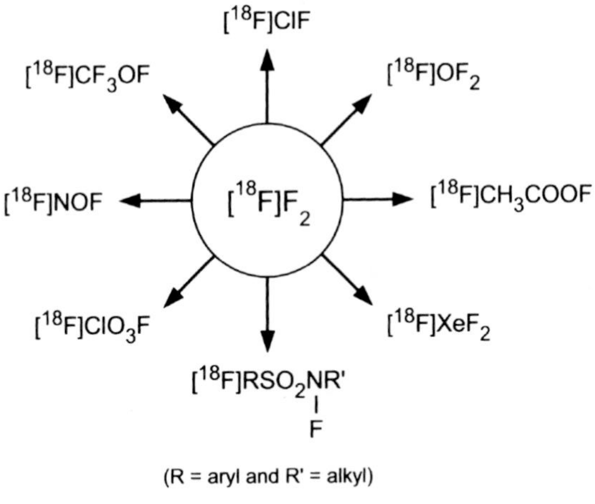

FIGURE 3-10. Common ^{18}F-labeled precursors derived from [^{18}F]F$_2$ for the synthesis of various classes of radiopharmaceuticals.

[^{18}F]ClF

[^{18}F]CF$_3$OF

[^{18}F]OF$_2$

[^{18}F]NOF

[^{18}F]F$_2$

[^{18}F]CH$_3$COOF

[^{18}F]ClO$_3$F

[^{18}F]XeF$_2$

[^{18}F]RSO$_2$NR'
|
F

(R = aryl and R' = alkyl)

TABLE 3-8. Selected ^{18}F-labeled Radiopharmaceuticals and Their Use in PET Studies[87–93]

^{18}F Radiopharmaceutical	Process or target
Carrier-added products	
6-[F-18]Fluoro-L-DOPA (FDOPA)	Presynaptic dopamine synthesis
4- and 6-[F-18]Fluoro-L-m-tyrosine (FMT)	Presynaptic dopamine synthesis
FDG	Glucose metabolism
5-[^{18}F]Fluorouracil	Tumor therapy to monitor metastases
8-[^{18}F]Fluoropenciclovir	Reporter gene expression
No-carrier-added products	
FDG	Glucose metabolism
[^{18}F]Fluoromisonidazole	Hypoxic cell
FESP	Dopamine D-2 receptor and D-2 reporter gene expression
4-[^{18}F]Fluorodexetimide	Muscarinic acetylcholine receptor
[^{18}F]Fluoroaltanserin	Serotonin S-2 receptor
6-[^{18}F]Fluoronorepinephrine	Adrenergic nerves
HBG	Reporter gene expression
3'-fluoro-3'-deoxythymidine ([F-18]FLT)	DNA synthesis
[^{18}F]Fluoroethyl or methyl choline	Choline uptake in prostate cancer

fluorides, resin-bound fluoride, and quaternary ammonium fluorides are readily produced from their corresponding carbonates, bicarbonates, or hydroxides by reacting them with ^{18}F$^-$. Others (Figure 3-11) are obtained by rapid synthetic methods.[89] [^{18}F]Fluoride ion is principally used in nucleophilic substitution reactions in aromatic and aliphatic systems. Among all these ^{18}F secondary precursors, K^{18}F and [^{18}F]tetra-n-butylammonium fluoride (nBu$_4$N^{18}F) are the most widely used in radiofluorination reactions.[87] The reactivity of K^{18}F is enhanced by complexing it with a cryptand called Kryptofix 2.2.2. The nucleophilic substitution reactions are conducted in dry polar aprotic solvents such as acetonitrile or dimethyl sulfoxide.

Substrates that are amenable to aromatic ^{18}F nucleophilic substitution reactions are those with leaving groups such as nitro and quaternary ammonium moieties located at the ortho or para position with reference to electron withdrawing functional groups like CN, CHO, or COCH$_3$. No-carrier-added

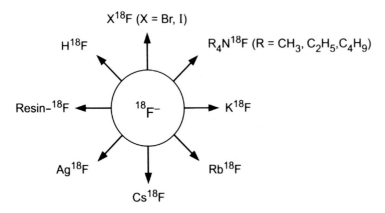

FIGURE 3-11. No-carrier-added ^{18}F labeled precursors obtained from ^{18}F$^-$ for the synthesis of various classes of radiopharmaceuticals.

K^{18}F/Kryptofix complex reacts with ease with such substrates and provides ^{18}F arylfluorides in 60% to 70% yields.[87] These ^{18}F arylfluorides are subsequently utilized in the synthesis of a variety of complex radiopharmaceuticals. Similarly, short chain [^{18}F]fluoroalkyl halides or sulfonates (e.g., [^{18}F]fluoromethyl bromide, [^{18}F]fluoroethyl tosylate) are prepared from alkyldihalides or sulfonates using K^{18}F/Kryptofix. These [^{18}F]fluoroalkyl halides or sulfonates find extensive use in the alkylation of nitrogen and oxygen centers in compounds of pharmaceutical interest.[87–89] [^{18}F]Fluoroalkyl groups, for example, can be used as relatively long-lived alternatives to ^{11}CH$_3$-alkylated derivatives. The most important ^{18}F nucleophilic synthesis involves the preparation of FDG which is produced in greater than 60% radiochemical yield on a routine basis in just about every PET center.[90] As expected, no-carrier-added ^{18}F nucleophilic substitution reactions provide products with high specific activity (1,000–10,000 Ci/mmol). Such high specific activity radiopharmaceuticals are generally required for receptor- and gene expression-related assays.[87] Table 3-8 provides certain important no-carrier-added ^{18}F radiopharmaceuticals used in PET studies.[27,82,85,87,89,91–93]

AUTOMATED SYNTHESIS MODULES

The success of PET in the long run depends on the availability of cyclotron-based synthesis systems with easy, simplified operations for repetitious and reliable radiopharmaceutical preparation.[11,94,95] PC-controlled automation of the synthetic process is highly desirable for the widespread use of PET. The rationale for automation of radiopharmaceutical synthesis includes: 1) reduction of radiation exposure to personnel, 2) efficient use of personnel by eliminating the need to do time-consuming syntheses, 3) better reproducibility of the synthetic method, and 4) overall cost savings. Furthermore, automation of the radiopharmaceutical synthesis would facilitate compliance with the U.S. Food and Drug Administration's (FDA's) upcoming new regulations mandated by U.S. FDA Modernization Act of 1997.[96]

Historically, two distinct approaches have been applied to the automation of radiopharmaceutical synthesis, namely, automated modules based on the principle of unit operations and robotics-based systems.[70,97] The unit operations approach is based on the philosophy that a complex process can be reduced to a series of simple operations or reactions, which are identical in fundamentals regardless of the labeled compound being prepared.[98,99] Synthetic methodologies based on this principle have remained the most popular technique for automation of PET radiopharmaceutical syntheses.[97]

Automatic systems based on both the unit operations approach[100–102] and robotics[103] have been used for the synthesis of nonradioactive compounds. For example, the first automated instrument for peptide synthesis using the unit operations approach was described in 1966.[104] Over the years, a number of new automated synthesizers based on this maxim, for peptides, DNA and RNA, and oligonucleotides have been developed by both academia and industry.[105–107] In the past 15 years, biotechnology companies have further advanced this methodology and have developed a variety of PC-controlled, bench-top automated systems for DNA, RNA, and peptide synthesis, as well as for small drug molecules in combinatorial chemical technology.[108] These versatile yet user-friendly systems are easy to operate and maintain and are extensively used in genome sequencing and mapping projects and a growing array of polymerase chain reaction (PCR) applications.

On the other hand, automated systems based on robotics are generally designed to perform a small set of manipulations many times (e.g., sample preparations) and not a large set of manipulations a few times (or once) as is normally required for a chemical synthesis.[109–111] Robots are invariably complicated and substantially expensive because they are mechanical devices and require a large work area to accommodate the hardware. Further, for the day-to-day operation of a robotics-based automated system, personnel with special training in computer programming and some engineering might be required.[112] In spite of these shortcomings, robots have been used in synthetic chemistry.[103,113] Described in this section is the utilization of automated modules based on unit operations as well as robotics for the routing synthesis of positron emitter-labeled radiopharmaceuticals.

Automated synthesizers based on unit operation principles

During the past 20 years, at the University of California, Los Angeles (UCLA), we have applied the principle of unit operations in the development of semi-automated and automated systems for the synthesis of a variety of positron-emitting radiopharmaceuticals.[114–120] A similar approach has also been utilized by other laboratories.[85] In this approach, a multistep synthetic process is broken down into the required unit operations (e.g., addition of reagent, removal of solvent, solvent extraction, chromatography and sterilization, and so on). These simple unit operations are performed in sequence on a remote, semiautomated basis where standard laboratory glassware and equipment are used in conjunction with solenoid valves. The interaction of a chemist is entirely remote and involves the addition of reagents, transfer of fluids by application of pressure or vacuum, and the initiation of each operation by actuating the appropriate combination of electrical switches controlling the solenoid valves. The reliability of this unit operation-based design approach is underscored by the record of several thousand production runs over the past two decades for the preparation of a host of positron-emitting labeled radiopharmaceuticals in our laboratories.[121] Such semiautomated systems were the prelude to achieving complete automation of the synthetic process with a PC.

To illustrate the versatile concept of an unit operations-based semiautomated synthesis system and its direct extension to a computer-controlled fully automated module, we chose the example of FDG synthesis.[90] A semiautomated system for the synthesis of FDG using the method described in the literature[90] was constructed early on (Figure 3-12) and thoroughly tested before embarking on the automation process. The complete synthetic process was broken down into appropriate unit operations and the basic steps were: 1) release of [^{18}F]fluoride ion from the cyclotron target, 2) nucleophilic fluorination of the precursor, 3) isolation of the intermediate product, 4) acid hydrolysis of protecting groups, 5) purification of FDG by ion-exchange chromatography, and 6) sterilization of FDG for human use.

These unit operations for the synthesis of FDG were automated under PC control at UCLA in collaboration with CTI, Inc. This fully automated module, termed Chemistry Process Control Unit (CPCU)[122] (Figures 3-12 and 3-13A), emulates the well-tested, semiautomated system developed in our laboratories based on unit operation principles. The initial module incorporated self-

Semi-automated

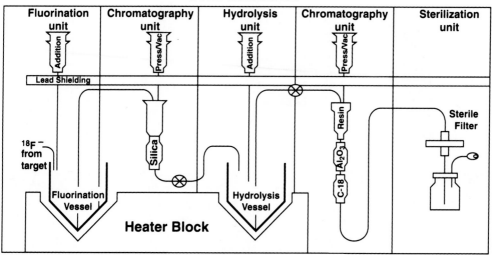

Automated

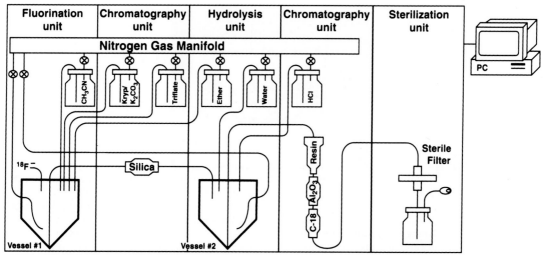

FIGURE 3-12. Schematics of semiautomated (top) and automated (bottom) FDG synthesis modules, both based on unit operation approach. The automated system consists of five unit operations (fluorination, chromatography, hydrolysis, chromatography, and sterilization) identical to those of the semiautomated system. The semiautomated system has manual operations and is assisted by pressure/vacuum for transfer of fluids from one reaction vessel to another while in the automated module, nitrogen gas pressure is utilized for analogous transfers. Vessels #1 and #2 in the automated system correspond to the fluorination and hydrolysis vessels, respectively, in the semiautomated system. The aluminum heater block in the semiautomated system is replaced by moving oil baths (not shown) in the automated system. Complete details on these systems have been reported.[122] (Reprinted from Satyamurthy N, Phelps ME, Barrio JR. Electronic generators for the production of positron-emitter labeled radiopharmaceuticals: Where would PET be without them? Clin Positron Imag. 1999;2:233–253, with permission from Elsevier.)

A.   B.   C.

D.

E.

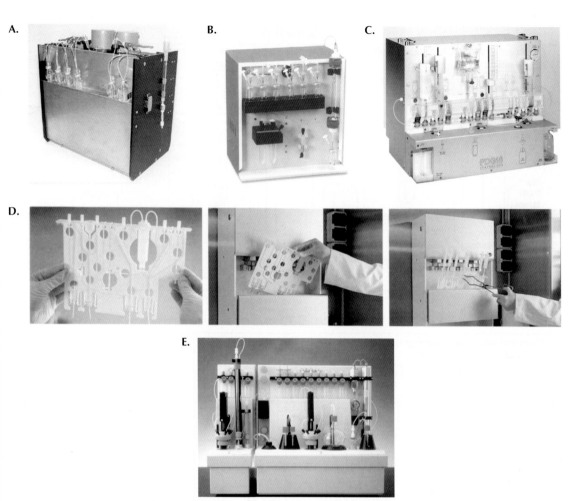

FIGURE 3-13. A: Automated FDG synthesis system based on the unit operations principle (Figure 3-12) as commercially available from CTI, Inc. of Knoxville, TN. This device is called Chemistry Process Control Unit (CPCU). (Courtesy of CTI.) B: Automated FDG synthesis module available from Jaltech. (Courtesy of Jaltech). C: Automated FDG synthesizer from Coincidence Technologies (GE Medical Systems). This system uses disposable components to ensure a clean operation and minimal time between synthesis. The highlight of this module is the fast synthesis of FDG (20 min) with high radiochemical yields (55–65%). (Courtesy of Coincidence Technologies, GE Medical Systems). D: GE automated FDG synthesis system. This device utilizes a fully disposable cassette containing reagent vials, tubings, and syringes (left). This cassette is loaded into the automated module (middle) for the synthesis of FDG. After the production run, the expired cassette is easily and rapidly removed (right) and a new one inserted for the next run. No manual cleaning between production runs is required minimizing greatly radiation exposure to personnel. (Courtesy of GE Medical Systems). E: Automated nucleophilic/electrophilic fluorination module from Nuclear Interface. This unit can be easily adapted for the synthesis of a number of ^{18}F-labeled radiopharmaceuticals. (Courtesy of Nuclear Interface, GE Medical Systems.)

diagnosis and feedback from sensors such as vapor pressure monitors, liquid level sensors, and so on. However, the system worked quite well with a simple series of on/off commands and timed waits from a PC. Thus, to maintain simplicity and reliability, the timing of various tasks that took place during the synthesis were determined, and a margin for variation was incorporated in the final program. However, to ensure mechanical stability, optical feedback limit switches as well as thermocouple feedback signals were utilized for the overall reliability of the system. The success rate of the synthesis of FDG with this automated chemistry module has been greater than 99%. Using this system, pure, sterile, and pyrogen-free FDG for human use is routinely obtained in an average radiochemical yield of greater than 60%. Currently, over 150 of these FDG modules are in daily use in the United States and Europe, attesting to the validity of the unit operation approach towards automating positron-emitting radiopharmaceutical synthesis.

Automated FDG modules based on the principles of unit operations are also commercially available from Jaltech (Figure 3-13B), IBA, and Nuclear Interface (GE Medical Systems). All these modules provide pure, sterile, and pyrogen-free FDG suitable for human use in good yields. Both GE (Figure 3-13D) and Coincidence Technologies (GE Medical Systems; Figure 3-13C) have developed unique FDG synthesizers based on this principle. These devices utilize disposable cassettes made of standard medical components containing all the required reagents for the synthesis of FDG. Interestingly, with the synthesizer developed by Coincidence Technologies, the complete FDG preparation, based on the alkaline hydrolysis of the radiolabeled glucose intermediate, can be performed in 20 min with a radiochemical yield of 54%. Thus, starting from 5.9 Ci of [^{18}F]fluoride ion delivered from the cyclotron, 3.3 Ci of FDG ready for human use can be obtained with this automated unit,[123] an attribute highly attractive to PET radiopharmaceutical distribution companies. In this regard, it is noteworthy that Nuclear Interface offers a radiopharmaceutical dose-dispensing unit. This fully automated computer-controlled module can dispense unit doses from a large batch (e.g., > 500 mCi) of PET tracer, under sterile conditions, vastly reducing radiation exposure to personnel.

Indeed, in addition to FDG, computer-controlled automated synthesizers have become commercially available for a variety of positron emitter-labeled radiopharmaceuticals. For example, Table 3-9 summarizes ^{11}C- and ^{18}F-labeled precursors that are commonly used for the production of PET tracers. Carbonation of Grignard reagents with [^{11}C]CO$_2$ and methylation of heteroatoms (e.g., nitrogen or oxygen) with [^{11}C]CH$_3$I are the most popular reactions for the preparation of ^{11}C-labeled radiopharmaceuticals as discussed in ^{11}C-labeled Precursors (p. 249). Likewise, [^{18}F]fluoride ion and [^{18}F]fluorine gas have been the reagents of choice for nucleophilic and electrophilic substitution reactions as described in ^{18}F-labeled Precursors (p. 250). Versatile automated modules for all these classes of reactions are readily available from several commercial sources. For example, Nuclear Interface has developed a generic nucleophilic/

TABLE 3-9. Examples of Radiolabeled Precursors, Generic Reactions, and Products for Automated Synthesizers

Precursor	Generic reaction	Example of product[a]
[^{11}C]CO$_2$	Carbonation of Grignard reagent	1-[C-11]acetate
[^{11}C]CH$_3$I	N-Alkylation	[^{11}C]Methylspiperone [^{11}C]WIN-35,428
[^{18}F]F$^-$	Nucleophilic substitution	FDG, [^{18}F]Fluoroethyl-spiperone
[^{18}F]F$_2$	Electrophilic substitution	FDOPA

[a]As described in sections ^{15}O-labeled Precursors, p. 248, and ^{13}N-labeled Precursors, p. 249 (both sections in this chapter) the other important PET tracer [^{13}N]ammonia is directly produced in the target while ^{15}O-labeled water, oxygen, carbon monoxide, and carbon dioxide are prepared via simple flow-through systems.

electrophilic fluorination module, based on the unit operations approach, (Figure 3-13E) that is suitable for the routine preparation of a variety of ^{18}F-labeled PET tracers. This module can easily be adapted to synthesize FDG and ^{18}F-labeled drugs such as fluoromisonidazole, fluoroestradiol, altanserine, 5-fluorouracil, and so on.[124] Similarly, the utility of the CPCU (Figure 3-13A) has readily been extended to the synthesis of 2-[^{18}F]fluoro-2-deoxymannose, [^{18}F]fluoroacetate, 2'-[^{18}F]fluoroethyl-spiperone, and FDOPA.[122,125]

All commercially available automated modules for the synthesis of PET radiopharmaceuticals have certain similarities among them. They are all generally compact, they occupy a space less than 20″ × 20″ × 20″, and, thus, they nicely fit inside a hot cell. The units are fully controlled by PCs with user-friendly menu-driven operating systems and allow a graphical visualization of the entire sequence of the synthetic operation. All the reaction parameters of the synthesis and other pertinent data are automatically saved for quality control documentation. Further, the software in all systems is quite flexible; therefore, users can easily modify and adapt the module for any future automation of new syntheses. Incidentally, most modules can also automatically self-clean between production runs. Most importantly, these automated synthesizers can easily be operated by technicians and are highly suitable for hospital-based PET centers and commercial radiopharmacies for day-to-day routine production of pure, sterile and pyrogen-free radiopharmaceuticals.

Robotics-based automated synthesizers

Automated modules for the synthesis of positron emitter-labeled radiopharmaceuticals based on robotics are still in the research domain.[97] Several ^{18}F- and ^{11}C-labeled PET tracers have been synthesized with robotic units.[97] However, routine synthesis of these products using robots in a clinical environment is yet to be realized. While every cyclotron manufacturer offers automated synthesizers based on the unit operation principle, none offers analogous modules based on robotics. Until easy-to-use and user-friendly robotic modules that do not require personnel with competence in computer programming and engineering for routine use are developed,[126,127] their utilization in a clinical PET facility for the synthesis of radiopharmaceuticals will be quite limited.

INTEGRATED AUTOMATED SYSTEM— ELECTRONIC GENERATOR

The integrated radiopharmaceutical production system, termed electronic generator, is a concept for the routine production of positron-emitting radiopharmaceuticals for commercial radiopharmacies, clinical service, and research.[11] An electronic generator has the following components: 1) a low-energy, single particle (proton only), preferably negative ion cyclotron; 2) small volume targets for an in-target or on-line production of positron emitter-labeled precursor molecules; and 3) automated synthesizers for the routine production of sterile and pyrogen-free radiopharmaceuticals. All these components are integrated as a single device with its operation fully controlled by a PC using simple menu-driven options chosen by a technician. A composite figure that represents an electronic generator is shown in Figure 3-14.

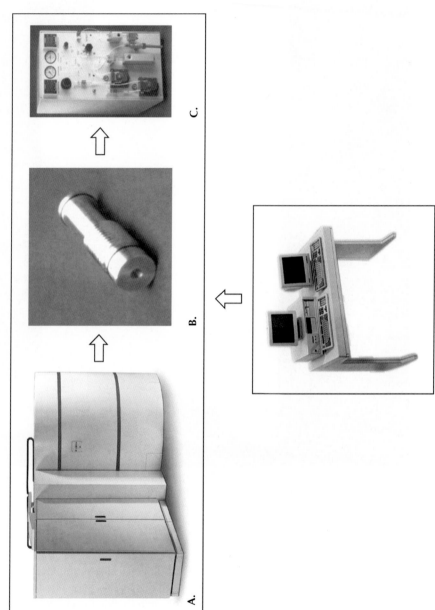

FIGURE 3-14. Electronic generator consisting of A) a low-energy negative ion cyclotron, B) a small volume target, and C) an automated radiopharmaceutical synthesizer. The target (B) is contained within the cyclotron (A). The operation of all these components is fully controlled by a PC.

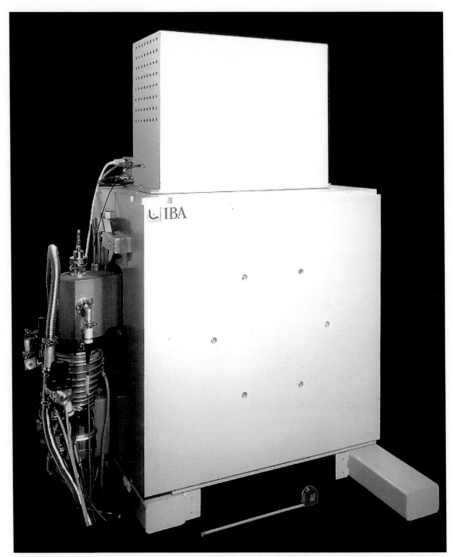

FIGURE 3-15. Classic example of an electronic generator, the Cyclone 3 system from IBA for the production of ^{15}O-labeled radiopharmaceuticals. This compact system (56.4" × 27.6" × 69.1") is shown here without the shields. (Courtesy of IBA Technology Group, Louvain-la-Neuve, Belgium.)

The most elegant example of an electronic generator is the Cyclone 3 system (Figure 3-15), developed by IBA more than 10 years ago. The heart of this generator is a small, 3.6-MeV deuteron-only self-shielded cyclotron capable of continously producing ^{15}O isotope via $^{14}N(d,n)^{15}O$ nuclear reaction. This simple and reliable electronic generator, aptly designed for the hospital environment, runs basically unattended after start-up by a technician. Whenever a study is required, a technician can simply draw out a dose similar to drawing a dose from a $^{99}Mo/^{99m}Tc$ generator. In this analogy, the electronic generator is substituted for ^{99}Mo, parent of ^{99m}Tc. Delivery of $[^{15}O]O_2$ (continuous flow: > 100 mCi/min), $[^{15}O]H_2O$ (batch: > 150 mCi), $[^{15}O]CO_2$ (continuous flow: > 80 mCi/min), and $[^{15}O]CO$ (continuous flow: > 60 mCi/min) is possible within 15 min of startup.[128] Four units of this electronic ^{15}O generator are currently in daily use in Europe.

In the 1990s, cyclotron manufacturers clearly developed systems that met the objectives of electronic generators. As discussed earlier, the latest generation of cyclotrons has a PC that controls all targets and automated synthesizers. The cyclotron manufacturers have seamlessly interfaced these three components of the electronic generator for low-cost production of PET radiopharmaceuticals. Currently using such electronic generators, PET radiopharmaceuticals such as FDG, $[^{13}N]$ammonia, and ^{15}O-labeled O_2 and H_2O, are routinely produced for clinical studies by technicians, literally with a few computer keystrokes. Thus, through inventions and innovations, what was once a handicap in the early days of PET, namely the cyclotron, has now become an advantage through the electronic production of PET radiopharmaceuticals. It is anticipated that relatively complex synthesis of ^{18}F-labeled tracers (e.g., FDOPA, 3-(2′-[^{18}F]fluoroethyl)-spiperone, 9-(4-[^{18}F]fluoro-3-hydroxymethylbutyl)guanine, FLT, and [^{18}F]fluoroethylcholine, and so on) will also be brought under the umbrella of electronic radiopharmaceutical generators in the near future.[125,129]

PET RADIOPHARMACIES AND CLINICAL PET

Although further technological advances will produce additional refinements, the concept of integrated, remote, automated systems for PET radiopharmaceuticals has now become a reality. The recent advancement of electronic generators for the reliable and routine production of commercial PET radiopharmaceuticals, especially FDG, has largely been responsible for the inception of regional distribution by national companies like P.E.T.Net® Pharmaceuticals, Inc. (Knoxville, TN), Syncor International Corp. (Woodland Hills, CA) Syncor Advanced Isotopes, LLC (Woodland Hills, CA), and Eastern Isotopes (Sterling, VA) and many small regional companies. The daily distribution of FDG to clinical PET centers is akin to the services provided by radiopharmaceutical companies that supply single photon-emitting radiopharmaceuticals to nuclear medicine practices. Thus, PET radiopharmaceuticals are available as an operating expense to a hospital involved in clinical service without the previous practical limitations and expense of on-site cyclotrons and their associated facility and personnel requirements. In the year 2003, PET radiopharmacies (Figure 3-16) are within 100 miles of 50% of the hospital beds in the United States.

Parenthetically, the versatility of the automated synthesizers provides an interesting avenue in PET radiopharmaceutical production. With the advent of the new microPET technology (Chapter 1), a current rapid integration of biology with molecular imaging exists for studying the biological nature of disease and developing molecular therapies in such models as genetically engineered mice and mice transplanted with cells of human disease. This integration has opened new avenues for PET radiopharmacies (Figure 3-16) originally designed to serve a clinical PET market. These new customers are biological scientists from academia and the pharmaceutical and radiopharmaceutical industries, interested

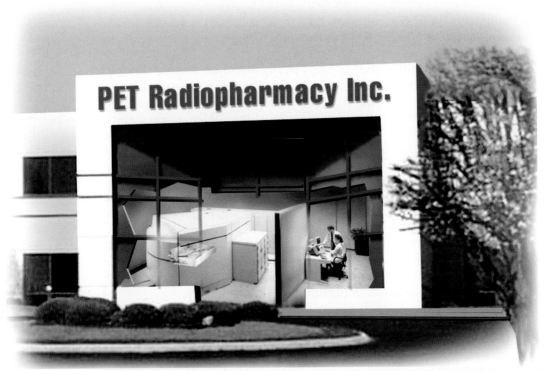

FIGURE 3-16. A conceptual picture of a PET radiopharmacy for the production and distribution of positron-emitting radiopharmaceuticals for clinical and research applications. PET Radiopharmacy, Inc. is a generic name. (Reprinted with permission from Satyamurthy N, Phelps ME, Barrio JR. Electronic generators for the production of positron-emitter-labeled radiopharmaceuticals: Where would PET be without them? *Clin Positron Imag.* 1999;2:233–253, with permission from Elsevier.)

in PET molecular imaging probes for research, generally aimed at specific protein and mRNA and DNA targets (Chapter 4). These potential customers may not necessarily be chemistry-driven or may not have the resources to open their own PET research centers. It is predicted, therefore, that custom synthesis of PET molecular imaging probes would be supplied for in-vivo studies much like ^{14}C-, ^{3}H-, and ^{32}P-labeled compounds are now provided for in-vitro applications.

Because commercially available automated modules can be stand-alone units easily adaptable to synthesize a variety of PET tracers, with the current availability of [^{18}F]fluoride ion from commercial radiopharmaceutical sources throughout the world, these automated synthesizers would also enable *in-situ* preparation of ^{18}F-labeled PET tracers without the need to have an in-house cyclotron and without the overhead resulting from sophisticated chemistry operations. This combination of initiatives and the availability of electronic generators will not only provide PET a range of molecular imaging probes but also increase in volume and lower the cost of production of radiopharmaceuticals. It will also provide further integration of nuclear medicine into the biological and pharmaceutical sciences.

The recent legislative action, the U.S. Food and Drug Administration Modernization Act of 1997,[96] has also opened a new era in PET radiopharmaceutical regulations. Working together with the PET radiopharmaceutical community, the FDA is currently embarked on the formulation of new PET radiopharmaceutical regulations and their clinical indications. This process involves the grandfathering of existing PET radiopharmaceuticals in current clinical use (e.g., FDG, [18F]fluoride, [13N]ammonia, [15O]water, and FDOPA) and implementation of efficient procedures to introduce new PET radiopharmaceuticals into the clinical domain (e.g., bibliography-based review vs. New Drugs Applications/Abbreviated New Drug Applications approaches). As part of this overall process, the FDA has recently approved the clinical use of FDG for all cancers, myocardial viability, and epilepsy. Further, [13N]ammonia was also approved as a myocardial perfusion agent. Working in partnership with the U.S. Pharmacopeia, the FDA is producing quality control standards for all these PET radiopharmaceuticals which are also being developed. It is also envisioned that the whole regulatory process for PET radiopharmaceutical development, including Radiation Drug Research Committee approvals and Investigational New Drug applications will be revamped as a recognition of the excellent record of safety of PET radiopharmaceuticals[130] and the mandate of the Modernization Act of 1997.[96]

The combination of technological and regulatory developments is opening a new era for PET. The future is bright and is filled with new opportunities, but the efforts to reach the goals are not trivial. These efforts involve both the clinical and research arena, and most specifically, the creation of a new vision, the PET radiopharmacy serving clinicians, researchers, and industry. The new regulatory atmosphere should also provide impetus to the creation of new PET molecular imaging probes for research and the clinic, new partnerships between academia and industry, new approaches for synthesis [e.g., combinatorial (radio)chemistry],[131] and more advanced technologies for automation and system integration.

The joint endeavor between academia and the cyclotron industry has led to the development of the novel concept of electronic generators, integrated systems consisting of a low-energy (e.g., 11-MeV proton), self-shielded negative ion cyclotron, small volume targets for the production of positron-emitting precursors, and automated synthesizers all under the control of a personal computer for the routine production of PET radiopharmaceuticals for clinical and research applications. The evolution of such systems had been envisioned more than a decade ago, as an important step for the widespread use of PET as a clinical tool.[121] Currently, electronic generators for the routine production of multiple doses of FDG, [13N]ammonia, and 15O-labeled radiopharmaceuticals are commercially available and the number of commercially available PET radiopharmaceuticals is expected to grow rapidly over the coming years. The hallmark of the electronic generators is the efficient, reliable, and cost-effective method for the production of PET radiopharmaceuticals. Thus, the implementation of the legislative action embodied in the Modernization Act of 1997 and the availability of electronic generators auger well for the success of clinical PET.

REFERENCES

1. Phelps ME, Hoffman EJ, Mullani NA, Ter-Pogossian MM. Application of annihilation coincidence detection to transaxial reconstruction. *J Nucl Med.*1975;16:210–224.

2. Phelps ME, Hoffman EJ, Mullani NA, Higgins CS, Ter–Pogossian MM. Design considerations for a positron emission transaxial tomography (PETT III). *IEEE Nucl Sci.* 1976;NS–23:516–522.
3. Hoffman EJ, Phelps ME, Mullani NA, Coble CS, Ter–Pogossian MM. Design and performance characteristics of a whole body positron transaxial tomography. *J Nucl Med.* 1976;17:493–502.
4. Phelps ME. Emission computed tomography. *Semin Nucl Med.* 1977;7:337–365.
5. Phelps ME, Hoffman EJ, Huang S-C, Kuhl DE. ECAT: A new computerized tomograph imaging system for positron-emitting radiopharmaceuticals. *J Nucl Med.* 1978;19:635–647.
6. Phelps ME, Huang SC, Hoffman EJ, Selin C, Sokoloff L, Kuhl DE. Tomographic measurement of local cerebral glucose metabolic rate in humans with (F-18) 2-fluoro-2-deoxy-D-glucose: Validation of method. *Ann Neurol.* 1979;6:371–388.
7. Reivich M, Kuhl D, Wolf A, Greenberg J, Phelps M, Ido T, Casalla V, Fowler J, Hoffman E, Mavi A, Som P, Sokoloff L. The [^{18}F]fluorodeoxyglucose method for the measurement of local cerebral glucose utilization in man. *Circ Res.* 1979;44:127–137.
8. Phelps ME. Positron computed tomography studies of cerebral glucose metabolism in man: Theory and application in nuclear medicine. *Semin Nucl Med.* 1981;11:32–49.
9. Proceedings of the Symposium on New Developments in Radiopharmaceuticals and Labeled Compounds. Vol. I and II. International Atomic Energy Agency, Vienna, Austria, 1973.
10. Phelps ME, Hoffman EJ. Role of cyclotrons and positron imaging in the future of nuclear medicine. In: Serafini AN, Beaver JE, eds. *Medical Cyclotrons in Nuclear Medicine. Progress in Nuclear Medicine.* Vol. 4. Basel: S. Karger; 1978:165–183.
11. Tilyou SM. Yesterday, today and tomorrow—The evolution of positron emission tomography. *J Nucl Med.* 1991;32:15N–26N.
12. Livingston MS. *High-energy Accelerators.* New York: Interscience Publishers, Inc.; 1954.
13. Evans RD. *The Atomic Nucleus.* New York: McGraw–Hill Book Company, Inc.; 1955.
14. Livingston MS. *Particle Accelerators: A Brief History.* Cambridge: Harvard University Press; 1969.
15. Livingston MS, Blewett JP. *Particle Accelerators.* New York: McGraw-Hill Book Company, Inc.; 1962.
16. Livingood JJ. *Principles of Cyclic Particle Accelerators.* Princeton, NJ: D. Van Nostrand Company, Inc.; 1961.
17. Persico E, Ferrari E, Segre SE. *Principles of Particle Accelerators.* New York: W.A. Benjamin, Inc.; 1968.
18. Kolomensky AA, Lebedev AN. *Theory of Cyclic Accelerators.* Amsterdam: North-Holland Publishing Company; 1966.
19. Kollath R, ed. *Particle Accelerators.* London: Sir Isaac Pitman and Sons Ltd.; 1967.
20. Scharf W. *Particle Accelerators and Their Uses.* Part I. Chur: Harwood Academic Publishers; 1986.
21. Humphries S Jr. *Principles of Charged Particle Acceleration.* New York: John Wiley & Sons; 1986.
22. Conte M, Mackay WW. *An Introduction to the Physics of Particle Accelerators.* Singapore: World Scientific; 1991.
23. Wolf AP, Jones WB. Cyclotrons for biomedical radioisotope production. *Radiochim Acta.* 1983;34:1–7.
24. Comar D, Crouzel C. Biomedical cyclotrons for radioisotope production. *Nucl Med Biol.* 1986;13:101–107.
25. Hoop B Jr, Laughlin JS, Tilbury RS. Cyclotrons in nuclear medicine. In: Hine GJ, Sorensen JA, eds. *Instrumentation in Nuclear Medicine.* Part 2. New York: Academic Press; 1974:407–457.
26. Wolf AP, Schlyer DJ. Accelerators for positron emission tomography. In: Burns HD, Gibson RE, Dannals RF, Siegel PKS, eds. *Nuclear Imaging in Drug Discovery, Development, and Approval.* Boston: Birkhauser; 1993:33–54.
27. Fowler JS, Wolf AP. Positron emitter-labeled compounds: Priorities and problems. In: Phelps ME, Mazziotta JC, Schelbert HR, eds. *Positron Emission Tomography and Autoradiography: Principles and Applications for the Brain and Heart.* New York: Raven Press; 1986:391–450.
28. Glasstone S. *Source Book on Atomic Energy.* New York: Van Nostrand Reinhold Company; 1967.

29. White HE. *Introduction to College Physics.* New York: Van Nostrand Reinhold Company; 1969.
30. Paul AC. *Variable Energy Extraction from a Negative Ion Cyclotron and Related Measurements.* Ph.D. Dissertation; University of California, Los Angeles; 1967.
31. Paul AC, Wright BT. Variable energy extraction from negative ion cyclotrons. *IEEE Trans Nucl Sci.* 1966;NS-13:74–83.
32. Richardson JR, Wright BT. The UCLA SF cyclotron; Progress and status, January 1966. *IEEE Trans Nucl Sci.* 1966;NS-13:495–499.
33. Lofgren EJ. Negative ions and charge neutralization in the cyclotron. *Rev Sci Instr.* 1951;22:321–323.
34. Judd DL. Electric dissociation of negative hydrogen ions in cyclotrons and synchrocyclotrons. *Nucl Instr Meth.* 1962;18,19:70–73.
35. Forrester AT. *Large Ion Beams. Fundamentals of Generation and Propagation.* New York: Wiley-Interscience Publication; 1988.
36. Weast RC, ed. *CRC Handbook of Chemistry and Physics.* 61st ed. Boca Raton: CRC Press, Inc.; 1980.
37. MacDonald NS. The UCLA biomedical cyclotron facility. In: Serafini AN, Beaver JE, eds. *Medical Cyclotrons in Nuclear Medicine. Progress in Nuclear Medicine.* Vol. 4. Basel: S. Karger; 1978;23–27.
38. Ter-Pogossian MM, Wagner HN Jr. A new look at the cyclotron for making short-lived isotopes. *Semin Nucl Med.* 1998;28:202–212.
39. Wagner HN Jr. A brief history of positron emission tomography (PET). *Semin Nucl Med.* 1998;28:213–220
40. Friesel DL, Smith W. Medical applications at the Indiana University cyclotron facility. In: Serafini AN, Beaver JE, eds. *Medical Cyclotrons in Nuclear Medicine. Progress in Nuclear Medicine.* Vol. 4. Basel: S. Karger; 1978;63–71.
41. Robinson GD Jr. Cyclotron-related radiopharmaceutical development program at UCLA. In: Serafini AN, Beaver JE, eds. *Medical Cyclotrons in Nuclear Medicine. Progress in Nuclear Medicine.* Vol. 4. Basel: S. Karger; 1978;80–92.
42. Sodd VJ. The cyclotron: Past, present, and future role in nuclear medicine. In: Freeman LM, Weissman HS, eds. *Nuclear Medicine Annual 1982.* New York: Raven Press; 1982; 291–317.
43. Ehrenkaufer R, Erdman K. Accelerators. In: Link JM, Ruth TJ, eds. *Proceedings of the Sixth Workshop on Targetry and Target Chemistry.* Vancouver: TRIUMF; 1995;23–25.
44. Shefer RE, Klinkowstein RE, Hughey BJ, Welch MJ. Production of PET radionuclides with a high current electrostatic accelerator. In: Weinreich R, ed. *Proceedings of the IVth International Workshop on Targetry and Target Chemistry.* Villigen: Paul Scherrer Institut; 1992;4–10.
45. Wangler TP, Cimabue AG, Merson J, Mills RS, Wood RL, Young LM. Superconducting RFQ linear accelerator. *Nucl Instr Meth.* 1993;B79:718–720.
46. Krohn KA, Link JM, Young P, Hagan WK, Pasquinelli R, Chrisman B, Bida GT. ^{3}He RFQ for PET isotope production. A brief progress report, August 1995. In: Link JM, Ruth TJ, eds. *Proceedings of the Sixth Workshop on Targetry and Target Chemistry.* Vancouver: TRIUMF; 1995;38–39.
47. Robinson GD Jr. Status of AccSys Technology's PULSAR™ System. In: Link JM, Ruth TJ, eds. *Proceedings of the Sixth Workshop on Targetry and Target Chemistry.* Vancouver: TRIUMF; 1995;34–36.
48. Swenson DA. Compact proton linac systems for medical and industrial applications. In: Link JM, Ruth TJ, eds. *Proceedings of the Sixth Workshop on Targetry and Target Chemistry.* Vancouver: TRIUMF; 1995;42–44.
49. Webster W. NHVG: A compact direct current accelerator. In: Link JM, Ruth TJ, eds. *Proceedings of the Sixth Workshop on Targetry and Target Chemistry.* Vancouver: TRIUMF; 1995;28–30.
50. Roberts AD, Nickles RJ, Davidson RJ. The UW Pelletron lab: PET radioisotope production with the NEC 9SDH tandem accelerator. In: Zeisler S, Helus F, eds. *Proceedings of the Seventh International Workshop on Targetry and Target Chemistry.* Heidelberg: German Cancer Research Center (DKFZ); 1997;42–43.
51. Friedlander A, Kennedy JW, Macias ES, Miller JM. *Nuclear and Radiochemistry.* 3rd ed. New York: John Wiley & Sons; 1981.

52. Browne E, Firestone RB. *Table of Radioactive Isotopes.* New York: John Wiley & Sons; 1986.

53. Keller KA, Lange J, Munzel H. *Landolt-Bornstein Numerical Data and Functional Relationships in Science and Technology. Group I: Nuclear and Particle Physics. Vol. 5: Q-values and Excitation Functions of Nuclear Reactions. Part C: Estimation of Unknown Excitation Functions and Thick Target Yields for p, d, ^{3}He and α Reactions.* Berlin: Springer-Verlag; 1974.

54. Helus F, Wolber G. Activation techniques. In: Helus F, Colombetti LG, eds. *Radionuclides Production.* Vol. I. Boca Raton: CRC Press, Inc.; 1983;57–120.

55. Wieland BW, Highfill RR. Proton accelerator targets for the production of ^{11}C, ^{13}N, ^{15}O, and ^{18}F. *IEEE Trans Nucl Sci.* 1979;NS-26:1713–1717.

56. Qaim SM. Nuclear data relevant to cyclotron produced short-lived medical radioisotopes. *Radiochim Acta.* 1982;30:147–162.

57. Williamson C, Boujot J, Picard J. Range-energy tables for charged particles. Centre D'Etudes Nucléaires de Saclay, Report No. CES-R3042; 1966.

58. Janni JF. Calculations of energy loss, range, path length, straggling, multiple scattering, and the probability of inelastic nuclear collisions for 0.1 to 1000-MeV protons. Technical Report No. AFWL-TR-65-150. Air Force Weapons Laboratory, Kirtland Air Force Base, New Mexico; 1966.

59. Gandarias-Cruz D, Okamoto K. Status on the compilation of nuclear data for medical radioisotopes produced by accelerators. IAEA Nuclear Data Section. Vienna; 1988.

60. Vaalburg W, Paans AMJ. Short-lived positron emitting radionuclides. In: Helus F, Colombetti LG, eds. *Radionuclides Production.* Vol. II. Boca Raton: CRC Press, Inc.; 1983; 47–101.

61. Nozaki T. Other cyclotron radionuclides. In: Helus F, Colombetti LG, eds. *Radionuclides Production.* Vol. II. Boca Raton: CRC Press, Inc.; 1983;103–124.

62. Clark JC, Buckingham PD. *Short-lived Radioactive Gases for Clinical Use.* London: Butterworths; 1975.

63. Wieland BW, Schmidt DG, Bida GT, Ruth TJ, Hendry GO. Efficient and economical production of oxygen-15 labeled tracers with low energy protons. *J Label Compd Radiopharm.* 1986;23:1214–1216.

64. Wieland BW, Hendry GO, Schmidt DG. Design and performance of targets for producing ^{11}C, ^{13}N, ^{15}O and ^{18}F with 11 MeV protons. *J Label Compd Radiopharm.* 1986;23: 1187–1189.

65. Wieland BW, Hendry GO, Schmidt DG, Bida GT, Ruth TJ. Efficient small volume ^{18}O water target for producing ^{18}F-fluoride with low energy protons. *J Label Compd Radiopharm.* 1986;23:1205–1207.

66. Qaim SM, Clark JC, Crouzel C, Guillaume M, Helmeke HJ, Nebeling B, Pike VW, Stocklin G. PET radionuclide production. In: Stocklin G, Pike VW, eds. *Radiopharmaceuticals for Positron Emission Tomography. Methodological Aspects.* Dordrecht: Kluwer Academic Publishers; 1993;1–42.

67. Alvord CW, Zigler SS. Target systems for the RDS-111 cyclotron. In: Link JM, Ruth TJ, eds. *Proceedings of the Sixth Workshop on Targetry and Target Chemistry.* Vancouver: TRIUMF; 1995;155–161.

68. Schlyer DJ, Bastos MAV, Alexoff D, Wolf AP. Separation of [^{18}F]fluoride from [^{18}O]water using anion exchange resin. *Appl Radiat Isot.* 1990;41:531–533.

69. Nickles RJ, Daube ME, Ruth TJ. An ^{18}O target for the production of [^{18}F]F$_2$. *Int J Appl Radiat Isot.* 1984;35:117–122.

70. Goodman MM. Automated synthesis of radiotracers for PET applications. In: Hubner KL, Collmann J, Buonocore E, Kabalka G, eds. *Clinical Positron Emission Tomography.* St. Louis: Mosby Year Book; 1992;110–122.

71. Tilbery RS, Gelbard AS. ^{11}C, ^{13}N, and ^{15}O tracers. In: Rayudu GVS, ed. *Radiotracers for Medical Applications.* Vol. I. Boca Raton: CRC Press, Inc.; 1983;275–291.

72. Clark JC. Production and application of oxygen-15; Radiopharmacy aspects. In: Schubiger PA, Westera G, eds. *Progress in Radiopharmacy.* Dordrecht: Kluwer Academic Publishers; 1992;91–107.

73. Wieland B, Bida G, Padgett H, Hendry G, Zippi E, Kabalka G, Morelle J-L, Verbruggen R, Ghyoot M. In-target production of [^{13}N]ammonia via proton irradiation of dilute aqueous ethanol and acetic acid mixtures. *Appl Radiat Isot.* 1991;42:1095–1098.

74. Baumgartner FJ, Barrio JR, Henze E, Schelbert HR, MacDonald NS, Phelps ME, Kuhl DE. ^{13}N Labeled L-amino acids for in vivo quantitative assesment of local myocardial metabolism. *J Med Chem.* 1981;24:764–766.

75. Henze E, Schelbert HR, Barrio JR, Egbert JE, Hansen HW, MacDonald NS, Phelps ME. Evaluation of myocardial metabolism with N-13 and C-11 labeled amino acids for positron computed tomography. *J Nucl Med.* 1982;23:671–681.

76. Langstrom B, Dannals RF. Carbon-11 compounds. In: Wagner HN Jr, Szabo Z, Buchanan JW, eds. *Principles of Nuclear Medicine.* 2nd ed. Philadelphia: W.B. Saunders Company; 1995;166–178.

77. Larsen P, Ulin J, Dahlstrom K, Jensen M. Synthesis of [^{11}C]iodomethana by iodination of [^{11}C]methane. *Appl Radiat Isot.* 1997;48:153–157.

78. Link JM, Krohn KA, Clark JC. Production of [^{11}C]CH$_3$I by single pass reaction of [^{11}C]CH$_4$ with I$_2$. *Nucl Med Biol.* 1997;24:93–97.

79. Jewett DM. A simple synthesis of [^{11}C]methyl triflate. *Appl Radiat Isot.* 1992;43:1383–1385.

80. O'Hagan D, Rzepa HS. Some influences of fluorine in bioorganic chemistry. *Chem Commun.* 1997;645–652.

81. Welch JT, Eswarakrishnan S. *Fluorine in Bioorganic Chemistry.* New York: John Wiley & Sons; 1991.

82. Zielinski M, Kanska M. Syntheses and uses of isotopically labelled organic halides. In: Patai S, Rappoport Z, eds. *The Chemistry of Halides, Pseudo-halides and Azides. Supplement D2. Part 1.* Chichester: John Wiley & Sons; 1995;403–533.

83. Ido T, Wan C-N, Casella V, Fowler JS, Wolf AP, Reivich M, Kuhl DE. Labeled 2-deoxy-D-glucose analogs. ^{18}F-Labeled 2-deoxy-2-fluoro-D-glucose, 2-deoxy-2-fluoro-D-mannose and ^{14}C-2-deoxy-2-fluoro-D-glucose. *J Label Compd Radiopharm.* 1978;14:175–183.

84. Bishop A, Satyamurthy N, Bida G, Hendry G, Phelps M, Barrio JR. Proton irradiation of [^{18}O]O$_2$: Production of [^{18}F]F$_2$ and [^{18}F]F$_2$ + [^{18}F]OF$_2$. *Nucl Med Biol.* 1996;23:189–199.

85. Fowler JS, Wolf AP. *The Synthesis of Carbon-11, Fluorine-18 and Nitrogen-13 Labeled Radiotracers for Biomedical Applications.* Publication: NAS-NS-3201. Virginia: National Technical Information Service; 1982.

86. Satyamurthy N, Bida GT, Phelps ME, Barrio JR. N-[^{18}F]Fluoro-N-alkylsulfonamides. Novel reagents for mild and regioselective radiofluorination. *Appl Radiat Inst.* 1990;41:733–738.

87. Stocklin G. Fluorine-18 compounds. In: Wagner HN Jr, Szabo Z, Buchanan JW, eds. *Principles of Nuclear Medicine.* 2nd ed. Philadelphia: W.B. Saunders Company; 1995;178–194.

88. Namavari M, Barrio JR, Toyokuni T, Gambhir SS, Cherry SR, Herschman HR, Phelps ME, Satyamurthy N. Synthesis of 8-[^{18}F]fluoroguanine derivatives: In vivo probes for imaging gene expression with positron emission tomography. *Nucl Med Biol.* 2000;27:157–162.

89. Kilbourn MR. *Fluorine-18 Labeling of Radiopharmaceuticals.* Nuclear Science Series NAS-NS-3203. Washington, D.C. National Academy Press; 1990.

90. Hamacher K, Coenen HH, Stocklin G. Efficient stereospecific synthesis of no-carrier-added 2-[^{18}F]-fluoro-2-deoxy-D-glucose using aminopolyether supported nucleophilic substitution. *J Nucl Med.* 1986;27:235–238.

91. Alauddin MM, Conti P. Synthesis and preliminary evaluation of 9-(4-[^{18}F]fluoro-3–hydroxymethylbutyl)guanine([^{18}F]FHBG): A new potential imaging agent for viral infection and gene therapy using PET. *Nucl Med Biol.* 1998;25:175–180.

92. Grierson JR, Shields AF. Radiosynthesis of 3′-deoxy-3′-[^{18}F]fluorothymidine: [^{18}F]FLT for imaging of cellular proliferation in vivo. *Nucl Med Biol.* 2000;27:143–156.

93. De Grado TR, Coleman RE, Wang S, Baldwin SW, Orr MD, Robertson CN, Polascik TJ, Price DT. Synthesis and evaluation of ^{18}F-labeled choline as an oncologic tracer for positron emission tomography: Intial findings in prostate cancer. *Cancer Res.* 2000;61:110–117.

94. Coleman RE. Clinical PET: A technology on the brink. *J Nucl Med.* 1993;34:2269–2271.

95. Deutsch E. Clinical PET: Its time has come? *J Nucl Med.* 1993;34:1132–1133.

96. Food and Drug Administration Modernization Act of 1997. Public Law 105-115-Nov. 21, 1997.

97. Crouzel C, Clark JC, Brihaye C, Langstrom B, Lemaire C, Meyer GJ, Nebeling B, Stone-Elander S. Radiochemistry automation for PET. In: Stocklin G, Pike VW, eds. *Radiopharmaceuticals for Positron Emission Tomography. Methodological Aspects.* Dordrecht: Kluwer Academic Publishers; 1993;45–79.

98. Foust AS, Wenzel LA, Clump CW, Maus L, Andersen LB. *Principles of Unit Operations.* 2nd ed. New York: John Wiley & Sons; 1980.

99. McCabe WL, Smith JC, Harriott P. *Unit Operations of Chemical Engineering.* 5th ed. New York: McGraw-Hill, Inc.; 1993.

100. Hayashi N, Sugawara T, Shintani M, Kato S. Computer-assisted automatic synthesis II. Development of a fully automated apparatus for preparing substituted N− (carboxyalkyl) amino acids. *J Automatic Chem.* 1989;11:212–220.

101. Hayashi N, Sugawara T, Kato S. Computer-assisted automatic synthesis III. Synthesis of substituted N− (carboxyalkyl) amino acid tert-butyl estser derivatives. *J Automatic Chem.* 1991;13:187–197.

102. Sugawara T, Kato S, Okamoto S. Development of fully-automated synthesis systems. *J Automatic Chem.* 1994;16:33–42.

103. Frisbee AR, Nantz MH, Kramer GW, Fuchs PL. Robotic orchestration of organic reactions: Yield optimization via an automated system with operator-specified reaction sequences. *J Am Chem Soc.* 1984;106:7143–7145.

104. Merrifield RB, Stewart JM, Jernberg N. Instrument for automated synthesis of peptides. *Anal Chem.* 1966;38:1905–1914.

105. Erickson BW, Lukas TJ, Prystowsky MB. Automated solid-phase peptide synthesis. In: Beers RF. Jr, Bassett EG, eds. *Polypeptide Hormones.* New York: Raven Press; 1980;121–134.

106. Hewick RM, Hunkapiller MW, Hood LE, Dreyer WJ. A gas-liquid solid phase peptide and protein sequenator. *J Biol Chem.* 1981;256:7990–7997.

107. Efcavitch JW. Automated system for the optimized chemical synthesis of oligodeoxyribonucleotides. In: Schlesinger DH, ed. *Macromolecular Sequencing and Synthesis. Selected Methods and Applications.* New York: Alan R. Liss; 1988;221–234.

108. Meldrum D. Automation for genomics, part one: Preparation for sequencing. *Genome Res.* 2000;10:1081–1092.

109. Plummer GF, Waterworth G, Roberts W. Six years of robots. *J Automatic Chem.* 1991;13: 29–37.

110. Weinstein DB, France DS. Jumping into the 20th century before it is too late: Is laboratory robotics still in its infancy? *J Automatic Chem.* 1992;14:59–63.

111. McGonigle EJ. Practical aspects of laboratory automation in pharmaceutical development. *J Automatic Chem.* 1993;15:3–8.

112. Rulon PW. Selection criteria for laboratory robotic application personnel. *J Automatic Chem.* 1992;14:51–53.

113. Hutchins B. Robotic applications: lessons on what constitutes success. *J Automatic Chem.* 1991;13:9–12.

114. Barrio JR, MacDonald NS, Robinson GD Jr, Najafi A, Cook JS, Kuhl DE. Remote, semiautomated production of ^{18}F-labeled 2-deoxy-2-fluoro-D-glucose. *J Nucl Med.* 1981;22: 372–375.

115. Padgett HC, Barrio JR, MacDonald NS, Phelps ME. The unit operations approach applied to the synthesis of [1-^{11}C]2-deoxy-D-glucose for routine clinical operations. *J Nucl Med.* 1982;23:739–744.

116. Padgett HC, Robinson GD, Barrio JR. [1-^{11}C]Palmitic acid: Improved radiopharmaceutical preparation. *Int J Appl Radiat Isot.* 1982;33:1471–1472.

117. Barrio JR, Keen RE, Ropchan JR, MacDonald NS, Baumgartner FJ, Padgett HC, Phelps ME. L-[1-^{11}C]Leucine: Routine synthesis by enzymatic resolution. *J Nucl Med.* 1983;24: 515–521.

118. Ropchan JR, Ricci A, Low G, Phelps ME, Barrio JR. An automated high pressure vessel for routine preparation of short-lived radiopharmaceuticals. *Appl Radiat Isot.* 1986;37: 1063–1068.

119. Luxen A, Perlmutter M, Bida GT, Van Moffaert G, Cook JS, Satyamurthy N, Phelps ME, Barrio JR. Remote semiautomated production of 6–[^{18}F]fluoro-L-dopa for human studies with PET. *Appl Radiat Isot.* 1990;41:275–281.

120. Satyamurthy N, Namavari M, Barrio JR. Making ^{18}F radiotracers for medical research. *Chemtech* 1994;24:25–32.
121. Barrio JR, Bida G, Satyamurthy N, Padgett HC, MacDonald NS, Phelps ME. A minicyclotron-based technology for the production of positron-emitting labeled radiopharmaceuticals. In: Greitz T, Ingvar DH, Widen L, eds. *The Metabolism of the Human Brain Studied with Positron Emission Tomography.* New York: Raven Press; 1985;113–121.
122. Padgett HC, Schmidt DG, Luxen A, Bida GT, Satyamurthy N, Barrio JR. Computer-controlled radiochemical synthesis: A chemistry process control unit for the automated production of radiochemicals. *Appl Radiat Isot.* 1989;40:433–445.
123. Morelle J-L. Coincidence technologies. Liege, Belgium. Private communication.
124. PET Trace Synthesizer Modules and PET Laboratory Equipment. Product information. Nuclear Interface, Munster, Germany.
125. Zhang ZY, Kabalka GW, Longford CPD, Padgett HC, Zigler SS. Automated production of 6–[18F]fluoro-L-dopa in a commercially available chemistry module. In: Link JM, Ruth TJ, eds. *Proceedings of the Sixth Workshop on Targetry and Target Chemistry.* Vancouver: TRIUMF; 1995;305–306.
126. Dessy R. Robots in the laboratory: Part I. *Anal Chem.* 1983;55:1100A–1114A.
127. Dessy R. Robots in the laboratory: Part II. *Anal Chem.* 1983;55:1232A–1242A.
128. Mackay DG, Steel CJ, Poole K, McKnight S, Schmitz F, Ghyoot M, Vebruggen R, Vamecq F, Jongen Y. Quality assurance for PET gas production using the cyclone 3D oxygen-15 generator. *Appl Radiat Isot.* 1999;51:403–409.
129. de Vries EFJ, Luurtsema G, Brussermann M, Elsinga PH, Vaalburg W. Fully automated synthesis module for the high yield one-pot preparation of 6-[18F]fluoro-L-DOPA. *Appl Radiat Isot.* 1999;51:389–394.
130. Silberstein EB, Pharmacopeia Committee of the Society of Nuclear Medicine. Prevalence of adverse reactions to positron emitting radiopharmaceuticals in nuclear medicine. *J Nucl Med.* 1998;39:2190–2192.
131. Terrett NK. *Combinatorial Chemistry.* Oxford: Oxford University Press; 1998.
132. McCarthy DW, Shefer RE, Klinkowstein RE, Bass LA, Margeneau WH, Cutler CS, Anderson CJ, Welch MJ. Efficient production of high specific activity ^{64}Cu using a biomedical cyclotron. *Nucl Med Biol.* 1997;24:35–43.
133. Vaidyanathan G, Wieland BW, Larsen RH, Zweit, J, Zalutsky MR. High-yield production of iodine-124 using the [125]Te (p, 2n) [124]I reaction. In: Link JM, Ruth TJ, eds. *Proceedings of the Sixth Workshop on Targetry and Target Chemistry.* Vancouver: TRIUMF; 1995;87–88.

CHAPTER 4

The Molecular Basis of Disease

Jorge R. Barrio

For as long as man has lived, he has been concerned with health and well being. Much of human history has revolved around uncontrollable diseases; many critical events, wars, and even the fate of many societies have been determined by human health. Medicine is as old as human history and has evolved from mystical and religious beginnings to the scientific discipline of today.

The boundaries of medical knowledge are continually expanding. A modern definition of disease as: *a disordered or incorrectly functioning organ, part structure, or system of the body resulting from the effect of genetic or developmental errors, infection, poisons, nutritional deficiency or imbalance, toxicity, or unfavorable environmental factors*[1] hints at the chemical basis of disease. We can further say that disease results from a disruption of the chemical homeostasis of the body or, in other words, a disruption of a tendency to dynamic stability in the normal body states of the organism. Alteration of chemical homeostasis can be induced by internal or external factors resulting in specific biochemical abnormalities that change normal organ function to the point that clinical symptoms are produced. Today, however, the technical elements of medical practice to diagnose and treat disease still are—for the most part—anatomical in nature. Practicing physicians order—and feel comfortable with—computerized tomography (CT), magnetic resonance imaging (MRI) scans, and ultrasound but have been slow to incorporate biological criteria from molecular imaging techniques such as positron emission tomography (PET) into their practice.

In classical medical practice, biological abnormalities are typically tested clinically and by determining biochemical parameters at a distance from the involved organ. Kidney function, for example, is assessed by measuring creatinine, phosphate, and urea plasma levels; liver function is similarly assessed with specific liver markers (e.g., transaminases) also in plasma. Moreover, from ancient times, physicians have ordered prescriptions for their patients that are attempts at restoring a disturbed chemical imbalance of disease. Drugs are used to reverse or control chemical imbalances by targeting key enzymes, transporters, and receptor systems. In sufficient amounts, drugs are used to either block or inhibit specific pathways in neurotransmission (e.g., neuroleptics binding to dopamine-

D2 receptors to control schizophrenic symptoms), supplement substrates when enzyme deficits exist [e.g., L-DOPA to treat Parkinson's disease where central dopaminergic aromatic amino-acid decarboxylase (AAAD) concentration is decreased], or inhibit specific tumor enzymes with the aim of destroying tumor cells (e.g., 5-fluorouracil to inhibit thymidylate synthetase).

If living organisms are governed by chemical homeostasis, some conclusions can be established:

1. Chemical disturbances will precede anatomical abnormalities in disease. It is now well established, for example, that genetic mutations or loss of regulated expression of genes will precede clinical symptoms of cancer by many years, perhaps decades. Similarly, Parkinson's disease and Alzheimer's disease have subclinical stages for years wherein the brain can control degenerative processes by adjusting function through compensating mechanisms of neuronal plasticity or through biochemical reserves controlling neuronal processes.

2. As a result of (1), above, diagnostic procedures using imaging probes aimed at detecting these biochemical abnormalities will permit earlier and informative detection of disease, sometimes many years ahead of conventional medical practice. This concept was demonstrated in Huntington's disease, a familial neurodegenerative disease that could be detected with PET studies of glucose metabolism seven years before symptoms develop.[2] More recently, preclinical assessment of Alzheimer's disease was also made possible using similar PET metabolic studies in patients with increased predisposition for the disease due to their carrying the APOE4 gene.[3]

3. Imaging probes (diagnostic) and drugs (therapeutics) share common concepts in structural design and principle of action because they target the same enzymes, receptors, and neurotransmitter systems. Drugs, through mass action, block or inhibit their targets and, thus, restore chemical imbalances conducive to control or diminish or remove clinical symptoms. Molecular imaging probes, at tracer levels, probe the same targets assessing their functional status. Thus, drugs and molecular imaging probes typically share structural requirements, being the same molecule or structural analogs of each other (Figure 4-1).

When using molecular imaging probes, it is always necessary to consider that the ultimate objective of a PET determination is quantitation of the process that is measured. Tracer kinetic techniques are generally used to monitor dynamic processes with PET, namely tissue perfusion, local metabolic processes (e.g., glucose metabolic rates in the brain, the heart, and tumors), synthesis processes (e.g., protein and neurotransmitter synthesis), receptor properties (e.g., their number and affinities), and so on (Chapter 2). Accurate estimation of quantitative parameters requires formulation of a tracer kinetic model according to the process to be measured and the biochemical or pharmacologic information available at the time.

Steps to develop a successful tracer kinetic model are:

1. Molecular probe design and synthesis.
2. Formulation of a workable model.
3. Model validation.
4. Model application.

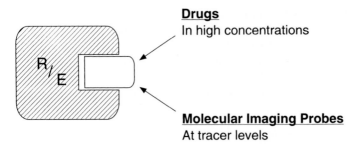

Drugs
In high concentrations

Molecular Imaging Probes
At tracer levels

FIGURE 4-1. Schematic diagram indicating common targets [e.g., enzyme (E) or receptor proteins (R)] for drugs and molecular imaging probes.

The process is iterative to achieve maximum accuracy and success. When the process is understood and demonstrated to be generally effective, other quantitative (or semiquantitative) approaches are developed to simplify the utilization of the procedure. Ultimately, the molecular imaging probe is introduced in the clinic for routine use. The best example of a positron-emitting molecular imaging probe going through this evolutionary pathway is 2-deoxy-2-[F-18]fluoro-deoxy-D-glucose (FDG). Other pharmaceuticals have also followed this pathway and are now entering the clinical arena, like [N-13] ammonia as a myocardial perfusion agent and 6-[F-18]fluoro-L-DOPA as a probe of central dopaminergic system integrity. Many other PET probes have been developed and thoroughly studied but have not yet become available for routine clinical use. This chapter will focus on molecular probe design to develop an understanding of the noninvasive biochemical or pharmacological process to be measured with PET. For all other mathematical aspects of tracer kinetic modeling, the reader is referred to Chapter 2 and other excellent publications in the field.[4]

MOLECULAR PROBE DESIGN: GENERAL PRINCIPLES

In order to obtain meaningful results, investigations of living organisms must be performed with a minimum of interference with the system under investigation. The introduction of radioactive molecules into the system is one of the preferred alternatives for the study of biological systems because it produces only minimal experimental disturbances, due to the extremely low mass of the probe, and thus allows one to distinguish the experimental components from the background (Figure 4-2). Most of the present knowledge of biochemistry, particularly metabolism, has been obtained by the use of radioactive (carbon-14 and tritium) and stable (deuterium, carbon-13, and nitrogen-15) isotopes. For a variety of reasons, however, these isotopes are not adequate for the noninvasive assessment of physiological and biochemical processes. Even though tracer techniques have led to the development of useful clinical applications (e.g., conventional nuclear medicine techniques), the development of PET has led the way in the development and use of quantitative assays of local biochemical and pharmacological processes in humans.

Properties of molecular imaging probes labeled with positron-emitting radioisotopes

Some important properties that make molecular imaging probes used with PET very valuable for the *in-vivo* assessment of biochemical and pharmacological processes in humans can be summarized as follows:

1. Compounds labeled with positron-emitting radioisotopes can be prepared with high-specific activity (Chapter 3) so that the process to be measured is not perturbed.
2. Gamma rays produced after positron annihilation allow for quantitative high resolution imaging (Chapter 1).
3. With cyclotron-produced positron-emitting radioisotopes of carbon (C-11; t 1/2 = 20.38 min), nitrogen (N-13; t 1/2 = 9.96 min), oxygen (O-15; t 1/2 = 2.03 min) and fluorine (F-18; t1/2 = 109.72 min) (Chapter 3), true molecular imaging probes matching the strict requirements of enzyme and/or receptor targets can be designed. The design of these molecular probes takes advantage of the following: (a) labeling with the most common positron-emitting radioisotopes, carbon-11, nitrogen-13, and oxygen-15, renders compounds biochemically indistinguishable from their natural counterparts; and (b) fluorine-18 can be used to provide labeled substrate analogs (e.g., FDG) or pharmacological agents (F-18-labeled spiperone) to trace biochemical or pharmacological processes in a predictable manner. Fluorine is an important element used to modify biologically active compounds (e.g., in drug design). Because of its small size and the strength of the C-F bond, fluorine is commonly used to replace H or OH on a molecule. This modification allows favorable interactions of the new molecule (e.g., molecular imaging probe, drug) with the target (e.g., enzyme, receptor) to occur without steric hindrance. Moreover, the presence of fluorine may block, with target enzymes, subsequent reactions in a given pathway.
4. The positron emitters carbon-11, nitrogen-13, oxygen-15, and fluorine-18 constitute the only externally detectable forms of carbon, nitrogen, oxygen,

FIGURE 4-2. Molecular imaging probes as reporters in *in-vivo* systems.

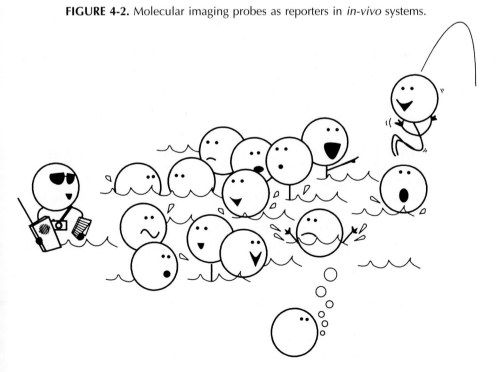

and fluorine, respectively. The time course of radioactive emission can be readily quantitated with PET, permitting the application of tracer kinetic techniques for the measurement of substrate concentrations, reaction rates, and receptor binding in tissue.

5. The short half-lives of these isotopes permit extension of these determinations to humans.

General criteria for selecting and using molecular imaging probes

The question of whether a specific compound can be labeled with a positron emitter, with the intention of using that probe as a molecular imaging agent, is often asked. There is, however, much more to the effective design of molecular imaging probes than this question alone. Indeed, it is the wrong question altogether if it is not preceded by a complete understanding of the structural requirements of the target enzyme or receptor and the process to be measured. To select a molecular imaging probe to measure a specific process or assess organ function, the probe should meet the following criteria:

1. Target specificity—ideally, the probe should be restricted to the target process.
2. High membrane permeability to reach target areas.
3. As a result of a specific interaction with a target molecule in tissue, trapping of the labeled molecule or labeled reaction product should occur in a slow turnover pool.
4. Use of analogs specific to one biochemical pathway to isolate one step or a few steps of the process—thus, the kinetics of only the administered compound is represented in the measured data.
5. Rapid turnover rates (small precursor pool) for the substrate precursor are desirable to allow reaction of the labeled molecule probe to proceed rapidly and, thus, reduce background signal rapidly. This implies high affinity of the molecular probe for its tissue target and rapid clearance of the probe from nonspecific areas.
6. Rapid blood pool clearance of the molecular imaging probe to reduce blood pool background at the tissue target (e.g., brain, heart, and tumor) and increase the rate of clearance of the probe from tissue as a result of the temporal decrease in probe concentration in blood.
7. No—or—slow peripheral metabolism of the probe to have the administered probe as the only—or—primary chemical entity in blood.
8. High-specific activity (low masses at the radioactivity concentrations used; Chapter 3) to trace the process under investigation without exerting mass effects on the target molecule.
9. Low nonspecific binding to increase target specificity and target-to-background ratios $>> 1$.
10. A small number of transport and biochemical reaction steps for the molecular imaging probe to allow tracer kinetic modeling to establish quantitative parameters for the imaging determination (Chapter 2).

TYPES OF MOLECULAR IMAGING PROBES

As indicated earlier, to assess biochemical disturbances (e.g., disease states) noninvasively using molecular imaging with PET, specific probes are designed and used to target the process to be investigated (e.g., glucose metabolism, neurotransmitter synthesis, neurotransmitter re-uptake, postsynaptic receptor binding, protein synthesis, gene expression, and so on). In general, these molecular probes should have specific properties. Based on the target molecule in tissue, PET imaging probes are divided into three large groups: 1) Probes based on enzyme-mediated transformations; 2) Probes based on stoichiometric binding interactions; and 3) Probes for determination of perfusion. With a few exceptions (e.g., [N-13]ammonia), the latter probes have no specific structural requirements, except for their high vascular membrane permeability without specific macromolecular targets in tissue. The reader is referred to Chapter 2 for review of the assays for tissue perfusion determinations.

Probes based on enzyme-mediated transformations

These probes are characterized by trapping in tissue the product of a specific interaction of the probe with an enzyme. This interaction will normally produce a chemical transformation of the original probe catalyzed by the enzyme that is being targeted. The product of the enzyme-mediated transformation (e.g., phosphorylated substrate) is impermeable to cell membranes and is, therefore, retained in tissue in proportion to the rate of reaction of the enzyme-mediated process. The process has been called metabolic trapping (Figure 4-3).

The best known examples of PET imaging probes acting through this mechanism are 1) hexokinase-mediated trapping of FDG-6-phosphate after FDG administration in the estimation of local glucose metabolic rates in tissue; 2) aromatic amino acid decarboxylase-mediated transformation of 6-[F-18]fluoro-L-DOPA (FDOPA) into 6-[F-18]fluorodopamine with subsequent storage in vesicles in central dopaminergic terminals; 3) the herpes simplex thymidylate kinase (HSV1-TK) model of gene expression that mediates trapping of radiofluorinated acycloguanosines and thymidine analogs to their corresponding 5′-phosphates; and 4) 3′-[F-18]fluoro-3′-deoxythymidine ([F-18]FLT) used in the assessment

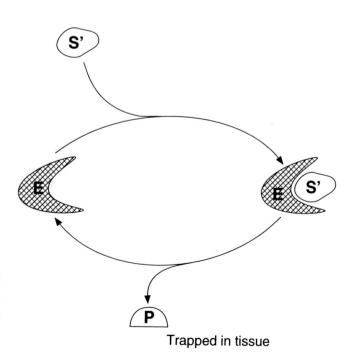

FIGURE 4-3. Diagrammatic representation of the enzyme (E)-mediated transformation of a molecular imaging probe (S′) into a product (P) that is trapped in tissue. An enzyme catalyzes a large number of molecular transformations amplifying the signal from the labeled end product of the reaction.

Trapped in tissue

of DNA replication the utilization of which is based on the specific mammalian thymidine kinase-mediated phosphorylation to its 5′-phosphate.

Probing enzyme function

In regards to structural requirements, enzyme-mediated probes are the ones with the strictest molecular constraints. Since enzymes have evolved over a period of millions of years, they have developed structural specificity for their substrates and have—for the most part—limited specificity to accommodate major modifications to the original substrate. Consider that enzymes are designed by evolution to accelerate chemical reactions decreasing the activation of the free energy barrier (G) between their natural substrate and product (Figure 4-4). For a general reaction:

$$A + B \rightleftarrows C + D \tag{4-1}$$

there are two ways to accelerate its rate: (1) by an increase in temperature (T), which increases motion and the probability for molecules to enter the transition state; and (2) by means of a catalyst (enzyme). By combining transiently with the reactants (e.g., A and B), the enzyme will lower the transition state energy for the reaction to occur. To understand this effect, we need to look at the fundamental relationship between a free energy change (ΔG) of a chemical reaction and its equilibrium constant (K), that is established as:

$$\Delta G = \Delta G° + RT \ln \frac{[C][D]}{[A][B]} \tag{4-2}$$

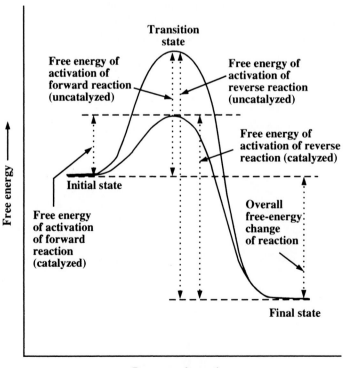

FIGURE 4-4. Energy diagram for a chemical reaction—catalyzed and uncatalyzed.

where R is the gas constant, T the absolute temperature and [A], [B], [C], and [D] the molar concentrations of solutes and, thus, [C][D]/[A][B] = K (equilibrium constant) and $\Delta G°$ is the standard free energy change of the reaction (e.g., at a concentration of 1 mol/L). At equilibrium, ΔG should be zero; then from Equation 4-2,

$$\Delta G° = -RT \ln K \qquad (4\text{-}3)$$

EXAMPLE 4-1

The estimated free energy of activation ΔG for the uncatalyzed and catalyzed (by catalase) decomposition of hydrogen peroxide at 20°C is 18 kcal/mol and 7 kcal/mol, respectively. How much catalase accelerates the rate of the reaction?

ANSWER

In Equation 4-3 the gas constant $R = 1.98 \times 10^{-3}$ kcal/mol and $T = 293°K$; thus, $\Delta G° = -1.33 \log K$.

Since the $\Delta G°$ difference between catalyzed (7 kcal/mol) and uncatalyzed reactions (18 kcal/mol) at 20°C is 11 kcal/mol, then:

$$\Delta G° = -11 \text{ kcal/mol} = -1.33 \log K$$

$$\therefore \log K = \frac{11}{1.33} = 8.24$$

Then, the reaction rate for the decomposition of peroxide increases 10^8-fold when the reaction is catalyzed by catalase.

EXAMPLE 4-2

The lowering of the energy of activation (ΔG) explains enzymatic catalytic power, but how is this catalytic feat accomplished?

ANSWER

Enzymes are composed of amino acid residues forming chains (polypeptide chains) allowing free rotations about C—C and C—N bonds at their backbone. These amino acid residues can directly interact with water molecules in a complex fashion, in general forming hydrogen bonds with: 1) charged groups in the protein; 2) polar, uncharged groups (e.g., carbonyl groups); and hydrogen bonds 3) organized around nonpolar protein residues. These protein-water interactions are very dynamic in nature with almost 80% to 90% of the protein backbone involved, resulting in protein motions from very short (femtoseconds) to slow (milliseconds-seconds).

Enzyme interactions with the solvent cannot be separated from enzyme-substrate interactions. The solvent, water, is always present as the third component of binding and, therefore, enzyme-substrate interactions are also a very dynamic process. Therefore, the multiplicity of interactions between enzyme, substrate, and solvent result not in one but in a large number of substates that are close in energy. As a result, the description of the act of enzyme catalysis (e.g., transformation of the substrate into a product at the enzyme binding site) is attributable to the structural mobility of the enzyme-substrate complex and its consequence in lowering the energy of the reaction. Upon binding, the substrate displaces the nonspecific presence of water at the binding site in a continuously interactive way. Indeed, enzymes are not static but dynamic, constantly shaking structures. This motion induces transient strains in the substrate resulting in enzyme substates favoring transformation of the substrate into a product.[5]

Let's analyze the principles of enzyme kinetics to understand the importance of some concepts in molecular imaging probe design and utilization:

As an oversimplification of the concepts stated above, we can say that enzyme reactions typically consist of two steps: 1) formation of the enzyme-substrate complex (ES) and 2) decomposition of ES with formation of product (P).

$$E + S \underset{k_2}{\overset{k_1}{\rightleftharpoons}} ES \overset{k_3}{\rightarrow} E + P \tag{4-4}$$

The rate of [ES] formation is determined by the difference between reactions leading to its formation and reactions leading to its disappearance:

$$d \frac{[ES]}{dt} = k_1[E][S] - k_2[ES] - k_3[ES] \tag{4-5}$$

Steady-state equilibrium assumes the concentration of [ES] is constant:

$$d \frac{[ES]}{dt} = 0 \tag{4-6}$$

To solve the equations, one should express them in terms of experimentally measurable quantities. For example:

$$[E_o] = [E] + [ES] \tag{4-7}$$

where E_o = initial or total enzyme concentration that is measurable.

Therefore, combining Equations 4–3 and 4–5 under conditions of steady-state equilibrium render:

$$k_1([E_o] - [ES])[S] = (k_2 + k_3)[ES]$$

Upon rearrangement:

$$[ES](k_2 + k_3 + k_1[S]) = k_1 E_o[S]$$

Solving for [ES] after dividing for k_1:

$$[ES] = \frac{E_o[S]}{K_m + [S]} \tag{4-8}$$

where $K_m = \dfrac{k_2 + k_3}{k_1}$ = Michaelis constant. The rate constants k_1, k_2, and k_3 control the formation and decomposition of [ES].

Thus, the velocity (V) of the enzymatic reaction is:

$$V = \frac{dP}{dt} = k_3[ES] = \frac{k_3[E_o][S]}{K_m + [S]} \tag{4-9}$$

When the enzyme is saturated, then the enzyme is mostly as the enzyme-substrate complex [ES] and $k_3[Eo]$ = maximal velocity of the reaction (Vm). The constant k_3 is also named k_{cat} (catalysis constant), representing the rate of decomposition of the enzyme-substrate complex [ES].

Thus, Equation 4-9 becomes:

$$V = \frac{V_m[S]}{K_m + [S]} \tag{4-10}$$

also called the Michaelis–Menten equation.

Thus, k_{cat}/K_m or V_m/K_m is a measure of the enzymatic catalytic efficiency. Therefore, in enzymatically catalyzed reactions, the formation and rate of decomposition of the enzyme-substrate complex to form product are essential parameters to determine the ability of a particular substrate [S] to be transformed into product [P].

EXAMPLE 4-3
How is the principle of enzyme kinetics applied to a kinetic determination made with PET?

ANSWER
The principle of competitive kinetics applies when two competing reactions between two different substrates are taking place with the same enzyme (i.e., glucose and FDG with hexokinase).

For the endogenous substrate:

$$E + [S] \underset{k_2'}{\overset{k_1'}{\rightleftarrows}} [ES] \overset{k_3}{\to} E + [P]$$

For the competitive substrate:

$$E + [S'] \underset{k_2'}{\overset{k_1'}{\rightleftarrows}} [ES'] \overset{k_3'}{\to} E + [P']$$

Under the steady-state assumption, $d\frac{[ES]}{dt} = 0$; thus, formation of [ES] is determined by:

$$[ES] = \frac{k_1}{k_2 k_3}(E_o - [ES] - [ES'])[S] \tag{4-11}$$

being E_o = total enzyme concentration and $k_1/k_2 + k_3 = 1/K_m$

Similarly,

$$[ES'] = \frac{k_1'}{k_2'K_3'}(E_o - [ES] - [ES'])[S'] \tag{4-12}$$

where $k_1'/k_2' + k_3' = 1/K_m'$

Thus:

$$[ES]K_m = E_o[S] - [ES][S] - [ES'][S] \tag{4-13}$$

and

$$[ES']K_m' = E_o[S'] - [ES][S'] - [ES'][S'] \tag{4-14}$$

Therefore,

$$[ES](K_m[S]) = E_o[S] - [ES'][S] \tag{4-15}$$

and

$$[ES] = \frac{E_o[S] - [ES'][S]}{K_m + [S]} \tag{4-16}$$

Replacing [ES] in Equation 14:

$$[ES']K_m' = E_o[S'] - \frac{E_o[S] - [ES'][S]}{K_m + [S]}[S'] - [ES'][S']$$

$$= [E_o][S'] = \frac{E_o[S][S']}{K_m + [S]} + \frac{[ES'][S][S']}{K_m + [S]} - [ES'][S'] \tag{4-17}$$

Rearranging terms:

$$[ES']\left(K_m' - \frac{[S][S']}{K_m + [S']} + [S']\right) = E_o[S'] - \frac{E_o[S][S']}{K_m + [S]} \tag{4-18}$$

Solving [ES']:

$$[ES'] = \frac{[E_o[S'] - \dfrac{E_o[S] + [S']}{K_m + [S]}]}{K_m' - \dfrac{[S][S']}{K_m + [S]} + [S']} \tag{4-19}$$

Rearranging terms:

$$[ES'] = \frac{E_o[S'](K_m + [S]) - E_o[S][S']}{K_m'(K_m + [S]) - [S][S'] + [S'](K_m + [S])}$$

$$= \frac{E_o K_m[S']}{K_m'K_m + K_m'[S] + K_m[S']}$$

$$[ES'] = \frac{\dfrac{E_o}{K_m'}[S']}{1 + \dfrac{[S]}{K_m} + \dfrac{[S']}{K_m'}} \tag{4-20}$$

Therefore, the velocity (V') of the reaction with a competitive substrate (S'') is:

$$V' = k_3'[ES'] = \frac{\dfrac{k_3'E_o}{K_m'}[S']}{1 + \dfrac{[S]}{K_m} + \dfrac{[S']}{K_m'}} \tag{4-21}$$

Since $V'_m = k_3'E_o$

$$V' = \frac{\dfrac{V'_m}{K_m'}[S']}{1 + \dfrac{[S]}{K_m} + \dfrac{[S']}{K_m'}} \tag{4-22}$$

If the competitive substrate concentration is very low ($[S'] \ll [S]$), as is always the case with PET determinations where the molecular imaging probe is used in tracer concentrations, Equation 4-22 can be simplified further:

$$V' = \frac{\dfrac{V'_m}{K_m'}}{1 + \dfrac{[S']}{K_m}}[S'] \qquad (4\text{-}23)$$

that is the reaction rate measured by PET:

$$V' = k_3'(PET)[S'] = \frac{\dfrac{V'_m}{K_m'}}{1 + \dfrac{[S]}{K_m}}[S'] \qquad (4\text{-}24)$$

where k3' (PET) is the rate constant of the enzyme reaction.

If we divide by V, or the original rate of the endogenous process unaffected by the presence of the tracer $[S']$:

$$\frac{V'}{V} = \frac{\dfrac{V'_m K_m'}{1 + [S]/K_m'[S']}}{\dfrac{V_m K_m}{1 + [S]/K_m}[S]} \qquad (4\text{-}25)$$

Rearranging terms:

$$\frac{V'}{V} = \frac{V_m'/K_m'[S']}{V_m/K_m[S]} \qquad (4\text{-}26)$$

Therefore, V, the rate of the endogenous reaction to be measured (i.e., local metabolic rate for glucose, LMRGlc) with the molecular imaging probe (i.e., FDG) and PET combining Equations 4-24 and 4-26 is:

$$V = k_3'(PET)[S']\frac{V_m/K_m[S]}{V_m'/K_m'[S']}$$

Thus:

$$V = k_3'(PET)\frac{V_m/K_m}{V_m'/K_m'}[S] \qquad (4\text{-}27)$$

In the case of glucose metabolic rate determinations with FDG, $V = LMRGlc$, $[S] = $ plasma glucose concentration and $\dfrac{V_m'/K_m'}{V_m/K_m} = $ lumped constant (LC) indicating the ratio of catalytic efficiency between the imaging probe and the endogenous substrate.[6] Thus, LC is derived from the principle of competitive kinetics to convert the measured reaction rate of a substrate analog to the reaction rate of the natural substrate. Unless this ratio is known, no absolute determination of the endogenous process can be made. It should be noted, however, that the LC does vary with the species of animal (Table 4-1)[7–13] and also changes in pathophysiological states, (e.g., severe hypoglycemia).[14]

TABLE 4-1. Values of the FDG Lumped Constant in Several Species

Species	Mean ± SD	Reference
Albino rat		
Conscious	0.464 ± 0.099[a]	Sokoloff, 1986[7]
Anesthetized	0.512 ± 0.118[a]	Sokoloff, 1986[7]
Conscious (5% CO_2)	0.463 ± 0.122[a]	Sokoloff, 1986[7]
Combined	0.481 ± 0.119	Sokoloff, 1986[7]
Rhesus monkey		
Conscious	0.344 ± 0.095	Sokoloff, 1986[7]
Cat		
Anesthetized	0.411 ± 0.013	Sokoloff, 1986[7]
Dog (beagle puppy)		
Conscious	0.558 ± 0.082	Sokoloff, 1986[7]
Sheep		
Fetus	0.416 ± 0.031	Sokoloff, 1986[7]
Newborn	0.382 ± 0.024	Sokoloff, 1986[7]
Mean	0.400 ± 0.033	Sokoloff, 1986[7]
Human		
Conscious	0.568 ± 0.105	Sokoloff, 1986[7]
Conscious	0.418 ± 0.058	Huang et al, 1980[8]
Conscious	0.520 ± 0.028	Reivich et al, 1985[9]
Conscious	0.660 ± 0.170[b]	Hasselbalch et al, 1997[10]
Conscious	0.670 ± 0.210[c]	Hasselbalch et al, 1997[10]
Conscious	0.810 ± 0.150	Hasselbalch et al, 1998[11]
Conscious	0.860 ± 0.140	Spence et al, 1998[12]
Conscious	0.670 ± 0.170	Wu et al, 2001[13]

[a]No statistically significant difference between normal conscious and anesthetized rats ($0.3 < p < 0.4$) and conscious rats breathing 5% CO_2 ($p > 0.9$); [b]Steady state; [c]Bolus injection.

When the principle of competitive enzyme kinetics is used with PET, the molecular imaging probe (i.e., FDG) will compete with the endogenous substrate (i.e., glucose) for the same sites at the catalytic enzyme (e.g., hexokinase). This competition between the newly designed imaging probe and the endogenous substrate for the same enzyme site immediately indicates that the imaging probe should have very favorable kinetic characteristics to trace the process under study. If the imaging probe has low Vm' and high Km' (low Vm'/Km'), it will compete unfavorably with the endogenous substrate, with two consequences: 1) a reduction in the probability of yielding a metabolic trapping product of the labeled analog and 2) as a result, a low PET signal. Therefore, favorable enzyme kinetic characteristics of the imaging probe permit competition with the endogenous substrate for successful formation of the radiolabeled trapping product leading to accumulation of the labeled product—an essential consideration in designing enzyme-mediated molecular imaging probes.

Using substrate analogs of enzyme function

To further understand the question of why knowledge of the target molecule in tissue is important, this chapter will analyze the example of hexokinase and the successful use of a radiolabeled substrate analog of enzyme function, FDG, as a molecular imaging probe to estimate local rates of glucose metabolism. FDG was found to retain the transport and enzymatic characteristics of 2-deoxy-D-glucose. Its utilization for the noninvasive determination of LMRGlc is then based on the general biochemical principle developed by Sokoloff et al[6] with [C-14]2-deoxy-D-glucose. Fluorination of carbon-2— that is, the replacement of the OH group in the 2-position of D-glucose with a fluorine—is successful for at least two reasons: First, it respects the steric characteristics of D-glucose without any substantial distortion in geometry, which is a requirement for preservation of its needed activity with hexokinase; and, second, it predictably assures that fluorodeoxyglucose-6-phosphate (FDG-6-P), the product of the hexokinase-mediated phosphorylation of FDG, will not be susceptible to further metabolism within the time-frame of the imaging determination (e.g., typically 45 min). The reason is that the next reaction in the glycolytic pathway after hexokinase is the freely reversible isomerization of glucose-6-phosphate to fructose-6-phosphate, in effect, a rearrangement of the carbonyl group from C-1 to C-2. The enzymatic transformation imposes structural and geometric requirements in the substrate that cannot be met by FDG due to the presence of fluorine substitution on carbon 2. All these factors make the accumulation of radioactivity in the use of FDG very specific to the measurement of glucose metabolic rates. At pharmacological doses, FDG can block phosphorylation of glucose due to inhibition of hexokinase by FDG-6-P. This mechanism was observed early when 2-deoxy-D-glucose was originally introduced as a therapeutic agent to inhibit glycolysis in tumors. Because of the high-specific activity of FDG (Chapter 3), there are no significant mass action effects of FDG-G-P on hexokinase when a PET determination is performed.

Consequently, the time-dependent accumulation of radioactivity as FDG-6-P is proportional to the rate of the hexokinase-mediated reaction in tissue. This biochemical trick, referred to as the principle of metabolic trapping, permits the biochemical isolation of the hexokinase reaction, whose rate under steady-state conditions is equal to the glycolysis rate or LMRGlc assuming no significant glycogen formation or breakdown. It has been estimated that only 3% of glucose is metabolized via the pentose phosphatase shunt, at least in normal rat brain.[15] Moreover, the radiofluorinated glucose analog is a poor substrate of glucose-6-phosphate dehydrogenase,[16] the first enzyme in the pentose phosphate shunt. Therefore, this pathway seems to contribute only minimally to the measure of LMRGlc. Similarly, the influence of the highly compartmentalized glucose-6-phosphatase to hydrolyze back FDG-6-P is low within the experimental period of the tomographic determination (e.g., 45 min)[17] (Chapter 2). Thus, FDG provides a measure of the rate of hexokinase-mediated glycolysis, independent of all subsequent reactions in the glycolytic pathway.

The *in vivo* kinetic properties of FDG as a substrate for hexokinase are in accord with the mechanism of hexokinase binding to its substrate and ATP to induce phosphorylation at carbon-6. In the design of a radiolabeled imaging probe targeting hexokinase to measure local glucose metabolic rates, it is important to know that hexokinase is particularly insensitive to modifications at carbon 2, including stereochemical modifications. In that regard, FDG and 2-deoxy-2-fluoro-D-mannose (FDM), which only differ in the fluorine atom configuration (e.g., the fluorine substitution can have two possible arrangements) at carbon-2, are both good substrates for hexokinase. By contrast, 1-fluoro-, 3-fluoro- and 4-fluorodeoxy-D-glucoses are poor substrates for hexokinase (Table

TABLE 4-2. Experimentally Determined Kinetic Constants of Fluorohexoses with Hexokinase

Compound	K_m (mM)	Relative V_{max}	K_m MgATP^{2-} (mM)	Calculated K'_m K_m (glucose)	Experimental K'_m K_m (glucose)
D-Glucose	0.17	1.00	0.20	1	1
2-Deoxy-D-*arabino*-hexose	0.59 ± 0.11	0.85	0.36 ± 0.11	—	—
2-Deoxy-2-fluoro-D-glucose	0.19 ± 0.03	0.50	0.26 ± 0.05	1.14	1.36 ± 0.37
2-Deoxy-2-fluoro-D-mannose	0.41 ± 0.05	0.85	0.66 ± 0.25	2.46	0.86 ± 0.75
2-Deoxy-2,2-difluoro-D-*arabino*-hexose	0.13 ± 0.02	0.53	0.21 ± 0.02	0.78	0.91 ± 0.47
3-Deoxy-3-fluoro-D-glucose	70 ± 30[a]	0.10	2.3 ± 0.3[b]	—	—
4-Deoxy-4-fluoro-D-glucose	84 ± 30[a]	0.10	1.9 ± 0.1[c]	—	—
2-Chloro-2-deoxy-D-glucose	2.1 ± 0.6	0.54	0.97 ± 0.33	12.6	9 ± 10

Source: Reprinted from Bessell et al.,[18] with permission from Biochemical Journal, © The Biochemical Society.

[a]Concentration of ATP, 4.1 mM.   [b]Concentration of 3-deoxy-3-fluoro-D-glucose, 10 mM.

[c]Concentration of 4-deoxy-4-fluoro-D-glucose, 10 mM.

Note: Compounds that are not substrates: α-D-glucopyranosyl fluoride, β-D-glucopyranosyl fluoride, 2-O-methyl-D-glucose, 2,2-dichloro-2-deoxy-D-*arabino*-hexose, 2-deoxy-2-fluoro-D-galactose, 2,3-anhydro-D-mannose (kindly provided by Professor J. G. Buchanan), 2-chloro-2-deoxy-D-mannose, 2-O-methyl-D-mannose. Compounds that are not inhibitors: α-D-glucopyranosyl fluoride, β-D-glucopyranosyl fluoride, 2-deoxy-2-fluoro-D-galactose, 2-deoxy-2,2-dichloro-D-*arabino*-hexose, 2,3-anhydro-D-mannose. Compounds that are inhibitors: 2-O-methyl-D-glucose (K_I 60mM), 2-O-methyl-D-mannose (K_I 7mM). Values are means ± SEM.

4-2).[18] Therefore, in the design of a successful molecular imaging probe, the issue is not only whether a radiolabeled fluorine atom can be introduced on a specific substrate, but also how to meet the biochemical requirements imposed by the target enzyme/receptor.

EXAMPLE 4-4

Is it possible to use other radiolabeled halogenated (i.e., I-123; Br-75) glucose analogs to adapt the same concept described above to single-photon emission tomography?

ANSWER

In most cases, it is easier to introduce synthetic iodine, bromine, or chlorine than fluorine to a given site in a molecule. Then it is not a question of whether the synthesis of halogenated probes is possible, but whether radiohalogenated probes, other than radiofluorinated probes, are useful for the intended purpose. Beyond the excellent physical qualities of fluorine-18 as a positron emitter, e.g., 97% positron decay mode, a convenient half-life (109.72 min), a short positron range (Chapter 1), and the capability of being prepared with high-specific activity, its importance resides in the fact that fluorine is the second smallest substituent, closely mimicking hydrogen in geometric requirements (the van der Waal's radii of fluorine and hydrogen atoms are very similar, 1.35 and 1.2 Å, respectively). The van der Waals radius of a group or atom is a measure of its size, and the larger the atom, the higher the probability of unfavorable interaction with another group or atom at the enzyme binding site. If this occurs—if, in other words, the electron clouds begin to penetrate each other—the interaction becomes repulsive. As a result, one can expect that C-F analogs will closely mimic the biological behavior of C-H derivatives. The high fluorine of electronegativity, however, introduces a polarity more akin to a hydroxyl substituent.[19] This explains why, when compared with glucose which contains an OH group at the 2 position, FDG binding affinity with hexokinase, as well as the chemical reactivity of the transition state intermediate during phosphoryl transfer, is not drastically affected (e.g., Vm'/Km' and Vm/Km are similar; Table 4-2). All other 2-radiohalogenated deoxyglucoses would not meet these criteria because of the larger van der Waal's radii of the other halogens (Cl, Br, and I). The geometric constraints imposed by these radiohalogenated deoxyglucose analogs drastically reduce their binding affinity with the enzyme (hexokinase). For example, the Km of 2-chloro-2-deoxy-D-glucose for hexokinase is 0.97 mM, about 5-fold higher than that of FDG.[20] For larger halogens, the apparent affinity for hexokinase drops even further. As a result, 2-radiohalogenated deoxyglucoses, other than FDG, cannot be effectively used as molecular imaging probes for LMRGlc.

Molecular imaging probes targeting tumor enzymes

The principle of the FDG method has been applied to the investigation of the biochemistry of cancer. It is currently applied extensively to the diagnosis and staging of the disease (Chapter 5). The knowledge obtained with FDG is centered on energy utilization by tumor cells *in vivo*, as a source of energy (e.g., adenosine triphosphate or ATP). Recently, approaches to target enzymes involved in biosynthetic processes in the tumor have been developed. The two most relevant examples are the development and use of: 1) fluorine-18-labeled 3'-fluoro-3'-deoxythymidine ([F-18]FLT) as a probe of DNA replication and, therefore, cell replication, targeting mammalian thymidylate kinase (TK); and 2) carbon-11-labeled choline and fluorine-18 labeled choline analogs to target choline kinase. Both enzymes are overexpressed in tumor tissue. Other approaches targeting tyrosine kinases in tumors are under development.

3'-[F-18]FLUORO-3'-DEOXYTHYMIDINE ([F-18]FLT)

Using [F-18]FLT as an imaging probe of DNA replication is based on early work on the use of 3'-fluoro-3'-deoxythymidine[21] as a candidate for an anti-AIDS drug in clinical trials.[22] Incorporation of FLT via mono-, di-, and triphosphates into the DNA of MT4 cells and other cell lines was demonstrated.[23] The ability of FLT to incorporate into DNA resides in the efficiency of its triphosphate, formed intracellularly following the thymidine kinase (TK)-mediated synthesis of its monophosphate, as a substrate of DNA polymerases.[24] It appears that within the time of the PET determination, however, [F-18]FLT-5'-monophosphate is the main product accumulating in tissue (Figure 4-5).

F-18 FLT[25,26] has been used in animal models and humans[27] and has been shown to be effective in the visualization of primarily nonsmall cell lung cancer and brain tumors as well as normal highly proliferating tissues such as bone marrow (Figure 4-6). [F-18]FLT has excellent properties as a molecular imaging probe in that it has specificity for mammalian TK and is essen-

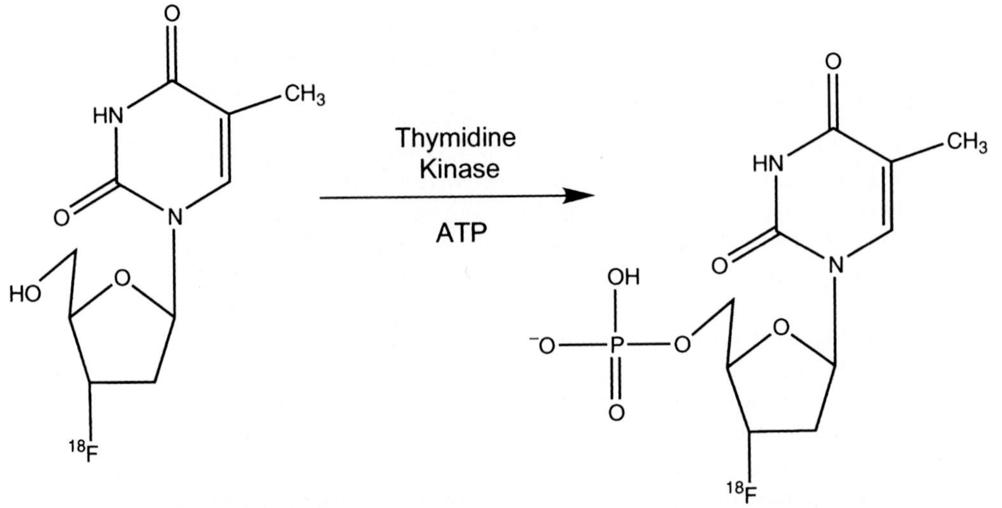

FIGURE 4-5. Description of the thymidine kinase-mediated phosphorylation of [F-18]FLT into its 5′-monophosphate that is metabolically trapped in tissue within the time of the experimental determination with PET (i.e., ≤ 2 h). With longer exposure times, the monophosphate would be subsequently phosphorylated by cellular kinases to the di- and tri-phosphate, and the latter incorporated into DNA.

tially not metabolized *in vivo* in dogs. However, it appears to have increased glucuronidation in humans, as evidenced by its accumulation in hepatocites.[27]

EXAMPLE 4-5
What would be necessary to know to quantify the mammalian TK-mediated phosphorylation of [F-18]FLT?

ANSWER
Similar to FDG, the use of [F-18]FLT is based on the principle of metabolic trapping mediated by mammalian TK (Figure 4-6). Because trapping is due to the initial phosphorylation of [F-18]FLT mediated by mammalian TK to [F-18]FLT-5′-monophosphate, a similar 3-compartment model can be used for the determination of k3′(PET), or the rate of accumulation of the probe in DNA. However, the determination of the absolute rate of DNA replication would require knowledge of the concentration of thymidine in tissue (i.e., tumor or bone marrow) and the determination of the transport and enzyme-mediated rate constants for [F-18]FLT and thymidine to act as substrates with TK (i.e., Vm′/Km′ and Vm/Km, respectively; Equation 4-27, p. 281). This information is not yet available for the substrate analog. Thus, [F-18]FLT is currently used only semiquantitatively to assess relative alterations in DNA replication.

RADIOLABELED CHOLINE AND FLUORINATED ANALOGS
These molecular imaging probes are used to target choline kinase, an enzyme elevated in tumor cells. These molecular imaging probes are particularly useful in prostate cancer because of their ability to be rapidly trapped in the prostate can-

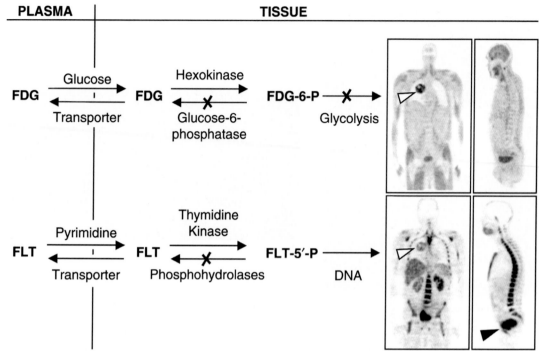

FIGURE 4-6. Tracer kinetic models for FDG and [F-18]FLT based on their biochemical similarities as molecular imaging probes. Arrows show forward and reverse transport between plasma and tissue and phosphorylation and dephosphorylation. Both FDG and [F-18]FLT phosphates are not significant substrates for dephosphorylation or further metabolism at normal imaging times of 40 min to 60 min after injection. Images are 6-mm-thick longitudinal tomographic sections of a patient with a lung tumor (arrows) that has high glucose metabolism and DNA replication. The rest of the images show normal distribution of glucose utilization and DNA replication, exceptions being the clearance of both tracers to the bladder (arrowhead) and in the case of [F-18]FLT glucuronidation by hepatocytes in the liver.

cer cells, coupled with their slow excretion rate via the kidney to the bladder, which can obscure the prostate gland. This results in clear visualization of primary prostate cancer, proximal lymphatic nodes, and local metastasis in humans, because no or little activity accumulates in the bladder in the first 10 minutes after intravenous administration of the radiolabeled probe (Chapter 5; Figure 4-7).[28]

Carbon-11 (methyl)-labeled choline[29] was utilized in the detection of brain tumors[30,31] prostate cancer,[32] and esophageal carcinoma[33] with good results. The target enzyme is choline kinase[34] that not only takes choline as a substrate but has sufficient binding flexibility at the binding site pocket to phosphorylate other analogs (Table 4-3).[34] The enzyme transforms choline into its phosphorylated form, which is then incorporated into membrane components of tumor cells (i.e., phospholipids). As a result of this essential activity in tumor cell proliferation, the enzyme has also been considered as a therapeutic target.[35]

Choline kinase seems to tolerate modifications in one of the methyl groups of choline well. Fluoromethyl- and fluoroethyl-choline-substituted analogs are good substrates for the enzyme (e.g., compare V_m/K_m to that of choline). Initial results in prostate cancer patients with an F-18-labeled fluoromethylcholine analog seem to confirm these expectations *in vivo*. It appears, however, that excretion via kid-

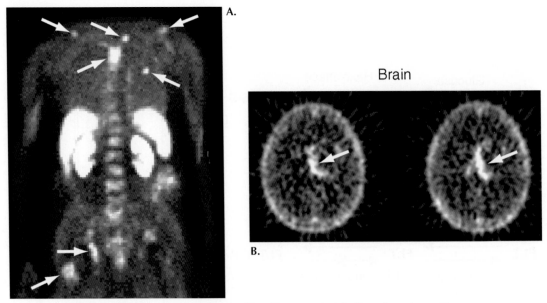

FIGURE 4-7. Whole-body image using [F-18]fluoromethylcholine of a patient with prostate cancer taken 5 min to 8 min after injection of the probe. A) Notice the presence (arrows) of tumor metastasis in the pelvic area and upper thorax, as well as the lack of activity in the bladder. B) Metastasis (arrows) is also observed in the brain of this patient. At later times, the radiolabeled probe is excreted via the kidney and fills the bladder.

ney is increased with the fluorinated analog when compared with C-11 choline,[28] which essentially shows no accumulation of activity in the bladder.

EXAMPLE 4-6
Do choline derivatives meet the necessary requirements for quantitation of choline kinase activity?

ANSWER
Initial studies have shown that choline and derivatives are fairly specific for the target enzyme, choline kinase. However, their significant peripheral metabolism *in vivo* may complicate the formulation of tracer kinetic modeling for quantitation of choline activity as a marker of phospholipid synthesis in the target tissue (e.g., tumor). Regardless, the qualitative use of labeled choline analogs to identify accelerated increases in phospholipid synthesis, that can be increased more than 10-fold in tumors, has been demonstrated. Moreover, as indicated above for [F-18]FLT, for quantification it is necessary to know: 1) the concentration of the endogenous substrate, choline (preferentially in the tissue target); and 2) the kinetic characteristics (Vm'/Km') of the radiolabeled probe. Vm/Km of choline are known.[34] It is obvious that the use of C-11 choline would simplify the quantification process because in Equation 4-27 $Vm/Km/Vm'/Km' = 1$. However, whenever possible, fluorinated choline analogs are more attractive for human use because of the longer half-life of F-18 compared with that of C-11.

TABLE 4-3. Acyclic, Alkyl Analogs of Choline as Substrates of Yeast Choline Kinase

$$R_1{-}\overset{\displaystyle R_2}{\underset{\displaystyle R_4}{N}}{-}R_3$$

Number	Compound R$_1$	R$_2$	R$_3$	R$_4$	Relative V_{max}*	Apparent K_m (μM)
1a	—CH$_3$	—CH$_3$	—CH$_3$	—CH$_2$CH$_2$OH	100 (100)	18 ± 2
b	—H	—H	—H	—CH$_2$CH$_2$OH	–(5 ± 1)	—
c	—H	—H	—CH$_3$	—CH$_2$CH$_2$OH	24 ± 2 (22 ± 1)	1107 ± 273
d	—H	—CH$_3$	—CH$_3$	—CH$_2$CH$_2$OH	37 ± 2 (37 ± 2)	66 ± 1
e	—CH$_2$CH$_3$	—CH$_3$	—CH$_3$	—CH$_2$CH$_2$OH	110 ± 6 (100 ± 5)	17 ± 1
f	—CH$_2$CH$_2$CH$_3$	—CH$_3$	—CH$_3$	—CH$_2$CH$_2$OH	116 ± 5 (80 ± 4)	33 ± 4
g	—CH$_2$CH$_2$CH$_2$CH$_3$	—CH$_3$	—CH$_3$	—CH$_2$CH$_2$OH	–(8 ± 2)	—
h	—CH$_2$CH$_3$	—CH$_2$CH$_3$	—CH$_3$	—CH$_2$CH$_2$OH	96 ± 8 (82 ± 3)	68 ± 15
i	—CH$_2$CH$_3$	—CH$_2$CH$_3$	—CH$_2$CH$_3$	—CH$_2$CH$_2$OH	38 ± 5 (21 ± 3)	652 ± 115
j	—CH$_3$	—CH(CH$_3$)$_2$	—CH(CH$_3$)$_2$	—CH$_2$CH$_2$OH	–(7 ± 1)	—
k	—CH$_3$	—CH$_3$	—CH$_3$	—CH$_2$CH$_2$CH$_2$OH	55 ± 4 (45 ± 2)	117 ± 14
l	—CH$_3$	—CH$_3$	—CH$_3$	—CH$_2$CH$_2$CH$_2$CH$_2$OH	–(<3)	—
m	—CH$_3$	—CH$_3$	—CH$_3$	—CH$_2$CH(CH$_3$)OH	–(<3)	—
n	—CH$_3$	—CH$_3$	—CH$_3$	—C(CH$_3$)$_2$CH$_2$OH	–(<3)	—
o	—CH$_3$	—CH$_3$	—CH$_3$	—CH(CH$_3$)CH$_2$OH	39 ± 4 (41 ± 1)	443 ± 28

Source: Reprinted from Clary et al.,[34] with permission from Elsevier.

Note: Each analog was compared with choline at a constant (10 mM) substrate concentration and a fixed, saturating concentration of ATP and magnesium to give a relative initial rate (choline = 100). For those analogs with a relative initial rate greater than 25% of that of choline, a relative apparent V_{max} and an apparent K_m (± SEM) were also determined. Compounds 1m and 1o are racemic mixtures. Compound 1a is choline.

*The values within the parentheses report the relative rate (± SEM) of the reaction obtained at a fixed substrate concentration (10 mM).

Probes based on stoichiometric binding interactions

Receptor-ligand binding: general principles

These imaging probes are radiolabeled drug derivatives or analogs that bind with a high degree of specificity to: 1) receptor systems, 2) neurotransmitter presynaptic reuptake carriers, or 3) enzymes. Unlike probes based on enzyme-mediated transformations, these probes do not experience chemical modifications as a result of this interaction. There are many examples in the literature of these kinds of drug-mimicking probes that have permitted extensive evaluation of central neurotransmission and other biochemical processes with PET in health and disease (Table 4-4). In contrast with probes for enzyme-mediated reactions, trapping of receptor-mediated probes is the result of stoichiometric binding to the target site (Figure 4-8). This trapping of the molecular imaging probe (or receptor ligand) is related to its specificity for the target site, the number of target sites (Bmax), and its affinity (KD) for the same target. Because the number of target sites is limited (typically in the nanomolar concentration) in tissue and the binding is stoichiometric, binding specificity is highly dependent on the specific activity (Chapter 3) of the PET imaging probe. When the probe specific activity decreases (mass of cold or unlabeled component increases per unit amount of radioisotope), receptor site occupancy may reach saturation affecting the accuracy of the determination by lowering the ratio of specific-to-nonspecific binding and, thus, image contrast. On the other hand, this very important property of receptor sites can be exploited using these molecular imaging

TABLE 4-4. Selected Imaging Probes and Their *In Vivo* Use with PET

Imaging probe	Use
6-[F-18]Fluoro-L-dopa	Presynaptic dopaminergic function
4-[F-18]Fluoro-L-m-tyrosine	Presynaptic dopaminergic function
6-[F-18]fluoro-L-m-tyrosine	Presynaptic dopaminergic function
2-[F-18]Fluoro-L-tyrosine	Protein synthesis, amino acid transport
[F-18]Long-chain fatty acids	β-Oxidation
[F-18]Misonidazole	Hypoxic cells
[F-18]N-Methylspiperone	D-2 Receptor
N-[F-18]Fluoroethylspiperone	D-2 Receptor
[F-18]Fluoroalkylbenzamides	D-2 Receptor
4-[F-18]Fluorodexetimide	Muscarinic acetylcholine receptor
MPPF	5-HT$_{1A}$ Receptor
N-[F-18]Fluoroethylketanserin	5-HT$_2$ Receptor
[F-18]Setoperone	5-HT$_2$ Receptor
[F-18]Altanserin	5-HT$_2$ Receptor
4-[F-18]Fluorofentanil	Opioid receptor
[F-18]3-Acetylcyclofoxy	Opioid receptor
[F-18]Fluoroethylflumazenil	Benzodiazepine receptor
6-[F-18]Fluoronorepinephrine	Adrenergic nervous system
5-[F-18]Fluorouracil	Tumor therapy control
16α-[F-18]Fluoroestradiol	Breast tumors
[F-18]FLT	DNA replication and cell proliferation
C-11- and F-18-labeled choline analogs	Phospholipid synthesis in tumors

Abbreviations: D-2, dopamine2 receptor; FLT, 3'-deoxy-3'-fluorothymidine; HT$_2$, serotonin type 2 receptor; MPPF, 4-[F-18]fluoro-N-{2-[4-(2-methoxyphenyl)piperazin-1-yl]ethyl}-N-pyridin-2-ylbenzamide.

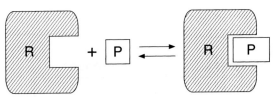

FIGURE 4-8. Schematic representation of the stoichiometric interaction of a molecular imaging probe (P) with a receptor (R). Similar interactions may exist with enzymes, mimicking enzyme inhibitor interactions commonly found with drugs.

probes to determine receptor occupancy by drugs [see Molecular Imaging in Drug Development (p. 310) and Chapter 2]. Therefore, PET imaging probes using receptors as targets should typically have very high-specific activity (1-10 Ci/μmol) to preclude mass effects during the *in-vivo* determination. This requirement can be met with probes for enzyme–mediated reactions, but is not critical. Enzyme-mediated probes can be successfully used even at specific activities 1,000 times lower (1-10 Ci/mmol) than the ones needed for receptor-mediated probes. Also, the binding affinity of these stoichiometric probes for their target should be high, typically in the nanomolar range. Low-binding affinities diminish the specificity of the determination because the measured radioactivity in tissue containing the receptor target may not be increased over that of tissue lacking receptors.[4A]

Imaging endogenous gene expression with radiolabeled oligonucleotides: a perspective from probe design

Imaging approaches directed to gene expression involve either externally transferred genes into cells (transgenes) or endogenous genes (Figure 4-9). The imaging approach involves extending reporter gene techniques used in biology to PET using a PET reporter gene (PRG) and a PET reporter probe (PRP). The PRG–PRP approach has used either an enzyme or a receptor gene as PRG. PRP is, therefore, either an imaging probe that is a substrate of the PRG-enzyme or a probe that is a ligand that binds to the PRG-receptor. In both approaches, the PRG is incorporated into the genome of an adenovirus, which, following intravenous injection into the mouse tail vein, mainly localizes (> 90%) in the liver. Thus, using microPET technology (Chapter 1), it is possible to determine the location, magnitude, and temporal changes of gene expression. In either case, the principle of utilization follows the general discussion above [e.g., 1) probes based on enzyme-mediated transformations[36–39] and 2) probes based on stoichiometric binding interactions.[38,40]] A detailed description of the assays, strategies, and procedures is found in Chapter 2.

Endogenous gene expression is generally directed at the transcription of genes into messenger RNA (mRNA). Single-stranded mRNA is encoded with four bases: adenine (A), cytosine (C), guanine (G), and uracil (U). Specific sequences are targeted for imaging using radiolabeled antisense oligonucleotides (RASON) with a sequence complementary to a specific sequence on the target mRNA molecule. Complementarity is established with the specific pairing of A and U (or thymidine, T, in DNA molecules) and C with G (Figure 4-10). Then, the approach is based on stoichiometric binding of the radiolabeled imaging probe with an endogenous target molecule as described above.

In Vivo Imaging of Gene Expression

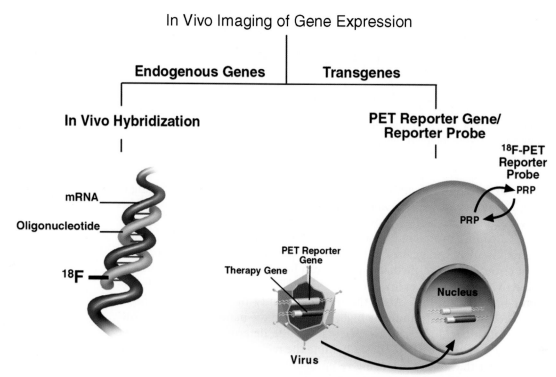

FIGURE 4-9. Two approaches to imaging gene expression *in vivo* with PET. The approach on the left images the expression of endogenous genes. *In situ* hybridization is translated to *in vivo* hybridization using F-18-labeled oligonucleotides that contain complementary sequences of mRNA to be imaged. The approach on the right images transgenes (transplanted genes) administered to the subject. The PET reporter gene (PRG) and therapy gene with common promoter are administered to the subject through a vehicle such as a virus. Virus transfers PRG and therapy gene to cells of the subject. Radiolabeled PET reporter probe (PRP) is then intravenously injected to determine whether gene expression is occurring from PRG.

EXAMPLE 4-7

Does imaging of endogenous gene expression satisfy the molecular probe requirements outlined above (under Molecular Probe Design: General Principles, p. 272)?

ANSWER

Let's analyze the major requirements:

1. Target specificity by the RASON is achieved by the pairing process (A-U and C-G) described above. mRNA is typically several hundred to several thousand nucleotide units, but only limited portions of the sequence are exposed for pairing to the radiolabeled probe because of the secondary and tertiary structures of the mRNA. It has been established that only 11 to 15 bases are necessary in the RASON for selective pairing of all mRNA expressed from the human genome[38] (Figure 4-9). The binding affinity of antisense molecules for mRNA is very

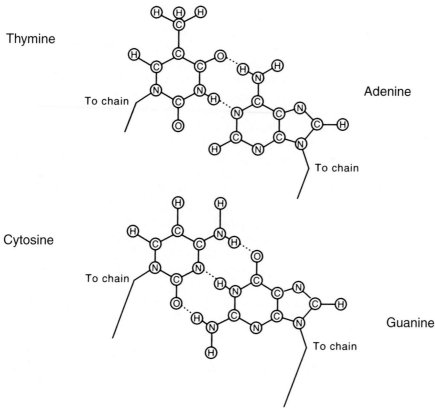

FIGURE 4-10. Hydrogen-bonded base pairs adenine-thymine and guanine-cytosine, the four common bases found in DNA.

high, but it can drop significantly, as much as 300-fold, with a single mismatch (e.g., when a U pairing with A is replaced by C, G, or A).[41] The pairing specificity and the strength of binding will ensure RASON trapping in a slow turnover pool upon binding to mRNA.

2. The stoichiometric basis of the binding to the target mRNA molecule imposes strict requirements of specific activity for RASON. Normal mRNA concentrations are 1 to 1,000 pmol/L, although in disease (i.e., cancer) mRNA can be expressed 100 to 10,000 times higher.[36,37,42] It has been estimated[42] that the lower limit of 1 pmol/L for mRNA concentrations will require RASON specific activities of 1 to 10 Ci/μmol that can be easily achievable with F-18 labeling.

3. Membrane permeability for RASON to access mRNA targets may be a limiting factor. Oligonucleotides are charged molecules that cross membranes using various transport mechanisms including receptor-mediated endocytosis, adsorptive endocytosis, and pinocytosis, but the rates of these processes are not well known. Clearly, oligonucleotides cannot cross the blood-brain-barrier, but delivery of RASON to the brain can be achieved using a brain drug targeting technology.[43] The ratio of specific binding to nonspecific bind-

ing occurring within cells as a function of time is related to the concentration of the target mRNA, to the concentration of nonspecific sites, and to the rate of back transport of RASON, but this will be less of a drawback with high mRNA expression.[43]

4. Peripheral metabolism should also be carefully considered when using RASON for imaging gene expression. Different structural variations of antisense imaging probes can be used: 3′,5′-phosphodiester oligonucleotides (PO–ODN); 3′,5′-phosphorothioate PS-ODN; and ODNs with a peptide backbone (PNA). PO–ODNs are rapidly degraded by endo- and exonucleases that break down the oligonucleotide throughout the body. This can severely limit their utility *in vivo*. 2′-Substituted PO–ODNs are better candidates because of their increased resistance to nuclease hydrolysis. PS–ODNs are not good substrates for nucleases, which dramatically increase their metabolic stability *in vivo*. However, their *in vivo* use has definite drawbacks resulting from high PS–ODN affinity for cellular and plasma proteins potentially resulting in high, nonspecific binding and reduced signal-to-noise. PNAs, having a peptide backbone, are completely stable to nucleases. However, they do not cross cell membranes well. RASON delivery technologies[43] and specific 2′-ODN modifications are being developed to overcome the important issues of membrane permeability and peripheral metabolism. This is an active area of research for imaging probes as well as drugs that are being developed to block translation of disease-mediating mRNAs into proteins.

Targeting enzymes without catalytic transformation of the molecular imaging probe

This chapter reviewed that tissue enzymes can be targeted with radiolabeled substrates and analogs for *in vivo* assessment of their functionality. This approach has been most successfully used with the application of the concept of metabolic trapping [see Using Substrate Analogs of Enzyme Function (p. 282); Figure 4-3]. However, enzyme localization and function can also be assessed with molecular imaging probes that bind to enzymes, either covalently or noncovalently in a process similar to the one described for receptor-ligand interactions (Figure 4-8). The most successful and elegant studies with PET were performed with C-11-labeled compounds (e.g., chlorgyline (N-[3-(2,4-dichlorophenoxy)propyl-N-methyl-2-propynylamine) and L-deprenyl [(−)-N, α-dimethyl-N-2-propynyl-phenethylamine] that irreversibly bind to monoamine oxidase (MAO) A and B, respectively.[44] The covalent binding to the enzyme itself by chlorgyline and L-deprenyl follows the principle frequently referred to as suicide enzyme inactivation.[45] The use of these radiolabeled molecular imaging probes with PET in humans was based on the original development and use of these MAO inhibitors as drugs. Because probes based on the principle of suicide enzyme inactivation selectively bind to the target enzyme only when active, they provide a means to assay the amount of enzyme in the functional state. PET studies with these suicide enzyme inactivation probes have allowed: 1) determination of the *in vivo* distribution of MAO A and B in the human brain, 2) understanding of the effect of antidepressant drugs and smoking on brain MAO activities, and 3) assessment of the rate of recovery of MAO activities in the human brain.

Probes targeting pathological deposition

When the tissue target is not an enzyme or receptor system, either endogenous or purposely introduced (see below, this chapter, *In vivo* Imaging of Transgenic Gene Expression, p. 298) but rather a protein or other tissue target resulting from the specific pathology, imaging probes can be designed to target them. The best known example is the targeting of radiolabeled antibodies to sites on the surface of tumor cells. This is discussed in Chapter 2 with the use of engineered minibodies and antibodies. Other examples of these imaging probes are now emerging together with a more complete understanding of the specific pathologies. One such example is the development of molecular imaging probes to target β-amyloid plaques and neurofibrillary tangles in the brain of patients with Alzheimer's disease. Common features in the brain of patients with familial or sporadic Alzheimer's disease include the presence of abundant intraneuronal neurofibrils (NFTs), extracellular amyloid rich β-amyloid plaques (APs), and neuronal loss.[46] The difficulty in finding such molecular imaging probes to target these pathologies resides mostly in the fact that most probes known to bind amyloid plaques (i.e., Congo red, chrysamine G) do not appreciably cross the blood-brain-barrier, making them essentially useless *in vivo*. A new generation of radiolabeled, highly hydrophobic naphthalene derivatives has been developed and used in humans.[47,48] These compounds have the ability to easily diffuse into the brain and bind to both β-amyloid plaques and neurofibrillary tangles with various degrees of specificity. Results were confirmed by brain autoradiography in the same brain specimens matching results with immunostaining (Figure 4-11).[49] Because these probes are fluorescent, binding is also demonstrated with confocal fluorescent microscopy and *in vitro* binding affinity measurements with β-amyloid neurofibrils. Moreover, the binding of several nonsteroidal anti-inflammatory drugs (NSAIDs; e.g., naproxen, ibuprofen) to the same β-amyloid site was demonstrated by competitive kinetics with the radiolabeled naphthalene probes[50] (see Molecular Imaging and Drug Development, p. 310).

EXAMPLE 4-8

Are amyloid molecular imaging probes analogous to receptor binding probes in their mode of binding?

ANSWER

In a way, they are. β-amyloid peptides aggregate by forming extended chains of cross β-sheets, which, in turn, form tubular, 30Å-diameter protofilaments, with three to five of these protofilaments constituting the amyloid fibril. Multiple fibril aggregates form amyloid plaques. Therefore, the amyloid fibril is organized as a tubular micelle with polar domains forming the outer wall of the amyloid fibril while the hydrophobic domain is at the center of the fiber (Figure 4-12). Thus, APs have multiple binding sites as evidenced by the presence of at least two kinetically distinguishable binding affinities with these probes.[50]

Drug mimicking imaging probes

There are few examples in PET that better illustrate the marriage of therapy (drug interventions and treatment) and diagnostics using molecular imaging than en-

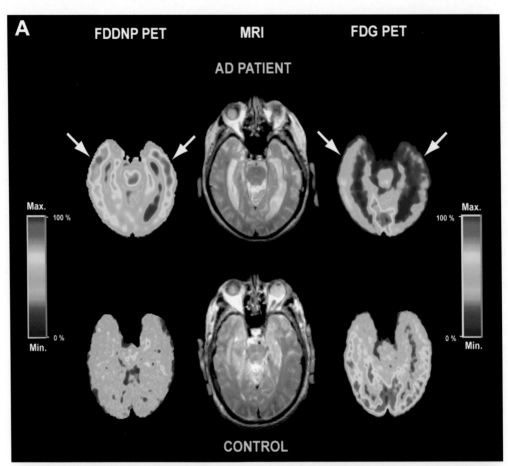

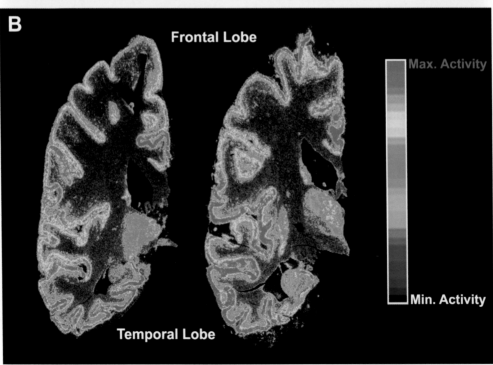

FIGURE 4-11. A direct comparison of *in-vivo* PET (A) and *in-vitro* digital autoradiography (B) for detection of β-amyloid senile plaques (SPs) and neurofibrillary tangles (NFTs) in the brain of a patient with Alzheimer's disease (AD). PET and autoradiography utilized the molecular imaging probe, 2-(1-{6-[2-[F-18]fluoroethyl)(methyl) amino]-2-naphthyl}ethylidene)malononitrile (-18]FDDNP). Subset A shows the FDDNP and FDG–PET images coregistered to their respective MRI images. Areas of FDG hypometabolism are matched with the localization of NFTs and APs resulting from FDDNP binding (marked arrows). The [18F]FDDNP images were obtained by summing frames 12 to 14, corresponding to 25 minutes to 54 minutes post-FDDNP administration. The FDG images were obtained by summing frames corresponding to 20 minutes to 60 minutes postFDG injection. The color bar represents the scaling of the FDDNP and FDG images. (Reprinted from Shoghi–Jadid et al,[48] with permission from the American Psychiatric Association.) Subset B demonstrates the power of autoradiography to map localization of NFTs and APs in brain specimens from patients with Alzheimer's disease.

dogenous gene expression with ODNs (see above) and transgenic expression determinations. For example, human gene therapy trials with exogenous genes (transgenes) can be significantly aided by the ability to locate, determine the magnitude of, and establish time-dependent changes in gene expression. Assay techniques are described in Chapter 2.

FIGURE 4-12. Schematic representation of β-amyloid plaque formation in brain tissue, a phenomenon associated with Alzheimer's disease. Because of their ambiphilic nature, amyloid peptides aggregate, forming simple microtubules that associate to form neurofibrils with multiple microtubules. Neurofibril aggregates form neurofibrillary plaques that frequently have cellular debris.

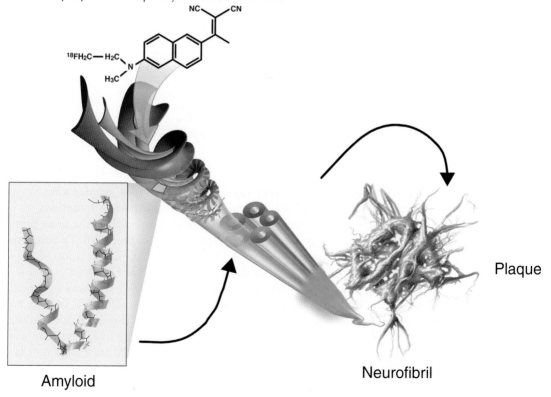

Amyloid

Neurofibril

Plaque

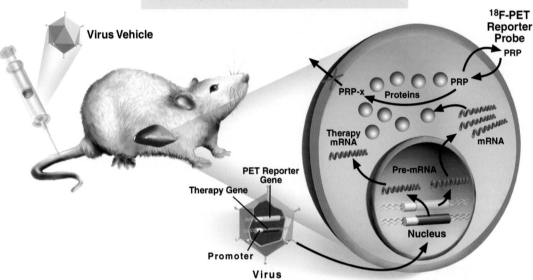

FIGURE 4-13. PET reporter gene-PET reporter probe (PRG–PRP) approach using either enzyme or receptor gene as PRG system. In this example, PRG reporter and therapy gene are placed in virus, which is injected into the tail vein of a mouse. Virus is delivered throughout the body via the bloodstream and localizes in the liver. Virus then transfers PRG and therapy gene to cells in the liver. Because of a common promoter, the expression of PRG corresponds to the expression of therapy gene. The PRG and therapy gene can also be connected together via a common promoter in a single construct (Chapter 2). PRG expression proceeds through transcription to mRNA and then translation to the protein product. In an enzyme example with herpes simplex virus thymidine kinase (HSV-1-tk) gene, the protein product is HSV-1-TK enzyme. The mouse then receives an intravenous injection with the PRP, [F-18]fluoroganciclovir, which diffuses into cells and is cleared to the bladder. If gene expression is present, HSV-1-TK enzyme phosphorylates [F-18]fluoroganciclovir, which is retained in the cell. In the receptor approach, [F-18]fluoroethylspiperone is used as PRP to bind to the D_2 receptor, which is the protein product of PRG.

In vivo *imaging of transgenic expression with herpes simplex virus thymidylate kinase (HSV1-TK): focus on probe-binding interactions*

Molecular imaging probes for HSV1-TK were developed on the same principles that produce metabolic trapping of the product of the HSV1-TK reaction, as phosphorylated substrate in a process similar to the phosphorylation of FDG by hexokinase (Figure 4-13). In terms of probe design, ideal reporter probes for HSV1-TK, the enzyme product of the reporter gene HSV1-tk, should be good substrates for the enzyme and poor substrates for mammalian TK (mTK), an endogenous cytosolic enzyme [e.g., kcat (or Vm)/Km for HSV1-TK $\gg$ kcat (or Vm)/Km for mTK]. It should also be understood that the imaging probe will have to compete *in vivo* with endogenous thymidine, a substrate with very favorable kinetics for HSV1-TK.[36]

To date, two main substrate groups have been developed as reporter probes for HSV1-TK: 1) pyrimidine analogs and 2) acycloguanosine derivatives (Figure 4-14; Table 4-5).[38,39,51–104] Pyrimidine analogs [e.g., 5-iodo-2′-fluoro-2′-deoxy-1-β-D-arabinofuranosyl-5-iodouracil (FIAU) radiolabeled with C-14, I-131 or I-124] have very high sensitivity as imaging agents because they are high affinity substrates for HSV1-TK. Their Vm and Km approach those of the endogenous substrate thymidine.[36] However, they are also excellent substrates of the endogenous mammalian TK, thus reducing their specificity for the HSV1-TK infected-target tissue. Some differences do exist, however, between the in vivo kinetics of the interaction of FIAU with HSV1-TK and mammalian-TK because some imaging specificity is obtained when clearance of the nontarget component of the label is allowed. For example,

FIGURE 4-14. Structures of thymidine, guanosine, and closely related analogs with affinity for HSV1-TK. Radiolabeled versions of these molecules produced molecular imaging probes used in the assessment of HSV1-tk mediated gene expression *in vivo* with PET.

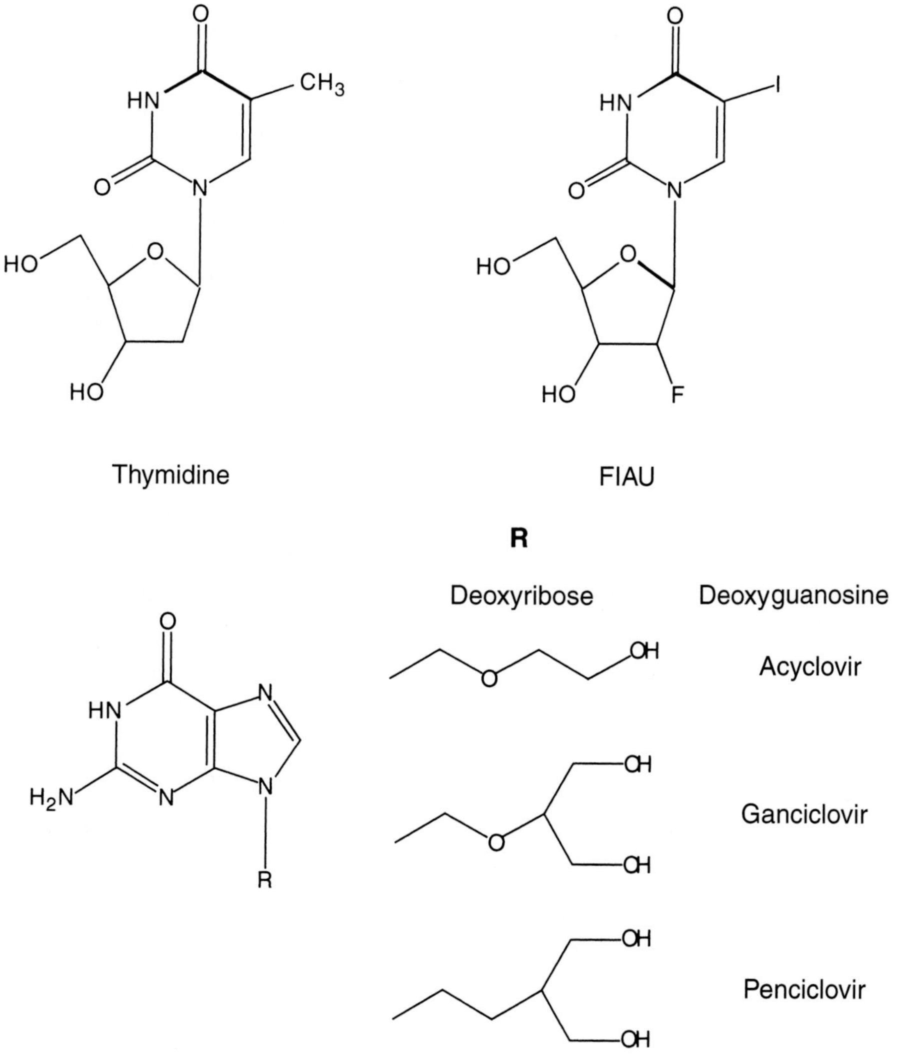

TABLE 4-5. Summary of Reporter Gene/probe Systems

Reporter gene	Mechanism	Imaging agents	Imaging	References
Cytosine deaminase	Deamination	[3H]-5-fluorocytosine	Cell culture study	Haberkorn et al. (1996)[52]
		[19F]-5 fluorocytosine	MRS	Stegman et al. (1993)[53]
Herpes-simplex virus type 1 thymidine kinase (HSV1-tk)	Phosphory-lation	[131I]FIAU, [14C]FIAU	SPECT, gamma camera	Tjuvajev et al. (1996)[54]
		[131I]FIAU	SPECT, gamma camera	Tjuvajev et al. (1999)[55]
		[124K]FIAU	PET	Tjuvajev et al. (1999)[56]
		[123/125]FIAU	Gamma camera	Haubner et al. (2002)[57]
		[125]IVDU, [125I]IVFRU, [125I]VFAU, [125I]IVAU	Cell culture	Morin et al. (1997)[58]
		[125I]FIAU, [125I]FIRU	Cell culture	Wiebe et al. (1999)[59]
		[3H]FFUdR	Cell culture	Germann et al. (1998)[60]
		[14C]GCV, [3H]GCV	Autoradi-ography	Gambhir et al. (1998)[61] Haberkorn et al. (1997)[62] Haberkorn et al. (1998)[63]
		[18F]GCV	PET	Gambhir et al. (1999)[37] Gambhir et al. (1998)[61]
		[18F]PCV	PET	Iyer et al. (2001)[64]
		[18F]FHPG	PET	Alauddin et al. (1996)[65] Alauddin et al. (1999)[66] de Vries et al. (2000)[67] Hospers et al. (2000)[68] Hustinx et al. (2001)[69]
		[18F]FHBG	PET	Alauddin and Conti (1998)[70] Yaghoubi et al. (2001)[71]
Mutant Herpes-simplex virus type 1 thymidine kinase (HSV1-sr39-tk)	Phosphory-lation	[18F]PCV	Cell culture, PET	Gambhir et al. (2000)[38] Sun et al. (2001)[72]
		[18F]FHBG		Yaghoubi et al. (2001)[71] Yu et al. (2000)[39]
Dopamine2 receptor	Receptor-ligand	[18F] FESP	PET	MacLaren et al. (1999)[73] Sun et al. (2001)[72] Yaghoubi et al. (2001)[74] Yu et al. (2000)[39]
Mutant Dopamine2 receptor	Receptor-ligand	[18F] FESP	PET	Liang, et al. (2001)[75]
Somatostatin receptor	Affinity binding	[111In]DTPA-D-Phe1-octreotide	Gamma camera	Rogers et al. (1999)[76]
		[64Cu]-TETA-octreotide	Tumor uptake study	Buchsbaum et al. (1999)[77]
		[188Re]-somatostatin analogue, 99mTc somatostatin analogue	Gamma camera	Rogers et al. (2000)[78] Zinn et al. (2000)[79]

TABLE 4-5. (continued)

Reporter gene	Mechanism	Imaging agents	Imaging	References
Oxotechnetate-binding fusion proteins	Binding via transchelation	[^{99m}Tc] Oxotechnetate	Autoradiography Gamma camera	Bogdanov et al. (1997)[80] Bogdanov et al. (1998)[81]
Gastrin-releasing peptide receptor	Affinity binding	[^{125}I]-mIP-Des-Met^{14}-bombesin (7-13)NH$_2$ [^{125}I]bombesin, [^{99m}Tc]-bombesin analogue	Cell culture Cell culture Cell culture	Baidoo et al. (1998)[82] Rogers et al. (1997)[83] Rogers et al. (1997)[84] Rosenfeld et al. (1997)[85]
Sodium/iodine symporter (NIS)	Active symport	[^{131}I]	Gamma camera	Boland et al. (2000)[86] Haberkorn et al. (2001)[87]
Tyrosinase	Metal binding to melanin	Synthetic metallomelanins [^{111}In], Fe	Cell culture/ MRI	Enochs et al. (1997)[88] Weissleder et al. (1997)[89]
Green fluorescent protein (GFP)	GFP gene expression resulting in fluorescence	Fluorescence	Fluorescence microscopy	Hasegawa et al. (2000)[90] Pfeifer et al. (2001)[91] Yang et al. (2000)[92] Yang et al. (2001)[93] Yang et al. (2000)[94] Yang et al. (1998)[95] Yang et al. (1999)[96]
Luciferase (firefly)	Luciferase–luciferin reaction in presence of oxygen, Mg^{2+} and ATP	Bioluminescence	CCD camera	Contag et al. (1997)[97] Contag et al. (1998)[98]
Luciferase (renilla)	Luciferase–luciferin reaction in presence of oxygen, no other cofactors required	Bioluminescence	CCD camera	Bhaumik and Ghambir (2001)[99]
Cathepsin D	Quenched NIRF fluorochromes	Fluorescence activation	CCD camera	Tung et al. (1999)[100] Tung et al. (2000)[101] Weissleder et al. (1999)[102]
β-galactosidase	Hydrolysis of β-glycoside bond	(1-(2-(β-galacto-pyranosyloxy) propyl)-4,7,10-tris (carboxymethyl)1,4,7,10 tetraazacyclodo-decane) gadolinium(III) or EgadMe	MRI	Louie et al. (2000)[103]
Engineered transferrin receptor (TfR)	Receptor-ligand, internalization	Superparamagnetic iron	MRI	Weissleder et al. (2000)[104]

Abbreviations: ATP, adenosine triphosphate; CCD, charged coupled device; MRI, magnetic resonance imaging; MRS, magnetic resonance spectroscopy; NIRF, near-infrared fluorescent probes; PET, positron emission tomography; SPECT, single photon emission computed tomography.

Source: Adapted from Ray et al,[51] with permission from Elsevier.

[I-124]FIAU has been successfully used with PET in animals with implanted tumors with various levels of HSV1-TK expression, but many hours (e.g., 30) were necessary to achieve the required specificity, namely, high ratios of specific (i.e., produced by the HSV1-TK-mediated phosphorylated product of [124I]FIAU) to nonspecific background activity.[54] Molecular probes have also been developed and used with other gene reporter systems (Table 4-5).[38,39,51–104]

Acycloguanosine derivatives have also been extensively investigated as PET reporter probes for HSV1-TK. A detailed description of their utilization in mice models using microPET technology is presented in Chapter 2. This chapter outlines the principles of their utilization based on their kinetic properties with HSV1-TK.

Using acycloguanosine derivatives as PET reporter probes with the HSV1-tk PET reporter gene is based on the utilization of acycloguanosines (most notably, acyclovir and ganciclovir) as therapeutic agents for herpes simplex virus infections and in gene therapy protocols, using the HSV1-TK/ganciclovir suicide system to treat many forms of cancers[105–107] and AIDS.[108,109]

9-[2-Hydroxyethoxymethyl]guanine (acyclovir) was shown 25 years ago to be specifically phosphorylated by HSV1-TK. This discovery constituted the basis of the successful treatment of Herpes simplex virus infection. Since then, other acycloguanosines (Figure 4-14) have been developed with even better efficacy as therapeutic agents. In all cases, the phosphorylated acycloguanosine derivatives are converted by cellular enzymes to their corresponding triphosphates which, upon incorporation into the viral DNA, produce chain termination and thereby interrupt the vital cycle of virus replication. The safety of acycloguanosines as therapeutic agents is predicated on the premise that they are poor substrates for mammalian TK. Therefore, phosphorylation only occurs in virus-infected cells, which minimizes toxic effects. The low affinity of acycloguanosines for mammalian TK and high affinity for HSV1-TK is also a very important property for utilization of these acycloguanosines as PET reporter probes to produce high specificity in the image.

There are no amino acid sequence similarities between HSV1-TK and mammalian TK.[110] However, both enzymes may share their ability to bind the natural substrate, thymidine, and some pyrimidine analogs very efficiently. HSV1-TK also phosphorylates purine as well as pyrimidine analogs. It also has low specificity for the ribosyl moiety in nucleoside, readily accepting cyclic and acyclic side chains. Therefore, the different characteristics of the binding sites of both enzymes permit exploitation of this feature in the design of radiolabeled acycloguanosine analogs as molecular imaging probes.

First, it is important to understand the binding characteristics of thymidine to HSV1-TK. The reported Km of thymidine for HSV1-TK is in the range 0.2 μm to 8.5 μM (most likely, submicromolar is the most accurate value) whereas thymidine plasma concentration is 0.05 μM to 0.5 μM. This presents thymidine as a formidable competitor for HSV1-TK sites *in vivo*, which necessitates imaging probes with high affinity and catalytic efficiency (high kcat/Km) for high signal-to-noise ratios in the tomographic images (see above). A map of the HSV1-TK active site obtained with X-ray crystallography (Figure 4-15) shows the binding characteristics of thymidine to HSV1-TK. Interaction of the pyrimidine ring is via its C-4 carbonyl and 3-NH group with the amide group of glutamine-

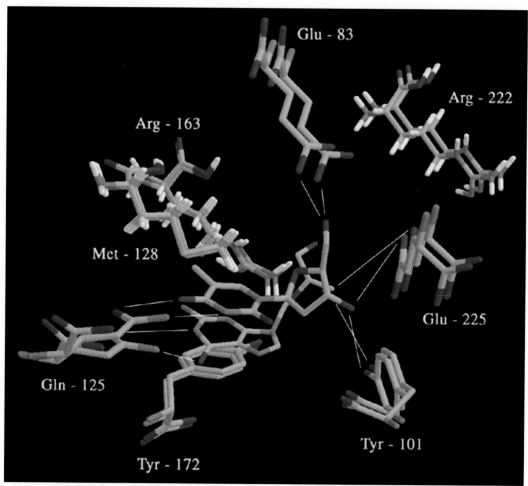

FIGURE 4-15. Binding modes of thymidine (dark gray bonds) and ganciclovir (light gray bonds) in the active site pocket of HSV-1-TK. Oxygen and nitrogen atoms are drawn as light and dark gray spheres, respectively. Hydrogen bonds are indicated as dashed lines. There is a remarkable overlap between amino acid side chains in the two active-site pockets. The only exception is glutamine-125, whose amide functionality is flipped approximately 180 between the two crystal forms in order to optimize hydrogen-bonding opportunities. See ref. 111 and 112

125 and arginine-176, via two water molecules. Also, the pyrimidine ring is sandwiched and fixed between methionine-128 and tyrosine-172. The 3′-OH in the deoxyribose moiety binds with tyrosine-101 and glutamate-225 and the 5′-OH with glutamate-83. The site also has a domain (LID domain) that closes[111] and is expected to undergo conformational changes upon substrate and ATP binding for phosphoryl-transfer.

Binary complexes of acycloguanosines (i.e., acyclovir, ganciclovir, and penciclovir) with HSV1-TK were also determined by X-ray crystallography at 2.37 Å resolution (Figure 4-15). The guanine base occupies approximately the same geometric plane as the pyrimidine (in thymidine). Similarly, the guanine NH-1 and 6-carbonyl groups form hydrogen bond pairing with glutamine-125 and arginine-176. The hydrogen bond with glutamine-125 involves a conformational shift of the side chain as well as a 180° rotation of the amide. There are only slight variations in the hydrogen-bonding pattern of the guanine moiety among these acycloguanosine analogs. The acycloriboside moiety (in acycloguanosines) and the deoxyribose (in thymidine) are similarly located at the binding site. The single hydroxyl of acyclovir [and the pro-(S)-groups of ganciclovir and penciclovir] mimics the 5'-OH interactions of ribose.[112]

The introduction of radiolabeled fluorine to acycloguanosines[70,113,114] produces structural features that modify their binding parameters (Km, kcat) as well as their catalytic efficiency (kcat/Km) and, as a result, their ability to act as molecular imaging probes (Table 4-6). A combination of two factors decreases substrate specificity for HSV1-TK: 1) Carbon-8 fluorine substitution destabilizes guanine binding by modifying aromatic ring stacking with tyrosine-172 and hydrogen bonding with glutamine-125 and arginine-176, and 2) the simultaneous presence of C-8 fluorine/C-2'-oxygen induces a shift from anti- to a preferred quasi-syn conformation, redirecting the 5'-OH (the phosphoryl acceptor) away from the ATP binding domain. When the fluorine is in the lateral chain, in both ganciclovir and penciclovir, guanine binding characteristics are preserved, and as a result, these compounds present the highest catalytic efficiency (particularly the fluorinated penciclovir analog, FHBG (Tables 4-5[38,39,51–104] and 4-6). These properties are matched by the ability of these radiofluorinated analogs to act as *in vivo* molecular imaging probes (see Chapter 2).

Moreover, the availability of HSV1-TK mutants (e.g., HSV1-sr39TK) with increased efficiency for acycloguanosines and decreased efficiency for endogenous thymidine makes this reporter gene/PET reporter probe system even more attractive for *in-vivo* gene expression determinations.[115]

Probing the functional integrity of neurotransmitter systems

The significance of the dopaminergic system in health and disease states, such as its well determined role in neurodegenerative disorders involving motor function (e.g., Parkinson's disease), emotional disorders (e.g., schizophrenia), and the effects of drugs of abuse (e.g., cocaine and m-amphetamine), has made it the best studied central neurotransmitter system *in vivo*. A plethora of molecular imaging probes have been developed in the last 20 years to evaluate the functional integrity of the dopaminergic system, involving probes of enzyme function acting as substrates (e.g., FDOPA, 4- and 6-[F-18]fluoro-L-m-tyrosine) or binding stoichioimetrically to enzymes (i.e., C-11 deprenyl), probes of the presynaptic dopamine reuptake carrier (e.g., WIN analogs, ritalin, and cocaine), and postsynaptic receptor probes (e.g., dopamine D1, D2, D3, and D4 probes) (Figure 4-16). The dopaminergic system is used in this chapter as an example of how multiple probes have been constructed to dissect the various biochemical components of a neurotransmitter-based cell communication. Reviews of molecular imaging probes for other neurotransmitter systems can be found elsewhere.[116]

Among molecular imaging probes of enzyme function, FDOPA has been exhaustively studied from a mechanistic perspective.[117] FDOPA has already demonstrated its value as a diagnostic tool for movement disorders and its utilization resulted in major discoveries in the neurodegenerative process leading

TABLE 4-6. The Efficiency of Radiolabeled Fluorine Bound to Acycloguanosines to Serve as Molecular Imaging Probes

Compound name	Compound number	R-2	R-6	R-9	R-8	Km (µM)	kcat (s-1)	Kcat/Km (s-1 M-1)	λmax (nm)	E (10-3 M/cm)	Relative imaging efficiency (in vivo) using PET and F-18-labeled substrate
Acyclovir	1	—NH2	—OH		—H	3.87	0.08	20763	250	13.53	NA
8-Fluoroacyclovir	2				—F	221.14	0.11	513	240	4.82	+
Ganciclovir	3				—H	10.23	0.26	25649	250	14.30	NA
8-Fluorogancyclovir	4				—F	396.39	0.4	1004	242	3.91	++
Penciclovir	6				—H	3.55	0.04	11745	252	11.97	NA
8-Fluoropenciclovir	7				—F	11.63	0.07	6452	242	3.23	+++
Rac-side-chain-fluorogancyclovir	5				—H	2.23	0.07	33290	250	13.98	++++
Rac-side-chain-fluoropenciclovir	8				—H	0.94	0.04	45428	250	11.84	+++++

*All compounds dissolved in 50 mM Tris-HCl buffer, pH 7.45. E(10^{-3} M/cm) for guanosine (λ_{max}: 252 nm) = 13.20

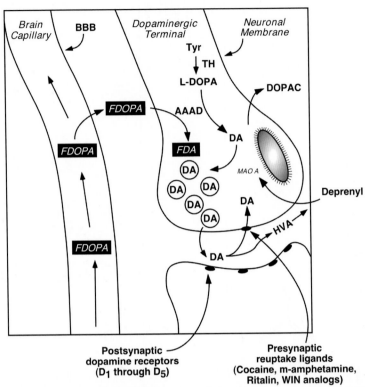

FIGURE 4-16. Schematic representation of a cellular dopaminergic terminal. The use of molecular imaging probes with PET for presynaptic function assessment (e.g., FDOPA) or presynaptic dopamine reuptake ligands (e.g., cocaine) or postsynaptic function (e.g., dopamine D_1-D_5 receptors) permits the biochemical dissection of the system. Abbreviations: AAAD, aromatic L-amino acid decarboxylase; BBB, blood-brain-barrier; DA, dopamine; DOPAC, dihydroxyphenylacetic acid; FDOPA, L-3,4-dihydroxy-6-[18F]fluoro-phenyl-alanine; HVA, homovanillic acid; L-DOPA, levodopa; MAO A, monoamine oxidase A; TH, tyrosine hydroxylase; Tyr, tyrosine.

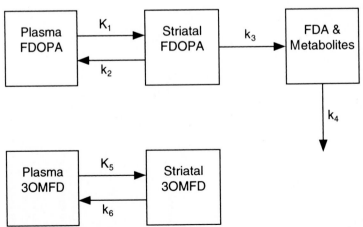

FIGURE 4-17. Compartmental model generally used to describe the tracer kinetics of 6-[18F]fluoro-L-DOPA (FDOPA) in brain tissue.

to Parkinson's disease progression (Chapter 7). As an analog of L-DOPA, FDOPA is decarboxylated by aromatic-L-aminoacid decarboxylase (AAAD) to 6-[F-18]fluorodopamine (FDA) that, like dopamine, accumulates in vesicles in the neurotransmitter terminal. This is a slow turnover rate functional pool with a turnover rate of 0.21 h^{-1}.[118,119] Thus, this trapping mechanism is a variation of the metabolic trapping via phosphorylation illustrated above with FDG/hexokinase and fluoroguanosines (or FIAU)/HSV1-TK. Based on this knowledge, various methods have been used to quantify accumulation of FDA, including simple specific-to-nonspecific ratios[120] and compartmental models with various degrees of complexity. Typically, these models represent reversible competitive transport of FDOPA across the blood-brain-barrier (K1/k2); AAAD-mediated decarboxylation and trapping (k3); and FDA vesicle release, metabolism, and tissue clearance (k4). The formation of peripheral metabolites (i.e., 3-O-methyl-[F-18]fluoro-L-DOPA, 3OMFD) is also represented in the mathematical model (Figure 4-17).

For analysis of the various tracer kinetic models, estimations, and constraints, the reader is referred to the above-mentioned references and Chapter 2.

EXAMPLE 4-9

How does FDOPA decarboxylation rate [k3 (PET)] relate to dopamine synthesis?

ANSWER

Under the conditions of uniform concentration of both enzyme and substrate, the competitive conversion of FDOPA (and L-DOPA) to FDA (or dopamine) follows the Michaelis–Menten equation as described in Equation 4-27. L-DOPA and FDOPA have similar Km and Vm for AAAD (see below), therefore the lumped constant Vm'Km/VmKm' = 1

As a result, Equation 4-27 can be simplified:

$$V = k'3 \ (PET)[S] \qquad (4\text{-}28)$$

Thus, the value of k'3 obtained for FDOPA in the PET determination can be used to estimate the decarboxylation rate of L-DOPA *in vivo*, if the concentration of L-DOPA in tissue is known. Using the average concentration of L-DOPA in striatum of 400 nM[121] and the FDOPA rate constant k'3 of 0.02/min (Table 4-7[114,122–135]), the calculated decarboxylation rate of L-DOPA in striatum is 8 pmol/min/g.

EXAMPLE 4-10

Is this determination reliable? Does the L-DOPA decarboxylation rate measured *in vivo* with PET compare with values?

ANSWER

The PET estimations of L-DOPA utilization rates using FDOPA in humans and nonhuman primates match determinations *in vivo* in rats.[133] They also correlate with AAAD activities in dopaminergic terminals[122] but are far below the 0.3 nmol/min/g rate experimentally measured for dopamine synthesis in rodents[133] and also significantly lower than determinations *in vitro* in the same animal species.[122] Several possible explanations may account for the discrepancy between *in vivo*- and *in*

TABLE 4-7. Summary of Reported *In-Vivo* Striatal Aromatic-L-amino Acid Decarboxylase (AAAD) Rates

Species	Assay description	AAAD activity $[k_3'$ (/min)]	Reference
Human	FDOPA PET	0.024	Gjedde et al. (1991)[123]
Human	FDOPA PET	0.041	Huang et al. (1991)[124,a]
Human	FDOPA PET	0.083	Hoshi et al. (1993)[125]
Human	FDOPA PET	0.021	Ishikawa et al (1996)[126]
Human	FDOPA PET	0.080	Kuwabara et al. (1995)[127]
Human	FDOPA PET	0.012	Nahmias et al. (1996)[128]
Human	6-FMT PET[a]	0.011	Nahmias and Wahl (1995)[129]
Monkey (*Macaca nemestrina*)	FDOPA PET	0.021	Barrio et al. (1990)[130]
Monkey (Vervet)	FDOPA PET	0.015	Barrio et al. (1996)[114]
Monkey (Rhesus)	L-[β-^{11}C]DOPA PET	0.012	Hartvig et al. (1993)[131]
Monkey (Rhesus)	L-[β-^{11}C]DOPA PET	0.011	Tsukada et al. (1996)[132]
Monkey (Vervet)	6-FMT PET[a]	0.033	Barrio et al. (1996)[114]
Rat (Sprague-Dawley)	FDOPA	0.010	Reith et al. (1990)[133]
Rat (Wistar)	[^{3}H]DOPA	0.260	Cumming et al. (1995)[134,b]
Rat (Long-Evans)	FDOPA	0.170	Cumming et al. (1994)[135,b]

Source: Reprinted with permission from Yee et al.[122]

Abbreviations: FDOPA, 6-[F-18]fluoro-L-DOPA; PET, positron emission tomography.

[a]6-FMT, 6-[^{18}F]fluoro-L-*m*-tyrosine.

[b]*Ex-vivo* experiments.

vitro-determined L-DOPA decarboxylation rates (Tables 4-7[114,122–135] and 4-8[122,133,135–143]). They have been summarized as follows:[122]

1. Estimated k_3' values can be impacted by partial volume effects when these determinations are performed in small animals (e.g., squirrel monkeys, total brain size = 25 g). These effects are important when the size of the object (in this case, the object is defined by the area of interest, namely the basal ganglia) is on the same order of the spatial resolution of the PET scanner. Corrections in spill-over may increase k_3' by 2- to 3-fold,[144] but they cannot account for the more than 10-fold underestimation in the k_3' determination.

2. The discrepancy between *in vitro* and *in vivo* decarboxylation rates may be the result of an overestimation of the *in vitro* AAAD activity in striatal tissue from the release of AAAD from nondopaminergic neurons.[145,146] However, only 15% to 20% of AAAD in striatum has nondopaminergic origin.[147]

3. Can differences of Km and Vm between L-DOPA (used *in vitro*) and FDOPA (used *in vivo*) as substrate for AAAD account for the differences? This is unlikely because Km and Vm determined for FDOPA against AAAD (101 μM and 150 nmol/min/g, respectively) are well within the range determined for L-DOPA (40-200 μM and 33-150 nmol/min/g, respectively). Equally important, *in vivo* PET determinations of k_3' with L-[β-C-11]DOPA are also within the range of k_3' values for FDOPA (Table 4-7[114,122–135]).

4. AAAD regulation *in vivo* may play a role because the enzyme needs a cofactor (pyridoxal phosphate) and its absence could be an inactivating mechanism for the enzyme.[148] Other biochemical and pharmacological modulating mechanisms have been identified in the

TABLE 4-8. Summary of Reported *In-Vitro* Aromatic-L-Aminoacid Decarboxylase (AAAD) Activity

Species	Brain region	AAAD activity (ml/min/g)	Reference
Cat	Caudate	0.215[a]	Kuntzman et al. (1961)[136]
Human (Postmortem)	Caudate	0.057	Mackay et al. (1978)[137]
Monkey (Green)	Putamen	—	Goldstein et al. (1969)[138]
Rat (Donryu)	Caudate	0.107	Rahman et al. (1981)[139]
Rat (Wistar)	Striatum	0.447	Broch and Fonnum (1972)[140]
Rat (Sprague–Dawley)	Striatum	0.075	Awapara and Saine (1975)[141]
Rat (Sprague–Dawley)	Striatum	0.090	Hefti et al. (1980)[142]
Rat (Hooded)	Striatum	1.800	Cumming et al. (1994)[135]
Rabbit	Caudate	0.155	McCaman et al. (1965)[143]

Source: Reprinted with permission from Yee et al.[122]

[a]Unit conversion was carried out by dividing AAAD activity determined by the average K_m for AAAD determined from pig kidney enzyme. The average K_m used was 165 μM as determined previously (Reprinted with permission from Reith et al.[133])

regulation of AAAD activity.[149] All these factors may be present *in vivo* and play a role in the down-regulation of AAAD.

5. Multiple compartmentalization of dopamine (and AAAD) within the neuron has been the subject of controversy.[150,151] Is it possible that because of this compartmentalization, the substrate (FDOPA) may have limited accessibility to AAAD *in vivo* and, therefore, the apparent k'_3 determined with PET underestimates the true value? There is considerable evidence for and against these hypotheses in the literature.

6. Is there a limitation on FDOPA access to intraneuronal AAAD? This possibility has been initially suggested[117] and later demonstrated using synaptosomal preparations.[122] Transport restriction rationalizations are supported by the observations that L-DOPA (and FDOPA) are transported competitively across dopaminergic neurons (main competing amino acids are aromatic amino acids, such as phenylalanine, tyrosine, tryptophan) with KD = 2-5 μM, well below the Km of either L-DOPA or FDOPA for AAAD (about 100 μM, see above). Furthermore, to a lesser extent, L-DOPA (and FDOPA) transport across dopaminergic neurons is also subjected to competition by neutral aliphatic amino acids, like leucine, isoleucine and valine.

Thus, even though possibility (4) and (5) above cannot be entirely dismissed, the following conclusions can be established:

1. k'3 (PET) AAAD decarboxylation determined with FDOPA-PET is limited by neuronal transport.

2. The specificity observed with FDOPA-PET for dopaminergic neurons in brain is determined in great measure by neuronal transport access to these terminals. Serotonin terminals also contain AAAD; however, the presence of the abundant aliphatic amino acids in plasma and brain tissue limits FDOPA access to these terminals.

3. These observations may explain results like the on-and-off phenomena in L-DOPA therapy in Parkinson's disease. This clinical effect relates to the apparent lack and resumption of response that Parkinson's patients may have to L-DOPA therapy, particularly af-

ter prolonged treatments. These phenomena may occur because delivery of L-DOPA to the remaining, active central dopaminergic terminals in these patients may be restricted by regulation of gene expression of neuronal aminoacid transporter proteins, coupled with severe competition with plasma amino acids, particularly at the level of the neuronal membrane.

MOLECULAR IMAGING AND DRUG DEVELOPMENT

Many examples of molecular probes used with PET and discussed above have originated from drugs developed by the pharmaceutical industry. The marriage of molecular diagnostics with molecular therapeutics in the field was mainly nurtured by the existence of excellent drugs that target enzymes and receptors that were later adapted as molecular imaging probes. As a result of this interaction, many drug-mimicking imaging probes were developed and their utilization with PET provided insight into their site of action and their time-dependent interaction with these sites. In this regard, earlier advances focused on the design of procedures to define the relationship between plasma levels of drugs and receptor occupancy at the site of action in tissue.[152,153]

Receptor occupancy has been defined as the fraction (%) of the receptor population that is occupied by the unlabeled drug.[152] Because the binding of the imaging probe is stoichiometric and based on saturation kinetics, at high-specific activity the radiolabeled probe occupies only a minimum number of receptor sites. Therefore, when a drug binding to the same site is present, binding of the site by the molecular imaging probe will be reduced based on the amount of unlabeled drug present, its binding affinity for the target (KD), and the number of receptor sites (Bmax).

Receptor occupancy determinations have been made with a number of neuroreceptor probes which have provided an accurate view of the necessary dose of a drug for optimal clinical efficacy and reduced toxicity (Table 4-9).[153] The method has been most extensively applied to the determination of antipsychotic drugs binding.[152] For example, as a result of the utilization of this technique with PET, it was determined that neuroleptic action requires 70% to 80% dopamine-D2 receptor occupancy. Higher receptor occupancy, associated with overdosing, is also frequently associated with side effects involving disturbances of the motor system (extrapyramidal syndromes). Therefore PET is an important tool to optimize patient dose by measuring the target receptor occupancy. Figure 4-18[152] illustrates this principle.

With the advent of microPET cameras (Chapter 1), the use of PET has expanded to drug development,[42] initiated by combining the resources of the pharmaceutical industry with those of the radiopharmaceutical industry, universities, and government facilities. It is anticipated that this continued effort will

TABLE 4-9. Neuroreceptor Quantitation and Occupancy Sites

Drug/Imaging probe	Receptor site
MDL-100, 907/N-[C-11]methylspiperone	5-HT2A receptors
Clomipramine/F-18 setoperone	5-HT2A receptors
Nalnefene/[C-11]carfentanil	Opiate receptors
SDZ MAR 327/[C-11] SCH 23390	Dopamine D_1 receptors

Source: Reprinted from Burns et al.,[153] with permission from Elsevier.

FIGURE 4-18. Suggested distinct thresholds for antipsychotic effects and extrapyramidal syndromes as induced by classical antipsychotic drugs, determined from PET measurement of receptor occupancy. Owing to the hyperbolic relationship between occupancy of the D_2 receptor and dose of antipsychotic drug (or plasma concentration), there is a rather narrow interval for optimal therapeutic treatment. Abbreviation: EPS, extrapyramidal syndromes. (Reprinted from Farde,[152] with permission from Elsevier.)

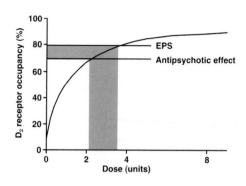

have a profound impact on the process of drug discovery and evaluation, reducing cost, and the time necessary to produce successful drugs for patient care. Such an approach is described in Figure 4-19.

Using the same technology as the one used to produce drugs (i.e., automated devices that perform combinatorial chemistry on solid support), combinatorial radiochemistry has proven effective in producing radiolabeled drugs. This technique, with a single radiolabeled reagent (i.e., C-11 methyl iodide), makes it possible to label large numbers of compounds identical to drug products or as analogs to be tested with microPET technology in mice and humans (Figure 4-20). These approaches will also be explored with other positron-emitting radioisotopes (e.g., F-18). Advantages of this approach include:

1. The solid-phase technology permits easy preparation of these radiolabeled drugs without purification because the only released product is the radiolabeled drug (i.e., Hoffman elimination).
2. MicroPET evaluation of drug candidates in mice (i.e., time-dependent organ distribution, plasma and cell membrane permeability, and mode of excretion) allows for the determination of structural predictors of *in-vivo* behavior based on specific physicochemical properties of these molecules (e.g., partition coeficient, a measure of the affinity of a compound for lipid environments).[154]

FIGURE 4-19. Model approach for discovery and evaluation of molecular imaging probes and drugs. A small number of animal models of disease are evaluated with microPET and molecular imaging probes and with direct biological assays and behavioral assessments. If results are positive, a small number of studies is performed in patients to assess the correlation between animal model and humans (A). In this case, a clinical PET scanner is used to perform the same assays in humans as were performed with microPET in animals. If the correlation is reasonable, larger numbers of animals are studied to better define the properties of the imaging probe or drug (B). A larger number of patient studies are then performed to evaluate an approach in humans with clinical PET (C), which could be used for evaluating drugs or molecular imaging probes.

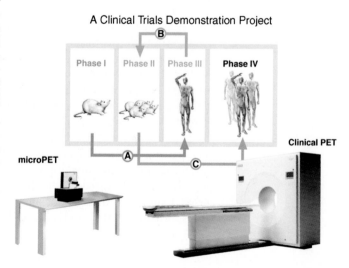

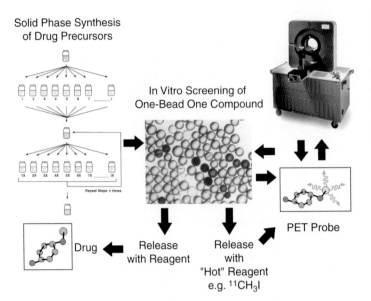

Solid Phase Synthesis
of Drug Precursors

In Vitro Screening of
One-Bead One Compound

PET Probe

Drug ← Release
with Reagent

Release
with
"Hot" Reagent
e.g. $^{11}CH_3I$

FIGURE 4-20. Schematic representation describing the marriage of combinatorial chemistry approaches in drug development and their use to produce radiolabeled versions of those drugs (PET probe) for *in vivo* evaluation with microPET in mice. This concept introduces PET in the early stages for *in vivo* evaluation of promising drug candidates.

It will also allow for the determination of the pharmacokinetic parameters associated with the mode of administration and the *in-vivo* affinity of drug candidates for tissue targets. By a commodity of methods used, microPET study paradigms are then translated to human patients with clinical PET scanners.

3. The data base on the *in-vivo* distribution of drug candidates will facilitate the computational design of new combinatorial libraries using, for example,

EXAMPLE 4-11
In addition to the examples given above, describe *specifically* how PET can be used in the process of drug discovery.

ANSWER
The genome and protein sequencing is increasing the number of targets (i.e., receptors, enzymes, messenger RNA, and genes) for pharmaceutical intervention. The pharmaceutical industry has addressed this challenge by developing combinatorial chemical technology that now permits the synthesis of millions of molecules for specific targets in short periods of time. Microarray and cell culture testing technology has been developed for *in-vitro* assay of the biological properties of these compounds for these targets. What is limiting the drug discovery process is high throughput *in-vivo* biological screening and *in-vivo* testing, a process complicated by the large number of compounds to be tested and the lack of technologies to perform biological screening in living mammals, from mice to humans. The use of labeled drugs and other molecular imaging probes to assess alterations in the biological process targeted by the drug provides the means through microPET and PET to evaluate pharmacokinetics, pharmacodynamics, transport from plasma to tissue, and tissue target occupancy.

pharmacophore fingerprinting[155] based on specific chemical features of the molecules. The application of computational tools to identify structural correlates of *in-vivo* data using various algorithms (i.e., computational informatics) will then: 1) enable the development of predictors of *in-vivo* behavior, 2) increase the likelihood of success when drug candidates are used in humans (clinical trials), and 3) accelerate the drug discovery process.

The combination of all these features, including rapid radiolabeling of thousands of molecules and their *in-vivo* evaluation in rodents, has the power to alter the dynamics of combinatorial chemistry design. It will also allow the rapid introduction of selective, promising drug candidates into rodents, nonhuman primates, and humans using the same radiolabeling concept. Therefore, the energy barrier for introduction of these drugs into clinical trials (Figure 4-19) will be reduced and, most importantly, a much more accurate and scientifically based selection and evaluation of candidate drugs will be achieved.

MAKING MOLECULAR IMAGING PROBES AVAILABLE VIA DISTRIBUTION CENTERS

In the late 1970s and early 1980s, enormous progress was made in the development of PET technology as a result of generous government support in the United States (i.e., Department of Energy and the National Institutes of Health) and abroad. This support resulted in: 1) the development of new cyclotron technology for biomedical use (Chapter 3); 2) synthesis of a wide array of biological imaging probes; 3) design and engineering of new automated synthesis integrated with the new cyclotron technology to yield a new concept of electronic generators (Chapter 3); and 4) new technological developments in instrumentation, leading to high-resolution tomographs (Chapter 1). Research in humans intensified and new observations on the biochemistry of disease, coupled with the technological innovations previously mentioned, paved the way for the clinical utilization of PET. The Food and Drug Administration Modernization Act of 1997[156] also provided the legal basis for a new regulatory paradigm for clinical PET and reimbursement for clinical applications of PET in cancer, as well as neurological and cardiovascular diseases.

Making PET available to patients would not have been possible without radiopharmacy distribution centers, a service that emerged in the mid 1990s and has grown very rapidly since then. Today, FDG, the main radiopharmaceutical used in clinical PET, is available throughout the United States and many parts of Canada, Europe, Japan, Asia, South America, and Australia because of the expansion of these radiopharmaceutical services. However, a new phenomenon is occurring as a result of progress in two major areas: 1) the development of microPET technology (Chapter 1), which has made PET accessible to biological scientists and physicians working on the molecular basis of disease; and 2) the aggressive introduction of the pharmaceutical industry in the field, alerted to the value of PET in the process of drug discovery. The relationship between PET and the pharmaceutical industry provides great value to each. To PET, the pharmaceutical industry provides access to their molecular syntheses, screening technologies, and molecular libraries. To the pharmaceutical industry, PET provides a means to biological screen and evaluate drugs in living mammals, from genetically engineered and human cell transplant models of disease to the ultimate laboratory setting of the patient.

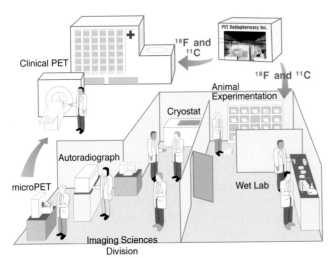

FIGURE 4-21. Relationship between clinical PET services and research and development of PET radiopharmaceuticals. In this model, PET radiopharmacy delivers Food and Drug Administration-approved PET radiopharmaceuticals to clinics. PET radiopharmaceuticals and radioisotopes are also delivered to imaging research laboratories with small-animal imaging modalities such as PET, MRI, single photon emission computed tomography (SPECT), CT, autoradiography, optical imaging systems, and wet laboratories for tissue, cell, and chemical analysis. These laboratories are in universities, radiopharmaceutical companies, or pharmaceutical companies and can focus on discovery of molecular imaging probes or pharmaceuticals or both together. Outcomes are translated into clinical research and, then, clinical practice.

Thus, the concept of integrated PET centers is evolving. The clinician operating a clinical PET service is no longer the only customer of the PET radiopharmacy. The need to make molecular imaging probes (i.e., for transgene expression determinations in animals or drug-mimicking probes) available through distribution centers has become indispensable for rapid growth of PET through biological and pharmacologic research in the new areas of molecular medicine. The delivery of positron-emitting radioisotopes and labeled compounds is indeed similar to the commercial delivery of C-14, H-3, P-32, and I-125 radioisotopes and labeled compounds to research laboratories.

In this new model, several alternatives are evolving, including availability and delivery of: 1) PET radiopharmaceuticals for diagnostic use; 2) imaging probes to research laboratories in hospitals, universities, and the pharmaceutical industry with microPET and PET tomographs for human use; and 3) chemistry precursors to these laboratories. The latter is a convenient avenue for sites that, having access to nearby PET radiopharmacies, may obtain the necessary radiolabeled precursor (i.e., fluoride ion) to prepare PET imaging probes or to labeled experimental probes. This process facilitates new investigations and opens novel pathways from probe discovery to clinical use (Figure 4-21).

REFERENCES

1. Webster's Encyclopedic Unabridged Dictionary of the English Language. New York: Gramercy Books; 1996;564.
2. Mazziotta JC, Phelps ME. In: Phelps ME, Mazziotta JC, Schelbert HR, eds. *Positron Emission Tomography Studies of the Brain in Positron Emission Tomography and Autography.* New York: Raven Press; 1986.
3. Small GW, Ercoli LM, Silverman DHS, et al. Cerebral metabolic and cognitive decline in persons at genetic risk for Alzheimer's disease. *Proc Natl Acad Sci USA.* 2000;97:6037–6042.
4. Huang S-C, Phelps ME. In: Phelps ME, Mazziotta JC, Schelbert HR, eds. *Positron Emission Tomography and Autoradiography: Principles and Applications.* New York: Raven Press; 1986;287–346.
4A. Huang S-C, Barrio JR, Phelps ME. Neuroreceptor assay with positron emission tomography: equilibrium versus dynamic approaches. *J Cereb Blood Flow Metab.* 1986;6:515–521.
5. Welch R, ed. *The Fluctuating Enzyme.* New York: John Wiley and Sons; 1986.

6. Sokoloff L, Reivich M, Kennedy C, et al. The [14C]deoxyglucose method for the measurement of local cerebral glucose utilization: theory, procedure, and normal values in the conscious and anesthetized albino rat. *J Neurochem*. 1977;28:897–916.

7. Sokoloff L. In: Phelps ME, Mazziotta JC, Schelbert HR, eds. *Positron Emission Tomography and Autoradiography*. New York: Raven Press; 1986;1–72.

8. Huang S-C, Phelps ME, Hoffman EJ, et al. Noninvasive determination of local cerebral metabolic rate of glucose in man. *Am J Physiol*. 1980;238:E69–E82.

9. Reivich M, Alavi A, Wolf A, et al. Glucose metabolic rate kinetic model parameter determination in humans: the lumped constants and rate constants for [18F]fluorodeoxyglucose and [11C]deoxyglucose. *J Cereb Blood Flow Metab*. 1985;5:179–192.

10. Hasselbalch SG, Knudsen GM, Madsen PL, et al. Calculation of the FDG lumped constants by extraction fractions of FDG and glucose. *J Cereb Blood Flow Metab*. 1997;17:S440.

11. Hasselbalch SG, Madsen PL, Knudsen GM, et al. Calculation of the FDG lumped constant by simultaneous measurements of global glucose and FDG metabolism in humans. *J Cereb Blood Flow Metab*. 1998;18:154–160.

12. Spence AM, Muzi M, Graham MM, et al. Glucose metabolism in human malignant gliomas measured quantitatively with PET, 1-[C-11]glucose and FDG: analysis of the FDG lumped constant. *J Nucl Med*. 1998;39:440–448.

13. Wu HM, Bergsneider M, Yeh E, et al. XXth International Symposium on Cerebral Blood Flow and Metabolism, Taipei, Taiwan, 2001.

14. Suda S, Shinohara M, Miyaoka M, et al. Local cerebral glucose utilization in hypoglycemia. *J Cereb Blood Flow Metab*. 1981;1:S62.

15. Siesjo BK. *Brain Energy Metabolism*. New York: John Wiley & Sons; 1978.

16. Bessell EM, Thomas P. The effect of substitution at C-2 of D-glucose 6-phosphate on the rate of dehydrogenation by glucose 6-phosphate dehydrogenase (from yeast and from rat liver). *Biochem J*. 1973;13:83–89.

17. Phelps ME, Huang SC, Hoffman EJ, et al. Tomographic measurement of local cerebral glucose metabolic rate in humans with (F-18)2-fluoro-2-deoxy-D-glucose: validation of method. *Ann Neurol*. 1979;6:371–388.

18. Bessell EM, Foster AB, Westwood JH. The use of deoxyfluoro-D-glucopyranoses and related compounds in a study of yeast hexokinase specificity. *Biochem J*. 1972;128:199–204.

19. Walsh C. In: Meister A, ed. *Advances in Enzymology*. New York: John Wiley & Sons; 1983;55:197–289.

20. Sols A, Crane RK. Substrate specificity of brain hexokinase. *J Biol Chem*. 1954;210:581–595.

21. Langen P, Etzold G, Hintsche R, et al. 3'-deoxy-3'-fluorothymidine, a new selective inhibitor of DNA-synthesis. *Acta Biol Med Ger*. 1969;23:759–766.

22. Kong X-B, Zhu Q-Y, Vidal PM, et al. Comparisons of anti-human immunodeficiency virus activities, cellular transport, and plasma and intracellular pharmacokinetics of 3'-fluoro-3'-deoxythymidine and 3'-azido-3'-deoxythymidine. *Antimicrob Agents Chemother*. 1992;36:808–818.

23. Matthes E, Lehmann CH, Scholz D, et al. Inhibition of HIV-associated reverse transcriptase by sugar-modified derivatives of thymidine 5'-triphosphate in comparison to cellular DNA polymerases alpha and beta. *Biochem Biophys Res Commun*. 1987;148:78–85.

24. Sundseth R, Joyner SS, Moore JT, et al. The anti-human immunodeficiency virus agent 3'-fluorothymidine induces DNA damage and apoptosis in human lymphoblastoid cells. *Antimicrob Agents Chemother*. 1996;40:331–335.

25. Grierson JR, Shields AF. Radiosynthesis of 3'-deoxy-3'-[(18)F]fluorothymidine: [(18)F] FLT for imaging of cellular proliferation in vivo. *Nucl Med Biol*. 2000;27:143–156.

26. Shields AF, Grierson JR, Muzik O, et al. Kinetics of 3'-deoxy-3'-[F-18]flurorthymidine uptake and retention in dogs. *Mol Imag Biol*. 2002;4:83–90.

27. Shields AF, Grierson JR, Dohmen BM, et al. Imaging proliferation in vivo with [F-18]FLT and positron emission tomography. *Natl Med*. 1998;4:1334–1336.

28. DeGrado TR, Coleman RE, Baldwin SW, et al. [18F]flurocholine (FCH) as an oncologic PET tracer: evaluation in murine prostate cancer xenograft model. *J Nucl Med*. 2000;41:231P.

29. Friedland RP, Mathis CA, Budinger TF, et al. Labeled choline and phosphorylcholine: body distribution and brain autoradiography: concise communication. *J Nucl Med*. 1983;24:812–815.

30. Hara T, Kosaka N, Shinoura N, et al. PET imaging of brain tumor with [methyl-11C]choline. *J Nucl Med*. 1997;38:842–847.

31. Shinoura N, Nishijima M, Hara T, et al. Brain tumors: detection with C-11 choline PET. *Radiology*. 1997;202:497–503.

32. Hara T, Kosaka N, Kishi H. PET imaging of prostate cancer using carbon-11-choline. *J Nucl Med*. 1998;39:990–995.

33. Kobori O, Kirihara Y, Kosaka N, et al. Positron emission tomography of esophageal carcinoma using (11)C-choline and (18)F-fluorodeoxyglucose: a novel method of pre-operative lymph node staging. *Cancer*. 1999;86:1638–1648.

34. Clary GL, Tsai C-F, Guynn RW. Substrate specificity of choline kinase. *Arch Biochem Biophys*. 1987;254:214–221.

35. Alcoceba HR, Saniger L, Campos J, et al. Choline kinase inhibitors as a novel approach for antiproliferative drug design. *Oncogene*. 1997;15:2289–2301.

36. Gambhir SS, Barrio JR, Herschman HR, et al. Assays for noninvasive imaging of reporter gene expression. *Nucl Med Biol*. 1999;26:481–490.

37. Gambhir SS, Barrio JR, Herschman HR, et al. Imaging gene expression: principles and assays. *J Nucl Cardiol*. 1999;6:219–233.

38. Gambhir SS, Bauer E, Black ME, et al. A mutant herpes simplex virus type 1 thymidine kinase reporter gene shows improved sensitivity for imaging reporter gene expression with positron emission tomography. *Proc Natl Acad Sci USA*. 2000;97:2785–2790.

39. Yu Y, Annala AJ, Barrio JR, et al. Quantification of target gene expression by imaging reporter gene expression in living animals. *Natl Med*. 2000;6:933–937.

40. MacLaren DC, Toyokuni T, Cherry SR, et al. PET imaging of transgene expression. *Biol Psychiatry*. 2000;48:337–348.

41. Crooke ST, Lebleu B. *Antisense and Application*. Ann Arbor: CRC Press; 1993;579.

42. Phelps ME. PET: the merging of biology and imaging into molecular imaging. *J Nucl Med*. 2000;41:661–681.

43. Shi N, Boado RJ, Pardridge WM. Antisense imaging of gene expression in the brain in vivo. *Proc Natl Acad Sci USA*. 2000;97:14709–14714.

44. Fowler JS, MacGregor RR, Wolf AP, et al. Mapping human brain monoamine oxidase A and B with ^{11}C-labeled suicide inactivators and PET. *Science*. 1987;235:481–485.

45. Abeles RH, Maycock AL. Suicide enzyme inactivators. *Acc Chem Res*. 1976;9:313.

46. Trojanowski JQ, Shin R-W, Schmidt ML. Relationship between plaques, tangles, and dystrophic processes in Alzheimer's disease. *Neurobiol Aging*. 1995;16:335–340.

47. Barrio JR, Huang S-C, Cole G, et al. PET imaging of tangles and plaques in Alzheimer's Disease with a highly hydrophobic probe. *J Label Compds Radiopharm*. 1997;42:S194–S195.

48. Shoghi-Jadid K, Small G, Agdeppa ED. Localization of neurofibrillary tangles and beta-amyloid plaques in the brains of living patients with Alzheimer disease. *Am J Geriatr Psychiatry*. 2002;10:24–35.

49. Agdeppa ED, Kepe V, Shoghi-Jadid K, et al. In vivo and in vitro labeling of plaques and tangles in the brain of an Alzheimer's Disease patient: a case study. *J Nucl Med*. 2001;42:65P.

50. Agdeppa ED, Kepe V, Petric A, et al. In vitro detection of (S)—naproxen and ibuprofen binding to plaques in the Alzheimer's brain using the PET molecular imaging probe [18F] FDDNP. *Neuroscience*. 2003;117:723–730.

51. Ray P, Bauer E, Iyer M, et al. Monitoring gene therapy with reporter gene imaging. *Semin Nucl Med*. 2001;31:312–320.

52. Haberkorn U, Oberdorfer F, Gebert J, et al. Monitoring gene therapy with cytosine deaminase: in vitro studies using tritiated-5-fluorocytosine. *J Nucl Med*. 1996;37:87–94.

53. Stegman LD, Rehemtulla A, Beattie B, et al. Noninvasive quantitation of cytosine deaminase transgene expression in human tumor xenografts with in vivo magnetic resonance spectroscopy. *Proc Natl Acad Sci USA*. 1999;96:9821–9826.

54. Tjuvajev JG, Finn R, Watanabe K, et al. Noninvasive imaging of herpes virus thymidine kinase gene transfer and expression: a potential method for monitoring clinical gene therapy. *Cancer Res*. 1996;56:4087–4095.

55. Tjuvajev JG, Chen SH, Joshi A, et al. Imaging adenoviral-mediated herpes virus thymidine kinase gene transfer and expression in vivo. *Cancer Res*. 1999;59:5186–5193.

56. Tjuvajev JG, Joshi A, Callegari J, et al. A general approach to the non-invasive imaging of transgenes using cis-linked herpes simplex virus thymidine kinase. *Neoplasia*. 1999;1:315–320.

57. Haubner R, Avril N, Hantzopoulos PA, et al. In vivo imaging of herpes simplex virus type 1 thymidine kinase gene expression: early kinetics of radiolabelled FIAU. *Eur J Nucl Med*. 2000;27:283–291.

58. Morin KW, Atrazheva ED, Knaus EE, et al. Synthesis and cellular uptake of 2′-substituted analogues of (E)-5-(2-[125I]iodovinyl)-2′-deoxyuridine in tumor cells trans-

duced with the herpes simplex type-1 thymidine kinase gene. Evaluation as probes for monitoring gene therapy. *J Med Chem.* 1997;40:2184–2190.

59. Wiebe LI, Knaus EE, Morin KW. Radiolabelled pyrimidine nucleosides to monitor the expression of HSV-1 thymidine kinase in gene therapy. *Nucleosides Nucleotides.* 1999; 18:1065–1066.

60. Germann C, Shields AF, Grierson JR, et al. 5-Fluoro-1-(2′-deoxy-2′-fluoro-beta-D-ribofuranosyl) uracil trapping in Morris hepatoma cells expressing the herpes simplex virus thymidine kinase gene. *J Nucl Med.* 1998;39:1418–1423.

61. Gambhir SS, Barrio JR, Wu L, et al. Imaging of adenoviral-directed herpes simplex virus type 1 thymidine kinase reporter gene expression in mice with radiolabeled ganciclovir. *J Nucl Med.* 1998;39:2003–2011.

62. Haberkorn U, Altmann A, Morr I, et al. Monitoring gene therapy with herpes simplex virus thymidine kinase in hepatoma cells: uptake of specific substrates. *J Nucl Med.* 1997;38:287–294.

63. Haberkorn U, Khazaie K, Morr I, et al. Ganciclovir uptake in human mammary carcinoma cells expressing herpes simplex virus thymidine kinase. *Nucl Med Biol.* 1998;25:367–373.

64. Iyer M, Barrio JR, Namavari M, et al. 8-[18F]Fluoropenciclovir: an improved reporter probe for imaging HSV1-tk reporter gene expression in vivo using PET. *J Nucl Med.* 2001;42:96–105.

65. Alauddin MM, Conti PS, Mazza SM, et al. 9-[(3-[18F]-fluoro-1-hydroxy-2-propoxy)-methyl] guanine ([18F]-FHPG): a potential imaging agent of viral infection and gene therapy using PET. *Nucl Med Biol.* 1996;23:787–792.

66. Alauddin MM, Shahinian A, Kundu RK, et al. Evaluation of 9-[(3-18F -fluoro-1-hydroxy-2-propoxy)methyl]guanine ([18F]-FHPG) in vitro and in vivo as a probe for PET imaging of gene incorporation and expression in tumors. *Nucl Med Biol.* 1999;26:371–376.

67. de Vries EFJ, van Waarde A, Harmsen MC, et al. [(11)C]FMAU and [(18)F]FHPG as PET tracers for herpes simplex virus thymidine kinase enzyme activity and human cytomegalovirus infections. *Nucl Med Biol.* 2000;27:113–119.

68. Hospers GAP, Calogero A, van Waarde A, et al. Monitoring of herpes simplex virus thymidine kinase enzyme activity using positron emission tomography. *Cancer Res.* 2000;60:1488–1491.

69. Hustinx R, Shiue CY, Alavi A, et al. Imaging in vivo herpes simplex virus thymidine kinase gene transfer to tumour-bearing rodents using positron emission tomography *Eur J Nucl Med.* 2001;28:5–12.

70. Alauddin MM, Conti PS. Synthesis and preliminary evaluation of 9-(4-[18F]-fluoro-3-hydroxymethylbutyl)guanine ([18F]FHBG): a new potential imaging agent for viral infection and gene therapy using PET. *Nucl Med Biol.* 1998;25:175–180.

71. Yaghoubi S, Barrio JR, Dahlbom M, et al. Human pharmacokinetic and dosimetry studies of [(18)F]FHBG: a reporter probe for imaging herpes simplex virus type-1 thymidine kinase reporter gene expression. *J Nucl Med.* 2001;42:1225–1234.

72. Sun X, Annala A, Yaghoubi S, et al. Quantitative imaging of gene induction in living animals. *Gene Ther.* 2001;8:1572–1579.

73. MacLaren DC, Gambhir SS, Satyamurthy N, et al. Repetitive, non-invasive imaging of the dopamine D2 receptor as a reporter gene in living animals. *Gene Ther.* 1999;6:785–791.

74. Yaghoubi SS, Wu L, Liang Q, et al. Direct correlation between positron emission tomographic images of two reporter genes delivered by two distinct adenoviral vectors. *Gene Ther.* 2001;8:1072–1080.

75. Liang Q, Satyamurthy N, Barrio JR, et al. Noninvasive, quantitative imaging in living animals of a mutant dopamine D2 receptor reporter gene in which ligand binding is uncoupled from signal transduction. *Gene Ther.* 2001;8:1490–1498.

76. Rogers BE, McLean SF, Kirkman RL, et al. In vivo localization of [(111)In]-DTPA-D-Phe1-octreotide to human ovarian tumor xenografts induced to express the somatostatin receptor subtype 2 using an adenoviral vector. *Clin Cancer Res.* 1999;5:383–393.

77. Buchsbaum DJ, Rogers BE, Khazaeli MB, et al. Targeting strategies for cancer radiotherapy. *Clin Cancer Res.* 1999;5:3048s–3055s.

78. Rogers BE, Zinn KR, Buchsbaum DJ. Noninvasive monitoring of gene transfer using a reporter receptor imaged with a high-affinity peptide radiolabeled with 99mTc or 188Re. *J Nucl Med.* 2000;41:887–895.

79. Zinn KR, Buchsbaum DJ, Chaudhuri TR, et al. Noninvasive monitoring of gene transfer using a reporter receptor imaged with a high-affinity peptide radiolabeled with 99mTc or 188Re. *J Nucl Med.* 2000;41:887–895.

80. Bogdanov A Jr., Petherick P, Marecos E, et al. In vivo localization of diglycylcysteine-bearing synthetic peptides by nuclear imaging of oxotechnetate transchelation. *Nucl Med Biol.* 1997;24:739–742.

81. Bogdanov A Jr., Simonova M, Weissleder R. Design of metal-binding green fluorescent protein variants. *Biochim Biophys Acta.* 1998;1397:56–64.

82. Baidoo KE, Scheffel U, Stathis M, et al. High-affinity no-carrier-added 99mTc-labeled chemotactic peptides for studies of inflammation in vivo. *Bioconjug Chem.* 1998;9:208–217.

83. Rogers BE, Curiel DT, Mayo MS, et al. Tumor localization of a radiolabeled bombesin analogue in mice bearing human ovarian tumors induced to express the gastrin-releasing peptide receptor by an adenoviral vector. *Cancer.* 1997;80:2419–2424.

84. Rogers BE, Rosenfeld ME, Khazaeli MB, et al. Localization of iodine-125-mIP-Des-Met14-bombesin (7-13)NH2 in ovarian carcinoma induced to express the gastrin releasing peptide receptor by adenoviral vector-mediated gene transfer. *J Nucl Med.* 1997;38:1221–1229.

85. Rosenfeld ME, Rogers BE, Khazaeli MB, et al. Adenoviral-mediated delivery of gastrin-releasing peptide receptor results in specific tumor localization of a bombesin analogue in vivo. *Clin Cancer Res.* 1997;3:1187–1194.

86. Boland A, Ricard M, Opolon, P, et al. Adenovirus-mediated transfer of the thyroid sodium/iodide symporter gene into tumors for a targeted radiotherapy. *Cancer Res.* 2000;60:3484–3492.

87. Haberkorn U, Henze M, Altmann A, et al. Transfer of the human NaI symporter gene enhances iodide uptake in hepatoma cells. *J Nucl Med.* 2001;42:317–325.

88. Enochs WS, Petherick P, Bogdanova A, et al. Paramagnetic metal scavenging by melanin: MR imaging. *Radiology.* 1997;204:417–423.

89. Weissleder R, Simonova M, Bogdanova A, et al. MR imaging and scintigraphy of gene expression through melanin induction. *Radiology.* 1997;204:425–429.

90. Hasgawa S, Yang M, Chishima T, et al. In vivo tumor delivery of the green fluorescent protein gene to report future occurrence of metastasis. *Cancer Gene Ther.* 2000;7:1336–1340.

91. Pfeifer A, Kessler T, Yang M, et al. Transduction of liver cells by lentiviral vectors: analysis in living animals by fluorescence imaging. *Mol Ther.* 2001;3:319–322.

92. Yang M, Baranov E, Jiang P, et al. Whole-body optical imaging of green fluorescent protein-expressing tumors and metastases. *Proc Natl Acad Sci USA.* 2000;97:1206–1211.

93. Yang M, Baranov E, Li XM, et al. Whole-body and intravital optical imaging of angiogenesis in orthotopically implanted tumors. *Proc Natl Acad Sci USA.* 2001;98:2616–2621.

94. Yang M, Hasegawa S, Jiang P, et al. Visualizing gene expression by whole-body fluorescence imaging. *Proc Natl Acad Sci USA.* 2000;97:12278–12282.

95. Yang M, Hasegawa S, Jiang P, et al. Widespread skeletal metastatic potential of human lung cancer revealed by green fluorescent protein expression. *Cancer Res.* 1998;58:4217–4221.

96. Yang M, Jiang P, Sun FX, et al. A fluorescent orthotopic bone metastasis model of human prostate cancer. *Cancer Res.* 1999;59:781–786.

97. Contag CH, Spilman SD, Contag PR, et al. Visualizing gene expression in living mammals using a bioluminescent reporter. *Photochem Photobiol.* 1997;66:523–531.

98. Contag PR, Olomu IN, Stevenson DK, et al. Bioluminescent indicators in living mammals. *Natl Med.* 1998;4:245–247.

99. Bhaumik S, Gambhir SS. Optical imaging of Renilla luciferase reporter gene expression in living mice. *Proc Natl Acad Sci USA.* 2002;99:377–382.

100. Tung CH, Bredow S, Mahmood U, et al. Preparation of a cathepsin D sensitive near-infrared fluorescence probe for imaging. *Bioconjug Chem.* 1999;10:892–896.

101. Tung CH, Mahmood U, Bredow S, et al. In vivo imaging of proteolytic enzyme activity using a novel molecular reporter. *Cancer Res.* 2000;60:4953–4958.

102. Weissleder R, Tung CH, Mahmood U, et al. In vivo imaging of tumors with protease-activated near-infrared fluorescent probes. *Nat Biotechnol.* 1999;17:375–378.

103. Louie AY, Huber MM, Ahrens ET, et al. In vivo visualization of gene expression using magnetic resonance imaging. *Nat Biotechnol.* 2000;18:321–325.

104. Weissleder R, Moore A, Mahmood U, et al. In vivo magnetic resonance imaging of transgene expression. *Natl Med.* 2000;6:351–355.

105. Shand M, Weber F, Mariani L, et al. A phase 1-2 clinical trial of gene therapy for recurrent glioblastoma multiforme by tumor transduction with the herpes simplex thymidine kinase gene followed by ganciclovir. GLI328 European-Canadian Study Group. *Human Gene Ther.* 1999;10:2325–2335.

106. Aghi M, Ting CC, Suling K, et al. Multimodal cancer treatment mediated by a replicating oncolytic virus that delivers the oxazaphosphorine/rat cytochrome P450 2B1 and ganciclovir/herpes simplex virus thymidine kinase gene therapies. *Cancer Res.* 1999;59:3861–3865.

107. Engelmann C, Panis Y, Bolard J, et al. Liposomal encapsulation of ganciclovir enhances the efficacy of herpes simplex virus type 1 thymidine kinase suicide gene therapy against hepatic tumors in rats. *Human Gene Ther.* 1999;10:1545–1551.

108. Kim B, Loeb LA. A screen in Escherichia coli for nucleoside analogs that target human immunodeficiency virus (HIV) reverse transcriptase: coexpression of HIV reverse transcriptase and herpes simplex virus thymidine kinase. *J Virol.* 1995;69:6563–6566.

109. Caruso M, Salomon B, Zhang S, et al. Expression of a Tat-inducible herpes simplex virus–thymidine kinase gene protects acyclovir-treated CD4 cells from HIV-1 spread by conditional suicide and inhibition of reverse transcription. *Virology.* 1995;206:495–503.

110. Bradshaw HD Jr., Deininger PL. Human thymidine kinase gene: molecular cloning and nucleotide sequence of a cDNA expressible in mammalian cells. *Mol Cell Biol.* 1984;4:2316–2320.

111. Pilger BD, Perozzo R, Albers F, et al. Substrate diversity of herpes simplex virus thymidine kinase. Impact of the kinematics of the enzyme. *J Biol Chem.* 1999;274:31967–31973.

112. Champness JN, Bennett MS, Wien F, et al. Exploring the active site of herpes simplex virus type-1 thymidine kinase by X-ray crystallography of complexes with aciclovir and other ligands. *Proteins.* 1998;32:350–361.

113. Alauddin MM, Conti PS, Mazza SM, et al. Synthesis of F-18 9-[(3-fluoro-1-hydroxy-2-propoxy)-methyl]-guanine (FHPG) for in vivo imaging of viral infection and gene therapy with PET. *J Nucl Med.* 1996;37:193P.

114. Barrio JR, Huang S-C, Yu D-C, et al. Radiofluorinated L-m-tyrosines: new in-vivo probes for central dopamine biochemistry. *J Cereb Blood Flow Metab.* 1996;16:667–678.

115. Herschman HR, Barrio JR, Satyamurthy N, et al. In: Curiel DR, Douglas JT, eds. *Monitoring Gene Therapy by Positron Emission Tomography.* New York: Wiley-Liss, Inc. 2002;661–689.

116. Pike VW, Halldin C, Wikstrom H, et al. Radioligands for the study of brain 5-HT(1A) receptors in vivo-development of some new analogues of way. *Nucl Med Biol.* 2000;27:449–455.

117. Barrio JR, Huang S-C, Phelps ME. Biological imaging and the molecular basis of dopaminergic diseases. *Biochem Pharmacol.* 1997;54:341–348.

118. Michael AC, Justice JB Jr., Neill DB. In vivo voltammetric determination of the kinetics of dopamine metabolism in the rat. *Neurosci Lett.* 1985;56:365–369.

119. Wood PL, Kim HS, Stocklin K, et al. Dynamics of the striatal 3-MT pool in rat and mouse: species differences as assessed by steady-state measurements and intracerebral dialysis. *Life Sci.* 1988;42:2275–2281.

120. Shoghi-Jadid K, Huang S-C, Stout DB, et al. Striatal kinetic modeling of FDOPA with a cerebellar-derived constraint on the distribution of volume of 30MFD: a PET investigation using non-human primates. *J Cereb Blood Flow Metab.* 2000;20:1134–1148.

121. Nissbrandt H, Carlsson A. Turnover of dopamine and dopamine metabolites in rat brain: comparison between striatum and substantia nigra. *J Neurochem.* 1987;49:959–967.

122. Yee RE, Huang S-C, Stout DB, et al. Nigrostriatal reduction of aromatic L-amino acid decarboxylase activity in MPTP-treated squirrel monkeys: in vivo and in vitro investigations. *J Neurochem.* 2000;74:1147–1157.

123. Gjedde A, Reith J, Dyne S, et al. Dopa decarboxylase activity of the living human brain. *Proc Natl Acad Sci USA.* 1991;88:2721–2725.

124. Huang S-C, Yu D-C, Barrio JR, et al. Kinetics and modeling of L-6-[^{18}F]fluoro-dopa in human positron emission tomographic studies. *J Cereb Blood Flow Metab.* 1991;11:898–913.

125. Hoshi H, Kuwabara H, Leger G, et al. 6-[^{18}F]fluoro-L-dopa metabolism in living human brain: a comparison of six analytical methods. *J Cereb Blood Flow Metab.* 1993;13:57–69.

126. Ishikawa T, Dhawan V, Chaly T, et al. Clinical significance of striatal DOPA decarboxylase activity in Parkinson's disease. *J Nucl Med.* 1996;37:216–222.

127. Kuwabara H, Cumming P, Yasuhara Y, et al. Regional striatal DOPA transport and decarboxylase activity in Parkinson's disease. *J Nucl Med.* 1995;36:1226–1231.

128. Wahl L, Nahmias C. Modeling of fluorine-18-6-fluoro-L-dopa in humans. *J Nucl Med.* 1996;37:432–437.

129. Nahmias C, Wahl L, Chirakal R, et al. A probe for intracerebral aromatic amino-acid decarboxylase activity: distribution and kinetics of [^{18}F]6-fluoro-L-m-tyrosine in the human brain. *Mov Disord.* 1995;10:298–304.

130. Barrio JR, Huang S-C, Melega WP, et al. 6-[^{18}F]fluoro-L-dopa probes dopamine turnover rates in central dopaminergic structures. *J Neurosci Res.* 1990;27:487–93.

131. Hartvig P, Tedroff J, Lindner KJ, et al. Positron emission tomographic studies on aromatic L-amino acid decarboxylase activity in vivo for L-dopa and 5-hydroxy-L-tryptophan in the monkey brain. *J Neural Transm Gen Sect.* 1993;94:127–135.

132. Tsukada H, Lindner KJ, Hartvig P, et al. Effect of 6R-L-erythro-5,6,7,8-tetrahydro-biopterin and infusion of L-tyrosine on the in vivo L-[beta-11C] DOPA disposition in the monkey brain. *Brain Res.* 1996;713:92–98.

133. Reith J, Dvye S, Kuwabara H, et al. Blood-brain transfer and metabolism of 6-[^{18}F]fluoro-L-dopa in rat. *J Cereb Blood Flow Metab.* 1990;10:707–719.

134. Cumming P, Kuwabara H, Ase A, et al. Regulation of DOPA decarboxylase activity in brain of living rat. *J Neurochem.* 1995;65:1381–1390.

135. Cumming P, Kuwabara H, Gjedde A. A kinetic analysis of 6-[^{18}F]fluoro-L-dihydroxy-phenylalanine metabolism in the rat. *J Neurochem.* 1994;63:1675–1682.

136. Kuntzman R, Shore PA, Bogdanshi D, et al. Microanalytical procedures for fluorometric assay if brain dopa-5HTP decarboxylase, norepinephrine, and seratonin, and a detailed mapping of decarboxylase activity in brain. *J Neurochem.* 1961;6:226–232.

137. Mackay AVP, Davis P, Dewar AJ, et al. Regional distribution of enzymes associated with neurotransmission by monoamines, acetylcholine and GABA in the human brain. *J Neurochem.* 1978;30:827–839.

138. Goldstein M, Anagnoste B, Battista AF, et al. Studies of amines in the striatum in monkeys with nigral lesions. The disposition, biosynthesis and metabolites of [3H]dopamine and [14C]serotonin in the striatum. *J Neurochem.* 1969;16:645–653.

139. Rahman MK, Nagatsu T, Kato T. Aromatic L-amino acid decarboxylase activity in central and peripheral tissues and serum of rats with L-DOPA and L-5-hydroxytryptophan as substrates. *Biochem Pharmacol.* 1981;30:645–649.

140. Broch OJ Jr., Fonnum F. The regional and subcellular distribution of catechol-O-methyl transferase in the rat brain. *J Neurochem.* 1972;19:2049–2055.

141. Awapara J, Saine S. Fluctuations in DOPA decarboxylase activity with age. *J Neurochem.* 1975;24:817–818.

142. Hefti F, Melamed E, Wurtman RJ. Partial lesions of the dopaminergic nigrostriatal system in rat brain: biochemical characterization. *Brain Res.* 1980;195:123–137.

143. McCaman RE, McCaman MW, Hunt JM, et al. Microdetermination of monamine oxidase and 5HTP decarboxylase activity in nervous tissue. *J Neurochem.* 1965;12:15–23.

144. Cumming P, Gjedde A. Compartmental analysis of dopa decarboxylation in living brain from dynamic positron emission tomograms. *Synapse.* 1998;29:37–61.

145. Arai R, Karasawa N, Geffard M, et al. Immunohistochemical evidence that central serotonin neurons produce dopamine from exogenous L-DOPA in the rat, with reference to the involvement of aromatic L-amino acid decarboxylase. *Brain Res.* 1994;667:295–299.

146. Mura A, Jackson D, Manley MS, et al. Aromatic L-amino acid decarboxylase immunoreactive cells in the rat striatum: a possible site for the conversion of exogenous L-DOPA to dopamine. *Brain Res.* 1995;704:51–60.

147. Melamed E, Hefti F, Pettibone DJ, et al. Aromatic L-amino acid decarboxylase in rat corpus striatum: implications for action of L-dopa in parkinsonism. *Neurology.* 1981;31:651–655.

148. Bowsher RR, Henry DP. In: Bowlton AA, Baker JB, and Yu PH, eds. *Neuromethods. Series 1: Neurochemistry, Neurotransmitter Enzymes.* Clifton, NJ: Humana Press; 1986;33–77.

149. Neff NH, Hadjiconstantinou M. Aromatic L-amino acid decarboxylase modulation and Parkinson's disease. *Prog Brain Res.* 1995;106:91–97.

150. Doteuchi M, Wang C, Costa E. Compartmentation of dopamine in rat striatum. *Mol Pharmacol.* 1974;10:225–234.

151. Groppetti A, Algeri S, Cattabeni F, et al. Changes in specific activity of dopamine metabolites as evidence of a multiple compartmentation of dopamine in striatal neurons. *J Neurochem.* 1977;28:193–197.

152. Farde L. The advantage of using positron emission tomography in drug research. *Trends Neuroscience.* 1996;19:211–214.

153. Burns HD, Hamill TG, Eng W, et al. Positron emission tomography neuroreceptor imaging as a tool in drug discovery, research and development. *Curr Opin Chem Biol.* 1999;3:388–394.

154. Lipinski CA, Lombardo F, Dominy BW, et al. Experimental and computational approaches to estimate solubility and permeability in drug discovery and development settings. *Adv Drug Deliv Rev.* 1997;23:3–25.

155. McGregor MJ, Muskal SM. Pharmacophore fingerprinting. 1. application to QSAR and focused library design. *J Chem Inform Comp Sci.* 1999;39:569–574.

156. Food and Drug Administration Modernization Act of 1997. Public Law 105–115-Nov. 21, 1997.

CHAPTER 5

Oncological Applications of FDG-PET

Johannes Czernin

In 1924, the German biochemist Otto Warburg and colleagues published their observations on the metabolism of cancer cells.[1] They posed the fundamental question of the metabolism of tumors as follows: "If the carcinoma problem is attacked in its relation to the physiology of metabolism, the first question is: In what way does the metabolism of growing tissue differ from the metabolism of resting tissue? The prospects of finding an answer are good."

Flexner and Jobling studied the metabolism of tumor cells in a rat model[2] and found that the glycolytic rates of tumors were 124 times greater than the glycolytic action of blood. Carcinoma tissue produced 200 times as much lactic acid as a resting frog's muscle and 8 times more than a working frog's muscle. They proceeded to evaluate the contribution of oxidative and cleavage (i.e., anaerobic) metabolism to overall tumor metabolism and observed that of 13 sugar molecules metabolized, only 1 was oxidized while the rest were fermented. From these and other observations, they concluded that the metabolism of rat tumor cells is predominantly one of glycolysis. They subsequently confirmed these findings in a variety of human cancer cells and uncovered that benign tumors also exhibited increased glycolytic activity but to a much smaller degree than malignant tumors. The marked amplification of glycolysis in tumor cells is necessary because oxidative metabolism is not increased, yet metabolic demand is.

Normally, 2 adenosine triphosphates (ATP) are generated from the metabolism of glucose to lactate (i.e., glycolysis), while 36 ATPs are generated by complete oxidation of a molecule of glucose in the tricarboxylic cycle (TCA). Thus, with loss of the TCA cycle, there is a 19-fold increase in glycolysis to yield an equivalent amount of ATP. In addition, accelerated rates of the hexose monophosphate pathway provide the carbon backbone for DNA and RNA synthesis in growing tumors.[3,4] To meet the high glycolytic rates, glucose transporters in tumor cell membranes and expression of hexokinase are also increased.[5,6] These alterations of cellular glucose metabolism are common to a wide variety of neoplastic cells.

Cancer is now understood as a systemic disease resulting from alterations in the interactions between oncogenes and tumor suppressor genes, which under physiological conditions control cell maturation, division, and migration. Traditionally, the diagnostic armamentarium for diagnosing, staging and restaging of patients with cancer relied on anatomic imaging with computed tomography (CT), magnetic resonance imaging (MRI), and ultrasound (US). These techniques cannot reliably discriminate between benign and malignant tumors or between post-therapeutic anatomical alterations such as scarring, inflammation or necrosis, and neoplastic processes. Further, these techniques are used to examine only certain arbitrary sections of the body, such as chest, abdomen, or pelvis rather than addressing cancer as a systemic disease of the whole human organism.

The biological alterations of tumor cells, uncovered more than 70 years ago together with more than 30 years of fundamental technical research since the original development of the positron emission tomography (PET) scanner,[7] have resulted in the emergence of molecular, whole-body imaging of disease with PET and the glucose analogue 2-deoxy-2-[F-18]fluoro-D-glucose [FDG].[8–12] After intravenous injection, FDG is taken up by tumor cells and phosphorylated by hexokinase to FDG-6-PO$_4$. Unlike glucose-6-PO$_4$, FDG-6-PO$_4$ is not metabolized further in the glycolytic pathway. It remains trapped intracellularly because tumor cells do not contain significant amounts of glucose-6-phosphatase to reverse this reaction during the time of the procedure. Therefore, the whole body distribution of FDG-6-PO$_4$ in normal and abnormal tissue can be imaged with PET (Figure 5-1).

The rate of glucose metabolism differs between benign and malignant neoplasia and has been shown to be inversely related to the degree of differentiation of tumor cells[13–15] (i.e., glucose metabolism increases with increasing neoplastic degeneration). Increased glucose metabolism is, however, not unique to malignant tissue. Some benign tumors such as adenomas, fibroids (Figure 5-2) inflammatory tissue (Figure 5-3), and normal tissue (Figure 5-4) can also exhibit accelerated rates of glucose metabolism. Thus, benign tumors, as well as

FIGURE 5-1. Tracer kinetic model for FDG illustrating forward and reverse transport between plasma and tissue, as well as hexokinase-mediated phosphorylation. The Xs denote that reactions do not significantly occur during the PET study time. A general exception to this is dephosphorylation of FDG-6-PO$_4$ in the liver during states in which glucose is being supplied to plasma from the liver and phosphatase activity is high. PET scans to the right are coronal and saggital images of a patient with nonsmall cell carcinoma of the lung (arrow). Black indicates the highest rate of glycolysis in this and all images in this chapter.

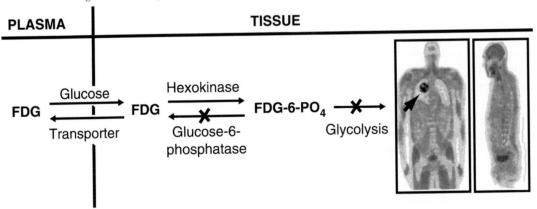

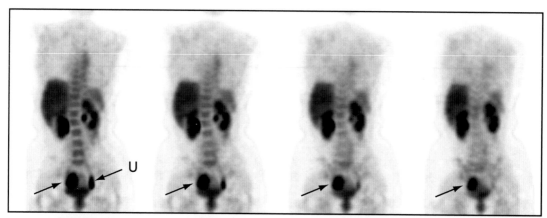

FIGURE 5-2. Whole-body PET obtained in a 57-year-old woman patient with lower p61487 abdominal pain. Images revealed increased glycolysis in the right lower pelvis, which was subsequently confirmed as uterine fibroid. Physiological urethral tracer activity (U) is present. Images from left to right are at levels more anterior to more posterior. This format is used throughout this chapter.

acute or chronic inflammation or physiologic processes, can result in false positive scan results. For instance, contracting striated muscle might result in false positive FDG–PET findings for cancer. With greater interpretive experience, however, increases in glycolysis in normal or benign tissue can very frequently be differentiated from malignancy.

This chapter reviews the clinical role and diagnostic accuracy of FDG–PET for diagnosing, staging, and restaging of the most important cancers in the context of

FIGURE 5-3. A 65-year-old patient with hemoptysis is evaluated for lung cancer. Intense FDG-uptake is present at the level of the subcarinal nodes bilaterally (LN). Subsequent histological and cytological evaluation revealed abundance of histiocytes and asbestos bodies. Thus, the diagnosis of asbestosis was established. Notice the physiologically increased cardiac tracer uptake (C). This occurs in up to 50% of all patients despite fasting. Prominent tracer accumulation in the bilateral kidneys (K) and the urinary bladder (B) is also observed.

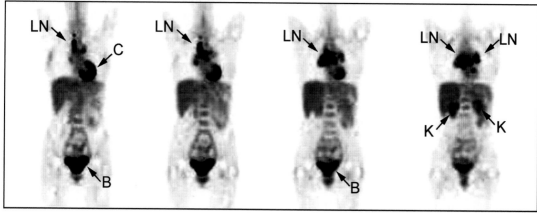

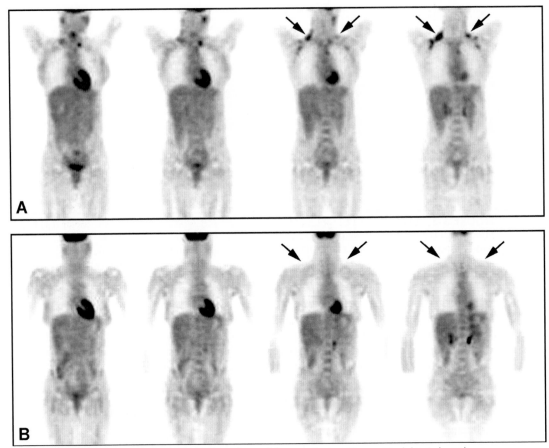

FIGURE 5-4. Whole body PET performed in a patient with nonHodgkin's lymphoma. A: Coronal images demonstrate intense and somewhat asymmetrical FDG-uptake in the bilateral supraclavicular region (arrows). Thus, residual lymphoma could not be ruled out with certainty. B: Patient was restudied after 1 mg of Ativan was administered intravenously. The bilateral supraclavicular uptake was no longer seen. Thus, increased neck muscle activity accounted for the increased FDG uptake in the neck.

other diagnostic imaging modalities. The use of PET for monitoring various cancer treatments will be discussed. When available, the prognostic value, cost-effectiveness, and impact on patient management of FDG–PET will be reviewed. It is acknowledged that a complete review of the published literature is beyond the scope of this chapter. Such a comprehensive review has recently been accomplished by Gambhir et al.[16] Every attempt is made, however, to include literature references that document the accuracy and value of PET in patient management.

CLINICAL PET IMAGING OF GLYCOLYSIS WITH FDG

State-of-the-art PET instrumentation is discussed in Chapter 1. It should be recognized however, that metabolic imaging can be accomplished with various scintillation cameras that are capable of coincidence imaging,[17–19] although with lower accuracy for smaller lesions.

Several groups have investigated the effects of dietary state and metabolic conditions on FDG uptake of tumors in cancer patients.[20,21] For these studies, patients were examined after fasting and again following an oral or intravenous glucose challenge. Both studies revealed higher semiquantitative indices of tumor-FDG uptake in the fasted state than after glucose loading. However, neither of the studies reported an effect of the dietary state on the diagnostic accuracy of PET. Another study[22] did report a reduced accuracy of FDG-PET for detecting liver metastases in patients with high serum glucose levels due to the retention of FDG-6-PO$_4$ in normal liver cells that results from low dephosphorylation by glucose-6-phosphatase in states of high plasma glucose. In this study, 6 of 20 metastatic liver lesions were missed when PET was performed during intravenous glucose application. The clinical benefit of intravenous insulin application in patients with elevated serum glucose levels remains controversial. Patients are routinely studied with PET after an overnight fast. Patients with diabetes mellitus are asked to continue their medication, and, if feasible, to remain in a fasting state. Despite fasting, considerable cardiac glucose metabolic activity is present in up to 50% of all patients (Figure 5-4). This increased myocardial FDG uptake would be further enhanced after insulin administration. No method has yet been found to consistently reduce the myocardial FDG uptake that potentially compromises the visualization of tumors in close proximity to the heart.

The commonly used intravenous dose of 0.21 mCi/kg is administered up to a maximum of 15 mCi. FDG-6-phosphate accumulation in tumors approaches its maximum at about 2 h after tracer injection with additional slow increase thereafter.[21,23,24] However, for practical purposes and to improve patient throughput, an uptake period of 45 minutes to 60 minutes usually suffices to achieve high tumor to background activity ratios (Figure 5-5).

After completion of the uptake period, patients are asked to void in order to allow for a better assessment of pelvic structures. Patients are subsequently

FIGURE 5-5. Patient with indeterminate solitary pulmonary nodule by CT was studied with PET. The solitary pulmonary nodule of the left upper lobe (arrows) exhibited increased metabolic activity. In addition, left hilar/mediastinal lymphadenopathy (arrow head) was identified by FDG-PET. This nodule was subsequently diagnosed by mediastinoscopy and biopsy as nonsmall cell lung cancer with ipsilateral lymph node involvement. Thus, the patient's stage was changed from I to IIIA.

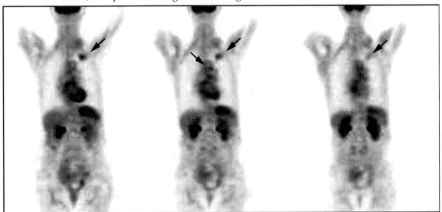

escorted to the imaging room and positioned on the imaging table in the supine position. The image acquisition sequence then commences.

Images are acquired for sufficient bed positions to cover the body from the mid thigh level to the base of the skull.[25] Transmission images are performed for each bed position to allow for appropriate attenuation correction. Image reconstruction is performed using either convolution-based or algebraic algorithms.[26,27]

On-line reconstruction allows for image review before patients leave the imaging suite. It is good medical practice to do this in every patient. For instance, substantial residual tracer activity in the bladder might obscure the view of the pelvic structures (see Figure 5-3). In this case, patients are asked to void, and the area of interest is re-imaged. In routine procedures, catheterization is not performed to reduce FDG activity in the bladder. Catheterization and irrigation of the bladder is used in some clinics for the imaging of primary prostate cancer.

Images are read on the computer screen, permitting the display of 3-dimensional (3-D) projection images, as well as of reoriented coronal, transaxial, and sagittal planes. Images are interpreted visually or semiquantitatively using indices such as the standardized uptake value [SUV = count activity per milliliter within region of interest (MBq^{-1})/[injected dose (MBq)/body weight $(kg \times 1000)$]. Lowe et al.[28] systematically analyzed the additional diagnostic value of these approaches in 107 patients with indeterminate solitary pulmonary nodules. Visual image analysis was as accurate as the semiquantitative approach for determining whether lung nodules were malignant or benign. These authors also investigated the usefulness of other semiquantitative approaches that included maximum and average activity ratios between pulmonary abnormalities and the contralateral, unaffected lung. As a limitation of their study, no correction for partial volume effects was performed. The authors concluded that none of the semiquantitative approaches helped to characterize pulmonary nodules with a higher diagnostic accuracy than visual analysis. Others confirmed these observations.[29] The fundamental limitations of these semiquantitative approaches have been discussed extensively.[24] However, SUVs might be useful to monitor the effects of therapeutic interventions if the interval from injection to image acquisition is identical, if regions of interest are placed in the exact same region, and if partial volume corrections are used.[30]

CURRENT CLINICAL APPLICATIONS OF FDG-PET IN ONCOLOGY

Solitary pulmonary nodules

Solitary pulmonary nodules (SPN) are defined as single, rounded lung lesions not associated with any other lung lesions or lymphadenopathy, measuring less than or equal to 3 cm in maximal diameter. Lesions larger than 3 cm are referred to as pulmonary masses. These nodules are most frequently detected incidentally by x-ray films or CT of the chest. Approximately 150,000 new solitary pulmonary nodules are diagnosed in the United States each year. The incidence of malignancy exceeds 40% in the large majority of reports on solitary pulmonary nodules.[31,32] Benign SPNs might represent granuloma, infections, carcinoid, adenoma, hamartoma, fibrosis, and others. Bronchogenic carcinoma represents the majority of malignant solitary pulmonary nodules. The considerable number of benign solitary pulmonary nodules implies that a large number of biopsies performed are unnecessary. For example, 20% to 40% of lung biopsies produce benign tissue but significant morbidity.[31,32]

Several morphological criteria have been used in conjunction with CT in an attempt to characterize SPNs as malignant or benign. These include size, calcification, shape, lobulation, cavitation, and others. Measurements of the density of the nodule by CT, which are based on the absorption coefficients in tissue expressed as Hounsfield units, provide a more quantitative analysis of SPNs but are rarely performed in routine clinical settings. However, even such sophisticated analysis results in a large number of indeterminate lung lesions which often are benign on histopathological evaluation.[33] Thus, improvements in diagnostic accuracy are desirable to reduce the number of unnecessary lung biopsies in patients who have benign solitary pulmonary nodules.

To our knowledge Kubota et al[34] were the first to evaluate the potential role of FDG–PET for characterizing solitary pulmonary nodules in 22 patients. The diagnostic accuracy of FDG-PET was 86%, with a sensitivity of 83% and a specificity of 90%. Two false negative cases occurred. Similar accuracy data were reported by others[28,29,34–41] (Table 5-1, Figure 5-5).

Dewan and coworkers[42] compared a standard Bayesian approach to establish the likelihood for malignancy which included patient age, history of smoking, history of previous malignancy, size and edge of the nodule by CT, and degree of calcification, to the probability of cancer based on PET findings. A positive PET scan was associated with a likelihood ratio for malignancy of 7.1 (95% confidence interval: 6.36–7.96) while the likelihood ratio for a negative PET was 0.06 (95% confidence interval: 0.05–0.07). PET alone was more accurate than the standard criteria in correctly classifying solitary pulmonary nodules in 55 patients. These and other data were used to determine the cost-effectiveness of PET for characterizing solitary pulmonary nodules.

The notion that PET imaging adds to the costs associated with the workup of patients with lung nodules was refuted by Gambhir et al.[43] These authors conducted a sophisticated decision-tree sensitivity analysis that takes into account the pretest likelihood for malignancy, costs of imaging tests as well as down-

TABLE 5-1. FDG–PET for Solitary Pulmonary Nodules

Author	Ref #	Year	N	SENS (%)	SPEC (%0	PPV (%)	NPV (%)	Criteria	ACC (%)
Kubota et al	34	1990	22	83	90	91	82	Visual	86
Dewan et al	35	1993	30	95	80	90	89	Visual	90
Patz et al	36	1993	51	89	100	100	77	SUR > 2.5	92
Lowe et al	28	1994	197	96	77	86	92	SUR>2.5	88
Duhaylongsod et al	37	1995	87	97	82	92	92	SUR > 2.5	92
Gupta et al	29	1996	61	93	88	92	82	Visual	92
Knight et al	38	1996	27	100	72	64	100	SUR>2.5	81
Bury et al	39	1996	50	100	88	94	100	Visual	96
Lowe et al	41	1998	89	92	90	90	92	SUR > 2.5	91
				98	69	—	—	Visual	89
Weighted Average				95	84	89	90		90

Abbreviations: ACC, accuracy; N, number of patients; NPV, negative predictive value; PPV, positive predictive value; SENS, sensitivity; SPEC, specificity; SUR, standardized uptake ratio; SUV, standardized uptake value; —, could not be determined.

stream costs associated with invasive and noninvasive procedures. This study provided evidence that a strategy combining chest CT and FDG–PET was most cost-effective for managing patients with SPN.

Because of its high diagnostic accuracy and cost-effectiveness, FDG–PET has been incorporated into the clinical workup of solitary pulmonary nodules. The current standard of practice is to perform FDG–PET in every patient with an indeterminate solitary pulmonary nodule. Referring physicians should, however, be cautioned that false-negative PET findings can occur if lung nodules are smaller than 1 cm. Because the sensitivity of FDG–PET is less than 100%, each negative PET study needs to be followed by CT within 3 months of the PET study to rule out morphological interval changes. Conversely, because of the high-positive predictive value of FDG–PET, each positive scan needs to be considered suspicious for malignancy until proven otherwise by histology.

Lung cancer

Clinical background

Lung cancer is the most common cancer in the world. Its incidence is increasing largely due to a continuing rise of smoking cigarettes in women. There were an estimated 180,000 new cases and around 160,000 cancer deaths in 1996. The 5-year survival rate of lung cancer patients remains disappointingly low at 13%. Surgical removal of the tumor represents the only curative treatment.[44]

A 4-point staging system based on the tumor stage at the time of diagnosis has been adopted worldwide. The outcome of patients can be predicted from the clinical stage with reasonable accuracy.[45] For instance, the 5-year survival of patients with mediastinal lymph node involvement is only about 10% while it is about 50% in patients without mediastinal node involvement. Patients with stage I through stage III A disease (i.e., those with only ipsilateral lymph node involvement) are considered surgical candidates while those with contralateral lymph node or lung involvement (stage III B) or distant disease (stage IV) are not.

Current anatomic imaging results in considerable numbers of patients who are understaged when compared to the findings at surgery.[46] Importantly, the size of lymph nodes cannot be used reliably to predict the presence of cancer metastases in lymph nodes.

McKenna et al[47] conducted a prospective study in 102 lung cancer patients to determine the accuracy of chest CT for mediastinal lymph node staging. Using pathological findings from thoracotomy and mediastinal nodal dissection, these authors reported an overall accuracy of CT of only 61%. The authors concluded that "enlarged nodes need not contain metastases and normal-appearing small nodes may harbor microscopic disease." Arita et al[48] examined the incidence of metastases in normal-sized lymph nodes as determined by CT in 90 patients with nonsmall cell lung cancer. These authors found lymph node metastases in 19 (21%) of their patients. Importantly, metastatic lymph nodes were of normal size in 14 (74%) of these 19 patients. Thus, size criteria fail to reliably identify lymph nodes that harbor cancer. The Radiologic Diagnostic Oncology Group[49] provided even more disappointing findings for mediastinal staging with CT and MRI. The sensitivity and specificity of CT was 52% and 48%, respectively, while for MRI it was 69% and 64%, respectively.

Histopathological findings obtained through mediastinoscopy are frequently used as the gold standard for staging of the mediastinum. Using surgical findings as the gold standard, the validity of mediastinoscopy was questioned by Dillemans and coworkers in 569 patients[50] with a presumed resectable nonsmall cell lung cancer. Using a cutoff point of 1.5 cm for defining lymph nodes as malignant, these authors reported sensitivity, specificity, and accuracy of 69%, 71%, and 71%, respectively, for CT. Importantly, the sensitivity of mediastinoscopy was also found to be only 72% and its negative predictive value was 84%. Thus, a considerable number of abnormal mediastinal lymph nodes are missed by mediastinoscopy.

Mediastinal staging with PET (Figure 5-6)

Dwamena et al[51] conducted a metaanalysis to compare the performance of PET and CT for mediastinal lymph node staging in lung cancer patients (Table 5-2). Using stringent selection criteria, this analysis included 514 lung cancer patients studied with PET (included in 14 published studies) and 2,226 patients evaluated with CT (derived from 29 published studies). They concluded that both sensitivity (79% versus 60%) and specificity (91% versus 77%) for correctly classifying mediastinal lymph nodes was higher for PET than for CT.

Fujuwara et al[52] were the first, to our knowledge, to report increased FDG uptake in malignant lung tumors of 6 patients. Nolop and coworkers[53] expanded these initial observations and demonstrated that the rate of uptake of FDG in tumor tissue was on the average more than 6 times higher than that of the contralateral, unaffected lung.

In a retrospective study[54] of 62 patients, FDG–PET correctly identified all but three primary tumors. The same group[55] subsequently compared CT and PET prospectively for staging of the mediastinum and concluded from their results in 27 patients that PET was significantly more accurate than CT (sensitivity 100% vs 67%, specificity: 98% vs 93%, positive predictive value: 91% vs 60%).

Several large retrospective and prospective trials have subsequently established the superiority of PET over CT for mediastinal lymph node staging.[37,56–58] More specifically, Patz and coworkers[59] reported a higher diagnostic accuracy of PET for mediastinal than for hilar/lobar lymph nodes. Importantly, these au-

FIGURE 5-6. Patient with known nonsmall cell lung cancer of the left midlung. FDG–PET revealed contralateral superior mediastinal lymph node involvement (LN), subsequently confirmed by biopsy. In addition, a small focus of increased uptake in the right upper posterior chest wall was diagnosed as metastasis of a posterior rib (R). The large primary tumor was located in the posterior left midlung field (P). Patient management was changed from surgery to chemotherapy and radiation treatment.

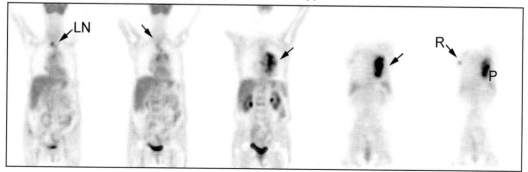

TABLE 5-2. Estimates of Accuracy and Predictive Values of FDG–PET for Mediastinal Lymph Node Staging

	PET	CT
SENS (%)	72	60
SPEC (%)	91	77
PPV (%)	90	50
NPV (%)	93	85
ACC (%)	92	75

Source: Data from Dwamena et al.[51]

Abbreviations: ACC, accuracy; CT, computerized tomography; NPV, negative predictive value; PET, positron emission tomography; PPV, positive predictive value; SENS, sensitivity; SPEC, specificity.

thors concluded that normal PET findings in regards to thoracic nodes obviate the need for mediastinoscopy. In another study of 35 patients,[60] the accuracy of PET for determining N0, N1, N2, and N3 disease was 100%, 60%, 82%, and 100%, respectively. These values were significantly higher than those reported for CT (75%, 40%, 54%, 50%, and 59%). The overall accuracy differed significantly between the two modalities ($p < 0.02$).

In a large retrospective analysis that included 100 consecutive patients with newly diagnosed bronchogenic carcinoma, Marom et al[61] compared the diagnostic accuracy of whole-body PET to that of conventional imaging that included chest CT, bone scintigraphy, and brain CT or MRI. The PET and CT findings were verified with biopsy or surgery. The stage derived with PET was correct in 83% as compared to 65% for all conventional anatomic imaging modalities combined ($p < 0.005$). These authors concluded that PET was superior to anatomical imaging and cost-effective for the staging of newly diagnosed lung cancer.

A diagnostic algorithm as proposed by Vansteenkiste et al[62] is shown in Figure 5-7. In this study, FDG–PET substantially reduced the number of staging mediastinoscopies.

Mediastinal staging with PET plus CT

Chin et al[63] reported a series of 30 patients studied with PET and CT to determine mediastinal lymph node involvement. They concluded that the combined information of PET and CT yielded the highest diagnostic accuracy (90%). Weng et al[64] also reported a higher diagnostic accuracy for PET plus CT than for PET or CT alone for lung cancer staging.

A similar study was conducted by Magnani et al.[65] Their study of 28 patients with nonsmall cell lung cancer used the coregistration of CT and PET images of the chest. Using histopathological findings as the gold standard, 25 of 28 patients were staged correctly with PET plus CT while only 21 and 22 patients were staged correctly with CT or PET alone. PET/CT image fusion resulted in a sensitivity of 78% and a specificity of 95% with a diagnostic accuracy of 89%.

Vansteenkiste et al[66] compared the accuracy of visually analyzed FDG–PET and CT images to that of computed tomography alone for the mediastinal staging of 68 lung cancer patients. State-of-the-art spiral CT and a dedicated whole-body PET scanner were used. Invasive surgical staging served as the gold standard in all patients for a total of 690 lymph node stations. Overall, the diagnostic accuracy was better for PET plus CT than CT alone (87% vs 59%). Importantly,

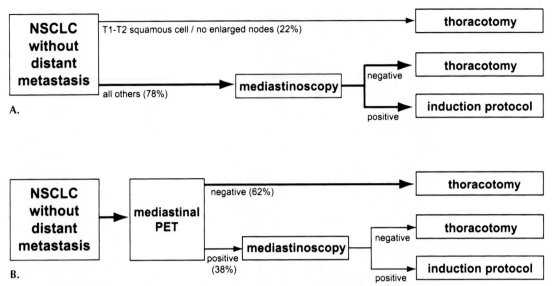

FIGURE 5-7. Proposed algorithm for the mediastinal staging of lung cancer patients: A: CT-based staging: T1/T2 tumors without enlarged lymph nodes (22% of the patients) undergo thoracotomy without the need for further mediastinoscopic evaluation. All others undergo mediastinoscopy followed by thoracotomy or induction protocol. B: PET-based algorithm: Patients with negative mediastinal PET (62% of the patients) proceed directly to thoracotomy. To avoid the consequences of a false positive PET study, all patients with mediastinal abnormalities by PET undergo mediastinoscopy. Notice that 62% of mediastinal PET studies but only 22% of mediastinal CT studies were negative. Thus, PET results in a significantly lower number of mediastinoscopies. (Reprinted from Vansteenkiste et al.,[62] with permission from Elsevier.)

PET plus CT was also superior to CT alone for detecting locally advanced disease (N2/N3). Sensitivity, specificity, and accuracy of CT alone were 75%, 63%, and 68% vs 93%, 95%, and 94% for PET plus CT, respectively (p = 0.0004). Based on their findings of a very high negative predictive value of PET, these authors reported that mediastinoscopy could have been omitted in 29 of 68 patients. On the other hand, although the positive predictive value of PET was high, patients should not be denied a chance for potentially curative surgery because of a potentially false positive PET. Thus, patients without mediastinal involvement by PET may be treated surgically without the need for staging mediastinoscopy. Those, with PET positive findings for mediastinal lymph node involvement should undergo mediastinoscopy to rule out false positive PET findings.

Clinical devices that combine PET and CT within a single device are undergoing initial testing[67,68] (Figure 5-8). These anatomical and biological imaging devices are likely to greatly facilitate the interpretation of metabolic and anatomical alterations and will result in improved staging of the mediastinum. Importantly, they will allow the most accurate biological and anatomical lung cancer staging in a single examination.

Staging for distant disease
Several authors addressed the role of PET for detecting distant metastatic disease. In a study of 99 lung cancer patients, Valk et al[69] identified distant dis-

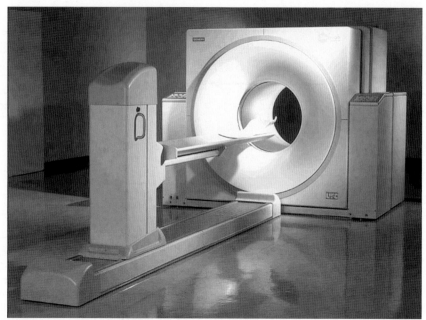

FIGURE 5-8. The combined lutetium oxyorthosilicate-positron emission tomography (LSO–PET) dual slice spiral CT device currently in use at the author's institution. PET/CT imaging allows for near ideal fusion between anatomical and molecular images. PET lesion localization is greatly facilitated by this device. Using a weight-based protocol, whole-body PET/CT studies are completed within 7 minutes to 25 minutes depending on patient weight.

ease unsuspected by conventional imaging in 11% of the patients. Unknown lesions were located in the skeleton (n = 5), liver (n = 3), periportal region (n = 1), and soft tissue (n = 2). In addition, PET and CT concordantly detected metastatic disease in 7% of the patients. In this study, PET yielded no false positive results while CT findings were false positive in 19% of the patients.[69]

Weder et al[70] examined 94 patients with stages less than or equal to IIIA for the presence of extrathoracic metastases. Using histology or radiological followup as the gold standard, these authors reported that FDG–PET uncovered unknown distant disease in 15% of all patients. The metastatic lesions detected by PET were located in the bones (n = 13), liver (n = 3), adrenal gland (n = 4), supraclavicular nodes (n = 3), and central nervous system (n = 1). Bury et al[71] expanded these observations by comparing the accuracy of all conventional imaging to that of PET in patients with nonsmall cell lung cancer. Specifically, they addressed the accuracy of these modalities for mediastinal staging and for determining distant metastatic disease in 109 patients. Conventional imaging included chest and abdominal CT and bone scintigraphy. FDG–PET was superior to a combination of conventional imaging for mediastinal staging (sensitivity: 89% vs 79%; specificity: 87% vs 71%; accuracy: 88% vs 75%). Importantly, all 59 sites of distant metastases were detected accurately with FDG–PET. There were no false negative findings. In contrast, 19 of the 59 metastatic sites were not detected by conventional imaging. The sensitivity of PET for distant metastases was 100% with a specificity of 91%. By contrast, conventional imaging had a sensitivity of 80% and a specificity of 90%. Thus, PET provided equivalent or better staging information than the combined use of conventional imaging.

Pieterman and coworkers[72] prospectively compared the standard CT approach for staging of the mediastinum to one involving PET in 102 patients prior to surgical resection. The sensitivity and specificity of PET for the detection of mediastinal metastases were 91% (95% CI: 81% to 100%) and 86% (95% CI: 78% to 94%), which was significantly more accurate than CT [sensitivity and specificity of 75% (95% CI: 60% to 90%) and 66% (95% CI: 55% to 77%)]. As an additional advantage, PET identified unknown distant metastases in about 10% of the patients. These authors concluded that PET "improves the rate of detection of local and distant metastases in patients with nonsmall-cell lung cancer."

Impact of PET on management of lung cancer patients

In a study of 97 patients,[73] PET correctly altered the clinical stage in 27% and detected distant unknown metastases in 13% of the patients. PET resulted in clinical management changes in 37% of all patients: surgery was cancelled in 15 patients while surgery was performed in 11 patients because findings suspected with PET correctly ruled out metastatic disease. Four patients had surgery because PET suggested lung cancer and 6 patients required further evaluation because of the PET findings.

Lewis et al[74] investigated whether FDG–PET improved the preoperative detection of metastases. To that aim, 34 patients with resectable nonsmall-cell lung cancer who underwent FDG–PET were analyzed. PET identified unknown metastatic lesions in 29% of the patients. Management changes occurred in 41% of the patients whereby 6 (18%) patients were deemed surgically nonresectable because of PET.

The impact of whole-body PET on staging and managing patients with lung cancer from the referring physician's perspective was recently investigated by Seltzer et al[75] (Figure 5-9 and 5-10). In their survey of more than 350 referring

FIGURE 5-9. Impact of FDG–PET on the staging of lung cancer and nonlung cancer from the referring physician's perspective. PET findings changed the staged in 44% of lung cancer patients (29% upstaged and 15% downstaged) and in 39% of nonlung cancer patients. Abbreviation: (n), number of the patients.

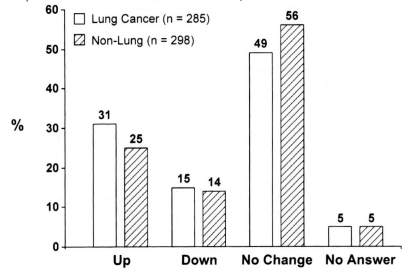

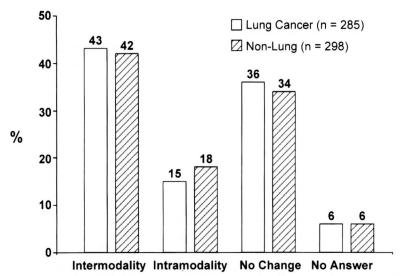

FIGURE 5-10. Impact of FDG–PET on the management of lung cancer and nonlung cancer from the referring physician's perspective. Intermodality changes are defined as changes between treatment modalities (e.g., from surgery to radiation or from radiation to medical treatment). Intramodality changes denote changes within a treatment modality (i.e., a different surgical or radiation approach). Notice that PET altered the treatment in 54% of lung cancer patients and in 60% of nonlung cancer patients. Abbreviation: (n) is the number of patients.

physicians, PET changed the clinical stage in 43% of 583 patients. Twenty-eight percent were upstaged, 15% downstaged, and 52% had no change in clinical stage. PET resulted in intermodality management changes (i.e., a management change from one therapeutic option such as chemotherapy to another one such as radiation therapy) in 40% of all patients.

A rigorous decision tree sensitivity analysis for cost-effectiveness of FDG–PET has also demonstrated that combining PET and CT for staging lung cancer is more economical than the conventional strategy of CT staging alone.[76]

These and other data provide convincing evidence that FDG–PET is the diagnostic imaging modality of choice for the staging and restaging of patients with lung cancer.

Cancers of the head and neck region

Head and neck cancer

CLINICAL BACKGROUND

Head and neck cancers comprise about 5% of all cancers worldwide. Physical examination, endoscopic techniques, MRI, and CT provide anatomical approaches to detection and staging but are limited in their ability to discriminate between benign structural alterations and malignancy. Most head and neck cancers are diagnosed at an advanced stage with only about 30% diagnosed at stage I or II. The diagnosis of recurrent and residual disease after surgical treatment, chemotherapy, or radiation is difficult using conventional anatomic imaging. This difficulty arises from the complex and variable anatomy of the head and neck region as well as from the high incidence of inflammatory changes with subsequent lymph node enlargement in the oropharyngeal and nasopharyngeal space. This situation is further complicated by unspecific post-therapeutic changes such as scarring, inflammation, and necrosis that render the differentiation between benign and malignant alterations difficult, if not impossible by CT and MRI. The key requirement for any imaging modality in head and neck cancer is its ability to accurately detect primary tumors, to stage for lymph node or distant organ involvement, and to reliably distinguish between treatment sequelae and residual or recurrent disease.

DIAGNOSIS, STAGING, AND RESTAGING (TABLE 5-3[77–83]; FIGURE 5-11)

Minn et al[84] were the first to demonstrate that head and neck cancers exhibit increased glucose metabolic activity. Jabour et al[77] reported that FDG–PET accurately detected primary tumors and correctly identified 25 of 34 positive lymph nodes. In this study of 12 patients with squamous cell carcinoma, FDG–PET was equivalent or better than MRI for detecting primary tumors and lymph node involvement. These findings were corroborated in a larger series by Rege et al[78] who studied 60 patients with biopsy-proven head and neck cancer. Of these, 34 were staged prior to treatment, 19 were evaluated for recurrent disease after radiation, and 7 were studied after laser excision. PET correctly identified the primary tumor in 29 of 30 patients, a finding superior to MRI results which identified 23 of 30 primary tumors. Further, PET correctly detected tumor recurrence in 9 of 10 patients while MRI only detected 6 of 10. PET and MRI correctly confirmed the presence or absence of lymph node involvement in 32 and 31 of 34 patients. Consistently, Lowe et al,[83] Faber et al,[82] and others[81] concluded that FDG–PET was useful for identifying primary and recurrent early stage laryngeal cancer.

A large retrospective study assessed the efficacy of FDG–PET imaging for distinguishing residual from recurrent tumor in 28 patients following radiation treatment.[82] Using histopathology and clinical followup as study endpoints, these authors reported a sensitivity and specificity of 86% and 93% and positive and negative predictive values of 92% and 87% for FDG–PET.

TABLE 5-3. FDG–PET in Head and Neck Cancer

Author	Ref #	Year	N	SENS (%)		SPEC (%)		PPV (%)		NPV (%)		ACC (%)	
				PET	CT	PET	CT	PET	CT	PET	CT	PET	CT
Jabour et al	77	1993	15	74	71	—	—	—	—	—	—	—	—
Rege et al[a]	78	1994	60	95	85	100	57	100	63	92	82	97	70
Benchaou et al	79	1996	48	86	86	90	84	86	78	90	90	89	85
Adam et al	80	1998	60	90	82	94	85	—	—	—	—	93	85
Paulus et al	81	1998	38	64	76	96	93	94	—	73	—	80	82
Faber et al	82	1999	28	86	71	93	33	92	—	87	—	89	—
Lowe et al	83	2000	44	100	38	93	85	—	—	—	—	—	—
Weighted Average				87	74	95	75	94	70	87	86	91	80

[a]MRI.

Abbreviations: ACC, accuracy; CT, computerized tomography; MR, magnetic resonance imaging; N, number of patients; NPV, negative predictive value; PET, positron emission tomography; PPV, positive predictive value; SENS, sensitivity; SPEC, specificity; —, could not be determined.

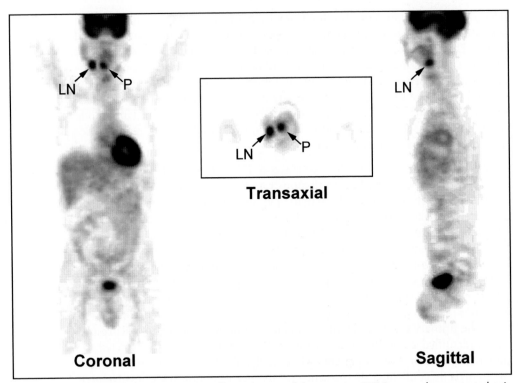

FIGURE 5-11. Squamous cell carcinoma of the tongue. PET images demonstrated primary tumor (P) and left inframandibular lymph node involvement (LN).

Hubner et al[85] who retrospectively studied 45 patients with head and neck cancer provided similar results. They reported a sensitivity of 97% and a specificity of 82% when clinical outcome and histological data were used as study endpoints. Importantly, the specificity of PET was superior to that of CT in patients with primary head and neck cancer (82% vs 31%) and those with recurrent disease (82% vs 31%). Similarly, Lapela et al[86] reported a sensitivity and specificity of 88% and 86% of PET for the presence of malignancy in 17 patients who were studied for recurrent head neck cancer. Regional lymph node involvement profoundly affects the survival of patients with head and neck cancer. Therefore, accurate determination of lymph node involvement is clinically important. The accuracy of FDG–PET for lymph node staging relative to that of conventional imaging was evaluated by Adam et al[80] in 60 patients with histologically proven squamous cell cancer of the head and neck. In this study, the sensitivity (90%), specificity (94%), positive (58%) and negative (99%) predictive values, and accuracy (93%) of PET was superior to that of CT, MRI, and ultrasound (Table 5-4). Benchaou et al[79] confirmed these findings in their study of 48 patients; that is, PET was more accurate for detecting lymph node involvement than CT and physical examination (89% vs 85% and 81%).

MONITORING TREATMENT

The effects of chemotherapy on tumor glucose metabolic activity were examined by Lowe et al[87] in 28 patients with advanced head and neck cancer. Tis-

TABLE 5-4. Comparison of ^{18}F-FDG–PET and Conventional Imaging Modalities with Histopathological Findings in Head and Neck Cancer

Method	SENS (%)	SPEC (%)	PPV (%)	NPV (%)	ACC (%)
PET	90	94	58	99	93
CT	82	85	35	98	85
MRI	80	79	27	98	79
Sonography	72	70	19	96	70

Source: Data reprinted with permission from Adam et al.[80]

Abbreviations: ACC, accuracy; CT, computerized tomography; MRI, magnetic resonance imaging; NPV, negative predictive value; PET, positron emission tomography; PPV, positive predictive value; SENS, sensitivity; SPEC, specificity.

sue biopsies were performed before and after chemotherapy. All followup PET studies were performed within 1 to 2 weeks after the end of treatment. The positive and negative predictive values of PET for treatment response were 95% and 71%, respectively. The overall accuracy of PET was 89%.

Importantly, the tumor SUV declined by 82% ± 5% in patients with complete response but only by 34% ± 29% in patients with residual disease. Thus, positive PET findings after treatment were indicative of tumor recurrence or poor therapeutic responses.

The same group evaluated the ability of FDG–PET[88] to detect recurrence of head and neck cancer prospectively in 44 patients with advanced disease. All patients had serial post-treatment FDG–PET scans at 2 months and 10 months following treatment. Based on tissue biopsies, patients were grouped into complete responders and those who had residual disease. In this study, PET had sensitivities and specificities of 100% and 93% while conventional imaging had a low sensitivity of 38% and a specificity of 85% for disease recurrence or residual disease. Physical examination had a specificity of 100% but, as expected, a sensitivity of only 44%.

The usefulness of PET to monitor the effects of radiation treatment on head and neck cancers were studied by Sakamoto et al.[89] These authors observed that tumor size as measured by CT was not affected by radiation treatment while FDG uptake was reduced 3 weeks to 4 weeks after the end of treatment. Patients without viable tumor cells following treatment had lower FDG uptake values than those with residual tumor viability. Further, the anatomical response to treatment did not correlate with metabolic tissue activity. These authors, therefore, concluded that FDG–PET was more accurate than anatomical imaging as it provides an independent indicator of clinical responses to treatment that includes radiation and chemotherapy or a combination of both.

Peng et al[90] investigated the use of FDG to assess tumor response to radiation therapy in patients with nasopharyngeal carcinoma. They studied 46 patients within 1 to 36 months of radiation treatment and reported a sensitivity and specificity of 80% and 87% for recurrent and residual cancer. If only those patients who underwent PET more than 6 months after treatment were included, their sensitivity and specificity improved to 92% and 100%. Thus, the predictive accuracy for treatment response might depend upon the time interval between the last treatment and PET.

In summary, the available literature indicates that PET is highly accurate for detecting primary head and neck tumors, staging lymph node involvement, and assessing tumor response to radiation therapy or chemotherapy.

Thyroid cancer

CLINICAL BACKGROUND

Thyroid cancers include a variety of histological types that are associated with different prognoses. For instance, the 10-year survival rate of patients with papillary and follicular cancer approaches 90% while nondifferentiated cancers have a 10-year mortality rate of close to 90%.[91] Thryoidectomy and surgical lymph node assessment is frequently followed by radioablation therapy with 131-iodine. Postsurgical management consists of monitoring serum thyroglobulin or calcitonin levels; patients routinely undergo whole-body scanning with radioactive iodine. This test, while highly specific for detecting recurrent disease, has a limited sensitivity that ranges from 40% to 60%. This is explained by the inability of undifferentiated thyroid cancers to trap iodine. Poorly differentiated thyroid tumors exhibit, however, increased rates of glucose metabolism, and thus, increased FDG uptake.[92–98] The inverse relationship between 131-iodine and FDG uptake has been termed the flip-flop phenomenon[99] (Figure 5-12). Yeo et al[95] evaluated the usefulness of FDG–PET imaging for detecting recurrent lymph node involvement in patients with negative 131-iodine scans. In their study of 22 patients with differentiated papillary thyroid carcinoma, the sensitivity and specificity of FDG–PET for lymph node metastases was 80% and 84%. A similar study[96] in 37 patients with differentiated, iodine negative thyroid carcinoma revealed a negative and positive predictive value of PET for disease recurrence of 93% and 92%. False negative findings were explained by minimal disease. PET affected patient management in 19 of the 37 patients. van Tol et al[100] who reported false positive findings in 64% of their 11 patients disputed these findings. This high rate of false positive findings might be explained by benign thyroid disorders such as autonomous adenoma, Graves' disease[101,102] or thyroiditis.[103]

A large multicenter trial that included 222 patients with differentiated thyroid carcinoma was conducted in Germany[97] (Table 5-5). Using anatomic im-

FIGURE 5-12. Flip–flop phenomenon in a patient with papillary thyroid cancer and rising serum levels of thyroglobulin. Notice that the 131-iodine whole-body scan (A) was normal, while FDG–PET (B) showed markedly increased glycolysis in the region of the thyroid (T). This was subsequently confirmed as local tumor recurrence.

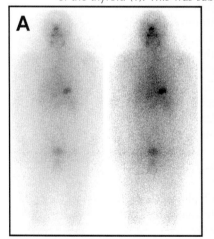
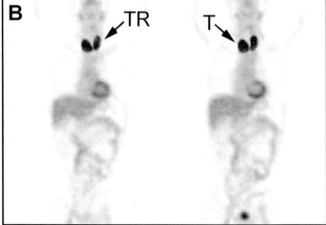

TABLE 5-5. Sensitivity, Specificity, Positive and Negative Predictive Values, and Accuracy of FDG–PET for the Various Subgroups of Thyroid Cancer

	SENS (%)	SPEC (%)	PPV (%)	NPV (%)	ACC (%)
Overall	75	90	88	79	83
WBS-positive	65	100	100	10	66
WBS-negative	85	90	81	93	89
Tg < 5 μg/L	77	87	61	94	85
Tg ≥ 5 μg/L	76	100	100	56	81
TSH < 5 mU/L	91	74	78	89	83
TSH ≥ 5 mU/L	67	94	89	82	84
Grading < G2	67	100	100	83	87
Grading ≥ G2	76	82	87	69	79
Papillary	73	86	78	82	81
Follicular	78	100	100	73	86
Hürthle cell	87	100	100	71	90

Source: Data used with permission from Grünwald et al.[97]

Abbreviations: ACC, accuracy; G2, grade 2; NPV, negative predictive value; PPV, positive predictive value; SENS, sensitivity; Tg, thyroglobulin; TSH, thyroid stimulating hormone; WBS, whole-body [131]iodine sensitivity.

aging and clinical outcome as gold standards, the overall sensitivity and specificity and diagnostic accuracy of PET was 75%, 90% and 83%, respectively. FGD–PET tended to perform best in patients with iodine negative tumors (sensitivity 85%, specificity 90%, accuracy 89%) while the sensitivity of PET was only 65% in patients with iodine positive tumors.

PET is, therefore, especially useful in patients with negative 131-iodine whole-body scans and high serum thyroglobulin levels.[92]

Wang et al[104] attempted to determine the ability of FDG–PET for identifying a subgroup of thyroid cancer patients with poor prognosis. The volume of FDG-avid disease was the strongest predictor of patient survival by multivariate analysis.

Thus, the published literature strongly supports the use of FDG–PET in those patients with thyroid cancer who have suspected disease recurrence but negative findings by conventional 131-radioiodine scanning.

Cancers of the gastrointestinal tract

Colorectal cancer

CLINICAL BACKGROUND

Around 160,000 new cases of colorectal cancer are diagnosed every year in the United States. It accounts for about 15% of all cancers in the United States. The mortality rate of colorectal cancer is, however, declining. This is attributed in part to improved screening techniques that allow for early detection and resectability of cancer and also to improved diet that is high in fiber content and low in saturated fat.[105] Screening with flexible sigmoidoscopy allows early detection of colorectal cancer.[106] Fecal occult blood testing (a simple noninvasive test to detect hemoglobin in stool samples) as well as digital rectal examinations, in addition to frequently rather vague symptoms, also leads to the diagnosis of colorectal cancer.

Computed tomography, ultrasound, MRI, and other noninvasive tests do not play a significant role for screening and diagnosing colorectal cancer. Similarly, FDG–PET imaging has not been examined systematically for its ability to detect primary colorectal cancer. Rather, imaging modalities are used to stage the disease prior to surgery and to restage it after therapeutical interventions.

INITIAL DIAGNOSIS AND STAGING OF COLORECTAL CANCER

In a pilot study conducted in 16 patients, Falk et al[107] compared the usefulness of FDG–PET to that of CT in the preoperative staging of colorectal cancer. The sensitivity of FDG–PET was higher than that of CT (87% vs 47%), but CT was more specific than PET (100% vs 67%). Importantly, the overall predictive accuracy of PET for primary tumor and metastatic lesions was significantly higher than that of CT (83% vs 56%; p < 0.05). In a subsequent study, Abdel–Nabi et al[108] correlated the presurgical PET findings with histopathological results and CT results in 48 patients with biopsy proven or suspected colorectal cancer. For primary tumors, FDG–PET had a sensitivity of 95%. The specificity was 40% due to several false positive PET findings including inflammatory bowel disease and postsurgical inflammation, both of which might be associated with markedly increased glucose metabolic activity.[109,110] Patient preparation including bowel cleansing with an isoosmotic solution together with bladder catheterization has been suggested to reduce physiological bowel and bladder uptake of FDG.[111] FDG detected lymph node metastases in only 4 (29%) of 14 patients. The specificity of PET for lymph node metastasis was, however, 96%. The comparative values for CT were 29% and 85%. The limited spatial resolution of PET might have accounted for the low sensitivity. Overall, PET correctly upstaged 4 (10.8%) of 37 patients with carcinoma from localized to metastatic disease. PET was more sensitive than CT for detecting liver metastases (88% vs 38%) while the specificity for liver lesions did not differ between the two modalities (100% vs 97%).

RESTAGING OF COLORECTAL CANCER

Extensive published data support the importance and usefulness of FDG–PET for diagnosing and restaging recurrent colorectal cancer (Figure 5-13).

FIGURE 5-13. Recurrent colorectal cancer in patients with rising serum CEA levels and negative findings on abdominopelvic CT. Notice the two foci of increased glycolysis in the right pelvis consistent with lymph node metastases (LN).

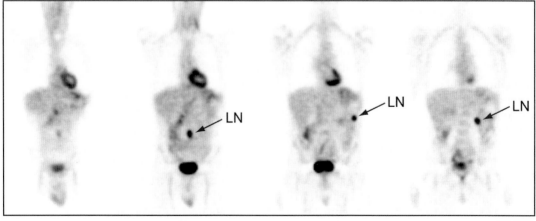

Strauss and coworkers[112] studied 29 patients with suspected local tumor recurrence. Because of limited spatial resolution of early generation PET imaging devices, this investigation was limited to tumors of greater than 1.5 cm in largest diameter. Using the standardized uptake ratio for FDG, these authors reported "lesion to soft tissue ratios" that significantly differed from those in scar tissue. Using O-15-labeled water as tracer of tumor perfusion yielded no further improvement in accuracy.

Schiepers et al[113] conducted a comparison between PET and conventional imaging in 76 consecutive patients presenting with suspected recurrent local or distant metastatic colorectal cancer. PET was compared to standard conventional imaging including CT of the pelvis, and CT and/or ultrasound of the liver. The accuracy of PET for local recurrence of 95% was superior to CT of the pelvis, which had an accuracy of only 65%. Similarly, the accuracy (98%) of PET for detecting liver metastases tended to be higher than that of conventional imaging (93%). PET detected unexpected extrahepatic metastases in 10 patients. Thus, PET improved the staging of apparently resectable recurrent disease.

Delbeke et al[114] studied 52 consecutive patients with PET, CT, portography, and CT plus portography. They reported a diagnostic accuracy of PET for intrahepatic lesions of 92% versus 78% for CT and 80% for portography. One false positive PET finding was due to an abscess while 9 false negative findings were due to a lesion size of less than 1 cm. The accuracy of PET for determining postsurgical recurrence of liver lesions was also investigated. Fourteen sites of postsurgical recurrence were identified. The diagnostic accuracy of PET, CT, and CT-portography was 86%, 64%, and 45%, respectively. PET was also superior to the other tests for identifying extrahepatic disease recurrence (92% vs 71% for CT). Similar accuracies were reported by others[115] and, more specifically, in rectal carcinoma.[116]

The role of PET for identifying sites of tumor recurrence in patients with unexplained rising plasma carcinoembryonic antigen (CEA) levels and negative findings by other imaging modalities was investigated by Flanagan et al.[117] PET detected abnormalities in 17 of 22 patients. All of these 17 patients had confirmed disease recurrence. Correctly identified sites of unknown metastatic disease included liver, lung, peritoneum, adrenal glands, lymph nodes, pancreas, spleen, and others.

A recent metaanalysis[118] (Table 5-6) of the literature that included 11 research articles selected by a-priori quality criteria evaluated the use of FDG–PET in the detection of recurrent colorectal cancer. This analysis yielded an overall sensitivity of 97% (95% confidence level, 95%–99%) and an overall specificity of 76% (95% confidence level, 64%–88%) of FDG–PET. Further, this study revealed that FDG–PET affected the clinical management in 29% (95% confidence level, 25%–34%) of the patients.

MONITORING OF TREATMENT WITH *PET*

Radiation treatment Haberkorn et al[119] used FDG–PET to determine the effectiveness of radiation treatment in 12 patients with recurrent colorectal cancer. Followup PET was performed in 9 patients early after a single treatment session, while 12 patients had a second followup scan 6 weeks later. Tumor glycolysis as imaged with FDG uptake declined in 11 cases while it remained unchanged in 7 and increased in 2 patients. Thus, a metabolic tumor response to radiation

TABLE 5-6. Metaanalysis of Sensitivity and Specificity of FDG–PET Data in Colorectal Cancer

Type	Calculation method	Patients/ lesions	N	TP	FP	TN	FN	Combined sensitivity (95% confidence interval)	Combined specificity (95% confidence interval)
Whole Body	Pooled Data	Patients	281	229	11	34	7	97% (95%–99%)	76% (63%–88%)
	Weighted Average							97%	77%
Hepatic Involvement	Pooled Data	Patients	393	182	2	202	7	96% (94%–99%)	99% (98%–100%)
	Weighted Average							96%	97%
Hepatic Involvement	Pooled Data	Lesions	182	130	1	38	13	91% (86%–96%)	97% (92%–100%)
	Weighted Average							91%	97%
Local/Pelvic	Pooled Data	Patients	366	137	5	214	8	94% (91%–98%)	98% (96%–100%)
	Weighted Average							95%	97%

Source: Data used with permission from Huebner et al.[118]

Abbreviations: FP, false positive; FN, false negative; N, number of patients; TN, true negative; TP, true positive.

therapy was observed in only about 50% of the patients. Several reasons might have accounted for this finding. First, radiation therapy can be associated with intense inflammatory changes resulting in increased glucose metabolic activity. Second, radiation therapy rarely results in complete cure of the disease. Thus, residual tumor might explain the residual and persistent glycolysis. The authors concluded that PET was a sensitive method to evaluate the effects of radiotherapy but that its specificity was limited by inflammatory responses that occur early after radiation treatment. They suggested performing followup PET scans 6 months after radiation treatment when most inflammatory effects have subsided.

Chemotherapy The effect of chemotherapy with fluorouracil on tumor glycolysis was measured with FDG by Findlay et al[120] 1 to 2 weeks and 4 to 5 weeks after initiation of treatment. Measurements of glycolysis in liver metastases (SUV and tumor to normal background ratio) were compared to morphological changes as determined by CT in 20 patients. Using CT criteria as a reference standard, these authors demonstrated that SUVs failed to discriminate between responders and nonresponders after 1 to 2 weeks of treatment. In contrast, SUVs differed significantly between responders and nonresponders 4 weeks to 5 weeks after initiation of chemotherapy. This finding suggests that FDG–PET might be useful in predicting treatment response earlier than anatomic imaging can. The use of CT criteria to judge responders from nonresponders is itself questionable. A similar study was conducted by Bender et al[121] in 10 patients with nonresectable liver metastases before and after treatment with 5-fluorouracil and folic acid. Their preliminary data suggested that changes in glucose metabolic activity after a single course of chemotherapy might be useful to predict therapeutic outcome.

Vitola et al[122] examined the role of PET for monitoring the effects of chemoembolization therapy in 4 patients with 34 liver metastases. Successful chemoembolization as evidenced by significant decreases in tumor markers was associated with highly significant reductions in tumor glycolysis with FDG ($p <$ 0.00001) while increases in glycolysis indicated failure of treatment.[122]

A more novel approach was used by Dimitrakopoulou et al[123,124] and Kissel et al.[125] These authors used F-18-labeled uracil, 5-fluorouracil (5-FU), to examine the tumor uptake of the most frequently used chemotherapeutic agent in colorectal cancer patients. These studies were carried out in patients with liver metastases. Such an approach might allow the prediction of tumor responses to chemotherapy. However, they reported that results of the first study showed variable uptake patterns of 5-FU in liver lesions.

Surgery Resection of liver metastasis is an accepted treatment for patients with advanced colorectal cancer. Because anatomic imaging modalities frequently fail to correctly characterize liver lesions, several groups have studied the role of FDG–PET in this setting. Fong et al[126] addressed this issue in 40 patients who were evaluated for possible resection of liver metastases. Patient management was altered in 23% of the patients, most of whom were upstaged by PET. The diagnostic accuracy of PET was superior to that of CT for detecting extrahepatic disease (sensitivity: 79% vs 32%; specificity: 91% vs 81%). In the liver, only 21% of lesions smaller than 1 cm but 87% of lesions ranging from 1.1 cm to 1.4 cm were correctly detected by FDG–PET. Overall, the sensitivity of PET for liver lesions was 71% and was not superior to CT or CT-portography. The authors provided biological and technological reasons for this relatively low sensitivity. First, normal liver tissue displays high hexokinase activity and therefore accumulates considerable amounts of FDG-6-phosphate. Thus, background tracer activity is high. This may be corrected by lowering serum glucose levels with intravenous insulin[22] or by waiting longer time periods before performing scans so that more FDG-6-PO$_4$ has been dephosphorylated and cleared from normal liver tissue. Second, the spatial resolution of PET is limited. The authors[126] concluded that PET was most useful in those patients considered for resection of liver metastases who have a high risk for extrahepatic disease. Lai et al[127] made similar observations regarding the usefulness of PET for detecting extrahepatic disease. This group found unsuspected extrahepatic disease in 32% of the patients who were evaluated for resectability of liver metastases causing the patients to be upstaged and removed as surgical candidates.

IMPACT OF PET ON MANAGING PATIENTS WITH RECURRENT COLORECTAL CANCER

Valk et al[128] reported potential cost savings resulting from using PET for preoperative staging in 155 patients with recurrent colorectal cancer. PET correctly identified sites of recurrence in 12 of 18 patients with elevated serum carcinoembryonic antigen levels and negative CT findings. A cost-effectiveness analysis was based on discussions with referring physicians and on the assumption that patients with more than one metastatic lesion were no longer surgical candidates. The costs of surgical procedures that were avoided because of PET were then compared to the cost of PET imaging. Unnecessary surgery would have been avoided in 32% of the patients with recurrent colorectal cancer. The authors concluded that $3000/patient could have been saved if PET had been included in the management algorithm.

Flamen et al[129] observed discordant staging information between PET and conventional imaging in 14% of their 103 patients. In 13 patients with inconclusive or negative findings by conventional staging, FDG–PET provided diagnostic results in 62% of the patients who had inconclusive or negative findings by conventional imaging. In 4 of another 37 patients with presumably resectable liver metastases, PET resulted in upstaging to nonresectability.

Delbeke et al[114] reported that PET changed patient management in 28% of patients with colorectal cancer.

In a recent survey[130] referring physicians indicated that FDG–PET changed the clinical stage and management in about 40% of their patients.

Thus, PET is superior to anatomical imaging for staging metastatic and recurrent colorectal cancer and for defining its operability. Further, FDG–PET has a considerable and cost-effective impact on patient management.

Esophageal cancer

CLINICAL BACKGROUND

Esophageal cancer is the ninth most common malignancy in the world, with the highest incidence seen in developing countries.[131] In the United States, esophageal cancer accounts for approximately 1% of all newly diagnosed cancers per year, afflicting 12,300 people and resulting in 12,100 deaths per year.[132] Overall, the incidence of esophageal cancer is increasing in the United States.[133] The accurate determination of the extent of local tumor invasion, tumor size, lymph node involvement, and the presence of metastases at the time of diagnosis provide valuable prognostic information and is required for selecting the appropriate treatment. Generally, 75% of the patients have lymph node involvement at initial presentation.[134] Conventional staging modalities include upper endoscopy, bronchoscopy, computed tomography of chest and abdomen, bone scanning, MRI, endoscopic ultrasonography, and exploratory laparotomy. The accuracy of CT for diagnosing mediastinal lymph nodes ranges from 51% to 70%.[134] Endoscopic ultrasonography and exploratory laparotomy improve the staging accuracy.[135–137] Endoscopic ultrasound is also more accurate than CT for nodal staging.[137] These methods are reported to provide a combined accuracy of 70% to 90% for identifying metastatic disease.[138] However, a substantial number of patients are found to have more advanced disease than indicated by the diagnostic workup at the time of surgery. Surgical treatment of esophageal cancer, whether curative or palliative, carries a mortality rate ranging from 5% to 20%.[139] The only solution for reducing this mortality rate is careful preoperative staging.

Fukunaga et al[140] demonstrated increased glycolysis with FDG in 48 patients with primary esophageal cancer. High SUVs were associated with adverse patient outcome suggesting that the rate of glycolysis as determined with FDG in tumors might be a useful prognostic marker.

DIAGNOSIS, STAGING, AND RESTAGING

The accuracy of PET and CT for diagnosing and staging of esophageal cancer has been compared by several authors.[141–144] All reported a higher accuracy of PET results than CT for determining the patient's stage of disease prior to surgery (Table 5-7[140–143,145–147]; Figure 5-14).

Neither CT nor PET can reliably predict tumor infiltration of the esophageal wall.[143] However, PET detects distant metastases with a significantly greater accuracy than CT.[141,146–149] This difference is due to CT's inability to distinguish postoperative tissue alterations from tumor recurrence.

Recently, Flamen et al[145] evaluated the utility of FDG–PET for evaluating tumor recurrence after surgical resection in 41 patients with esophageal cancer.

TABLE 5-7. FDG–PET for Staging Esophageal Cancer

Author	Ref #	Year	N	SENS (%)		SPEC (%)		ACC (%)		Criteria
				PET	CT	PET	CT	PET	CT	
Fukunaga et al	140	1998	46	—	—	—	—	98	—	SUV > 2.0
Flamen et al[a]	145	2000	33	95	85	72	86	84	86	Visual
Kole et al[b]	143	1998	26	96	81	88	100	—	—	—
Nodal stage				—	—	—	—	90	62	—
Block et al[b]	142	1997	58	96	—	—	—	—	—	Visual
Nodal stage				45	21	90	92	74	62	—
Flanagan et al	141	1997	36	100	—	—	—	—	—	—
Nodal stage				72	28	82	73	76	45	Visual
Rankin et al	146	1998	25	100	96	—	—	—	—	—
Nodal stage				37	50	—	—	—	—	—
Luketich et al	147	1999	91	69	46	93	74	84	63	Visual
Weighted Average				75	66	87	81			

[a]Conventional imaging. [b]Primary tumor detection.

Abbreviations: ACC, accuracy; CT, computerized tomography; N, number of patients; PET, positron emission tomography; SENS, sensitivity; SPEC, specificity; SUV, standardized uptake value; —, could not be determined.

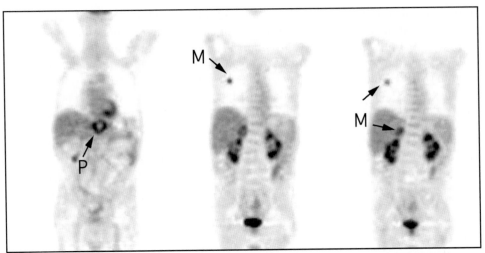

FIGURE 5-14. Sixty-three-year-old patient who was evaluated for resectability of cancer of the gastroesophageal junction (P). Whole-body PET revealed additional right upper lobe lung metastasis (M; middle panel) and a right adrenal lesion (M; right panel). Both were subsequently confirmed to be metastatic disease.

These authors found 40 sites of recurrence in 33 patients. In this study, the accuracy of conventional imaging and PET was comparable for detecting local recurrence. PET provided additional important staging information in 11 (27%) of 41 patients.

Thus, as a whole-body technique and because of its high accuracy for detecting mediastinal lymph node involvement, FDG–PET is superior to anatomic imaging for the presurgical staging of esophageal cancer.

Pancreatic cancer

CLINICAL BACKGROUND

Pancreatic cancer causes approximately 27,000 cancer deaths per year and was the fifth leading cause of cancer death in the United States in 1995. The 5-year survival rate is abysmal at 1% to 4%.[150,151] Clinical symptoms such as pain or jaundice due to biliary obstruction most frequently lead to the diagnosis. Surgical resection is curative in only a small number of patients.[152]

Because up to 40% of the patients with presumably resectable pancreatic cancer are found to have extensive disease, accurate staging is critical to identify patients with a potential survival benefit from surgery.[153] Imaging procedures such as ultrasound, CT, and MRI and endoscopic techniques such as retrograde cholangiopancreatography are used to diagnose and stage the disease.

DIAGNOSING, STAGING, AND RESTAGING

The performance of FDG-PET for characterizing pancreatic masses and for diagnosing and staging of pancreatic cancer has been assessed in several studies.

Diagnosis of pancreatic cancer (Figure 5-15) Pancreatic cancer cells are known to overexpress the glucose transporter 1 resulting in and exhibiting increased glycolysis as imaged with FDG in pancreatic cancer tissue.[154] The increased glycolysis has been shown to be best imaged with FDG 2 h after injection.[155] Us-

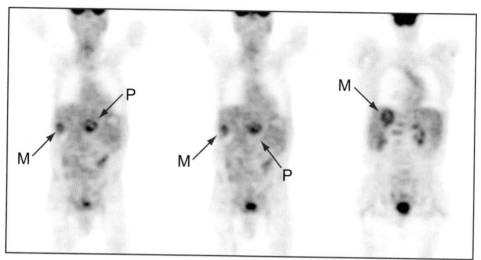

FIGURE 5-15. Fifty-eight-year-old patient referred for an FDG–PET evaluation of a pancreatic mass. The hypermetabolic was consistent with pancreatic malignancy (P). M indicates liver metastases.

ing an SUV cut-off point of 2.5 and a tracer retention index (i.e., the ratio between changes in SUV from the first to the second hour after injection, divided by the SUV obtained at 1 h), the accuracy of PET for diagnosing pancreatic cancer was 91.5%.

Using a similar image acquisition protocol, Imdahl et al[156] tested the diagnostic accuracy of PET in 48 patients (12 patients with chronic pancreatitis, 3 with acute pancreatitis, 27 with pancreatic cancer and 6 controls). A threshold for SUV of greater than 4.0 provided a sensitivity and specificity of 96% and 100% for correctly diagnosing pancreatic cancer.

Stollfuss et al[157] studied 73 patients with suspected pancreatic cancer with PET and CT within 8 weeks prior to surgery. In this study group with a greater than 50% prevalence of pancreatic cancer, the sensitivity and specificity of PET were superior to those of CT (93% vs 80% and 93% vs 74%, respectively). Less encouraging results were provided by Sendler et al[158] who compared helical CT, ultrasound, and PET for differentiating benign from malignant pancreatic masses. The authors concluded from the modest diagnostic accuracy of 69%, that PET could not exclude malignancy and that a combination of anatomic and PET imaging is required to optimize the diagnostic accuracy.

In a study of 106 patients, Zimny et al[159] diagnosed pancreatic cancer correctly in 63 of 74 patients and correctly ruled out malignancy in 27 of 32 patients. Sensitivity, specificity, and diagnostic accuracy for PET were 85%, 84%, and 85%, respectively. Friess et al[160] reported sensitivity and specificity of 94% and 88% in patients with suspected pancreatic cancer. False positive findings were explained by portal vein thrombosis or were related to a pancreatic pseudocyst.

Diederichs et al[161] and Zimny et al[159] emphasized the importance of normal serum glucose levels for detecting pancreatic cancer. Hyperglycemia reduced the sensitivity of PET from 86% to 42%.[161]

When staging pancreatic cancer, it is important to identify those patients who would benefit from surgical tumor resection. The ability of FDG–PET to identify hepatic involvement was studied by Fröhlich et al[162] in 168 patients. PET correctly identified liver involvement in 15 of 22 patients and identified 28 of 29 lesions larger than 1 cm. The specificity of PET was 95%. False positive findings occurred in patients with bile duct dilation and intrahepatic cholestasis.

Mertz et al[163] compared the sensitivity of endoscopic ultrasound, PET, and CT for pancreatic disease and that of CT and PET for metastatic disease in 35 patients with pancreatic cancer. In this study, the sensitivity of endoscopic ultrasound (91%) and PET (87%) was higher than that of CT (53%). Importantly, PET detected 7 of 9 distant metastatic lesions while CT only documented 3 of 9.

Impact on management and prognostic implications Rose et al[164] studied the diagnostic accuracy and impact of FDG–PET on managing patients with suspected or recurrent pancreatic carcinoma. The sensitivity and specificity of PET for diagnosing pancreatic cancer were superior to that of CT (92% vs 65% and 85% vs 62%). Clinical management changes occurred in 43% of the patients with suspected primary pancreatic cancer.

MONITORING TREATMENT

Maisey et al[165] studied the effects of chemotherapy in 11 patients with pancreatic cancer. Patients without residual tumor FDG uptake after chemotherapy had a better median survival rate (319 vs 139 days) and quality of life than those with residual tumor glycolytic activity. Zimny et al[166] corroborated these findings in 52 patients. Patient survival was 9 months for those with low tumor SUV with FDG but only 5 months in those with high SUVs.

Thus, PET provides important diagnostic, staging, and prognostic information in patients with pancreatic cancer.

Lymphoma

Clinical background

Lymphoma, i.e., Hodgkin's disease (HD), and nonHodgkin's lymphoma (NHL) are the fifth most common type of cancer diagnosed and the third most common form causing cancer deaths in the United States.[167] In the past 15 years, NHL has shown an approximate 50% increase in incidence.[168]

Tumor differentiation and FDG imaging

Determining the degree of glycolysis with FDG within lymphomatous tissue might allow prediction of tumor grade to establish the prognosis of lymphoma patients. Newman et al[169] investigated the relationship between tumor grade and glycolytic rate with FDG in 16 patients and found no significant difference between low- and high-grade lymphoma suggesting that the diagnostic accuracy of PET is not affected by tumor grade. Contradictory results were provided by Lapela et al[170] who studied the relationship between glycolytic rate with FDG and tumor grade in 22 patients with untreated nonHodgkin's lymphoma. These authors concluded that high glycolytic rate as determined with FDG metabolism is associated with high-grade malignancy of lymphoma, a notion supported by Okada et al[171] who conducted a study in 21 untreated patients with lymphoma of the head and neck region. Tumor glycolytic rates were determined using a tumor to background ratio and measured quantitatively by the Patlak graphical analysis.[172,173] These authors reported that patients with lymphoma of high glycolytic rates tended to have a poor prognosis. The same group[174] evaluated the relationship between tumor glycolytic rate and proliferative tumor activity by mitotic count rates. Lymphoma with a high mitotic count tended to be associated with higher glycolytic rates.

These findings have clinical implications: High-grade lymphoma is likely detected by FDG–PET with a higher sensitivity than low-grade lymphoma.

Staging and restaging

Correct staging is important for selecting the appropriate treatment for lymphoma patients. In addition to a patient's medical history, physical examination, and laboratory data, clinical staging, restaging after treatment, and detection of recurrence depend to a large degree on imaging studies, including CT, MRI, and 67-Gallium scintigraphy.

An early study by Paul[175] conducted in a group of 6 patients suggested that FDG–PET may be superior to 67-Gallium citrate for the detection of non-Hodgkin's lymphoma. A standard gamma camera was used to image patients with 67-Gallium and FDG. In this study, only 2 of 5 tumors were detected by Gallium imaging while 4 of 5 tumors were detected with FDG. This prompted more extensive research into the potential role of FDG–PET for diagnosing and staging of lymphoma as well as for monitoring the effects of therapeutic interventions.

Hoh and coworkers[176] compared the accuracy of PET for staging lymphoma to that of conventional imaging which included bone scans, CT, chest films, and others. In this pilot study that included 18 patients, PET staged lymphoma with similar or higher accuracy compared to conventional imaging. In a simple analysis of health care expenditures, these authors concluded that staging with PET alone would provide equivalent diagnostic information at a markedly lower cost and suggested that a whole-body PET based algorithm may be an accurate and cost-effective method for staging and restaging HD and NHL.

Moog et al[177] concluded from their study of 60 consecutive patients with Hodgkin's or nonHodgkin's lymphoma that FDG–PET was more accurate for detecting lymph node involvement than CT. Stumpe et al[178] arrived at the same conclusion when they compared the accuracy of FDG–PET for staging lymphoma to that of CT. As expected, the diagnostic sensitivity did not differ between PET and CT. However, the specificity of PET was 96% for Hodgkin's disease and 100% for nonHodgkin's lymphoma while the corresponding values were only 41% and 67% for CT.

Two studies[179,180] reported a high accuracy of PET for determining bone marrow involvement in lymphoma patients. Importantly, Moog et al[179] concluded that nuclear medicine bone scans and whole-body FDG–PET yielded a similar sensitivity for bone involvement, but that FDG–PET was more specific than bone scans. Similar results were provided by Carr et al.[180] These authors concluded from their study in 50 patients with nonHodgkin's lymphoma (n = 38) and Hodgkin's disease (n = 12), that visual interpretation of marrow glycolysis with FDG could identify bone marrow involvement with a comparable accuracy to that of bone marrow biopsy.

Prognosis and treatment monitoring (Figure 5-16[181] and 5-17; Table 5-8[181–184])

Using FDG-PET, Römer et al[185] assessed the effects of chemotherapy on changes in tumor glycolysis as determined by standardized uptake values and glucose metabolic rates utilizing a Patlak graphical analysis[172] in patients with nonHodgkin's lymphoma. FDG–PET was performed in 11 patients at 1 week and then again 6 weeks after initiation of chemotherapy. Patients who remained in complete remission had significantly lower tumor glycolysis as determined by SUV compared to those who relapsed. The authors concluded that longterm prognosis is better assessed when FDG–PET is performed after two full cycles of chemotherapy (6 weeks after initiation of chemotherapy).

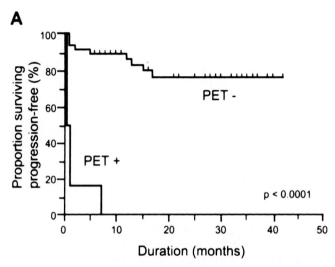

A

Panel A. Kaplan-Meier estimate of PFS in 6 patients with positive [18F]FDG-PET compared with 48 patients with negative [18F]FDG-PET.

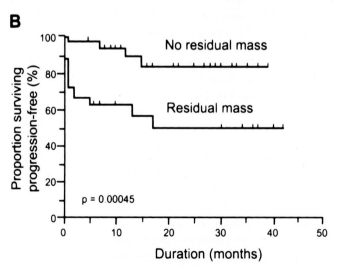

B

Panel B. Kaplan-Meier estimate of PFS in 24 patients with residual masses on CT compared with 30 patients without residual masses on CT.

5-16. Predictive value of FDG–PET in lymphoma patients. A, B: The negative predictive value of PET and CT was equally high. A positive PET was, however, diagnostic for residual and recurrent disease while positive findings with CT had a predictive value of only 40%. This finding is explained by the inability of CT to discriminate between anatomical alterations that occur after treatment (necrosis, scarring, fibrosis, and inflammation) of malignancy. (Reprinted with permission from Jerusalem et al.[181])

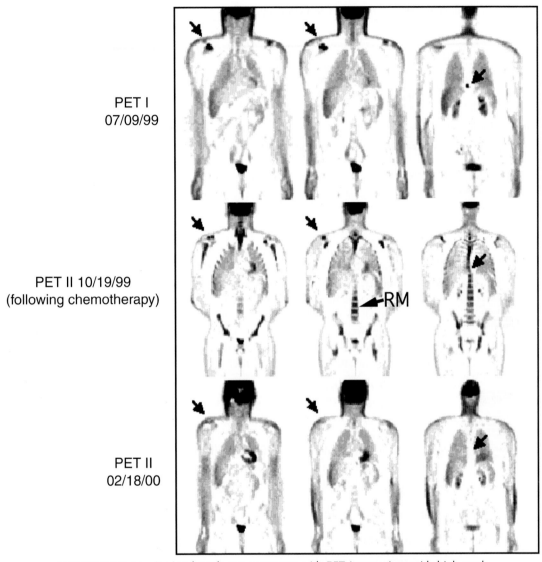

FIGURE 5-17. Monitoring lymphoma treatment with PET in a patient with high-grade large cell lymphoma. PET I: Notice 2 foci of glycolysis located in the right shoulder and distal T-spine (arrows). PET II: The second PET scan revealed marked improvement but not complete resolution after chemotherapy. Notice the increased bone marrow glycolytic activity consistent with regenerating bone marrow (RM) that is observed early after chemotherapy. PET III: The third PET scan revealed complete remission of disease. This patient has been free of disease for more than 18 months.

Jerusalem et al[181] (Figure 5-16) compared the predictive value of a residual mass on CT to that of glycolysis by FDG–PET in the post-treatment evaluation of 54 patients with Hodgkin's disease and nonHodgkin's lymphoma. These authors reported similar negative predictive values of FDG–PET and CT of 83% and 87% for disease recurrence but a significantly lower positive predictive value of CT than of PET (40% vs 100%). Others confirmed these findings.[183,184] The

TABLE 5-8. Predictive Value of FDG–PET in Lymphoma

Author	Ref #	Year	N	PPV (%) PET	PPV (%) CT	NPV (%) PET	NPV (%) CT	ACC (%) PET	ACC (%) CT	Criteria
Spaepen et al[a]	182	2001	93	100	50[b]	83	64[b]	—	—	Visual
Jerusalem et al[a]	181	1999	54	100	42	83	87	85	—	Visual
Zinzani et al[a]	183	1999	44	100	—	97	100	89	—	Visual
De Witt et al[c]	184	1999	44	57	19[b]	100	50[b]	80	21	Visual
Weighted Average				93	48	89	72	87	N/A	

Abbreviations: ACC, accuracy; N, number of patients; N/A, not assessed; NPV, negative predictive value; PPV, positive predictive value; —, could not be determined.

[a]Hodgkin's disease and nonHodgkin's lymphoma.

[b]Conventional imaging.

[c]NonHodgkin's disease only.

largest study to examine the prognostic value of FDG–PET in nonHodgkin's lymphoma included 93 patients who were studied within 1 to 3 months after chemotherapy.[182] Clinical outcome served as the reference gold standard. Twenty-six of the 93 patients had positive PET findings and all of these patients relapsed after a median disease-free survival of only 73 days. There were no false positive PET findings. In contrast, 56 of the 67 patients with negative PET studies remained in complete remission after a median followup period of 653 days. The remaining patients with negative PET relapsed after a median disease-free interval of 404 days.

Impact on management

The impact of PET on managing patients with lymphoma was investigated by Schöder et al.[186] PET changed stage and management in 46% and 48% of their 46 patients.

The scientific evidence, therefore, implies that PET is more accurate than conventional imaging for staging and restaging of lymphoma, provides important prognostic information, and is useful for monitoring the effects of treatment.

Cancers of the Skin

Melanoma

CLINICAL BACKGROUND

Melanoma, the most aggressive of all skin cancers, causes more than 75% of all skin cancer deaths. It is increasing in frequency, particularly among white people in areas of high sun exposure. The incidence of malignant melanoma is rising at a faster rate than any other malignancy in the United States with an estimated 44,000 new cases of melanoma in the year 2000.[187] Early detection and accurate staging is, therefore, crucial to identify the best treatment strategy for melanoma patients. This is especially important because melanoma tends to metastasize early and in an unpredictable pattern.[188]

Staging   Schwimmer et al[189] used a-priori quality criteria of published research articles to perform a metaanalysis addressing the role of PET for the management of melanoma patients. This analysis yielded a sensitivity of 92% (95% confidence level: 88%–96%) and a specificity of 90% (95% confidence level: 83%–96%) of FDG–PET for detecting recurrent melanoma (Table 5-9).[189]

TABLE 5-9. Metaanalysis of Sensitivity and Specificity Data for FDG–PET in Melanoma

Type	Calculation method	Patients/lesions/ LN basins	N	TP	FP	TN	FN	Combined sensitivity (95% confidence interval)	Combined specificity (95% confidence interval)
Whole Body	Pooled Data	Lesions	290	187	9	78	16	92% (88%–96%)	90% (83%–96%)
	Weighted Average							92%	87%
Whole Body	Pooled Data	Patients	274	68	12	174	20	77% (69%–86%)	94% (90%–97%)
	Weighted Average							78%	94%
Regional LN	Pooled Data	LN Basins	127	21	4	85	17	55% (40%–71%)	96% (91%–100%)

Source: Data used with permission from Schwimmer et al.[189]

Abbreviations: FN, false negative; FP, false positive; LN, lymph node; N, number of patients; TN, true negative; TP, true positive.

Rinne et al[190] prospectively studied 100 patients with melanoma using whole-body FDG–PET. On a lesion-by-lesion analysis, PET had a sensitivity and specificity of 92% and 94% while conventional imaging resulted in a low sensitivity and specificity of 58% and 45%. Similar results were reported by Steinert et al,[191] who found a sensitivity of 95% for detecting metastatic lesions with PET and a specificity of 100% if PET images were read with full knowledge of clinical findings. Macfarlane et al[192] confirmed these findings by reporting a high diagnostic accuracy of PET and only a small number of false positive and negative PET results. Postsurgical inflammatory changes and small lesion size accounted for false positive and false negative findings.

An important contribution to the understanding of lesion detectability in melanoma patients was made by Crippa et al.[193] The overall accuracy of PET for detecting lymph node involvement was 91%. PET detected all metastases greater than 10 mm in size, 81% of lymph nodes measuring 5 mm to 10 mm, and 21% of nodes smaller than 5 mm. Thus, while the overall diagnostic accuracy of PET for lymph node staging is high, PET, like all other imaging procedures, cannot detect subclinical, microscopic disease.

IMPACT ON MANAGEMENT

Eigtved et al[194] reported that 34% of 38 patients would have been staged incorrectly by conventional methods possibly resulting in unnecessary surgery. Similarly, a retrospective study[195] concluded that PET resulted in avoidance of unnecessary surgery in 8% of their patients. Wong et al[196] examined the impact of PET on staging and managing 51 patients with melanoma from the referring physician's point of view. FDG–PET changed the clinical stage and management in 29% of all melanoma patients.

In summary, FDG–PET stages melanoma with a higher diagnostic accuracy than any other imaging modality and has a considerable impact on patient management.

Breast Cancer

Clinical background

Approximately 183,000 women are diagnosed with breast cancer each year in the United States.[132] Breast cancer is the leading cancer and the second leading cause of mortality in women. The following section will discuss the potential contribution of FDG–PET for diagnosing, staging, and restaging breast cancer patients.

Diagnosis of breast cancer

Over the last decade, the mortality rate from breast cancer has declined which is largely ascribed to mammographic screening of large segments of the population. Despite these advances, the considerable mortality and morbidity associated with breast cancer poses a formidable challenge to the health care system. The public frequently assumes a near 100% sensitivity of mammography for the detection of breast cancer. This assumption is not supported by data. Rosenberg et al[197] investigated the effects of age, breast density, ethnicity, and estrogen replacement therapy on the sensitivity of mammography for detecting breast cancer. Their analysis of a population-based database of 183,134 screening mammograms yielded 807 cancers. The screening sensitivity of mammography was only minimally affected by age and ranged from 77% for women aged 40 to 49 years to 81% in women older than 65 years. Ethnicity did not significantly affect the screening sensitivity. Mammography, however, performed poorly in women with dense breasts with sensitivity of only 68% and especially in women aged 50 to 64 years who had dense breasts and had undergone estrogen replacement therapy (sensitivity of 55%). Importantly, the sensitivity of mammography did not exceed about 80% in any segment of the population studied. Thus, mammography results in a considerable number of missed cancers, especially in women with dense breasts.

Mandelson et al[198] investigated the relationship between breast density and risk for interval cancer defined as cancer occurrence within 24 months of a normal or benign mammogram. Using the American College of Radiology Breast Imaging Reporting and Data System[199] (BI-RADS system) for classifying breast density (1 = almost entirely fat; 2 = scattered fibroglandular tissue; 3 = heterogeneously dense; 4 = extremely dense), this study revealed sensitivities for breast cancer detection of 80%, 59%, and 30% in women with predominantly fatty breast tissue, those with heterogeneously dense, and those with extremely dense breasts. The authors concluded, "breast density is one of the strongest, if not the strongest, predictor of the failure of mammographic screening to detect cancer." Foxcroft et al[200] reported similar limitations of mammographic screening and recommended that women with dense breasts should undergo different screening tests.

The risk of not detecting breast cancer with mammography in dense breasts cannot be solely explained by the masking of cancer with dense tissue. John Wolfe[201] was the first to establish a relationship between breast density and breast cancer risk. He classified (Wolfe scale) breast tissue into four different groups according to breast density and uncovered that the cancer risk was lowest in radiolucent breasts and highest in dense breasts. This finding has been reproduced in many studies. Boyd et al[202] found that women with dense breasts are at a 4 to 6 times higher risk of developing breast cancer than those with predominantly fatty breasts. The reasons for the independent association between breast density and cancer risk are not completely understood. However, increased mitogenesis and damage to the DNA of dividing cells have been proposed as underlying mechanisms.

The less than desirable overall sensitivity of mammography is not completely explained by difficult-to-image breasts. Defining false negative mammographic findings with a pathological diagnosis of breast cancer within 1 year of a negative mammogram, Bird et al[203] reported that 77 (24%) of 320 cancers were missed by screening mammography. Reasons for missed breast cancers included misinterpretation of the mammograms (40/77 cases), overlooked cancers (33/77), and suboptimal technique (4/77 cases).

Thus, the sensitivity of mammography is considerably lower than 100% and probably close to 75% in the overall screened population. Its sensitivity drops to as low as 30% in women with extremely dense breasts. This decline is of particular importance because breast density is an independent cancer risk factor. The clinical practice of screening women with dense breasts with mammography is, therefore, simply inadequate in this population that is at increased risk for breast cancer.

A second important limitation of mammography is its low specificity. That is, the majority (60% to 80%) of breast biopsies reveal benign pathology. The American College of Radiology[199] that has established guidelines for the interpretation of mammographic findings has acknowledged this. The BI-RADS have been prospectively used to determine whether improvements in specificity can be achieved. Based on morphological criteria, breast lesions are defined as 0; if more imaging tests are required, II for benign appearance, III for probably benign, IV for suspicious, and V for highly suspicious. While BI–RADS classes II and V lesions are almost diagnostic for benignity or malignancy, class IV yields a positive predictive value of only 30%.[204] Thus, even after applying stringent mammographic criteria for malignancy, a large number of breast biopsies are unnecessary, which is associated with considerable and potentially avoidable costs. In fact, approximately 30% of the total costs of breast carcinoma screening are caused by open surgical biopsy for benign disease.[205]

Thus, mammographic breast cancer screening reduces breast cancer mortality but results in a considerable number of missed cancers and a large number of unnecessary breast biopsies. Most critical is that women with dense breasts who are at increased risk for breast cancer are subjected to tests with low diagnostic accuracy in a population of women who are also at high risk for cancer. Because of these shortcomings, other imaging modalities such as ultrasound, Doppler flow velocity measurements, and MRI have been proposed as additional diagnostic tools for improving breast cancer detection. These techniques might increase the sensitivity but will likely further reduce the specificity for breast cancer detection.

FDG–PET is not proposed as a screening test for breast cancer. However, because malignant breast tissue has high glycolytic rates, this test might serve as a problem solver in women with difficult to image breasts, for instance, in women with dense or scarred breasts, breast implants, or those at high risk for breast cancer or breast cancer recurrence. Thus, the question as to whether PET can contribute to the diagnosis of primary breast cancer needs to be posed differently. For instance, are cancerous breast lesions metabolically active? Does PET aid in the diagnosis of breast lesions of unknown character? Can patients at risk for breast cancer or breast cancer recurrence be identified that cannot reliably be screened with mammography and, therefore, would benefit from an FDG–PET study?

Glucose metabolic activity in malignant breast tissue

Avril et al[206] evaluated the degree of glycolysis with FDG in breast lesions that were categorized as suspicious by physical examination or mammography in 144 patients. Different means of semiquantitative, quantitative, and visual analysis were used to determine glycolysis with FDG and diagnostic accuracy of FDG–PET. Visual image interpretation followed a 3-point scale from: 1) unlikely malignant, 2) probably malignant, to 3) definitely malignant. All pathological specimens were histologically evaluated. In this study, 132 malignant and 53 benign breast tumors were evaluated in the 144 patients. If definite and probable malignancy were combined, the sensitivity and specificity of visual PET analysis for characterizing breast lesions were 80% and 75%. The positive predictive value of sensitive reading was 89.1%. If only definite PET findings were considered indicative for malignancy, the sensitivity dropped to 64.4% while the specificity increased to 94.3%. Sensitivity also depended upon tumor size and histological tumor type with a lower sensitivity for lobular carcinomas.

Thus, breast cancer exhibits increased glycolysis as seen with FDG that is more prominent in infiltrating ductal than in lobular carcinomas.[207] Further, high-grade tumors exhibit higher glycolysis with FDG than low-grade tumors. Also, patients with p53 > 0.5 ng/mg protein had higher glycolysis with FDG than those with p53 < 0.5 ng/mg protein.[207]

Thus, glycolysis imaged with FDG uptake in breast cancer is increased and the degree of glycolysis correlates with histological characteristics of breast tumors.

CHARACTERIZATION OF BREAST MASSES (TABLE 5-10[206,208–213]; FIGURES 5-18 AND 5-19)

In 1989, Kubota et al[214] reported focally increased glycolysis with FDG in one breast cancer patient. In a subsequent pilot study, Wahl et al[215] proved the principle that breast cancer exhibits increased glucose metabolic activity in 12 patients with primary tumors larger than 3 cm. In this study, FDG–PET correctly detected all primary tumors. The median tumor to background ratio was 8:1. Tse et al[216] and Nieweg et al[217] confirmed these findings in small study groups.

Adler et al[213] evaluated the accuracy of FDG–PET in a patient group with high prevalence of breast cancer. The sensitivity and specificity of PET was 97% and 100% in these 28 patients. The largest prospective study to date addressing the diagnostic sensitivity of PET included 124 patients with known breast cancer.[218] Seventy-nine of the patients had tumors of less than 3 cm in largest diameter. All primary tumors were clearly visualized by FDG–PET resulting in a sensitivity of 100%.

TABLE 5-10. FDG–PET in Primary Breast Cancer

Author	Ref #	Year	N	SENS (%) PET	SENS (%) AI	SPEC (%) PET	SPEC (%) AI	ACC (%) PET	ACC (%) AI	PET Criteria
Schirrmeister et al	208	2001	117	93	—	75	—	89	—	Visual
Avril et al	206	2000	144	64–80	—	75–94	—	73–79	—	Visual
Yutani et al	209	2000	40	79	76[b]	—	—	—	—	Visual
Rostom et al	210	1999	93	91	—	83	—	89	72[a]	Visual
Noh et al	211	1998	27	96	78[a]	100	35[a]	97	67	Visual
Scheidhauer et al	212	1996	30	91	86[a]	86	17[a]	90	—	Visual
Adler et al	213	1993	35	96	—	100	—	—	—	Visual
Weighted Average				88	80	81	55	84–86	70	

Abbreviations: ACC, accuracy; AI, anatomical imaging; N, number of patients; PET, positron emission tomography; SENS, sensitivity; SPEC, specificity; —, could not be determined.

[a]Mammography.

[b]With ^{99}Tc sestamibi.

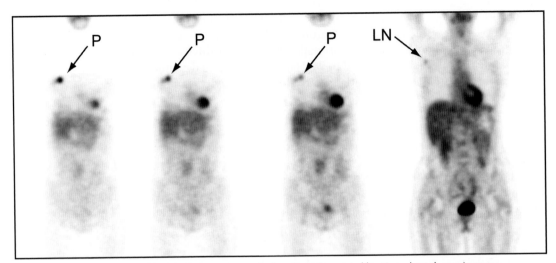

FIGURE 5-18. Characteristic pattern of glycolysis in an infiltrating ductal carcinoma. The primary tumor (P) was 1.8 cm in the largest diameter. PET detected axillary lymph node involvement (LN). This was subsequently confirmed by sentinel node biopsy.

The accuracy of FDG–PET was compared to that of mammography in several studies. Bassa et al[219] reported a sensitivity of 100% for PET, 62.5% for mammography, and 87.5% for ultrasound. The tumors evaluated in this study ranged in size from 1.7 cm to 9 cm.

In a large retrospective study,[210] sensitivity, specificity, and accuracy of PET were 91%, 83%, and 89%. False negative scans occurred in patients with carcinoma in situ, Paget's disease of the areola, and in 1 patient with a small tumor of 0.5 cm. Importantly, the overall accuracy of PET determined in 86 patients was better than that of mammography (90% vs. 72%; p < 0.0003).

Noh et al[220] reported a diagnostic accuracy of FDG–PET for detecting primary breast cancer of 97%. This compared favorably to mammography that had an accuracy of 67% and with physical examination with an accuracy of 78%. While the sensitivity of mammography, physical examination, and FDG–PET were similar, PET specificity was superior. The authors also observed a significant correlation between standardized uptake values and the number of metastatic axillary lymph nodes. That is, primary tumors with high glycolytic rates, and presumably more malignant, had greater degrees of metastases to lymph nodes.

Schirrmeister et al[208] studied 117 patients who were selected because of palpable lesions or suspicious mammographic or ultrasonic findings. Sensitivity and specificity of FDG–PET for primary tumors were 93% and 75%. Importantly, FDG–PET was twice as sensitive for detecting multifocal breast disease as the combination of ultrasound and mammography (63% vs. 32%).

POSTSURGICAL BREAST EVALUATION

Wahl et al[221] investigated the potential role of FDG–PET for detecting breast cancer in two patients after breast augmentation mammoplasty. Abnormal glycolysis with FDG consistent with malignancy was correctly identified in both patients. Noh et al[211] studied 8 patients after breast augmentation

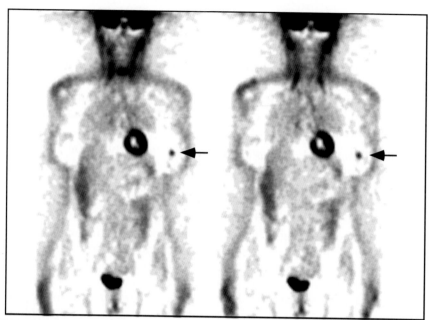

FIGURE 5-19. FDG–PET as a problem solver. Patient with palpable lymph node in the left axilla that was excised. Histological findings strongly suggested breast cancer. Several imaging tests (including mammography, MRI, and ultrasound) failed to identify the primary tumor. FDG–PET identified a hypermetabolic focus in the breast (arrow). Despite its limited anatomical resolution, PET was used as guidance for lumpectomy in this patient who had been scheduled for mastectomy.

who had equivocal findings on other imaging tests. FDG–PET correctly identified all cancers while mammography only uncovered 1 of 3 cases of cancer in this group. Four of 5 patients with negative tissue findings also had a negative FDG–PET scan.

Image acquisition protocols might affect the diagnostic accuracy of FDG–PET in breast cancer. Boerner et al[222] imaged 29 patients in the prone position 1.5 h and then again 3 h after FDG injection. They observed that tumor to background ratios increased significantly from 1.2 ± 0.6 after 1.5 h to 6.1 ± 3.0 3 h after tracer injection. At the same time, the tumor to normal breast ratio increased significantly from 3.4 ± 1.3 to 14.7 ± 6.8. The lesion detectability increased from 83% to 93%. The authors suggested that the diagnostic accuracy for FDG–PET for characterizing breast tumors could be improved if patients were imaged 3 h after FDG injection.

Yutani et al[223] who imaged breast cancer patients in the prone and in the supine position made another important procedural observation. In this study, FDG–PET detected 17 of 18 primary breast cancers (vs 13/17 detected by mammography and 16/17 by ultrasound). While the SUVs and tumor to background ratios were higher with patients in the prone position, the overall detectability of breast cancer was unaltered by patient positioning.

Attenuation correction might also alter the diagnostic accuracy of PET.[224] In a study that included 189 lesions (primary lesions, axillary lymph nodes, and distant metastases) in 28 patients, 5 small lesions were missed after correction for photon attenuation and iterative image reconstruction. While this study did not prove statistical evidence for superiority of noncorrected images, no additional diagnostic accuracy was gained by attenuation correction.

In summary, FDG–PET characterizes breast masses with a high diagnostic accuracy. PET is, therefore, specifically useful in women with difficult to image breasts by anatomical imaging, women with scared breasts or after breast augmentation, and in women who are at high risk for primary breast cancer, multifocal, or recurrent disease.

Axillary lymph node staging (Table 5-11[208–210,218,220,225–230]; Figure 5-20)

Axillary lymph node staging provides important prognostic information. Both patients with and without lymph node involvement have a reported survival benefit after undergoing chemotherapy. Thus, the therapeutic impact of axillary lymph node staging is limited. Sentinel node scintigraphy followed by biopsy assesses lymph node involvement with an accuracy of 90%. The accuracy of FDG–PET for lymph node staging is therefore measured against this modestly invasive procedure. The prognostic significance of axillary node staging by FDG–PET has not been determined. Several groups, however, have investigated the diagnostic accuracy of FDG–PET for lymph node staging. A comparable accuracy of FDG–PET and sentinel node biopsy for lymph node staging would infer a similar prognostic accuracy of these techniques.

Tse et al[216] were among the first to evaluate the ability of FDG–PET to identify tumor involved axillary lymph nodes. Seven of the 14 patients enrolled in this study had pathological evidence of axillary lymph node involvement. PET correctly identified 4 of these but missed 3. The lymph node status was correctly identified in 11 of 14 patients with FDG–PET.

TABLE 5-11. Axillary Lymph Node Staging with FDG–PET

Author	Ref #	Year	N	SENS (%) PET	AI	SPEC (%) PET	AI	PPV (%) PET	AI	NPV (%) PET	AI	ACC (%) PET	AI	Criteria
Greco et al	225	2001	167	94	—	86	—	84	—	84	—	90	—	Visual
Schirrmeister et al	208	2000	117	79	41	92	96	89	—	82	—	91	—	Visual
Ohta et al	226	2000	32	82	79a	—	—	—	—	—	—	—	—	Visual
Yutani et al	209	2000	40	50	37b	100	100b	84	—	73	69	79	74b	Visual
Rostom et al	210	1999	74	86	—	100	—	100	—	80	—	90	—	Visual
Crippa et al	227	1998	72	85	—	91	—	—	—	—	—	89	—	Visual
Noh et al	220	1998	24	100	100c	92	55c	—	—	—	96	60c	—	Visual
Smith et al	228	1998	45	88	—	97	—	93	—	93	—	93	—	Visual
Adler et al	229	1997	50	95	—	66	—	63	—	95	—	77	—	Visual
Crippa et al	230	1997	66	84	—	85	—	84	—	85	—	84	—	Visual
Utech et al	218	1996	124	100	—	75	—	69	—	100	—	88	—	Visual
Weighted Average				88		87	87	83	87	79	87	74		

Abbreviations: ACC, accuracy; AI, anatomical imaging; N, number of patients; PET, positron emission tomography; SENS, sensitivity; SPEC, specificity; —, could not be determined.

[a]Ultrasound.

[b]MIBI-SPECT (single photon emission tomography).

[c]Mammography.

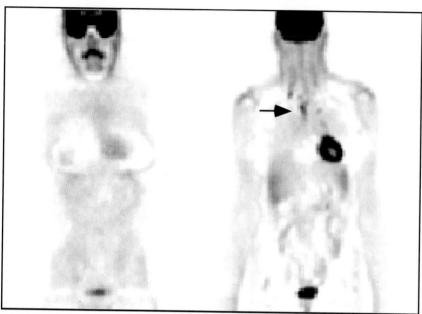

FIGURE 5-20. Internal mammary node involvement (arrow) on FDG–PET in a patient with negative PET and sentinel node biopsy of the axilla. Internal mammary node involvement, not detectable by sentinel node biopsy, is a powerful prognostic marker and occurs in up to 20% of breast cancer patients with negative axillary lymph nodes.

A larger, more systematic study included evaluated lymph node involvement in 28 patients with suspicious breast masses of greater than 1 cm in diameter.[213] All patients were studied prior to chemotherapy. Eighteen of the patients underwent axillary lymph node dissection. No false positive PET findings occurred. Eight of the nine patients with positive nodes had FDG–PET findings classified as probably or definitely positive. Thus, the sensitivity and specificity of FDG–PET were 90% and 100%. While the presence of lymph node involvement was determined with a high diagnostic accuracy, the number of individual nodes could not be established. In fact, only 28 of 95 abnormal lymph nodes were identified. The same group prospectively enrolled 50 patients prior to axillary lymph node dissection.[229] The authors observed only one false negative scan that occurred in an obese patient whose PET images were of poor quality. Thus, the sensitivity of PET was 95%. However, the specificity was lower because of several false positive findings later explained by sinus histiocytosis, mild plasmacytosis, and hemosiderin-laden macrophages that are known to have accelerated rates of glycolysis.

In a comparative study,[214] FDG-PET detected axillary or infra-clavicular node involvement with a sensitivity of 77% and a specificity of 100%. Ultrasound was more sensitive (87%) but less specific (50%) than PET.

The largest prospective study included 124 patients with a diagnosis of breast cancer.[219] FDG–PET correctly identified all 44 tumor involved lymph nodes resulting in a sensitivity of 100%. Further, all pathologically proven normal lymph nodes in 60 patients had normal PET findings. However, in 20 additional patients, PET showed increased glycolysis that remained unexplained by pathology in 18.

Reactive inflammation likely accounted for increased glycolysis in 2 patients. Thus, the overall specificity of PET was 75%. The authors provided no pathological explanation for the false positive scans. However, extravasation at the injection site with subsequent lymphatic drainage of the tracer, lack of attenuation correction, or other factors might have accounted for the false positive findings.

The National Cancer Institute of Milan, Italy studied 68 patients with findings suspicious for breast cancer with FDG–PET.[230] Most patients underwent axillary lymph node dissection after PET. Histological evaluation revealed that 31 of 83 patients had lymph node involvement. The overall sensitivity, specificity, and accuracy of PET were 84%, 85%, and 84%. PET was positive in 15 of 16 patients with fewer than 3 lymph nodes involved and positive in 11 of 15 of those with more than 3 lymph nodes involved. The sensitivity of PET was lower in patients without, than in those with, palpable axillary lymph nodes. In a subsequent study, these authors more specifically and prospectively addressed the accuracy of FDG–PET for lymph node staging in 68 patients with breast cancer.[227] Sensitivity, specificity, and diagnostic accuracy of PET was 85%, 91%, and 89%, respectively. The highest diagnostic accuracy was observed in patients with N1a disease.

Smith et al[231] reported a similar diagnostic performance in 50 patients and concluded "that FDG–PET appears to be the most accurate and reliable noninvasive method for determining axillary lymph node involvement in patients with breast cancer."

In another study, PET correctly classified the lymph node status in 67 of 74 patients.[210] All false negative cases occurred in patients with micrometastatic lymph node involvement.

Less encouraging findings were reported by Yutani et al,[209] who compared FDG–PET with MIBI–Single photon emission tomography (SPECT) for detecting primary breast cancer and axillary node involvement in 40 women with suspected breast cancer. While the overall accuracy of FDG–PET for axillary lymph node involvement tended to be better than MIBI–SPECT (79% vs 73%), the negative predictive value and sensitivity (50% vs 38%) were unacceptably low for both diagnostic tests. It is noteworthy that all 8 lymph node metastases missed by PET were smaller than 10 mm.

A higher sensitivity of PET than of ultrasound for detecting axillary lymph node involvement was reported by Ohta et al[226] in 32 patients.

Schirrmeister et al[208] studied 117 women and reported a sensitivity and specificity of FDG–PET of 79 and 92%. This compared favorably with physical examination of the axilla. False negative PET findings were usually explained by tumor involvement of nodes smaller than 1 cm. Nevertheless, because of the relatively low sensitivity, the authors concluded that PET could not replace the histopathological evaluation of axillary lymph nodes.

The largest study to date was recently published in the *Journal of the National Cancer Institute*.[225] This study involved 167 consecutive patients with breast cancer. All underwent axillary lymph node dissection after FDG–PET. Only patients with tumors smaller than 50 mm were included in the study. The authors reported a sensitivity, specificity, and diagnostic accuracy of PET of 94%, 86%, and 90%. Importantly, the accuracy of PET was not affected by the size of the primary tumors.

Thus, PET determines axillary lymph node involvement with a higher diagnostic accuracy than any other noninvasive imaging test. Importantly, the accuracy of PET is similar to that of sentinel node biopsy. PET determines presence or absence of lymph node involvement but cannot determine accurately the number of involved lymph nodes. Finally, micrometastatic disease cannot be detected with PET. Future studies need to determine whether PET and sentinel node biopsy provides equivalent prognostic information.

Staging for distant disease (Figure 5-21)

Accurate staging of breast cancer patients is required to optimize patient management. Patients undergo a variety of noninvasive and invasive tests to determine the extent of disease prior to and after treatment. These include bone scanning, x-ray techniques, CT, MRI, ultrasound, and tissue biopsy. As a whole-body technique, FDG–PET alone might provide staging information of similar accuracy compared to all other tests together.

An early pilot study by Wahl et al[215] that included 12 patients reported that FDG–PET correctly identified 10 of 10 bone metastases. In addition, PET correctly detected 5 known soft tissue metastases. Thirty patients with inconclusive breast findings by ultrasonography and mammography were studied by Scheidhauer et al.[212] Using histology as the gold standard, FDG–PET accurately classified 21 of 23 primary breast lesions and accurately uncovered the presence of multifocal disease in 1 patient. The accuracy of PET was 90% for primary breast cancer lesions and 94% for axillary lymph node involvement. PET correctly detected all 8 distant metastases in 23 patients without false positive findings. The authors suggested that FDG–PET provided important additional diagnostic and staging information to that obtained through other imaging approaches. They concluded that qualitative FDG–PET could be used for the preoperative staging in patients with highly suspicious breast findings to aid therapy planning.

In another study, whole-body FDG–PET staging revealed unknown distant disease in 2 of 50 patients with untreated breast cancer.[231]

Vranjesevic et al[232] recently investigated the predictive accuracy of FDG–PET in 63 women who also underwent various conventional restaging procedures. In fact, women averaged more than 3 conventional imaging procedures within 3 months of the PET study. This study revealed a significantly higher accuracy

FIGURE 5-21. Extensive metastatic disease in a patient with breast cancer. Whole-body FDG–PET identified carcinomatosis of the pleura (P), as well as, mediastinal lymph node (LN) and bone (B) involvement.

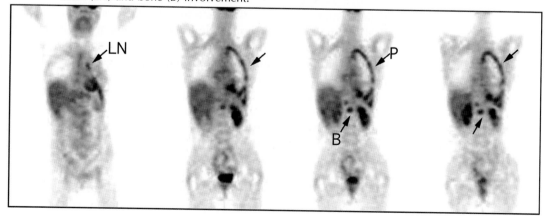

with PET than with conventional imaging for predicting the disease-free survival rate. This implies a higher accuracy of FDG–PET than combined conventional imaging for restaging of breast cancer.

The accuracy of PET for detecting recurrent or metastatic breast cancer was also investigated by Moon et al. In this study, the sensitivity and specificity of FDG–PET for detecting metastatic sites was 93% and 78%, respectively. Reasons for false positive interpretations were unspecific muscle uptake of FDG and inflammatory changes. Nevertheless, the authors concluded that PET accurately identifies metastatic disease.

Rostom et al[210] reported that all known distant metastatic lesions in 18 patients were accurately detected by FDG–PET. Importantly, only the combination of ultrasound, CT, and bone scanning achieved the same accuracy. An accuracy of 100% with FDG–PET for detecting distant disease was also reported by Schirrmeister et al.[208] PET resulted in upstaging 3 (2.6%) of the patients.

Monitoring Treatment

An early study by Minn et al[84] addressed the accuracy of FDG–PET for staging and treatment follow up in 17 patients with breast cancer. Ten patients were reimaged within 2 months to 25 months after treatment. Five of 7 patients with progressive disease had residual increased glycolysis as seen with FDG. Of the 2 remaining patients, 1 had developed new liver metastases while 1 patient with progressive disease did not exhibit increased glycolysis.

Wahl et al[215] subsequently utilized FDG–PET for monitoring breast cancer chemohormonotherapy in 11 women with newly diagnosed breast cancer larger than 3 cm. A baseline and 4 followup PET scans were performed. In patients with partial or complete pathologically determined response, the tumor diameter remained unchanged during the first 3 cycles of chemotherapy. Thus, treatment response could not be determined using anatomic criteria. In contrast, FDG–uptake declined to 78% of baseline already at day 8 after initiation of chemotherapy. After 9 weeks, tumor glycolysis was reduced to 52% of the baseline value. Importantly, no such decline was observed in those patients who did not achieve a partial or complete pathologically determined response.[233] Anecdotal evidence to support these initial findings was provided by Bruce et al[234] who observed decreasing glycolysis with FDG after a single chemotherapy cycle in 4 of 4 tumors with pathologic response.

Jansson et al. evaluated the metabolic tumor response to polychemotherapy using C-11 methionine and FDG–PET. Sixteen patients were enrolled in this study. Clinical response was determined clinically or radiographically but not histologically in this study. PET showed a decrease in tumor glycolysis in all clinical responders. In agreement with Wahl's observations,[233] a glycolytic response was discernible 1 to 2 weeks after initial chemotherapy in 11 of 12 clinical responders. Importantly, all early responders later exhibited clinical tumor regression.

Similar observations were made by Bassa et al[216] who studied 16 patients prior to and 13 patients between the end of the first cycle and the midpoint of chemotherapy, and in 14 patients again prior to surgery. Tumor glycolysis as expressed by the standardized uptake value declined from the pretreatment to both post-treatment FDG–PET studies. This study failed, however, to find a correlation between tumor response and patient outcome. Nevertheless, high residual glycolysis was associated with residual tumor. In other words, the negative predictive value of PET was low but the positive predictive value was high, suggesting that early changes in treatment might be warranted if high tumor glycolysis persists. Dehdashti et al[235] evaluated the glycolytic tumor response to tamoxifen treatment. These authors used fluorinated estradiol and FDG in 11 postmenopausal women with biopsy-proven, estrogen-positive metastatic breast cancer. Based on clinical followup, these authors identified 7 responders and 4 nonresponders. Clinical followup was used to determine the predictive value of PET. In this study, all responders had a glycolytic flare-response, i.e., increased tumor glycolysis as evidenced by a mean increase in SUV of 1.4 ± 0.7. No such flare-response was observed in nonresponders that exhibited a decreased glycolysis with a decline of SUV by 0.1 ± 0.4. In addition, baseline F-18 estradiol uptake was higher in responders than in nonresponders. Thus, a glycolytic flare predicted the responsiveness to antiestrogen treatment in patients with estrogen receptor positive breast cancer.

FDG–PET was used to monitor the efficacy of chemotherapy in 22 patients with 24 breast carcinomas.[236] This study included only patients with locally advanced breast cancer scheduled to undergo combination chemotherapy. Clinical response to treatment was assessed by comparing initial with preoperative tumor size as determined by MRI. Treatment responders were grouped into those with complete histologically proven response and those with residual scattered tumor foci. Changes in glycolysis during treatment differed significantly between these two groups ($p < 0.05$). Using receiver operating characteristic (ROC) curve analysis, patients with decreases of SUV to less than 55% of baseline discriminated best between responders and nonresponders. This resulted in a sensitivity of 100% and a specificity of 85% of PET for predicting treatment response. The predictive accuracy was 88%. After the second treatment course, the predictive accuracy was 91% when the threshold of 55% of baseline SUV was used as cutoff point. The authors concluded that monitoring treatment with FDG–PET might be useful in predicting responses early during the course of treatment.

In another study that included 30 patients with locally advanced noninflammatory breast cancer, FDG–PET predicted the treatment response with a sensitivity of 90% and a specificity of 74%.[228] In this study, all primary tumors and 11 of 11 pathologic axillary lymph nodes were detected by FDG–PET. The primary breast lesions that exhibited a complete clinical response after completion of chemotherapy had a significantly greater reduction in glycolysis after a single dose of chemotherapy than lesions without such response. Similarly, those with a pathologically proven response had a greater reduction in glycolysis after the first chemotherapeutic cycle ($p = 0.013$). Using a 10% reduction in FDG uptake, predicted treatment response had a sensitivity and specificity of 82% and 67%. Using 20% reduction of the differential uptake ratio, an index of tracer uptake in the tumor as cutoff, a complete pathological response after the first treatment cycle was predicted with a sensitivity of 90% and a specificity of 74%. The authors suggested that FDG–PET provides very useful information for predicting the treatment response of patients with locally advanced breast cancer.

Thus, FDG–PET is emerging as a powerful new tool for monitoring the response of breast cancer to chemotherapy.

Impact on management

Yap et al[237] recently investigated the impact of FDG–PET on managing 50 patients with breast cancer. In their survey of referring physicians, PET changed the clinical stage in 36% (28% upstaged, 8% downstaged) and altered the clinical management in about 40% of the patients.

The published literature therefore demonstrates that the fundamental alterations of glucose metabolism that are common to cancer also occur in breast cancer. FDG–PET diagnoses and stages breast cancer with a high diagnostic accuracy. It uniquely permits not only the accurate characterization of primary tumors and staging of axillary and mediastinal lymph node involvement but also the detection of distant metastases in a single whole-body examination. With regards to monitoring the effects of chemotherapy, FDG–PET seems ideally suited to predict therapy outcome of patients with locally advanced breast cancer.

Unknown Primary Cancer

Clinical background

Patients with cancer of unknown primary site represent 5% to 10% of all cancers.[238] These patients present with symptoms related to the metastatic site, but the primary tumors remain undetected despite extensive workup with conventional imaging techniques. Treatment of unknown primary cancer frequently involves empiric chemotherapy.[238] Identification of primary tumors is therefore important for more appropriate patient management.

Several groups have evaluated the ability of FDG–PET for detecting unknown primary cancers.[239] In 27 of 723 patients, the primary tumor could not be identified by conventional diagnostic procedures.[240] PET correctly uncovered the site of primary cancer in 7 (26%) of these patients. In another study,[241] PET correctly identified the known site of metastatic involvement in 28 of 29 patients and detected 5 additional unknown metastases. The unknown primary tumor was identified in 24% of the patients. A detection rate of 21% for primary tumors metastasizing to the head and neck region was reported in 14 patients.[242]

In a study of 53 patients with metastases to the head and neck region, FDG–PET identified the site of primary disease in 51% of the patients.[243]

The usefulness of PET for detecting occult primary tumors was, however, questioned in another study.[244] PET detected the unknown primary in only 1 (8%) patient but provided false positive results in 46% of 13 patients with metastases to the head and neck region. Multiple endoscopic tests identified the primary site in 46% of the patients.

Thus, the majority of studies suggest that FDG–PET results in a modest but clinically important improvement in the detectability of unknown primary cancers. While more studies are required that compare conventional imaging to PET, the current data indicate that PET can identify primary tumors in about 20% of all patients with unknown primary tumor.

Gynecologic Cancers

Ovarian cancer

CLINICAL BACKGROUND

Epithelial cancers of the ovaries continue to be a major health problem in the United States accounting for 4% of all cancers and 5% of all cancer deaths.

Approximately 28,000 new cases of ovarian cancer occur annually in the United States and about 60% of women with ovarian cancer will succumb to this disease within 5 years of the diagnosis. Ovarian cancer is currently the sixth most common cancer in the United States and the fourth most common cause of female cancer deaths, ranking behind lung, breast, and colon cancer. Five-year survival rates have been disappointingly stable at a low level of about 35% to 40% despite the use of aggressive chemotherapy, second-look surgery, and salvage therapies including radiation, intraperitoneal chemotherapy, and investigational drugs. Patients with stage I cancer (confined to ovary) have an excellent 5-year survival rate of 90%. However, the combined 5-year survival rate for stage III and IV patients is only 15% to 20%. Because there are no reliable screening tests, ovarian cancer is most frequently diagnosed at an advanced clinical stage. Only about 30% to 40% of all suspicious adnexal masses identified by ultrasound and CT are diagnosed as malignant during laparoscopy or laparotomy, indicating that 60% to 70% of all surgical explorations are unnecessary. The evaluation of adnexal masses has largely relied on the ultrasonic evaluation. Different size and morphological criteria have been established to determine the nature of adnexal masses.[245,246] Bromley et al[247] evaluated the diagnostic accuracy of ultrasound and Doppler flow velocity measurements to predict the nature of adnexal masses. While the sensitivity of transvaginal ultrasound was high (91%), its specificity was unacceptably low (52%).

Thus, early detection of ovarian cancer and a correct presurgical diagnosis are important to avoid unnecessary exploratory laparotomy or laparoscopy. Several studies have addressed the role of FDG–PET in this setting.

DIAGNOSIS, STAGING, AND RESTAGING

Fenchel et al[248] studied 85 patients with asymptomatic adnexal masses with FDG–PET. In this population with a 10% incidence of malignancy, the sensitivity and specificity of PET were 50% and 85%, respectively. False positive PET findings included Schwannoma, teratoma, and cystadenoma. False negative PET studies occurred in patients with borderline and early cancers. Grab et al[249] studied 102 patients with asymptomatic adnexal masses with FDG–PET, MRI, and ultrasound. The incidence of cancer was again low (< 10%) in this study. Ultrasound had the highest sensitivity (92%) but the lowest specificity (60%). The specificity of MRI and PET was better at 82% and 80%, respectively. However, the sensitivity of these two tests was lower than that of ultrasound. These authors concluded that PET could not replace surgical evaluation of patients with adnexal masses. Kubich–Huch et al[250] concluded from a study in 19 patients with primary or recurrent ovarian carcinoma that neither PET, CT, nor MRI were sufficiently accurate to obviate the need for surgical exploration in these patients. Zimny et al[251] arrived at the same conclusion after studying 26 patients with primary or recurrent ovarian cancer using FDG–PET. Römer et al[252] reported false positive FDG–PET studies in patients with inflammatory processes that resulted in a low specificity of FDG–PET of only 54% in 19 patients with adnexal masses.

Hubner et al[253] reported positive and negative predictive values of FDG–PET for ovarian cancer of 86% and 76% in 51 patients with suspected ovarian cancer prior to laparotomy. They concluded that PET might be useful in the diagnosis of ovarian cancer.

In summary, the current literature suggests that FDG–PET has a limited sensitivity and specificity for characterizing adnexal masses and diagnosing disease recurrence. FDG–PET cannot replace the surgical evaluation of adnexal masses and, because of its limited sensitivity, is unlikely to replace the second-look surgery for determining recurrent disease. Other important indications such as monitoring the effects of various treatment strategies with FDG–PET in ovarian cancer have not been studied extensively.

Cancers of the Genitourinary System

Renal cell cancer

CLINICAL BACKGROUND

Renal cell cancer is diagnosed in about 30,000 patients per year and accounts for 3% of the malignancies in adults in the United States. Advanced renal cell cancer carries a poor prognosis.[151] New treatment strategies such as immunotherapy are being used in an attempt to delay the progression of disease but remain controversial. Noninvasive tests for diagnosing, staging, and monitoring the course of disease would be desirable. The current procedures for staging and restaging of patients with renal cell cancer consist primarily of anatomic imaging modalities.

DIAGNOSIS, STAGING, AND RESTAGING

Several investigations have used FDG–PET for characterizing primary renal tumors (Figure 5-22). Bachor et al[254] studied 29 patients with solid renal masses, all of whom underwent FDG–PET before surgery. PET results were compared to surgical pathologic findings in 26 patients who had a histologic diagnosis of renal cell carcinoma. PET was true positive for malignancy in 20 patients but was falsely negative in 6 patients. Three patients with benign pathology (angiomyolipoma, pericytoma, and pheochromocytoma) were false positive by PET, indicating that some benign lesions have increased glycolysis.

Goldberg et al[255] performed 26 FDG–PET studies in 21 patients. They evaluated the ability of FDG–PET to characterize solid renal masses (n = 10 patients) and indeterminate renal cysts (n = 11 patients) as malignant or benign. PET correctly classified solid lesions as malignant in 9 of 10 patients subsequently confirmed histologically by surgery or biopsy (6 renal cell carcinoma, 3 lymphoma). One patient with bilateral renal cell carcinoma was false negative by PET. PET correctly classified indeterminate renal cysts as benign in 7 of 8 patients confirmed by surgery or needle aspiration. PET was false negative in 1 patient with a 4-mm papillary neoplasm. The authors suggested that a positive FDG–PET scan in the appropriate clinical setting might obviate the need for cyst aspiration in indeterminate renal masses.

More recently, Montravers et al[256] performed FDG–PET scans in 13 patients with renal masses who subsequently had nephrectomy or surgical resection. PET correctly characterized all but one of the malignant tumors and gave a false positive in 1 patient with renal tuberculosis, true negative in 3 patients with benign masses (1 angiomyolipoma, 2 indeterminate renal cysts), and false negative in 1 patient with a 3-cm renal cell carcinoma.

In order to investigate why some renal malignancies do not exhibit increased glycolysis, Miyauchi et al[257] compared several biological characteristics of renal tumors to the degree of glycolysis determined with FDG uptake. They studied 11 patients with newly diagnosed renal cell carcinoma and compared the results of FDG–PET to the expression of glucose transporters (Glut-1, 2,4,5), tumor

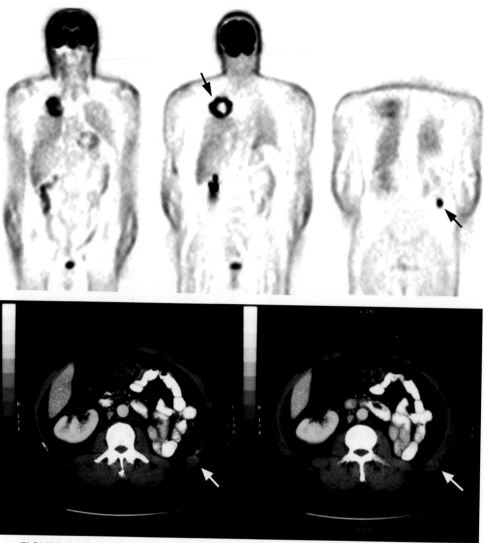

FIGURE 5-22. Patient with renal cell cancer underwent restaging with FDG-PET. The large right upper lung lesion (left and middle panel) with central necrosis was seen on both CT and PET images. A second focus (right panel) was located in the left flank. This was only retrospectively detected on CT (bottom panel). Biopsy demonstrated metastatic renal cell cancer.

size, and tumor grade. From this, they concluded that renal cancers that are well visualized by FDG–PET have higher tumor grades and Glut-1 expression and tend to be larger than poorly imaged tumors.

In addition to the biological characteristics of renal malignancies, the normal renal excretion of FDG results in residual parenchymal activity as well as the pooling of excreted tracer in the pelvicalyceal system, which may limit the ability of PET to visualize renal malignancies. Furthermore, lesions less than 1 cm in size or cystic lesions with mural malignancy may be below the spatial resolution of existing PET scanners (currently, approximately 8 mm).

The high positive predictive value of PET suggests that it is useful for non-invasive characterization of indeterminate renal masses in patients in whom surgical resection or biopsy is not feasible.

Kocher et al[258] performed presurgical staging with FDG–PET in 10 patients with renal cancer and found that PET predicted the presence or absence of lymph node metastases in all cases (3 positive, 7 negative). Bachor et al[254] reported that FDG–PET correctly identified regional lymph node metastases in 3 of 26 patients. Finally, Montravers et al[256] reported that PET correctly staged 11 of 12 patients (4 true positive, 7 true negative). The sites of positive PET findings were in the bone (n = 3), lung (n = 1), and lymph nodes (n = 1).

Safaei et al[259] assessed the utility of FDG–PET for restaging 36 patients with advanced renal cell carcinoma (RCC). In this retrospective study, the authors evaluated the additional value of whole-body PET to conventional imaging (including CT, MRI, ultrasound, plain radiography, and bone scintigraphy). In a patient-based analysis, PET correctly classified the clinical stage in 32 (89%) of 36 and was incorrect in (11%) 4 patients. In a lesion-based analysis, PET correctly classified 21 (81%) of 25 lesions that were subsequently biopsy proven. PET was true positive in 14, true negative in 7, false positive in 1, and false negative in 3 lesions resulting in a sensitivity of 82%, specificity of 88%, and diagnostic accuracy of 81%.

Testicular cancer

CLINICAL BACKGROUND

Testicular cancers are the most common solid tumors in men between the ages of 20 and 35 years. Testicular cancer is a diverse group of cancers with seminoma accounting for about 50%. Other testicular cancers include seminoma, embryonal carcinoma, teratoma, and others.[260]

Clinical staging of testicular cancers is usually performed using CT and measurement of serum tumor markers. However, these methods understage testicular cancer in up to 30% of all patients.[261]

Several studies have investigated whether FDG–PET can improve the staging of patients with testicular cancer. Cremerius et al[262] staged 50 patients with diagnosed testicular cancer using PET, CT, and tumor markers. During clinical followup, PET and CT had a sensitivity of 87% and 73% while both had a specificity of 94% for detecting metastatic involvement. Both PET and CT failed to identify small retroperitoneal lymph nodes.

Cremerius et al[263] also compared the role of FDG–PET to that of CT for detecting and restaging of metastatic germ-cell tumors in 33 patients prior to and after chemotherapy. Histology and clinical followup served as gold standards. The accuracy of PET and CT was similar for cancer detection. However, PET was superior to CT for assessing residual and recurrent tumor late but not early after treatment. The notion that FDG–PET is most useful in the post-therapeutic assessment of patients was supported by Müller–Mattheis et al[264] in a prospective study of 54 patients with testicular cancer. PET was not useful for evaluating teratoma and did not add staging information in patients with stage I seminoma. PET was, however, superior to CT in assessing the tumor response to treatment. Hain et al[265] made similar observations in 55 patients who were studied after treatment. The positive and negative predictive value of FDG–PET for disease recurrence was 96% and 90%.

FDG–PET only modestly improved staging of 37 patients with stage I and II testicular germ cell tumors.[266] PET and CT staged 34 of 37 and 29 of 27 patients correctly (p = NS). Again, PET did not identify teratoma and lesions smaller than 5 mm.

Thus, the available data suggest that PET stages testicular cancer with a good diagnostic accuracy. PET might be most useful for determining disease recurrence after treatment.

Prostate cancer

Prostate cancer is the most commonly diagnosed cancer in American men and is the second leading cause of cancer death in men. In 1999, there will be an estimated 179,000 new cases and 37,000 deaths due to prostate cancer.[151] The treatment of prostate cancer depends on the stage of the disease at the time of diagnosis. The likelihood of cure for confined tumors with specific local treatments such as surgery or radiation therapy is very high. Unfortunately, a high percentage of patients who present with newly diagnosed prostate cancer have disease that is not organ confined and is, therefore, unlikely to be cured with local therapies. Current imaging modalities used for evaluating the presence of metastatic disease include bone scintigraphy for determining the presence of osseous metastases, and CT of the pelvis to determine the presence of regional lymph node metastases. While bone scintigraphy is a highly sensitive test for detecting bone metastases, it is often nonspecific; positive findings may be related to degenerative joint disease or to benign bone disease. For the assessment of regional pelvic lymph node metastases, CT or MRI is not routinely performed due to their generally low sensitivity.

Because FDG–PET is a whole-body imaging technique, it might be useful for diagnosing local cancer recurrence and distant disease (Figure 5-23, left panel). However, the existing literature suggests that FDG–PET has a limited

FIGURE 5-23. FDG and [C-11] acetate uptake pattern in prostate cancer. FDG clears through the kidney to the bladder while [C-11] acetate is either incorporated into lipids or oxidized to [C-11] CO_2 that dilutes throughout the body. Thus, [C-11] acetate does not accumulate in the urinary bladder (BL). Notice that the local recurrence (LR) was easily detected on [C-11] acetate images, while it was difficult to differentiate from bladder activity with FDG. Both tracers identified lymph node involvement (LN).

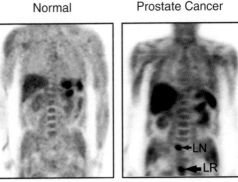

role for detecting the primary prostate tumor.[267] This is largely explained by the kinetics of FDG that undergo renal clearance with subsequent tracer accumulation in the bladder. This renders the detection of primary or recurrent prostate cancer difficult. In addition, increased glycolysis with FDG also occurs in benign prostate hypertrophy. More recently, Liu et al[268] also concluded that FDG–PET was not a useful test in the evaluation of organ-confined prostate cancer. In this study, PET correctly identified only 1 of 24 primary cancers. These results were obtained after intravenous hydration and furosemide administration to lower FDG activity in the urinary bladder.

The utility of FDG–PET for detecting metastatic disease in newly diagnosed prostate cancer patients was investigated by Shreve et al.[269] In this study, the authors evaluated 22 untreated prostate cancer patients with 202 osseous metastases detected by bone scintigraphy. When compared to bone scintigraphy, the sensitivity of PET was 65%. FDG–PET, however, had a high positive predictive value of 98% for the presence of metastatic tumor.

Yeh et al.[270] also reported that only approximately 18% of the lesions detected by conventional bone scanning exhibited high glycolysis with FDG in patients with androgen-independent prostate cancer. They suggested that prostate cancer tissue might utilize substrates other than glucose for energy production. It should be noticed however, that the glycolytic activity of bone lesions by FDG–PET may provide different prognostic information than the secondary osteoblastic reaction seen on conventional bone images.

Seltzer et al[15] investigated the ability of FDG–PET to detect lymph node metastases in 45 patients with rising serum prostate-specific antigen (PSA) levels after primary local therapy. This study demonstrated that FDG–PET can detect the presence of lymph node metastases in patients with recurrent prostate cancer. The detection rate of metastases by FDG–PET was, however, dependent on the level of the serum PSA and on the rate of change of the serum PSA level over time (PSA velocity). FDG–PET was positive for lymph node metastases in 50% of patients with a PSA greater than 4 ng/ml or a PSA velocity greater than 0.2 ng/ml/month. In contrast, FDG–PET was positive for distant disease in only 4% of patients with a PSA level less than 4 ng/ml or a PSA velocity less than 0.2 ng/ml/month. The low detection rate of metastases by FDG–PET in patients with a low PSA or low PSA velocity may be ascribed to the low incidence of metastases in this group of patients. Alternatively, small volume lesions might have precluded detectability with FDG–PET. This study also compared the imaging results of FDG–PET to conventional imaging with helical computed tomography of the abdomen and pelvis and to the monoclonal antibody scan, ProstaScint. In this comparison, the detection rate of metastases was similar for PET and helical CT—50% of patients with a high PSA or PSA velocity had a positive PET and CT scan—but both, CT and PET were superior to ProstaScint for the detection of lymph node metastases.

The present data, therefore, suggest that FDG–PET provides only limited diagnostic and staging information in patients with prostate cancer. The use of new tracers such as [C-11] acetate (Figure 5-23, right panel) or F-18 labeled choline, discussed in the following section, promise to improve the clinical usefulness of PET in prostate cancer.[271,272]

FUTURE APPLICATIONS OF PET IMAGING

PET technology is rapidly advancing (Chapter 1).[12] Among the most exciting developments is the emergence of combined PET and CT imaging devices[67] (Figure 5-24). The combination of molecular and anatomic imaging has several advantages: First, biologic and anatomic whole-body staging can be performed in one examination. Second, because of limited patient motion due to the near simultaneous acquisition of PET and CT images, near ideal fusion of biologic and anatomic images can be achieved. Third, anatomic landmarks provided by CT will greatly facilitate the assignment of biological abnormalities to anatomical structures in which disease exists. Finally and importantly, difficult-to-image regions of the body such as head and neck, mediastinum, and the postsurgical abdomen will be evaluated with a high diagnostic accuracy due to improved anatomical assignment of biologically identified disease. The first commercial PET/CT devices became available for clinical testing in the later part of 2001 (Chapter 1). The PET/CT will dramatically change the planning of radiation therapy and the monitoring of surgical, medical, and radiation treatments. Technological advances such as the introduction of the LSO detector technology allow for rapid imaging protocols. The author is currently using a weight-based protocol whereby patients who weigh less than 130 pounds are imaged with emission scans of 1 minute, and those who weight from 130 to 180 pounds with scans of 2 minutes per bed position. Three- and four-minute emission scans are used for patients who weigh above 180 and 250 pounds, respectively (Figure 5-24). Thus, whole-body PET/CT images can be completed in as little as 7 minutes and are usually performed within 15 minutes.

The development of new tracers that target specific biological properties of cancer cells is another important line of current research. Several new tracers are currently being tested for their clinical usefulness in cancer patients. For instance, [C-11] acetate and ^{18}F fluoromethylcholine are being tested to identify lipid synthesis that is increased 10- to 20-fold in prostate cancer,[271] (Figure 5-23, right panel; Chapter 4). FDG–PET detects distant prostate cancer metastases with high diagnostic accuracy in patients with moderately to severely elevated PSA levels. FDG, however, undergoes renal clearance and accumulates in the urinary bladder, which tends to obscure the prostate bed. Although this can be reduced by catheterization and irrigation of the bladder, this complicates the procedure and limits its usefulness for assessing primary and locally recurrent prostate cancer. Renal clearance of activity is eliminated in the case of Carbon-11 acetate because the [C-11] label is in the acid (COOH) group of acetate. Thus, when [C-11] acetate is oxidatively metabolized, the labeled product is $[C-11]-CO_2$ that is diluted through the body in the bicarbonate pool and, therefore, does not undergo renal clearance. The labeled product retained in tissue is in the form of lipids that are rapidly synthesized in prostate cancer cells. This represents a strategy of placing a positron label in a specific location in the molecular imaging probe to improve its diagnostic accuracy.

A different strategy is used with F-18 labeled choline. It has been shown that the synthetic reaction involving choline in prostate cancer is faster than the renal clearance of the tracer. Thus, the prostate bed can be imaged before tracer accumulation in the bladder occurs. Initial studies with [C-11] acetate by Seltzer

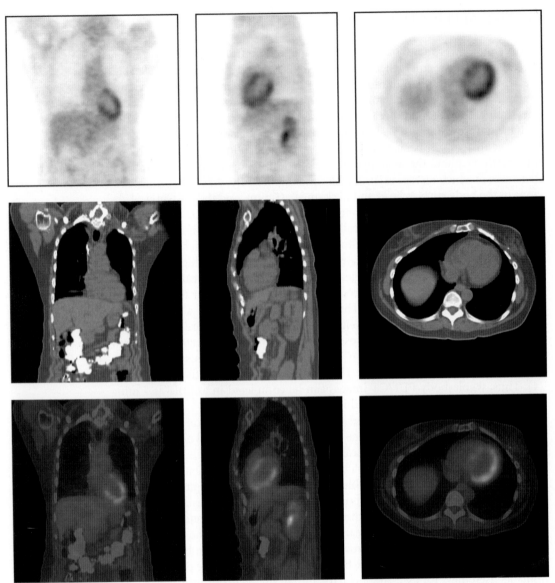

FIGURE 5-24. PET and CT image with the LSO-PET/CT system in a patient who was treated for Hodgkin's disease. The study was completed in 8 minutes. One minute was required for the CT portion and 7 minutes for PET (1 minute/bed position). The upper row displays coronal, saggital, and axial PET images. The same projections for CT are shown in the middle row. Fused PET/CT images are seen at the bottom. No abnormalities were identified.

et al[271] and with ^{18}F-fluoro methylcholine by DeGrado et al[272] suggest that these tracers detect primary and recurrent prostate cancer with a good diagnostic accuracy.

Shields et al[273] used FLT, to image DNA replication and cell proliferation of tumors in vivo. FLT is retained in proliferating tissues through the enzyme thymidine kinase 1 (Figure 5-25) that phosphorylates FLT to FLT-1-PO_4 that is

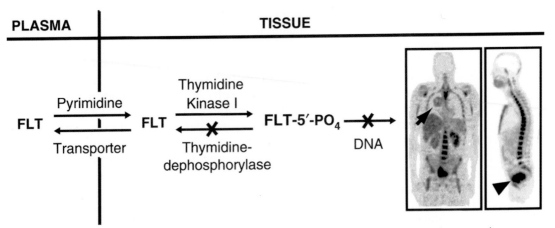

FIGURE 5-25. Tracer kinetic model for FLT. FLT is transported between plasma and tissue by thymidine-facilitated transport carriers and phosphorylated by thymidine kinase 1 to FLT-5'PO_4 which is either dropped into cells since it is not significantly dephosphorylated during the time of a PET study or is incorporated into and trapped in DNA. Images to the right are coronal and sagittal images of a patient with a nonsmall cell lung carcinoma (arrow) with a high DNA replication rate. Notice normal high DNA replication for cell proliferation in the skeletal system and clearance of FLT to the bladder (arrowhead). High activity in the liver is due to glycoronidation of FLT. These images are of the same patient as shown in Figure 5-1.

trapped in cells, much like FDG-6-PO_4. The authors obtained high target to background images of tumor cell proliferation in patients. A similar approach using[11]C-thymidine has also been used to investigate its value for monitoring the tumor response to chemotherapy.[274]

The novel and elegant concept of *in-vivo* imaging of gene expression with PET was recently introduced by Tjuvajev et al,[275] Gambhir et al,[276] and MacLaren et al[277] (Chapter 2). Gambhir et al[276] use a PET reporter-gene/reporter probe imaging approach using the herpes simplex type 1 virus thymidine kinase (HSV1-tk) gene, while MacLaren et al[277] use the dopamine type 2-receptor (D2R) gene as reporter genes for imaging gene expression in vivo. In this approach, a PET reporter gene is connected to another gene (i.e., a therapy gene), and this genetic construct is administered to the subject via a viral vector. The reporter gene product is a protein. This protein is the target of the PET reporter probe that can be administered at any time to image the location and degree of the reporter gene expression and, therefore, the expression of the other gene attached to it. This allows *in-vivo* monitoring of the gene therapy dosing at the site of action within cells of the target organs. The approach can also be used to image the expression of endogenous genes as they initiate disease processes.[12,278] In addition, a new high-resolution PET technology, microPET[279] (Chapter 1), has been developed for imaging genetically engineered and human disease cell transplant models of disease in mice. This technology provides the means to perform modern biology and genetic experiments in the living mouse by assessing such processes as metabolism, cell communication and gene expression. The microPET technology will also provide new technologies to dramatically improve the resolution of clinical PET scanners.

In summary, molecular imaging of the biological nature of disease with PET and FDG has arrived as a clinical tool for diagnosing, staging and restaging of most cancers.

PET radiopharmacies have been started throughout the United States to provide FDG and other imaging probes to hospitals and private radiology groups (Chapter 3). PET also represents the entry of molecular imaging of the fundamental biology of disease as a paradigm shift in diagnostic imaging. In this way, the importance of PET reaches far beyond characterizing glucose metabolism of tumors, as important as this is in its own right. New molecular imaging probes as well as technological advances will provide a powerful armamentarium for specifically characterizing and targeting the biological properties and genetics of tumor cells in vivo, monitoring the response to treatment, and establishing prognostic information. PET will play an important role in molecular medicine in the post genome era and will allow biologically directed and monitored therapeutic interventions to correct the molecular errors of disease.

REFERENCES

1. Warburg O, Posener K, Negelein E. VIII. The metabolism of cancer cells. *Biochem Zeitschr.* 1924;152:129–169.
2. Flexner S, Jobling S. Studies upon a transplantable rat tumour. *Monographs on Medical and Allied Subjects.* Rockefeller Institute for Medical Research, New York, 1910, pp. 1–51.
3. Weber G. Enzymology of cancer cells (Part 1). *N Engl J Med.* 1977;296:541–555.
4. Weber G. Enzymology of cancer cells (Part 2). *N Engl J Med.* 1977;296:541–555.
5. Flier J, Mueckler M, Usher P, Lodish H. Elevated levels of glucose transport and transporter messenger RNA are induced by ras and sarc oncogenes. *Science.* 1987;235:1492–1495.
6. Weber G, Banaejee G, Morris H. Comparative chemistry of hepatomas 5123. *Cancer Res.* 1961;21:933–937.
7. Phelps M, Hoffmann E, Mullani N, TerPogossian M. Application of annihilation coincidence detection to transaxial reconstruction tomography. *J Nucl Med.* 1975;16:210–224.
8. Valk PE, Pounds TR, Tesar RD, Hopkins DM, Haseman MK. Cost-effectiveness of PET imaging in clinical oncology. *Nucl Med Biol.* 1996;23:737–743.
9. Silverman D, Hoh C, Seltzer M, et al. Evaluating tumor biology and oncological disease with positron emission tomography. *Semin Radiat Oncol.* 1998;8:183–196.
10. Conti PS, Lilien DL, Hawley K, et al. PET and 18-F-FDG in oncology: a clinical update. *Nucl Med Biol.* 1996;23:717–735.
11. Rigo P. Positron emission tomography using 18F-fluorodeoxyglucose in oncology. *Bull Mem Acad R Med Belg.* 1997;152:353–361.
12. Phelps M. Positron emission tomography provides molecular imaging of biological processes. *PNAS.* 2000;97:9226–9233.
13. Rodriguez M, Rehn S, Ahlstrom H, Sundström C, Glimelius B. Predicting malignancy grade with PET in non-Hodgkin's lymphoma. *J Nucl Med.* 1995;36:1790–1796.
14. Feine U, Lietzenmeier R, Hanke J, et al. Fluorine-18-FDG and iodine-131-iodide uptake in thyroid cancer. *J Nucl Med.* 1996;37:1468–1472.
15. Seltzer M, Barbaric Z, Belldegrun A, et al. Comparison of helical computerized tomography, positron emission tomography and monoclonal antibody scans for evaluation of lymph node metastases in patients with prostate specific antigen relapse after treatment for localized prostate cancer. *J Urol.* 1999;162:1322–1328.
16. Gambhir S, Czernin J, Schwimmer J, et al. A tabulated summary of the FDG-PET literature. *J Nucl Med.* 2001;42:1S–71S.
17. Kunze W, Baehre M, Richter E. PET with dual head coincidence camera: spatial resolution, scatter fraction, and sensitivity. *J Nucl Med.* 2000;41:1067–1074.

18. Delbeke D, Patton J, Martin W, Sandler MP. FDG PET and dual head gamma camera positron coincidence detection imaging of suspected malignancies and brain disorders. *J Nucl Med.* 1999;40:110–117.
19. Landoni C, Gianolli L, Lucignani G, et al. Comparison of dual head coincidence PET versus ring PET in tumor patients. *J Nucl Med.* 1999;40:1617–1622.
20. Langen K, Braun U, Kops E, et al. The influence of plasma glucose levels on fluorine-18-fluorodeoxyglucose uptake in bronchial carcinomas. *J Nucl Med.* 1993;34:355–359.
21. Lindholm P, Minn H, Lekinen-Salo S, et al. Influence of the blood glucose concentration on FDG uptake in cancer—a PET study. *J Nucl Med.* 1993;34:1–6.
22. Crippa F, Gavazzi C, Bozzetti F, et al. The influence of blood glucose levels on [18F] fluorodeoxyglucose PET imaging. *Tumori.* 1997;83:748–752.
23. Wahl RL, Hutchins G, Buchsbaum D, et al. 18F-2-deoxy-2-fluoro-D-glucose uptake into human tumor xenografts. *Cancer.* 1991;67:1544–1550.
24. Fischman A, Alpert NM. FDG-PET in oncology: There's more to it than looking at pictures. *J Nucl Med.* 1993;34:6–11.
25. Dahlbom M, Hoffman EJ, Hoh CK, et al. Whole-body positron emission tomography: Part I. Methods and performance characteristics. *J Nucl Med.* 1992;33:1191–1199.
26. Meikle S, Hutton B, Bailey D, Hooper P, Fulham M. Accelerated EM reconstruction in total-body PET: potential for improving tumor detectability. *Phys Med Biol.* 1994;39:1689–1704.
27. Meikle SR, Dahlbom M, Cherry SR. Attenuation correction using count-limited transmission data in positron emission tomography. *J Nucl Med.* 1993;34:143–50.
28. Lowe V, Hoffman J, DeLong D, Patz E, Coleman R. Semiquantitative and visual analysis of FDG-PET images in pulmonary abnormalities. *J Nucl Med.* 1994;35:1771–1776.
29. Gupta N, Maloof J, Gunel E. Probability of malignancy in solitary pulmonary nodule using fluorine-18-FDG and PET. *J Nucl Med.* 1996;37:943–948.
30. Hoffman EJ, Huang SC, Phelps ME. Quantitation in positron emission computed tomography. *J Comput Assist Tomogr.* 1979;3:299–308.
31. Khouri N, Meziane M, Zerhouni E, Fishman E, Siegelman S. The solitary pulmonary nodule: Assessment, diagnosis and management. *Chest.* 1987;91:128–133.
32. Keagy B, Starek P, Murray G, et al. Major pulmonary resection for suspected but unconfirmed malignancy. *Ann Thorac Surg.* 1984;38:314–316.
33. Siegelman S, Zerhouni E, Leo R, Khouri N, Stitik F. CT of the solitary pulmonary nodule. *AJR.* 1980;135:1–13.
34. Kubota K, Matsuzawa T, Fujiwara T, et al. Differential diagnosis of lung tumor with positron emission tomography: a prospective study. *J Nucl Med.* 1990;31:1927–1933.
35. Dewan N, Gupta N, Redepennig L, Phalen J, Frick M. Diagnostic efficacy of PET-FDG imaging in solitary pulmonary nodules; potential role in evaluation and management. *Chest.* 1993;104:997–1002.
36. Patz E, Lowe V, Hoffman J, et al. Focal pulmonary abnormalities: evaluation with F-18 fluorodeoxyglucose PET scanning. *Radiology.* 1993;188:487–490.
37. Duhaylongsod F, Lowe V, Patz E, et al. Detection of primary and recurrent lung cancer by means of F-18 fluorodeoxyglucose positron emission tomography. *J Thorac Cardiovasc Surg.* 1995;110:130–140.
38. Knight S, Delbeke D, Stewart J, Sandler M. Evaluation of pulmonary lesions with FDG-PET: comparison of findings in patients with and without a history of prior malignancy. *Chest.* 1996;109:982–988.
39. Bury T, Dowlati A, Paulus P, et al. Evaluation of the solitary pulmonary nodule by positron emission tomography imaging. *Eur Respir J.* 1996;9:410–414.
40. Worsely D, Celler A, Adam M, et al. Pulmonary nodules: differential diagnosis using 18F-fluorodeoxyglucose single photon emission tomography. *AJR.* 1996;168:771–774.
41. Lowe V, Fletcher J, Gobar L, et al. Prospective investigation of positron emission tomography in lung nodules. *J Clin Oncol.* 1998;16:1075–1084.
42. Dewan N, Shehan C, Reeb S, et al. Likelihood of malignancy in a solitary pulmonary nodule: comparison of Bayesian analysis and results of FDG-PET scan. *Chest.* 1997;112:416–422.
43. Gambhir SS, Shepherd JE, Shah BD, Hart E, Hoh CK, et al. Analytical decision model for the cost-effective management of solitary pulmonary nodules. *J Clin Oncol.* 1998;16:2113–2125.

44. American Cancer Society. Cancer facts and figures. Atlanta, GA, 1996; pp. 12–13.
45. Mountain C. A new international staging system for lung cancer. *Chest.* 1986;89:225.
46. Mountain C. Value of the new TNM staging system for lung cancer. *Chest.* 1989;97:935.
47. McKenna R, Libshitz H, Mountain C, McMurtey M. Roentgenographic evaluation of mediastinal lymph nodes for pre-operative assessment in lung cancer. *Chest.* 1985;88:206–210.
48. Arita T, Kuramitsu T, Kawamura M. Bronchogenic carcinoma: incidence of metastases to normal sized lymph nodes. *Thorax.* 1995;50:1267–1269.
49. Webb R, Gatsonis C, Zerhouni E, et al. CT and MRI imaging in staging non-small cell bronchogenic carcinoma: report of the radiologic diagnostic oncology group. *Radiology.* 1991;178:705–713.
50. Dillemans B, Deneffe G, Verschakelen J, Decramer M. Value of computed tomography and mediastinoscopy in pre-operative evaluation of mediastinal nodes in non-small cell lung cancer. *Eur J Cardio-thorac Surg.* 1994;8:37–42.
51. Dwamena B, Sonnan S, Angobaldo J, Wahl RL. Metastases from non-small cell lung cancer: mediastinal staging in the 1990s—meta analytic comparison of PET and CT. *Radiology.* 1999;213:530–536.
52. Fujiwara T, Matsuszawa T, Ito M. F-18-deoxy-D-glucose positron emission tomography of human lung tumors. *Cyclotron and Radio-isotope Center Annual Report.* 1984:264–269.
53. Nolop K, Rhodes C, Brudin L, Beaney R, Krausz T, et al. Glucose utilization by human pulmonary neoplasms. *Cancer.* 1987;60:2682–2689.
54. Scott W, Schwabe J, Gupta N, et al. Positron emission tomography of lung tumors and mediastinal lymph nodes using [18F]Fluorodeoxyglucose. *Ann Thorac Surg.* 1994;58:698–703.
55. Scott W, Gobar L, Terry J, Dewan N, Sunderland J. Mediastinal lymph node staging of non-small-cell lung cancer: a prospective comparison of computed tomography and positron emission tomography. *J Thorac Cardiovasc Surg.* 1996;111:642–648.
56. Sazon D, Santiago S, Soo Hoo G, et al. Fluorodeoxyglucose-positron emission tomography in the detection and staging of lung cancer. *Am J Respir Crit Care Med.* 1996;153:417–421.
57. Sasaki M, Ichiya Y, Kuwabara Y, et al. The usefulness of FDG positron emission tomography for the detection of mediastinal lymph node metastases in patients with non-small cell lung cancer: a comparative study with x-ray computed tomography. *Eur J Nucl Med.* 1996;23:741–747.
58. Steinert H, Hauser M, Aleman F, et al. Non-small cell lung cancer: nodal staging with FDG-PET versus correlative lymph node mapping and sampling. *Radiology.* 1997;202:441–446.
59. Patz E, Lowe V, Goodman P, Herndon J. Thoracic nodal staging with PET imaging with 18-FDG in patients with bronchogenic carcinoma. *Chest.* 1995;108:1617–1621.
60. Guhlmann A, Storck M, Kotzerke J, et al. Lymph node staging in non-small cell lung cancer: evaluation by [18F]FDG positron emission tomography (PET). *Thorax.* 1997;52:438–441.
61. Marom E, McAdams H, Erasmus J, et al. Staging non-small cell lung cancer with whole body PET. *Radiology.* 1999;212:803–809.
62. Vansteenkiste J, Mortelmans L. FDG-PET in the locoregional lymph node staging of non-small cell lung cancer: a comprehensive review of the Leuven lung cancer group experience. *Mol Imag Biol.* 1999;4:223–231.
63. Chin R, Ward R, Keyes J, et al. Mediastinal staging of non-small-cell lung cancer with positron emission tomography. *Am J Respir Crit Care Med.* 1995;152:2090–2096.
64. Weng E, Tran L, Rege S. Accuracy and clinical impact of mediastinal lymph node staging with FDG-PET imaging in potentially resectable lung cancer. *Am J Clin Onc.* 2000;23:47–52.
65. Magnani P, Carretta A, Rizzo G, et al. FDG/PET and spiral CT image fusion for mediastinal lymph node assessment of non-small cell lung cancer patients. *J Cardiovasc Surg.* 1999;40:741–748.
66. Vansteenkiste J, Stroobants S, De Leyn P, et al. Lymph node staging in non-small-cell lung cancer with FDG-PET scan: a prospective study on 690 lymph node stations from 68 patients. *J Clin Oncol.* 1998;16:2142–2149.

67. Beyer T, Townsend D, Brun T, et al. A combined PET/CT scanner for clinical oncology. *J Nucl Med.* 2000;41:1369–1379.

68. Patton J, Delbeke D, Sandler M. Image fusion using an integrated, dual-head coincidence camera with X-ray tube-based attenuation maps. *J Nucl Med.* 1996;41:1364–1368.

69. Valk P, Pounds T, Hopkins D, et al. Staging non-small cell lung cancer by whole body positron emission tomographic imaging. *Ann Thorac Surg.* 1995;60:1573–1582.

70. Weder W, Schmid R, Bruchhaus H, et al. Detection of extrathoracic metastases by positron emission tomography in lung cancer. *Ann Thorac Surg.* 1998;66:886–892.

71. Bury T, Dowlati A, Paulus P, et al. Whole-body 18FDG positron emission tomography in the staging of non-small cell lung cancer. *Eur Respir J.* 1997;10:2529–2534.

72. Pieterman R, van Putten J, Meuzelaar J, et al. Preoperative staging of non-small-cell lung cancer with positron-emission tomography. *N Engl J Med.* 2000;343:254–261.

73. Saunders C, Dussek J, O'Doherty J. Evaluation of fluorine-18-fluorodeoxyglucose whole body positron emission tomography imaging in the staging of lung cancer. *Ann Thorac Surg.* 1999;67:790–797.

74. Lewis P, Griffin S, Marsden P, et al. Whole-body 18F-fluorodeoxyglucose positron emission tomography in preoperative evaluation of lung cancer. *Lancet.* 1994;344:1265–1266.

75. Seltzer M, Valk P, Wong C, et al. The impact of PET on the management of lung cancer: the referring physician's perspective. *J Nucl Med.* 2002;43:752–756

76. Gambhir SS, Hoh CK, Phelps ME, Madar I, Maddahi J. Decision tree sensitivity analysis for cost-effectiveness of FDG-PET in the staging and management of non-small-cell lung carcinoma. *J Nucl Med.* 1996;37:1428–1436.

77. Jabour B, Choi Y, Hoh C, et al. Extracranial head and neck: PET imaging with 2-[F-18]fluoro-2-deoxy-D-glucose and MR Imaging correlation. *Radiology.* 1993;186:27–35.

78. Rege S, Maas A, Chaiken L, et al. Use of positron emission tomography with fluorodeoxyglucose in patients with extracranial head and neck cancers. *Cancer.* 1994;73:3047–3058.

79. Benchaou M, Lehmann W, Slosman D, et al. The role of FDG-PET in the preoperative assessment of N-staging in head and neck cancer. *Acta Otolaryngol.* 1996;116:332–335.

80. Adam S, Baum R, Stuckensen T, Bitter K, Hör G. Prospective comparison of 18F-FDG PET with conventional imaging modalities (CT, MRI, US) in lymph node staging of head and neck cancer. *Eur J Nucl Med.* 1998;25:1255–1260.

81. Paulus P, Sambon A, Vivegnis D, et al. 18FDG PET for the assessment of primary head and neck tumors: clinical, computed tomography, and histopathological correlation in 38 patients. *Laryngoscope.* 1998;108:1578–1583.

82. Faber L, Benard F, Matchay M, et al. Detection of recurrent head and neck squamous cell carcinomas after radiation therapy with 2-18F-fluoro-2-deoxy-D-glucose positron emission tomography. *Laryngoscope.* 1999;109:970–975.

83. Lowe V, Kim H, Boyd J, et al. Primary and recurrent early stage laryngeal cancer: Preliminary results of 2-[fluorine 18]fluoro-2-deoxy-D-glucose PET imaging. *Radiology.* 1999;212:799–802.

84. Minn H, Paul R, Ahonen A. Evaluation of treatment response to radiotherapy in head and neck cancer with fluorine-18 fluorodeoxyglucose. *J Nucl Med.* 1989;29:1521–1525.

85. Hubner K, Thie J, Smith G, et al. Clinical utility of FDG-PET in detecting head and neck tumors: a comparison of diagnostic methods and modalities. *Clin Posit Imag.* 2000;3:7–16.

86. Lapela M, Grenman R, Kurki T, et al. Head and neck cancer: Detection of recurrence with PET and 2-[F-18]fluoro-2-deoxy-D-glucose. *Radiology.* 1995;197:205–211.

87. Lowe V, Dunphy F, Varvares M, et al. Evaluation of chemotherapeutic response in patients with advanced head and neck cancer using [F-18] fluorodeoxyglucose positron emission tomography. *Head Neck.* 1997;19:666–674.

88. Lowe V, Boyd J, Dunphy F, et al. Surveillance for recurrent head and neck cancer using positron emission tomography. *J Clin Oncol.* 2000;18:651–658.

89. Sakamoto H, Nakai Y, Ohaqshi Y, et al. Monitoring of response to radiotherapy with Fluorine-18 deoxyglucose PET of head and neck squamous cell carcinomas. *Acta Otolaryngol (Stockh).* 1998;538:254–260.

90. Peng N, Yen S, Liu W, Tsay D, Liu R. Evaluation of the effect of radiation therapy to nasopharyngeal carcinoma by positron emission tomography with 2-[F-18]fluoro-2-deoxy-D-glucose. *Clin Posit Imag.* 2000;3:51–56.

91. Hundahl S, Fleming I, Fremgen A, Menck H. A national cancer database report on 53,856 cases of thyroid carcinoma treated in the US. *Cancer.* 1998;83:2638–2648.
92. Altenvoerde G, Lerch H, Kuwert T, et al. Positron emission tomography with F-18 deoxyglucose in patients with differentiated thyroid carcinoma, elevated thyroglobulin levels, and negative iodine scans. *Langenbeck's Arch Surg.* 1998;383:160–163.
93. Schlüter B, Grimm-Riepe C, Beyer W, et al. Histological verification of positive fluorine-18 fluorodexoyglucose findings in patients with differentiated thyroid cancer. *Langenbeck's Arch Surg.* 1998;383:187–189.
94. Conti PS, Durski J, Bacqai F, Grafton S, Singer P. Imaging of locally recurrent and metastatic thyroid cancer with positron emission tomography. *Thyroid.* 1999;9:797–804.
95. Yeo J, Chung J, So Y, et al. F-18 fluorodeoxyglucose positron emission tomography as presurgical evaluation modality for I-131 scan-negative thyroid carcinoma patients with local recurrence in cervical lymph nodes. *Head Neck.* 2000;23:94–103.
96. Wang W, Macapinlac HA, Larson S, et al. 18F-2-fluoro-2-deoxy-D-glucose positron emission tomography localizes residual thyroid cancer in patients with negative diagnostic 131-I whole body scans and elevated serum thyroglobulin levels. *J Clin Endocrinol Metab.* 1999;84:2291–2302.
97. Grünwald F, Kälicke T, Feine U, et al. Fluorine-18 fluorodeoxyglucose positron emission tomography in thyroid cancer: results of a multicenter study. *Eur J Nucl Med.* 1999; 26:1547–1552.
98. Grünwald F, Menzel C, Bender H, et al. Comparison of 18FDG-PET with 131-Iodine and 99mTc-seatamibi scintigraphy in differentiated thyroid cancer. *Thyroid.* 1997;7:327–335.
99. Feine U, Lietzenmaurer R, Hanke J, Held J, Wohrle H. Fluorine-18-FDG and iodine-131 uptake in thyroid cancer. *J Nucl Med.* 1996;37:1468–1472.
100. van Tol K, Jager P, Dullaart R, Links T. Follow-up in patients with differentiated thyroid carcinoma with positive 18F-fluoro-2-deoxy-D-glucose-positron emission tomography results, elevated thyroglobulin levels, and negative high-dose 131-post-treatment whole body scan. *J Clin Endocrinol Metab.* 2000;85:2082–2083.
101. Boerner A, Voth E, Theissen P, Wienhard K, Schicha H. Glucose metabolism of the thyroid in autonomous goiter measured by F-18-FDG-PET. *Exp Clin Endocrinol Diabetes.* 2000;108:191–196.
102. Boerner A, Voth E, Theissen P, et al. Glucose metabolism of the thyroid in Graves' disease measured by F-18 fluoro-deoxyglucose positron emission tomography. *Thyroid.* 1998;8:765–772.
103. Yasuda S, Shohtsu A, Ide M, et al. Chronic thyroiditis: Diffuse uptake of FDG at PET. *Radiology.* 1998;207:775–778.
104. Wang W, Larson SM, Fazzari M, et al. Prognostic value of 18F fluorodeoxyglucose positron emission tomography scanning in patients with thyroid cancer. *J Clin Endocrinol Metab.* 2000;85:1107–1113.
105. Giovannucci E, Stampfer M, Colditz G. Relationship of diet to risk of colorectal cancer. *J Natl Cancer Inst.* 1992;84:91.
106. Ujszaszy L, Pronay G, Nagy G. Screening for colorectal cancer in a Hungarian county. *Endoscopy.* 1985;17:109.
107. Falk P, Gupta N, Thorson A, et al. positron emission tomography for pre-operative staging of colorectal carcinoma. *Dis Colon Rectum.* 1994;37:153–156.
108. Abdel-Nabi H, Doerr RJ, Lamonica DM, et al. Staging of primary colorectal carcinomas with fluorine-18 fluorodeoxyglucose whole-body PET: correlation with histopathologic and CT findings. *Radiology.* 1998;206:755–760.
109. Meyer M. Diffusely increased colonic F-18 FDG uptake in acute enterocolitis. *Clin Nucl Med.* 1995;20:434–435.
110. Hannah A, Scott AM, Akhurst T, et al. Abnormal colonic accumulation of fluorine-18-FDG in pseudomembranous colitis. *J Nucl Med.* 1996;37:1683–1685.
111. Miraldi F, Vesselle H, Faulhaber PF, Adler LP, Leisure GP. Elimination of artifactual accumulation of FDG in PET imaging of colorectal cancer. *Clin Nucl Med.* 1998;23:3–7.
112. Strauss L, Clorius J, Schlag P, et al. Recurrence of colorectal tumors: PET evaluation. *Radiology.* 1989;170:329–332.
113. Schiepers C, Penninckx F, De Vadder N, et al. Contribution of PET in the diagnosis of

recurrent colorectal cancer: comparison with conventional imaging. *Eur J Surg Oncol.* 1995;21:517–522.

114. Delbeke D, Vitola JV, Sandler MP, et al. Staging recurrent metastatic colorectal carcinoma with PET. *J Nucl Med.* 1997;38:1196–1201.

115. Vitola JV, Delbeke D, Sandler MP, et al. Positron emission tomography to stage suspected metastatic colorectal carcinoma to the liver. *Am J Surg.* 1996;171:21–26.

116. Ito K, Kato T, Ohta T, et al. Fluorine-18 fluoro-2-deoxyglucose positron emission tomography in recurrent rectal cancer: relation to tumour size and cellularity. *Eur J Nucl Med.* 1996;23:1372–1377.

117. Flanagan FL, Dehdashti F, Ogunbiyi OA, Kodner IJ, Siegel BA. Utility of FDG-PET for investigating unexplained plasma CEA elevation in patients with colorectal cancer. *Ann Surg.* 1998;227:319–323.

118. Huebner R, Park K, Shepherd J, et al. A meta-analysis of the literature for whole-body FDG PET detection of recurrent colorectal cancer. *J Nucl Med.* 2000;41:1177–1189.

119. Haberkorn U, Strauss LG, Dimitrakopoulou A, et al. PET studies of fluorodeoxyglucose metabolism in patients with recurrent colorectal tumors receiving radiotherapy. *J Nucl Med.* 1991;32:1485–1490.

120. Findlay M, Young H, Cunningham D, et al. Noninvasive monitoring of tumor metabolism using fluorodeoxyglucose and positron emission tomography in colorectal cancer liver metastases: correlation with tumor response to fluorouracil. *J Clin Oncol.* 1996;14:700–708.

121. Bender H, Bangard N, Metten N, et al. Possible role of FDG-PET in the early prediction of therapy outcome in liver metastases of colorectal cancer. *Hybridoma.* 1999;18:87–91.

122. Vitola JV, Delbeke D, Meranze SG, Mazer MJ, Pinson CW. Positron emission tomography with F-18-fluorodeoxyglucose to evaluate the results of hepatic chemoembolization. *Cancer.* 1996;78:2216–2222.

123. Dimitrakopoulou A, Strauss LG, Clorius JH, et al. Studies with positron emission tomography after systemic administration of flourine-18-uracil in patients with liver metastases from colorectal carcinoma. *J Nucl Med.* 1993;34:1075–1081.

124. Dimitrakopoulou-Strauss A, Strauss LG, Schlag P, et al. Fluorine-18-fluorouracil to predict therapy response in liver metastases from colorectal carcinoma. *J Nucl Med.* 1998;39:1197–1202.

125. Kissel J, Brix G, Bellemann ME, et al. Pharmacokinetic analysis of 5-[18F] fluorouracil tissue concentrations measured with positron emission tomography in patients with liver metastases from colorectal adenocarcinoma. *Cancer Res.* 1997;57:3415–3423.

126. Fong Y, Saldinger P, Akhurst T, et al. Utility of 18F-FDG positron emission tomography scanning on selection of patients for resection of hepatic colorectal metastases. *Am J Surg.* 1999;178:282–287.

127. Lai DT, Fulham M, Stephen MS, et al. The role of whole-body positron emission tomography with [18F] fluorodeoxyglucose in identifying operable colorectal cancer metastases to the liver. *Arch Surg.* 1996;131:703–707.

128. Valk P, Abella–Columna E, Haseman M, et al. Whole-body PET imaging with [18F]fluorodeoxyglucose in management of recurrent colorectal cancer. *Arch Surg.* 1999;134:503–11.

129. Flamen P, Stroobants S, Van Cutsem E, et al. Additional value of whole-body positron emission tomography with fluorine-18-2-fluoro-2-deoxy-D-glucose in recurrent colorectal cancer. *J Clin Oncol.* 1999;17:894–901.

130. Meta J, Seltzer MA, Schiepers C, et al. Impact of 18F-FDG PET on managing patients with colorectal cancer: the referring physician's perspective. *J Nucl Med.* 2001;42:586–590.

131. Day N, Varghese C. Esophageal cancer. *Cancer Surv.* 1994;20:43–54.

132. Greenlee R, Murray T, Bolden S, Wingo P. Cancer statistics, 2000. *CA Cancer J Clin.* 2000;50:7.

133. Blot W, Devesa S, Kneller R, Fraumeni R. Rising incidence of adenocarcinoma of the esophagus and gastric cardia. *JAMA.* 1991;265:1287–1289.

134. Rankin S. Esophageal cancer. In: Husband J, Reznek RH, eds. *Imaging in Oncology.* Oxford: Isis Medical Media; 1998:93–110.

135. Botet J, Lightdale C, Zauber A. Preoperative staging of gastric cancer: comparison of endoscopic US and dynamic CT. *Radiology*. 1991;181:426–432.
136. Lightdale C. Staging of esophageal cancer. I: Endoscopic ultrasonography. *Semin Oncol*. 1994;21:438–46.
137. Souquet J, Napoleon B, Pujol B, et al. Endosonography-guided treatment of esophageal carcinoma. *Endoscopy*. 1992;24:Suppl 1:324–328.
138. Chandawarkar R, Kakegawa T, Fujita H, Yamana H, Hayabuthi T. Comparative analysis of imaging modalities in the preoperative assessment of nodal metastasis in esophageal cancer. *J Surg Oncol*. 1996;61:214–217.
139. Fok M, Law S, Stipa F, Cheng S, Wong J. A comparison of transhiatal and transthoracic resection for esophageal carcinoma. *Endoscopy*. 1993;25:660–663.
140. Fukunaga T, Okazumi S, Koide Y, Imazeki K. Evaluation of esophageal cancers using fluorine-18 fluorodeoxyglucose PET. *J Nucl Med*. 1998;39:1002–1007.
141. Flanagan F, Dedashti F, Siegel B, et al. Staging of esophageal cancer with 18F-fluorodeoxyglucose positron emission tomography. *Am J Roentgenol*. 1997;168:417–424.
142. Block M, Patterson G, Sundaresan R. Improvement in staging of esophageal cancer with the addition of positron emission tomography. *Ann Thorac Surg*. 1997;64:770–776.
143. Kole A, Plukke RJ, Nieweg O, Vaalburg W. Positron emission tomography for staging of esophageal and gastroesophageal malignancy. *Br J Cancer*. 1998;78:521–527.
144. Skehan S, Brown A, Thompson M, et al. Imaging features of primary and recurrent esophageal cancer at FDG-PET. *Radiographics*. 2000;20:713–723.
145. Flamen P, Lerut A, Van Cutsem E, et al. The utility of positron emission tomography for the diagnosis and staging of recurrent esophageal cancer. *J Thorac Cardiovasc Surg*. 2000;120:1085–1092.
146. Rankin S, Taylor H, Cook G, Mason R. Computed tomography and positron emission tomography in the pre-operative staging of esophageal carcinoma. *Clin Radiol*. 1998;53:659–665.
147. Luketich J, Friedman D, Weigel T, et al. Evaluation of distant metastases in esophageal cancer: 100 consecutive positron emission tomography scans. *Ann Thorac Surg*. 1999;68: 1133–1136.
148. McAteer D, Wallis F, Couper G. Evaluation of 18F-FDG positron emission tomography in gastric and esophageal cancer.
149. Luketich J, Schauer P, Meltzer C, et al. Role of positron emission tomography in staging esophageal cancer. *Ann Thorac Surg*. 1997;1997:765–769.
150. Williamson R. Pancreatic cancer: the greatest oncological challenge. *Br Med J*. 1991;296: 445–449.
151. Wingo P, Tong T, Bolden S. Cancer Statistics. *CA Cancer J Clin*. 1995;45:8.
152. Nitecki S, Sarr M, Colvy T. Long-term survival after resection for ductal adenocarcinoma of the pancreas. *Ann Surg*. 1995;221:59–66.
153. Warshaw A, Fernandez-Del Castillo C. Pancreatic carcinoma. *N Engl J Med*. 1992;326: 455–465.
154. Reske S, Grillenberger K, Glatting G, et al. Overexpression of glucose transporter 1 and increased FDG uptake in pancreatic cancer. *J Nucl Med*. 1997;38:1344–1348.
155. Nakamoto Y, Higashi T, Sakahara H, et al. Delayed (18)F-fluoro-2-deoxy-D-glucose positron emission tomography scan for differentiation between malignant and benign lesions in the pancreas. *Cancer*. 2000;84:253–262.
156. Imdahl A, Nitzsche E, Krautmann F, et al. Evaluation of positron emission tomography with 2-[18F]fluoro-2-deoxy-D-glucose for the differentiation of chronic pancreatitis and pancreatic cancer. *Br J Surg*. 1999;86:194–199.
157. Stollfuss J, Glatting G, Friess H, et al. 2-(fluorine-18)-fluoro-2-deoxy-D-glucose PET in detection of pancreatic cancer: value of quantitative image interpretation. *Radiology*. 1995;195:339–344.
158. Sendler A, Avril N, Helmberger H, et al. Preoperative evaluation of pancreatic masses with positron emission tomography using 18F-fluorodeoxyglucose: diagnostic limitations. *World J Surg*. 2000;24:1121–1129.
159. Zimny M, Bares R, Frass J, et al. Fluorine-18 fluorodeoxyglucose positron emission tomography in the differential diagnosis of pancreatic carcinoma: a report of 106 cases. *Eur J Nucl Med*. 1997;24:678–682.

160. Friess H, Langhans J, Ebert M, et al. Diagnosis of pancreatic cancer by 2[18F]-fluoro-2-deoxy-D-glucose positron emission tomography. *Gut.* 1995;36:771–777.

161. Diederichs C, Staib L, Glatting G. Elevated plasma glucose reduces both uptake and detection rate of pancreatic malignancies. *J Nucl Med.* 1998;39:1030–1033.

162. Fröhlich A, Diederichs C, Staib L, et al. Detection of liver metastases from pancreatic cancer using FDG-PET. *J Nucl Med.* 1999;40:250–255.

163. Mertz H, Sechopoulos P, Delbeke D, Leach S. EUS, PET, and CT scanning for evaluation of pancreatic adenocarcinoma. *Gastrointest Endosc.* 2000;52:367–371.

164. Rose D, Delbeke D, Beauchamp R, et al. 18Fluorodeoxyglucose-positron emission tomography in the management of patients with suspected pancreatic cancer. *Ann Surg.* 1999;229:729–737.

165. Maisey N, Webb A, Flux G, et al. FDG-PET prediction of survival of patients with cancer of the pancreas: a pilot study. *Br J Cancer.* 2000;83:287–293.

166. Zimny M, Fass J, Bares R, et al. Fluorodeoxyglucose positron emission tomography and the prognosis of pancreatic cancer. *Scand J Gastroenterol.* 2000;35:883–888.

167. Landis S, Marray T, Bolden S, Wingo P. Cancer Statistics 1999. *CA: Cancer J Clin.* 1999; 49:8–31.

168. Devesa S, Fears T. Non-Hodgkin's lymphoma time trends: United States and international data. *Cancer Res.* 1992;52:5432S-5439S.

169. Newman J, Francis I, Kaminski M, Wahl RL. Imaging of lymphoma with PET with 2-[F-18]-fluoro-2-deoxy-D-glucose: Correlation with CT. *Radiology.* 1994;190:111–116.

170. Lapela M, Leskinen S, Minn H, et al. Increased glucose metabolism in untreated non-Hodgkin's lymphoma: a study with positron emission tomography and fluorine-18-fluorodeoxyglucose. *Blood.* 1995;9:3522–3527.

171. Okada J, Yoshikawa K, Imazeki K, et al. The use of FDG-PET in the detection and management of malignant lymphoma: correlation of uptake with prognosis. *J Nucl Med.* 1991;32:686–691.

172. Patlak C, Blasberg R, Fenstermacher J. Graphical evaluation of blood-to-brain transfer constants from multiple-time uptake data. *J Cereb Blood Flow Metab.* 1983;3:1–7.

173. Gjedde A, Wienhard K, Hess W. Comparative regional analysis of 2-fluorodeoxyglucose and methylglucose uptake in brain of four stroke patients. With special reference to the regional estimation of the lumped constant. *J Cereb Blood Flow Metab.* 1985;5:163–178.

174. Okada J, Yoshikawa K, Itami M, et al. Positron emission tomography using fluorine-18-fluorodeoxyglucose in malignant lymphoma: a comparison with proliferative activity. *J Nucl Med.* 1992;33:325–329.

175. Paul R. Comparison of fluorine-18-2-fluorodeoxyglucose and gallium-67 citrate imaging for detection of lymphoma. *J Nucl Med.* 1987;28:288–292.

176. Hoh C, Glaspy J, Rosen P, et al. Whole-body FDG-PET imaging for staging of Hodgkin's disease and Lymphoma. *J Nucl Med.* 1997;38:343–348.

177. Moog F, Kotzerke J, Reske S. FDG PET can replace bone scintigraphy in primary staging of malignant lymphoma. *J Nucl Med.* 1999;40:1407–1413.

178. Stumpe K, Urbinelli M, Steinert H, et al. Whole-body positron emission tomography using fluorodeoxyglucose for staging of lymphoma: effectiveness and comparison with computed tomography. *Eur J Nucl Med.* 1998;25:721–728.

179. Moog F, Kotzerke J, Reske SN. FDG PET can replace bone scintigraphy in primary staging of malignant lymphoma. *J Nucl Med.* 1999;40:1407–1413.

180. Carr R, Barrington S, Madan B, et al. Detection of lymphoma in bone marrow by whole-body positron emission tomography. *Blood.* 1998;91:3340–3346.

181. Jerusalem G, Beguin Y, Fasotte M, et al. Whole body positron emission tomography using 18 F-fluorodeoxyglucose for post-treatment evaluation in Hodgkin's disease and non-Hodgkin's Lymphoma has higher diagnostic and prognostic value than classical computed tomography scan imaging. *Blood.* 1999;94:429–433.

182. Spaepen K, Stoobants S, Dupont P, et al. Prognostic value of positron emission tomography with fluorine-18 fluorodeoxyglucose ([18F]FDG) after first line chemotherapy in non-Hodgkin's lymphoma: Is [18F]FDG-PET a valid alternative to conventional diagnostic methods? *J Clin Oncol.* 2001;19:414–419.

183. Zinzani P, Magagnoli M, Chierichetti F, et al. The role of positron emission tomography (PET) in the management of lymphoma patients. *Ann Oncol.* 1999;10:1181–1184.

184. de Witt M, Bumann D, Herbst K, Clausen M, Hossfeld D. Whole body positron emission tomography for diagnosis of residual mass in patients with lymphoma. *Ann Oncol.* 1997;8:S57–S60.

185. Römer W, Hanauske A, Ziegler S, et al. Positron emission tomography in non-Hodgkin's lymphoma: Assessment of chemotherapy with fluorodeoxyglucose. *Blood.* 1998;91:4464–4471.

186. Schöder H, Meta J, Yap C, et al. Effect of whole body 18F-FDG PET imaging on clinical staging and management of patients with malignant lymphoma. *J Nucl Med.* 2001;42:1139–1134

187. Rigel D, Kopf A, Friedman R. The rate of malignant melanoma in the US: are we making an impact. *J Am Acad Dermatol.* 1987;17:1050–1055.

188. Lee Y. Malignant melanoma: patterns of metastasis. *CA Cancer J Clin.* 1980;30:137–141.

189. Schwimmer J, Essner R, Patel A, et al. A review of the literature for whole-body FDG PET in the management of patients with melanoma. *Q J Nucl Med.* 2000;44:153–167.

190. Rinne D, Baum R, Hör G, Kaufman R. Primary staging and follow up of high risk melanoma patients with whole body 18F-fluorodeoxyvglucose positron emission tomography. *Cancer.* 1998;82:1664–1671.

191. Steinert HC, Huch RA, Buck A, et al. Malignant melanoma: staging with whole-body positron emission tomography and 2-[F-18]-fluoro-2-deoxy-D-glucose. *Radiology.* 1995;195:705–709.

192. Macfarlane DJ, Sondak V, Johnson T, Wahl RL. Prospective evaluation of 2-[18F]-2-deoxy-D-glucose positron emission tomography in staging of regional lymph nodes in patients with cutaneous malignant melanoma. *J Clinical Oncol.* 1998;16:1770–1776.

193. Crippa F, Leutner M, Belli F, et al. Which kinds of lymph node metastases can FDG PET detect? A clinical study in melanoma. *J Nucl Med.* 2000;41:1491–1494.

194. Eigtved A, Andersson A, Dahlstrom K, et al. Use of fluorine-18 fluorodeoxyglucose positron emission tomography in the detection of silent metastases from malignant melanoma. *Eur J Nucl Med.* 2000;27:70–75.

195. Jadvar H, Johnson D, Segall G. The effect of fluorine-18 fluorodeoxyglucose positron emission tomography on the management of cutaneous malignant melanoma. *Clin Nucl Med.* 2000;25:48–51.

196. Wong C, Silverman DH, Seltzer M, et al. The impact of 2-Deoxy-2[18F] fluoro-D-glucose whole body positron emission tomography for managing patients with melanoma: The referring physcian's perspective. *Mol Imag Biol* 2002;4:185–190.

197. Rosenberg R, Hunt W, Williamson M, et al. Effects of age, breast density, ethnicity, and estrogen replacement therapy on screening mammographic sensitivity and cancer stage at diagnosis: review of 183,134 screening mammograms in Albuquerque, New Mexico. *Radiology.* 1998;209.

198. Mandelson M, Oestreicher N, Porter P, et al. Breast density as a predictor of mammographic detection: Comparison of interval and screen-detected cancers. *J Natl Cancer Inst.* 2000;92:1081–1087.

199. Orsi C. The American College of Radiology Mammography Lexicon: an initial attempt to standardize terminology. *AJR.* 1996;166:779–780.

200. Foxcroft L, Evans E, Joshua H, Hirst C. Breast Cancer invisible on mammography. *Aust N Z J Surg.* 2000;70:162–167.

201. Wolfe J. Breast patterns as an index of risk for developing breast cancer. *Am J Roentgenol.* 1976;126:1130–1139.

202. Boyd N, Lockwood G, Byng J, Tritchler D, Yaffe M. Mamographic breast densities and breast cancer risk. *Cancer Epidemiol, Biomarkers Prev.* 1998;7:1133–1144.

203. Bird R, Wallace T, Yankaskas B. Analysis of cancers missed at screening mammography. *Radiology.* 1992;184:613–617.

204. Orel S, Kay N, Reynolds C, Sullivan D. BI-RADS categorization as a predictor of malignancy. *Radiology.* 1999;211:845–850.

205. Cyrlak D. Induced costs of low-cost screening mammography. *Radiology.* 1988:661–663.

206. Avril N, Rose M, Schelling M, et al. Breast imaging with fluorine-18 fluorodeoxyglucose: use and limitations. *J Clin Oncol.* 2000;18:3495–3502.

207. Crippa F, Seregeni E, Agresti R, et al. Association between [18F]fluorodeoxyglucose uptake and postoperative histopathology, hormone receptor status, thymidine labeling in-

dex and p53 in primary breast cancer: a preliminary observation. *Eur J Nucl Med.* 1998;25:1429–1434.

208. Schirrmeister H, Kühn T, Guhlman A, et al. Fluorine-18 2-deoxy-2-fluoro-D-glucose PET in the preoperative staging of breast cancer: comparison with the standard staging procedures. *Eur J Nucl Med.* 2001;28:351–358.

209. Yutani K, Shiba E, Tatsumi M, et al. Comparison of FDG-PET with MIBI-SPECT in the detection of breast cancer and axillary lymph node metastasis. *J Comp Assist Tomogr.* 2000;24:274–280.

210. Rostom A, Powe J, Kandil A, et al. Positron emission tomography in breast cancer: a clinicopathological correlation of results. *Br J Radiol.* 1999;72:1064–1068.

211. Noh D, Yun I, Kang H, et al. Detection of cancer in augmented breasts by positron emission tomography. *Eur J Surg.* 1999;165:847–851.

212. Scheidhauer K, Scharl A, Pietrzyk U, et al. Qualitative [18F] FDG positron emission tomography in primary breast cancer: clinical relevance and practicability. *Eur J Nucl Med.* 1996;23:618–623.

213. Adler L, Crowe J, al-Kaisi NK, Sunshine J. Evaluation of breast masses and axillary lymph nodes with [F-18] 2 deoxy-2-fluoro-D-glucose PET. *Radiology.* 1993;187:743–750.

214. Kubota K, Matsuzawa T, Amemiya A, et al. Imaging of breast cancer with [f18]Fluorodeoxyglucose and positron emission tomography. *J Comput Asst Tomogr.* 1989;13:1097.

215. Wahl R, Cody R, Hutchins G, Mudgett E. Primary and metastatic breast carcinoma: initial clinical evaluation with the radiolabeled glucose analogue 2-[F-18]-fluoro-2-deoxy-D-glucose. *Radiology.* 1991;179:765–770.

216. Tse N, Hoh C, Hawkins R, et al. The application of positron emission tomographic imaging with fluorodeoxyglucose to the evaluation of breast disease. *Ann Surg.* 1992;7:27–34.

217. Nieweg O, Kim E, Wong W, et al. Positron emission tomography with fluorine-18-deoxyglucose in the detection and staging of breast cancer. *Cancer.* 1993;71:3920–3925.

218. Utech C, Young C, Winter P. Prospective evaluation of fluorine-18 fluorodeoxyglucose positron emission tomography in breast cancer for staging of the axilla related to surgery and immunocytochemistry. *Eur J Nucl Med.* 1996;23:1588–1593.

219. Bassa P, Kim E, Inoue T, Wong F, et al. Evaluation of pre-operative chemotherapy using PET with fluorine-18-fluorodeoxyglucose in breast cancer. *J Nucl Med.* 1996;37:931–938.

220. Noh D, Yun I, Kim S, et al. Diagnostic value of positron emission tomography for detecting breast cancer. *World J Surg.* 1998;22:223–228.

221. Wahl RL, Helvie M, Chang A, Andersson I. Detection of breast cancer in women after augmentation mammoplasty using fluorine-18-fluorodeoxyglucose-PET. *J Nucl Med.* 1994;35:872–875.

222. Boerner A, Weckesser M, Herzog H, et al. Optimal scan time for fluorine-18 fluorodeoxyglucose positron emission tomography in breast cancer. *Eur J Nucl Med.* 1999;26:226–230.

223. Yutani K, Tatsumi M, Uehara T, Nishimura T. Effect of patients' being prone during FDG PET for the diagnosis of breast cancer. *AJR.* 1999;173:1337–1339.

224. Bleckmann C, Dose J, Bohuslavizki K, et al. Effect of attenuation correction on lesion detectability in FDG PET of breast cancer. *J Nucl Med.* 1999;40:2021–2024.

225. Greco M, Crippa F, Agresti R, et al. Axillary lymph node staging in breast cancer by 2-fluoro-2-deoxy-D-glucose-positron emission tomography: clinical evaluation and alternative management. *J Natl Cancer Inst.* 2001;93:630–637.

226. Ohta M, Tokuda Y, Saitoh Y. Comparative efficacy of positron emission tomography and ultrasonography in preoperative evaluation of axillary lymph node metastases in breast cancer. *Breast Cancer.* 2000;7:99–103.

227. Crippa F, Agresti R, Seregni E, et al. Prospective evaluation of fluorine-18-FDG PET in presurgical staging of the axilla in breast cancer. *J Nucl Med.* 1998;39:4–8.

228. Smith I, Welch A, Hutcheon A, et al. Positron emission tomography using [18F]-fluorodeoxy-D-glucose to predict the pathologic response of breast cancer to primary chemotherapy. *J Clin Oncol.* 2000;18:1676–1688.

229. Adler L, Faulhaber P, Schnur K, Al-Kasai N, Shenk R. Axillary lymph node metastases: screening with [F-18]2 deoxy-2-D-glucose (FDG) PET. *Radiology.* 1997;203:323–327.

230. Crippa F, Agresti R, Delle Donne V, et al. The contribution of positron emission tomography (PET) with 18F-fluorodeoxyglucose (FDG) in the pre-operative detection of axillary metastases of breast cancer: the experience of the national cancer institute of Milan. *Tumori.* 1997;83:542–543.

231. Smith I, Ogston K, Whitford P, et al. Staging of the axilla in breast cancer: accurate in vivo assessment using positron emission tomography with 2-(fluorine-18)-fliuoro-2-deoxy-D-glucose. *Ann Surg.* 1998;228:220–227.

232. Vranjesevic D, Filmont JE, Meta J, et al. Whole body 18F-FDG PET and conventional imaging for predicting outcome in previously treated breast cancer patients. *J Nucl Med.* 2002;43:325–329.

233. Wahl RL, Zasadny KR, Helvie M, et al. Metabolic monitoring of breast cancer chemohormonotherapy using positron emission tomography: initial evaluation. *J Clin Oncol.* 1993;11:2101–2111.

234. Bruce D, Evans N, Heys S, H, et al. Positron emission tomography: 2-deoxy-2-[18F]-fluoro-D-glucose uptake in locally advanced breast cancers. *Eur J Surg Oncol.* 1995;21:280–283.

235. Dehdashti F, Flanagan FL, Mortimer J, et al. Positron emission tomographic assessment of "metabolic flare" to predict response of metastatic breast cancer to anti-estrogen therapy. *Eur J Nucl Med.* 1998;26:51–56.

236. Schelling M, Avril N, Nährig J, et al. Positron emission tomography using [18F] fluorodeoxyglucose for monitoring primary chemotherapy in breast cancer. *J Clin Oncol.* 2000;18:1689–1695.

237. Yap CS, Valk P, Seltzer M, et al. Impact of whole body 18F-FDG PET on staging and imaging patients with breast cancer: the referring physician's perspective. *J Nucl Med.* 2002;42:1334–1337.

238. Greco A, Hainsworth J. Cancer of unknown primary site. In: DeVita V, Hellman S, Rosenberg S, eds. *Cancer: Principles & Practice of Oncology.* Philadelphia: Lippincott-Raven Publishers; 1997, pp 2423–2444.

239. Braams J, Pruim J, Kole A, et al. Detection of unknown primary head and neck tumors by positron emission tomography. *Int J Oral Maxillofac Surg.* 1997;26:112–115.

240. Jungehülsing M, Scheidhauer K, Damm M, et al. 2[F]-fluoro-2-deoxy-D-glucose positron emission tomography is a sensitive tool for the detection of occult primary cancer (carcinoma of unknown primary syndrome) with head and neck lymph node manifestation. *Otolaryngol—Head Neck Surg.* 2000;123:294–301.

241. Kole AC, Nieweg OE, Pruim J, et al. Detection of unknown occult primary tumors using positron emission tomography. *Cancer.* 1998;82:1160–1166.

242. Safa A, Tran L, Rege S, et al. The role of positron emission tomography in occult primary head and neck cancers. *Cancer J Sci Am.* 1999;5:214–218.

243. Bohuslavizki K, Klutmann S, Kröger S, et al. FDG PET detection of unknown primary tumors. *J Nucl Med.* 2000;41:816–822.

244. Greven K, Keyes J, Williams D, McGuirt W, Joyce W. Occult primary tumors of the head and neck: lack of benefit from positron emission tomography imaging with 2-[F-18]fluoro-2-deoxy-D-glucose. *Cancer.* 1999;86:114–118.

245. Parker W, Levine R, Howard F, Sansone B, Berek J. A multicenter study of laparoscopic management of selected cystic adnexal masses in postmenopausal women. *J Am Coll Surg.* 1994;179:733–737.

246. Shalev E, Eliyahu S, Peleg D, Tsabari A. Laparoscopic management of adnexal cystic masses in postmenopausal women. *Obstet Gynecol.* 1994;83:594–596.

247. Bromley B, Goodman H, Benacerraf B. Comparison between sonographic morphology and Doppler waveform for the diagnosis of ovarian malignancy. *Obstet Gynecol.* 1994;83:434–437.

248. Fenchel S, Kotzerke J, Stöhr I, et al. Preoperative assessment of asymptomatic adnexal tumors by positron emission tomography and F 18 fluorodeoxyglucose. *Nuklearmedizin.* 1999;38:101–107.

249. Grab D, Flock F, Stöhr I, et al. Classification of asymptomatic pelvic masses by ultrasound, magnetic resonance imaging, and positron emission tomography. *Gynecol Oncol.* 2000;77:454–459.

250. Kubich-Huch R, Dörffler W, von Schulthess G, et al. Value of (18F)-FDG positron emis-

sion tomography, computed tomography, and magnetic resonance imaging in diagnosing primary and recurrent ovarian carcinoma. *Eur Radiol.* 2000;10:761–767.

251. Zimny M, Schröder W, Wolters S, et al. [18F-fluorodeoxyglucose PET in ovarian carcinoma: methodology and preliminary results]. *Nuklearmedizin.* 1997;36:228–233.

252. Römer W, Avril N, Dose J, et al. Metabolic characterization of ovarian tumors with positron-emission tomography and F-18 fluorodeoxyglucose. *Rofo.* 1997;166:62–68.

253. Hubner K, McDonald T, Niethammer J, et al. Assessment of primary and metastatic ovarian cancer by positron emission tomography (PET) using 2-[18F] deoxyglucose (2-[18F] FDG). *Gynecol Oncol.* 1993;51:197–204.

254. Bachor R, Kotzerke J, Gottfried H, et al. Positron emission tomography in diagnosis of renal cell carcinoma. *Urologe; Ausgabe A.* 1996;35:146–150.

255. Goldberg M, Mayo-Smith W, Papanicolaou N, Fischman A, Lee M. FDG PET characterization of renal masses: preliminary experience. *Clin Radiol.* 1997;52:510–515.

256. Montravers F, Grahek D, Kerrou K, et al. Evaluation of FDG uptake by renal malignancies (primary tumor or metastases) using a coincidence detection gamma camera. *J Nucl Med.* 2000;41:78–84.

257. Miyauchi T, Brown R, Grossman H, Wojno K, Wahl R. Correlation between visualization of primary renal cancer by FDG-PET. *J Nucl Med.* 1996;37 Suppl:64P.

258. Kocher F, Grimmel S, Hautmann R, Reske S. Positron emission tomography. Introduction of a new procedure in diagnosis of urologic tumors and initial clinical results. *J Nucl Med.* 1994;35:223P.

259. Safaei A, Figlin R, Hoh C, et al. The Usefulness of F-18 deoxyglucose whole body Positron Emission Tomography (PET) for re-staging of renal cell cancer. *Clin Nephrol.* 2002;57:56–62.

260. Bosl G, Sheinfeld J, Bajorin D, Motzer R. Cancer of the testis. In: DeVita V, Hellman S, Rosenberg S, eds. *Principles & Practice of Oncology.* Philadelphia: Lippincott-Raven; 1997, pp 1397–1425.

261. Gatti J, Stephenson R. Staging of testis cancer: combining serum markers, histologic parameters and radiographic imaging. *Urol Clin North Am.* 1998;25:397–403.

262. Cremerius U, Wildberger H, Borchers H, et al. Does positron emission tomography using 18-fluoro-2-deoxyglucose improve clinical staging of testicular cancer?—Results of a study in 50 patients. *Urology.* 1999;54:900–904.

263. Cremerius U, Effert P, Adam G, et al. FDG PET for detection and therapy control of metastatic germ cell tumor. *J Nucl Med.* 1998;39:815–822.

264. Müller-Mattheis V, Reinhardt M, Gerharz C, et al. Positron emission tomography with [18F]-2-fluoro-2-deoxy-D-glucose (18FDG-PET) in diagnosis of retroperitoneal lymph node metastases of testicular tumors. *Urologe Ausgabe A.* 1998;37:609–620.

265. Hain S, O'Doherty M, Timothy AR, et al. Fluorodeoxyglucose positron emission tomography in the evaluation of germ cell tumours at relapse. *Br J Cancer.* 2000;83:863–869.

266. Albers P, Bender H, Yilmaz H, et al. Positron emission tomography in the clinical staging of patients with Stage I and Stage II testicular germ cell tumors. *Urology.* 1999;53:808–811.

267. Effert P, Bares R, Handt S, et al. metabolic imaging of untreated prostate cancer by positron emission tomography with 18fluorine-labeled deoxyglucose. *J Urol.* 1996;155:994–998.

268. Liu J, Zafar M, Lai Y, Segall G, Terris M. Fluorodeoxyglucose positron emission tomography studies in diagnosis and staging of clinically organ confined prostate cancer. *Urology.* 2001;57:108–111.

269. Shreve P, Grossmann H, Gross M, Wahl R. Metastatic prostate cancer: initial findings of PET with 2-deoxy-2-[F-18] fluoro-D-glucose. *Radiology.* 1996;199:751.

270. Yeh S, Imbriaco M, Larson S, et al. Detection of bony metastases of androgen-independent prostate cancer by PET-FDG. *Nucl Med Biol.* 1996;23:693–697.

271. Seltzer M, Barbaric Z, Belldegrun A, et al. Comparison of helical computerized tomography, positron emission tomography and monoclonal antibody scans for evaluation of lymph node metastases in patients with prostate specific antigen relapse after treatment for localized prostate cancer. *J Urol.* 1999;162:1322–1328.

272. DeGrado T, Coleman R, Wang S, et al. Synthesis and evaluation of18F-labeled choline as an oncologic tracer for positron emission tomography: initial findings in prostate cancer. *Cancer Res.* 2001;6:110–117.

273. Shields A, Grierson J, Dohmen B, et al. Imaging proliferation in vivo with [F-18]FLT and positron emission tomography. *Nature Med.* 1998;4:1334–1336.
274. Shields A, Mankoff D, Link J, et al. Carbon-11-thymidine and FDG to measure therapy response. *J Nucl Med.* 1998;39:1757–1762.
275. Tjuvajev J, Chen S, Joshi A, et al. Imaging adenoviral-mediated herpes virus thymidine kinase gene transfer and expression in vivo. *Cancer Res.* 1999;59:5186–5193.
276. Gambhir S, Barrio J, Wu L, et al. Imaging of adenoviral-directed herpes simplex virus type 1 thymidine kinase reporter gene expression in mice with radiolabeled ganciclovir. *J Nucl Med.* 1998;39:2003–2011.
277. MacLaren D, Toyokuni T, Cherry S, et al. PET imaging of transgene expression. *Biol Psychiat.* 2000;48:337–348.
278. Gambhir S, Herschman H, Cherry S, et al. Imaging transgene expression with radionuclide imaging technologies. *Neoplasia.* 2000;2:118–138.
279. Chatziioannou A, Cherry S, Shao Y, et al. Performance evaluation of microPET: a high resolution lutetium oxyorthosilicate PET scanner for animal imaging. *J Nucl Med.* 1999;40:1164–1175.

CHAPTER 6

Positron Emission Tomography of the Heart: Methodology, Findings in the Normal and the Diseased Heart, and Clinical Applications

Heinrich R. Schelbert

Studies of myocardial blood flow and substrate metabolism of the human heart with positron emission tomography (PET) have proved clinically useful in patients with coronary artery disease (CAD). The studies allow a comprehensive characterization of the extent and severity of CAD, detection of preclinical coronary disease, and, most importantly, identification of myocardial viability. More broadly, PET provides important novel insights into the physiology and biology of the normal and the diseased heart and explores beneficial effects of new therapeutic interventions and pharmaceuticals. The continued growth of an already large body of scientific literature on cardiac PET is fully acknowledged. However, a complete and well-deserved account of all these accomplishments is beyond the scope of this chapter. If some of these accomplishments are not included, this by no means implies judgment about their quality or relevance but is dictated by the need for brevity. Accordingly, the following chapter focuses on technical aspects of PET that are important for and are unique to the study of the human heart, it reviews observations made with PET in the normal heart and in cardiac disease, and it closes with a discussion of current clinical indications.

REQUIREMENTS FOR PET STUDIES OF THE HEART

Methodological aspects

The very anatomical and functional features of the heart offer advantages but also add complexities to the evaluation and, especially, quantification of regional functional processes. Advantages include the ability to directly and noninvasively measure radiotracer concentrations in arterial blood for determining radiotracer-input function as an essential component of tracer kinetic models for quantifying regional functional processes. Complexities pertain to cardiac and respiratory motion; the relatively thin-walled myocardium; the proximity of radiotracer in the myocardium, blood, and adjacent anatomical structures; and the asymmetric, off-center location and orientation of the cardiac chambers.

Cardiac and respiratory motion

Figure 6-1 depicts myocardial images of the normal human heart. Cardiac and respiratory motion causes blurring and, thus, degrades the quality of myocardial radiotracer uptake images. This blurring effect can be reduced by synchronizing the image acquisition with the respiratory and the cardiac cycles. Most PET systems allow gated image acquisition which can enhance the quality of myocardial images and, at the same time, offer measurements of regional and global left ventricular (LV) function. Indeed, systolic wall thickening and motion and LV volumes can be determined.[1–6] For example, LV volumes calculated from gated ^{18}F-deoxyglucose PET images ranged from 72 ml to 233 ml in end-diastole and from 24 ml to 203 ml in end-systole.[5] Left ventricular ejection fractions (LVEF) derived from gated PET images have been found to correlate closely with those from LV angiography and multiple-gated equilibrium blood pool imaging (MUGA).[5–7] Further, LVEFs by both techniques, gated PET and MUGA, were highly correlated over a range from 15% to 77% ($r^2 = 0.82$). The advantages of gated images are, to some extent, offset by longer image acquisition times, which, for most tracers of MBF with physical halftimes ranging from 75 sec to 10 min, are associated with images of low count densities and, hence, lower reconstructed image resolution. Longer acquisition times are also more susceptible to patient motion and, hence, additional image artifacts. Therefore, most laboratories acquire ungated cardiac PET images. The use of more efficient scintillation detector materials and

FIGURE 6-1. Reoriented myocardial 2-deoxy-2-[F-18]fluoro-D-glucose (FDG) uptake images in a normal volunteer. Panel A depicts the short axis images beginning on the left with the apex and proceeding to the base (right). Panel B depicts the vertical long axis cuts, proceeding from (left to right) the intraventricular septum to the lateral wall. Panel C depicts the corresponding horizontal long axis images, proceeding from inferior to superior.

A. **Short Axis Cuts**

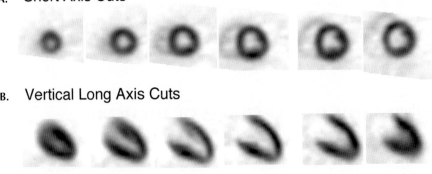

B. **Vertical Long Axis Cuts**

C. **Transaxial Cuts**

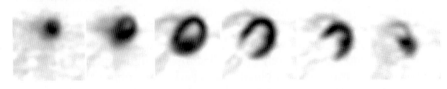

three-dimensional (3-D) image acquisition with new PET systems will overcome these limitations.

MYOCARDIAL WALL THICKNESS

As described in Chapter 1, regional tracer activity concentrations observed on PET images depend on the spatial resolution of the imaging device and the size of the imaged object, that is, in the case of the heart, the thickness of the myocardial wall (see Chapter 1).[8] According to this partial volume effect, the tracer activity concentrations observed on the PET images equal the true tracer activity concentrations only if the size of the object or the thickness of the myocardium exceeds two times the spatial resolution (full-width half-maximum, FWHM) of the imaging device. In the normal human heart, the thickness of the LV myocardium ranges from 8 mm to 12 mm as compared to an effective spatial resolution of about 10 mm (depending on count density and the type of reconstruction filter). Accordingly, most current PET systems consistently underestimate the true myocardial tracer activity concentration.

Corrections for partial volume related underestimations are possible. In animal experiments, for example, the regional myocardial wall thickness was measured with echocardiography or gated magnetic resonance imaging (MRI).[9] Also, algorithms have been developed for determining the wall thickness and the internal diameter of the LV chamber directly from gated cardiac images (Figure 6-2).[4,9,10] From the nonlinear relationship between object size and the observed tissue activity concentration, unique to each PET system, a recovery coefficient that corrects for the underestimation can be derived. For most current imaging systems with an effective spatial resolution of about 10 mm FWHM, for example, this recovery coefficient is about 0.65 to 0.75 so that true myocardial tracer activity concentrations are underestimated by about 25% to 35%.

For practical purposes, some laboratories assume a uniform wall thickness of 1 cm for the normal LV myocardium. Such an assumption might introduce some error in the estimates of the true tissue activity concentrations but appears to be reasonable especially when responses to physiological or pharmacological interventions during the same study session are examined because potential errors will cancel out between studies. It is important however, to keep in mind that hemodynamic changes associated with such interventions produce changes in heart rate and blood pressure that can affect the average wall thickness and, hence, might introduce some measurement errors. Use of an assumed wall thickness is, however, limited in patients with cardiac disease. It would overestimate the true tissue concentrations in, for example, patients with LV hypertrophy. The thicker myocardial wall is associated with an underestimation related to a lesser partial volume. Therefore, direct measurements of wall thickness in such patients are necessary if absolute values of tissue activity concentrations are required.[11,12]

As an important consideration, LV wall thickness represents an average between thickness in diastole and systole and, hence, depends on the duration of diastole and, thus, on heart rate. It also depends on the degree of wall thickening. Different from the normally functioning LV, wall thickening will be reduced in patients with enlarged LVs and low LVEFs. Of notice, the average wall thickness declines in dysfunctional, noncontracting myocardial regions, causing an

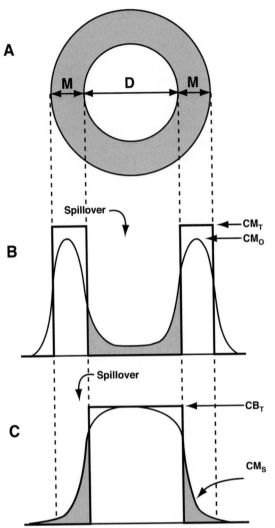

FIGURE 6-2. Diagrammatic representation of correction for partial volume effect and spillover of activity from the myocardium into the blood pool. Panel A depicts schematically a short axis cut through the LV myocardium. Panel B depicts the activity profile of the cross section shown in Panel A. Panel C depicts an activity profile of the same cross section when activity in arterial blood is high and myocardial tracer uptake is low. The bold lines in B and C reflect the true and the fine lines the observed tissue activity profiles. Because M is less than twice the spatial resolution of the tomography, CM_O is less than CM_T. CM_O can be corrected for the recovery coefficient if M is known. In arterial blood, the observed tissue concentrations approximate CB_T because the diameter of the blood pool is more than twice the spatial resolution. Misplacement of activity from myocardium to blood is shown in B and from blood into myocardium in C. The spillover fraction can be determined from the blood pool images from the ratio of activity in myocardium due to CM_S and CB_T. Abbreviations: CB_T, observed blood pool activity concentration; CM_O, observed myocardial concentration; CM_S, spillover of activity from the blood pool into the myocardium; CM_T, true myocardial activity concentration; D, internal diameter; LV, left ventricle; M, myocardial wall thickness.

artifactual reduction in regional tracer uptake even if the true tracer activity concentration is normal and not reduced.[13]

Tracer activity in the myocardium and in blood

Tissue activity concentrations derived from regions of interest (ROI) assigned to the LV myocardium or the LV blood pool are contaminated by bidirectional cross contamination of activity between the two structures. For example, early after radiotracer administration when blood activity is high, there is considerable spillover of activity from the LV blood pool into the myocardium. Conversely, late after tracer injection, when myocardial tracer uptake is high and blood pool activity is low, there may be considerable spillover of activity from the myocardium into the LV cavity. Spillover of activity from blood into the myocardium is augmented further by radiotracer activity in blood in the relatively large vascular space of the myocardium. In canine hearts, for example, the vascular space ranges from 8% to 11% (average 9.8%) of the total myocardial volume.[9]

Corrections for such activity spillover and blood activity in the vascular compartment including corrections for partial volume are possible (see Figure 6-2). One approach, for example, requires knowledge of the tomograph's performance, specifically its spatial resolution, and, thus, of the relationship between the recovery coefficient and object size, myocardial wall thickness, and LV cavity dimensions.[4,9] The principles of this correction approach and its effects on the determination of tracer tissue concentrations from the PET images are illustrated in Figure 6-2. Further, the contribution of activity from the vascular compartment to the myocardial activity can be corrected by incorporating the vascular compartment into the tracer kinetic model by adding a term that represents an adjustable weighting factor and the measured arterial input function.

Image reorientation and image display

PET systems, like most other tomographic imaging devices, image the heart in a transaxial orientation or perpendicular to the long axis of the body. The long axis of the LV cavity, pointing anteriorly and to the left, deviates from the body's long axis. The transaxially oriented images therefore slice through the LV myocardium at different oblique angles leading to partial, volume-related artifactual heterogeneities in the observed regional myocardial tracer activity concentrations.[14] This then necessitates reorientation of the transaxially acquired image sets along the major axes of the LV. The transaxially acquired images are reoriented into short, vertical, and horizontally long axis slices, that, by convention, are displayed from the apex to the base, from inferior to superior and from right (septum) to left (lateral wall; Figure 6-1).[15] Standardized models of segmentation of the LV myocardium are used for localizing and grading tracer uptake defects and their extent and severity (Figure 6-3). Individual segments are assigned to each of the three major vascular territories. The severity of regional tracer uptake reductions is usually graded as mild, moderate, and severe. Total uptake defect scores are calculated from the number of abnormal segments and defect severity scores from the sum of the severity grades and the number of segments with reduced tracer uptake.

Quantitative image analysis programs with polar map displays are also used. The relative distribution of myocardial tracer concentrations in a patient is compared to a database of normal values. The analysis program identifies location, extent and severity of uptake defects as well as changes between interventions as, for example, between stress and rest. Several quantitative image analysis programs are available (Figure 6-4).[15,16] Also, parametric polar maps of regional functional processes have been developed in which the color scale encodes functional processes in absolute units of substrate per minute per gram of myocardium.[17,18] Some laboratories utilize surface-rendered 3-D displays of the LV myocardium with more recently developed methods that merge the coronary anatomy and its abnormalities with the corresponding geographic map of myocardial tracer uptake.[19–21]

Image analysis for estimating functional processes

Measurements of functional processes like myocardial blood flow (MBF), metabolism of glucose, and free fatty acid (FFA), or of oxygen consumption, require the acquisition of serial (dynamic) images that begins at the time of the intravenous administration of the radiotracer. Image acquisition sequence, sampling rate, and total duration are tailored to each tracer. After reconstruction of

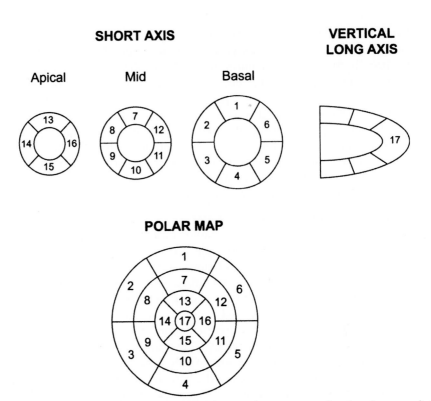

FIGURE 6-3. Standard 17-segment model for visual assessment of regional myocardial tracer activity concentrations. The segmentation approach is shown for the short and long axis cuts through the left ventricle and displayed in the form of a polar map.

the serially acquired transaxial image sets, the images are reoriented, which is accomplished by using the image set that visualizes best the LV myocardium as, for example, the final, static image of ^{13}N-ammonia for MBF measurements. This image is used for defining the reorientation parameters (i.e., the spatial orientation of the long axes of the LV) that are then copied to the serially acquired transaxial image sets. Adjustments for individual frames may become necessary for changes in patient position. Typically, several analytical approaches with different degrees of operator interaction are used:

1. *Multiple LV Regions of Interest:* The operator assigns multiple ROI to the short axes slices of the LV myocardium as well as a ROI to the LV blood pool. The latter ROI should be small (about 25 mm^3) in order to minimize contaminations from spillover of activity from the myocardium. The blood pool ROI is usually assigned to the LV slice with the largest diameter (i.e., the most basal slices) but can also be assigned to the left atrium, the descending or the ascending thoracic aorta. Time activity curves are then generated from the serially acquired short axis slices for the LV blood pool (arterial tracer input function) and the LV myocardium (myocardial tissue response). Modifications to this approach include assignments of a preset number of sectorial ROIs to the myocardium by dividing the circumference of the LV short axis image. The analysis program then searches for the peak

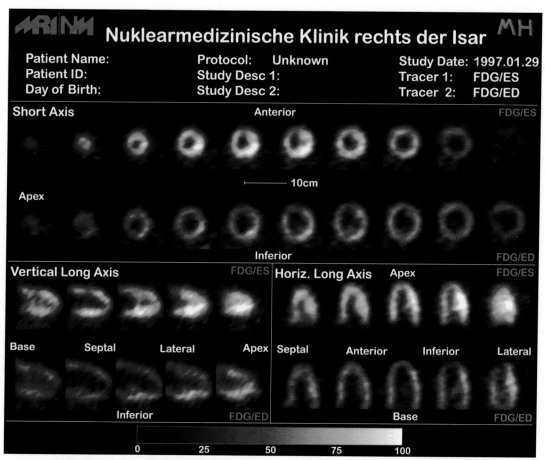

FIGURE 6-4. Gated myocardial FDG images as displayed by the Munich Heart Program software package. (Courtesy of S. Mekolla, Department of Nuclear Medicine, Technical University of Munich, Munich, Germany.)

myocardial counts in each sector and assigns automatically a 3- to 4-pixel wide ROI about the peak activity along that sector.[14]

2. *Polar Map Regions of Interest:* The software algorithm automatically searches all short axis slices for the circumference with the highest counts, assigns a 3- to 4-pixel wide circumferential ROI about the peak count and assembles the circumferential activity profiles into a polar map. A template with ROIs, corresponding, for example, to each of the 3 coronary artery territories, is then superimposed on the polar map for generating myocardial time activity curves for each vascular territory. Again, a separate ROI is assigned manually to the LV blood pool.[14,15]

3. *Factor Analysis:* This more recently developed analytical approach uses factor analysis for specifically delineating the changing tracer activity concentrations in the LV blood pool and the myocardium (see Chapter 1).[22,23] While promising, this approach has remained confined to the research environment, although initial testing for measurements of MBF with the [15]O water technique has been encouraging in the clinical setting.[24]

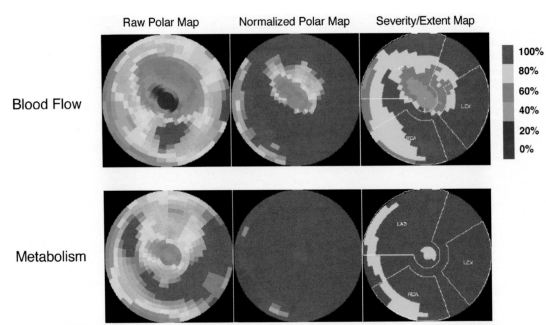

FIGURE 6-5. Polar map display of myocardial blood flow (upper panel) and myocardial metabolism (lower panel) imaged with ^{18}F-deoxyglucose in a patient with ischemic cardiomyopathy. Notice on the raw polar map the reduction in blood flow in the anterior wall and the LV apex, which is also seen on the normalized polar map (center). The polar map on the right was generated after being compared with a database of normal values and indicates for the 3 coronary artery territories (LAD, left anterior descending coronary artery; LCX, left circumflex coronary artery; RCA, right coronary artery) the reduction of regional tracer activity concentrations in percentages below 2 standard deviations below the normal mean. The lower panel depicts the polar maps for FDG uptake in the same patient and, after normalization and comparison to a database of normal values, does not indicate significant deviations from normal values.

Several comprehensive analysis programs for cardiac PET studies have now become available, including Tool Box at Emory University, Atlanta, GA; the PET Software developed at the University of Texas at Houston, TX; and the Munich Heart Program at the Technical University Munich, Munich, Germany. These software packages include routines for image reorientation, polar map displays, estimates of size and severity of regional tracer uptake defects (Figure 6-5), and generations of parametric images such as MBF or exogenous glucose utilization.

ASSESSMENT OF MYOCARDIAL BLOOD FLOW AND SUBSTRATE METABOLISM

This section describes tracer approaches for the evaluation and quantification of regional MBF, exogenous glucose utilization, FFA metabolism, and myocardial oxygen consumption (MVO_2).

Myocardial blood flow
Several positron-emitting tracers are available for evaluating the relative distribution of MBF and for measuring regional MBFs in absolute units of milliliters

TABLE 6-1. Tracers of Myocardial Blood Flow

Tracer	Half-life	E vs MBF	Investigation
^{15}O-Water	2.4 min	$E = 0.96 \pm 0.05$	Bergmann et al, 1984
^{13}N-Ammonia	9.8 min	$E = 1 - 0.607e^{-1.25/F}$	Schelbert et al, 1981
^{82}Rubidium	78 sec	$E = 1 - 0.73e^{-0.593/F}$	Glatting et al, 1994
^{62}Cu-PTSM	9.7 min	$E = 1 - 0.89e^{-0.45/F}$	Beanlands et al, 1992
^{38}Potassium	7.7 min	NA	

Abbreviations and Terms: E, first pass retention fraction; F and MBF, myocardial blood flow; Half-life, physical half life; NA, not available.

of blood per minute per gram of myocardium (Table 6-1). The section focuses on the most widely used flow tracers, ^{15}O-water, ^{13}N-ammonia, and ^{82}Rb but also includes several currently emerging tracers of MBF and describes their myocardial tissue kinetics and corresponding tracer kinetic models and, finally, lists for each tracer currently used study protocols.

General considerations

The ideal flow tracer accumulates in or clears from myocardium proportionally linear to MBF. The relationship between uptake and clearance of the tracer and MBF should be constant and independent of MBF, of physiological and pathophysiological changes of the myocardial tissue state, and of myocardial metabolism. However, most tracers of MBF do not fully meet these requirements.

Tracers of MBF share several common features. The concentration of a flow tracer in myocardium (Q_T) at time T after injection can be described as follows:

$$Q_t = E \cdot F \cdot \int_0^t C_a(t)dt \qquad (6\text{-}1)$$

where E is the first-pass, unidirectional extraction fraction of tracer, F is MBF, and C_a is the concentration of radiotracer in arterial blood at time t. In a given heart, the arterial input function and its integral to time T are identical for all myocardial regions. Therefore, regional differences in myocardial tracer concentration depend only on E and regional MBF. If the extraction fraction E were 1, then regional differences in tracer concentrations would depend on MBF only and be related linearly to regional differences in MBF.

The first-pass unidirectional extraction fraction E is the fraction of tracer that exchanges across the capillary membrane during a single transit of a pulsed tracer bolus through the coronary circulation. For most diffusible tracers, E is less than 1 and declines with increasing MBF because higher flow velocities in the capillaries shorten the time for the exchange of tracer across the capillary membrane. Assuming a model of rigid cylindrical tubes, Renkin[25] and Crone[26] described this relationship with:

$$E = 1 - e^{-PS/F} \qquad (6\text{-}2)$$

where P is the capillary permeability (cm $\cdot$ min^{-1}) and S the exchangeable surface area (cm$^2 \cdot$ g^{-2}). The product of P and S (the permeability-surface area product) is unique to each tracer. The term PS/F is defined as the extraction coefficient and reflects the competitive rates between extraction in tissue and clearance by blood.

Experimentally measured first-pass extraction fractions do not conform fully to the Renkin–Crone model (Equation 2). Measured values at higher flow exceed the values predicted by the equation, implying that the PS product is not constant but increases with flow. Recruitment of capillaries may account for a flow-dependent increase in the PS product, which can be accommodated in the flow extraction fraction relationship by modifying the original Renkin–Crone equation to:

$$E = 1 - e^{-(a+b/F)/F} \tag{6-3}$$

where a and b are derived from the best fit of the experimentally obtained data. The term $(a + b/F)$ represents the flow-dependent PS product. The single-capillary transit extraction fraction must be distinguished from the steady-state extraction fraction (also called extraction ratio), which is defined as the ratio of the difference between tracer concentrations in arterial (C_a) and coronary sinus blood (C_{CS}) over the concentration of tracer in arterial blood (C_a) at a steady state:

$$E_s = \frac{C_a - C_{cs}}{C_a} \tag{6-4}$$

where E_s reflects the net extraction of forward minus reverse transmembranous transport of tracer and is, therefore, usually lower than the first-pass unidirectional extraction fraction. As an example, the first-pass extraction fraction for the 16-carbon chain fatty acid palmitate averages in canine myocardium about 0.68 for resting MBFs of 0.8 ml $\cdot$ min^{-1} $\cdot$ g^{-1} while the steady state extraction fraction for total free fatty acid was only about 0.25.[27,28] The difference between first-pass and steady-state extractions is similar to that observed for palmitate in human myocardium where the steady-state extraction fraction for palmitate was 40 $\pm$ 9% and was significantly lower than the isotopic extraction fraction of 52 $\pm$ 9% for ^{14}C-labeled palmitate.[29]

The first-pass extraction fraction, E, should be distinguished from the first-pass retention fraction, R or the fraction of tracer that is effectively retained in myocardium after a transit of a tracer bolus through the coronary circulation. As illustrated in Figure 6-6, E and R may differ significantly. After tracer ex-

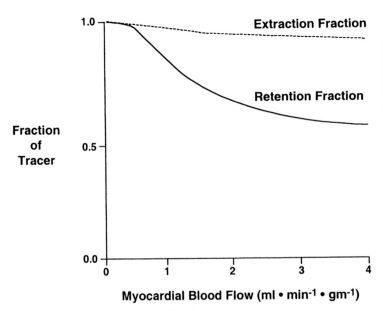

FIGURE 6-6. First-pass extraction fraction (dotted line), the first-pass retention fraction (solid line), and myocardial blood flow. The extraction fraction denotes the fraction of tracer that exchanges across the capillary and cell membranes during a singular capillary transitive tracer whereas the retention fraction is metabolically retained in myocardium. Metabolic trapping competes with flow-dependent back diffusion of tracer; this competition accounts for the progressive decline in retention fractions with increase in blood flows. The data shown were obtained for ^{13}N-ammonia in dog experiments.[41]

changes across the capillary membrane and enters the interstitial space, its subsequent transport across the cell membrane and trapping in the cell competes with back-diffusion of tracer into the vascular space and blood. The rate of back-diffusion normally depends on MBF. At higher flows, a greater fraction of tracer returns from the extravascular space into the blood and lowers the retention fractions.

Lastly, different mechanisms account for exchange of tracer across the capillary and sarcolemmal membranes and, hence, the PS product. The tracer can exchange across membranes via passive diffusion along a concentration gradient. Facilitated transport involves a protein transporter and a decreasing concentration gradient in the direction of transport and is saturable. Glucose transporters serve as an example of such facilitated transmembranous exchange systems. Conversely, tracers can be transported actively through energy [adenosine triphosphate (ATP)]-requiring processes against concentration gradients across the sarcolemmal membranes. The latter mechanism accounts, for example, for the transmembranous exchange of cations like $^{38}K^+$ or $^{82}Rb^+$ and their retention in myocardium.

Oxygen-15-labeled water

GENERAL CONSIDERATIONS

^{15}O-labeled water meets most closely the criteria of an ideal tracer of MBF. It is virtually freely diffusible, its first-pass extraction fraction approaches unity and is independent of MBF, without being affected by changes in the myocardium's metabolic state. Water labeled with the short-lived positron-emitting ^{15}O (120-sec physical half-life) readily diffuses across the capillary and sarcolemmal membranes.[30,31] The concentration of ^{15}O-labeled water in myocardium relative to that in blood depends further on the volume of distribution of water in myocardium and blood. This relation is frequently defined as the tissue-to-blood partition coefficient, represents the ratio of the tracer concentrations in myocardium to those in blood at equilibrium, and depends on the water content in myocardium and blood. The latter strictly represents the plasma water content and, therefore, depends on the hematocrit.

The advantages of ^{15}O-labeled water are offset partly by physical and physiological properties. The rapid physical decay of radioactivity results in low-count and, at times, diagnostically unsatisfactory images. Importantly, the tracer also distributes into blood and lung tissue. Although blood pool imaging and image subtraction can remove this activity, it further reduces image count statistics. This subtraction is accomplished by labeling red blood cells with ^{15}O-labeled carbon monoxide. Inhaled during a single breath, ^{15}O-labeled carbon monoxide firmly binds to hemoglobin by forming ^{15}O-carboxyhemoglobin. The carbon monoxide blood pool images are normalized to and then subtracted from the ^{15}O-labeled water images. Because of the relatively limited diagnostic quality of the resulting MBF images, few laboratories use ^{15}O-labeled water to evaluate the relative distribution of MBF but use it instead for measuring MBF in absolute units.

QUANTIFICATION OF MYOCARDIAL BLOOD FLOW

Estimates of MBF can be obtained with ^{15}O-labeled water from the myocardial influx rate K_1 or from the washout rate constant k_2. The washout approach has become more uniformly accepted because it is independent of the amount of tissue that is being interrogated and, thus, the partial volume effect. Further, ^{15}O-labeled water can be administered over a longer intravenous infusion period or by inhalation of ^{15}O-labeled carbon dioxide that carbonic anhydrase converts to ^{15}O-labeled water in the lung or, finally, as an intravenous bolus injection. Comparison studies indicate that the intravenous bolus administration yields the most accurate flow estimates so that this approach has become the preferred one.[32,33]

Measurements of MBF with ^{15}O-labeled water are based on a single tracer compartmental model (Figure 6-7). The model lumps the concentrations of tracer in tissue and blood into a single functional compartment and assumes immediate and complete equilibration of the tracer between plasma and tissue. Differences in tracer concentrations between blood and tissue are then a function of the respective distribution volumes that depend in blood on the hematocrit and in tissue on its water content. Applied to the ^{15}O-labeled water model, it is assumed that: 1) the tracer freely exchanges across the capillary membrane and instantaneously achieves equilibrium, and 2) the partition coefficient between plasma and myocardium is constant. Reported first-pass extraction fractions of 0.95 or greater support the first assumption of a negligible barrier effect of the capillary and sarcolemmal membranes to the exchange of water. According to Equation 1, the tracer concentration in myocardium, Q_T at time T is equal to the product of the integral of the arterial tracer concentrations from zero to time T and MBF corrected for the flow-dependent first-pass extraction fraction, E. The latter is assumed to be 1. By rearranging Equation 1, MBF or F, is then obtained by:

$$F = \frac{Q}{\int_0^t C_a(t)dt \cdot \lambda} \tag{6-5}$$

where λ is the partition coefficient. The volume of distribution in myocardium is assumed to equal the myocardial water content (0.7 g water/1.0 g myocardium).[30,31]

Animal experimental studies support the validity of the ^{15}O-labeled water approach for measurements of regional MBF. In canine myocardium, estimates of MBF correlate linearly with simultaneously performed independent microsphere MBF measurements over a range of flows from 0.3 to 5.0 ml $\cdot$ min^{-1} $\cdot$ g^{-1}.[30,31,34] Importantly, the slope of the regression line approaches unity (1.096; r = 0.95). In

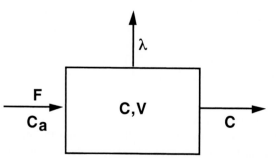

FIGURE 6-7. One-compartment model for ^{15}O-labeled water. Abbreviations: C, tracer concentration; C_a, tracer concentrations in arterial blood; F, blood flow; λ, physical decay constant for ^{15}O; V, volume of distribution in tissue.

healthy human volunteers, estimates of MBF at rest averaged 0.90 ± 0.22 ml $\cdot$ min$^{-1} \cdot$ g^{-1} and increased after intravenous dipyridamole to 3.55 ± 1.15 ml $\cdot$ min$^{-1} \cdot$ g^{-1}.[31]

WATER PERFUSABLE TISSUE INDEX

The search for novel strategies for solving the partial volume effect resulted in the concept of the perfusable tissue fraction.[35] The term describes the fraction of the myocardium that exchanges water rapidly. It is derived by subtraction of blood pool images, obtained with ^{15}O-labeled carbon monoxide, from the transmission images, which yields the extravascular myocardial tissue volume. A large ROI is assigned to the LV myocardial wall. The portion of this volume that on imaging with ^{15}O-labeled water exchanges water rapidly is referred to as the water perfusable tissue fraction. Theoretically, this fraction should be unity in normal myocardium because all myocytes are assumed to rapidly exchange water. Yet, in infarcted myocardial regions, the perfusable tissue fraction should decline in proportion to the fraction of necrotic myocardium or scar tissue if, as postulated, these tissues do not freely and rapidly exchange water. Indeed, an inverse correlation between the perfusable tissue index and the extent of tissue fibrosis as determined morphometrically has been observed in dog experiments.[36]

The perfusable tissue index approach offers two advantages: 1) a measure of the amount of fibrotic tissue in a given myocardial region, and 2) the fraction of viable myocardium to which functional processes can be related. Findings in early postinfarction patients and in patients with chronic CAD imply that the perfusable tissue index does, in fact, provide a measure of the extent of necrosis or fibrosis, or both, which at the same time contains prognostic information regarding the longterm outcome in regional contractile function. When more than 30% of a given myocardial segment no longer exchanges water rapidly, contractile function was found to be impaired irreversibly.[37,38]

Unfortunately, the water-perfusable tissue index is not without shortcomings. First, one relates to the low count and, thus, statistically noisy images that diminish the certainty with which regional processes can be determined. Second, corrections for spillover of activity from the blood pool into the myocardium, especially in the interventricular septum, which is affected by activity originating from both the left and the right ventricular cavities, remain resolved only incompletely. Third, separation of the activity in the anterior wall of the LV from that in the anterior chest wall remains incomplete. All three limitations may adversely affect estimates of MBF and of the perfusable tissue fraction, thus diminishing the confidence in individual regional measurements.

STUDY PROTOCOL

Determination of the perfusable tissue fraction has now become an integral part of MBF measurements with ^{15}O-labeled water. Transmission images are acquired first followed by acquisition of a blood pool image. The subject inhales ^{15}O-labeled carbon monoxide at a concentration of 3 MBq $\cdot$ ml^{-1} at a flow rate of 500 ml $\cdot$ min^{-1} for a total time of 4 minutes. After allowing 1 minute for equilibration with blood, a single 9-minute frame is acquired. ^{15}O-labeled water (550 to 1000 MBq) is then administered as a 20-second intravenous bolus. Acquisition of a 30-second background image precedes the bolus administration, followed immediately by acquisition of twelve 5-second, fifteen 10-second, and six 30-second image sets for a total acquisition time of 7 minutes. The amount of the radioactivity injected is tailored to the patient's weight and the performance characteristics of the PET system in order not to exceed 30% system deadtime.

Subtraction of the blood pool image from the transmission image results in an image of the myocardial tissue volume or, if corrected for specific gravity, myocardial mass. The image of myocardial mass is then related to that of the myocardial water content or MBF and yields information on the fraction of the myocardial mass that rapidly exchanges water. From a ROI assigned to the myocardium, defined on the ^{15}O-labeled carbon monoxide blood pool and ^{15}O-labeled water subtraction image, MBF is then calculated for the water exchanging tissue fraction.

Nitrogen-13 ammonia

GENERAL·CONSIDERATIONS

In blood, ^{13}N-ammonia (NH$_3$) exists in a rapidly exchanging equilibrium between NH$_3$ and NH$_4{}^+$, with equilibrium favoring the ionic species, the ammonium ion (NH$_4{}^+$).[39] The ammonium ion can substitute for K$^+$ on the sodium-potassium transmembranous exchange system in red blood cells[40] and may, therefore, be actively transported into myocardium. The second and probably primary route of exchange is diffusion of the lipid soluble ^{13}N-ammonia across the capillary and sarcolemmal membranes.[41] If the tracer leaves the vascular space in the form of ammonia, it then must be rapidly replenished by conversion of NH$_4{}^+$ to NH$_3$. Equilibrium between both species is achieved within about 19 microseconds, which is fast enough to permit almost complete extraction of ^{13}N-ammonia during a 2-second to 3-second transit through the coronary circulation.

Several metabolic routes are available to the cell for fixation of ^{13}N-ammonia. Foremost are the α-ketoglutarate-glutamate and the glutamate-glutamine reactions. The latter reaction appears to be the predominant one because inhibition of glutamine synthetase with L-methionine sulfoximine abolishes the retention of tracer in myocardium.[41–43] Because of a large intracellular pool of glutamine and its slow turnover rate, the ^{13}N label clears slowly from myocardium (clearance half-times ranges from 100 to 400 min in canine myocardium). Therefore, for the duration of the imaging study, ^{13}N-ammonia becomes effectively trapped in myocardium.

Residue function measurements in canine myocardium have demonstrated that as much as 95% to 100% of tracer initially crosses the capillary membrane (see Figure 6-6). Metabolic fixation in the cell competes with back-diffusion of tracer into the vascular space. The rate of back-diffusion depends on MBF so that the fraction of tracer that is ultimately retained in myocardium declines with higher flows. This relationship as defined by Equation 2 can be described by:

$$E = 1 - 0.607e^{-1.25/F} \tag{6-6}$$

where E is the first-pass retention fraction, and F is MBF. Equation 6-6 predicts for a flow of 1 ml $\cdot$ min^{-1} $\cdot$ g^{-1} a first-pass retention fraction of 0.83, that declines with higher flow and averages 0.60 at flows of 3 ml $\cdot$ min^{-1} $\cdot$ g^{-1}. The net retention of ^{13}N-ammonia as the product of first-pass retention fraction and flow and its relationship to MBF are shown in Figure 6-8 and compared with net retention of other diffusible tracers. The nonlinear relationship describes an initial steep rise of the net extractions in response to MBF. Further increases are,

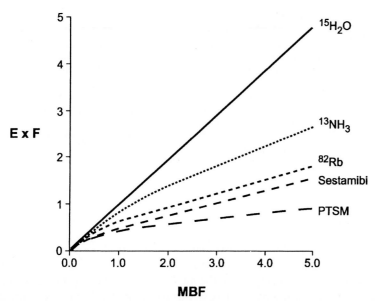

FIGURE 6-8. Myocardial net uptake of tracers of myocardial blood flow. The solid line represents the line of unity. The ideal tracer of blood flow would have a net uptake of 1 for a myocardial blood flow of 1 ml/min/g. Moreover, the net uptake would increase linearly with higher blood flows. Because the first-pass extraction fractions of commonly used tracers of myocardial blood flow declines with increase in blood flows, the relationship of myocardial blood flow to the net uptake is less than unity and correlates nonlinearly with myocardial blood flow (see text). Abbreviations: E, first-pass extraction fractions; F, blood flow; MBF, myocardial blood flow; PTSM, pyruvaldehyde bis(N4-methylthiosemicarbazonato)-copper (II).

however, associated with successively smaller increments in the net retention and thus in tracer tissue concentrations.

Although tracer is trapped metabolically in myocardium, changes in cardiac work and in inotropic state, as well as in myocardial metabolism, do not significantly perturb the observed relationship between tracer tissue concentrations and MBF.[41] Only unphysiologically low plasma pH levels and acute myocardial ischemia have been found to moderately but significantly lower the retention fraction of ^{13}N-ammonia, without invalidating its utility as a flow tracer.

STUDY PROTOCOL

For evaluations of the relative distribution of MBF at rest or during stress, 555 MBq to 1110 MBq of ^{13}N-ammonia are injected intravenously. Imaging commences 4 minutes to 7 minutes later, when the tracer has cleared from the blood to less than 5% of peak activity. Uptake of ^{13}N-ammonia is usually low in lung tissue. Occasionally, lung uptake may be high in patients with poor LV function or with pulmonary disease and in smokers. Because the tracer clears more rapidly from the lungs than from myocardium, longer time intervals between tracer injection and imaging may improve the myocardium-to-background signal ratios.

MEASUREMENTS OF MYOCARDIAL BLOOD FLOW

Two tracer compartment model configurations are used (Figure 6-9). One consists of 2,[14,44] and the other one of 3 functional compartments.[45] The

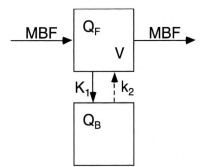

FIGURE 6-9. Two-compartment tracer kinetic model for the measurement of myocardial blood flow with ^{13}N-ammonia. Compartment 1 reflects a functional pool of freely exchangeable ^{13}N-ammonia that combines with the ^{13}N activity in the vascular and extravascular spaces. Compartment 2 reflects the ^{13}N activity that has become metabolically trapped. The sum of activity in both compartments at any time after tracer injection reflects the total activity present in the myocardium. Abbreviations: K_1 and k_2, forward and reverse rate constants, respectively; MBF, myocardial blood flow; Q_F and Q_B, trace activity concentrations; V, volume of distribution.

3-compartment configuration resembles the anatomical pools of the tracer (vascular, extravascular, and metabolic pools), whereas the 2-compartment model lumps the freely diffusible tracer in the intravascular and extravascular spaces into 1 functional compartment. First-pass extraction fractions of ^{13}N-ammonia of about 1 support the latter configuration (see Figure 6-6), because it implies the absence of a true barrier effect on the transmembranous exchange of the freely diffusible ^{13}N-ammonia. Both model approaches do not differ in principle; in the 3-compartment approach, the tracer mass flux rate from compartment 1 to compartment 2, defined as K_1, represents the MBF rate and thus acknowledges the absence of a true barrier effect of the capillary wall or between the 2 compartments.[45]

Because of this similarity, the following discussion focuses on the 2-compartment model, used initially in humans and subsequently validated in animal experiments.[14,44] As mentioned above, the model consists of 1 compartment of freely diffusible ^{13}N-ammonia that lumps the intravascular and extravascular spaces into one functional pool (Figure 6-9) and a second compartment that represents the metabolically trapped ^{13}N label in the myocardium, mainly in the forms of glutamate and mostly glutamine. The rate constant K_1 describes the rate of the glutaminase reaction, e.g., the incorporation of the labeled amino group into glutamate and glutamine. Trapping of the ^{13}N label in the myocardium is considered unidirectional because the clearance of tracer label from the myocardium is very slow (average half-time, 273 min) and because the operational equation derived from the model is applied to only the first 2 minutes of image data.

STUDY PROTOCOL

The study protocol entails an intravenous 30-second bolus injection of ^{13}N-ammonia (555 to 1110 MBq) and serial acquisition of ten 12-second images, followed by acquisition of 2 frames of 30 seconds each, 1 frame of 60 seconds, and 1 frame of 900 seconds (Figure 6-10). Again, the total activity administered should be such as not to exceed 30% of the imaging system's deadtime. This is one reason for spreading out the intravenous tracer bolus injection over 30 seconds so that peak activities remain lower. A second reason is to achieve a better match between the rate of temporal sampling and the curve-fitting routines, essential for deriving estimates of MBF. The third reason is that the 9-minute static image of the myocardial ^{13}N activity concentration reflects the relative dis-

RV LV

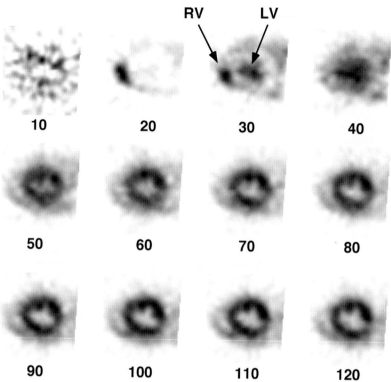

10 20 30 40

50 60 70 80

90 100 110 120

FIGURE 6-10. Serially acquired images following the intravenous injection of ^{13}N-ammonia in a dog experiment. Ten-second images are shown. Notice on the second image (20) the activity in the right ventricular cavity, visualization of the LV blood pool on the following image, and accumulation of the tracer in the myocardium and clearance from blood on the subsequent images. Abbreviations: LV, left ventricle; RV, right ventricular cavity.

tribution of MBF and is used for defining the image reorientation parameters. Time-activity curves are derived from the serially acquired reoriented short axis images (as described above) for the LV blood pool and the LV myocardium (Figure 6-11). The time-activity curves are corrected for physical decay of ^{13}N, for partial volume effects and spillover of activity from the blood pool into the myocardium and for blood activity in the myocardium's vascular space. When compared with independent measurements of MBF with the microsphere technique, the noninvasive ^{13}N-ammonia approach accurately tracks regional MBF. The ^{13}N-ammonia flow estimates obtained with the 2-compartment model correlated in canine myocardium linearly with independently measured flows. Over a range of flows from 0.3 ml · min^{-1} · g^{-1} to 5.0 ml · min^{-1} · g^{-1}, the noninvasive estimates correlated linearly with the corresponding microsphere measured flows (Figure 6-12).[14,46] The slope of the regression line between the two MBF measurement approaches in these animal experimental studies consistently approached unity.

Equally accurate estimates of regional MBF are obtained with the 3-compartment model.[45] Different from the 2-compartment model that uses only the first 2 minutes of image data, the 3-compartment model fits the serial im-

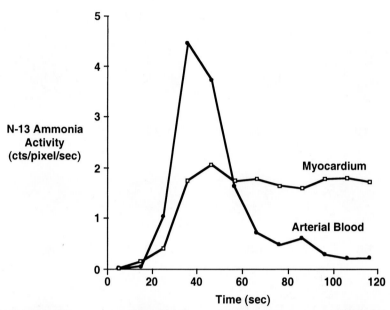

FIGURE 6-11. Time-activity curves of the tracer activity concentration in arterial blood and in myocardium derived from ROIs assigned to the LV blood pool and the LV myocardium on the images shown in Figure 6-10. Abbreviations: LV, left ventricle; ROIs, regions of interest.

FIGURE 6-12. Validation of noninvasive measurements of regional myocardial blood flow with ^{13}N-ammonia in canine myocardium. Notice the close correlation of the noninvasive estimates of myocardial blood flow with the independent measurements obtained by the standard microsphere technique. The correlation was obtained in 12 dog experiments. The error bars indicate the standard deviation of regional blood flow measurements and are an index of the total flow heterogeneity as a function of the spatial-, temporal-, and method-related heterogeneity. (Reproduced with permission from Kuhle et al.[14])

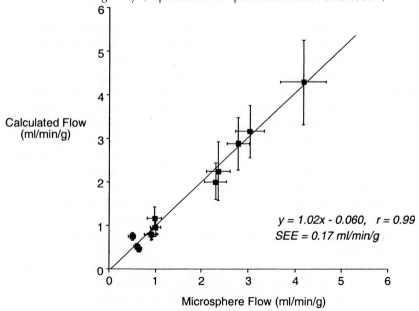

age data recorded for up to 19 minutes after the intravenous ^{13}N-ammonia bolus injection. Again, when compared to simultaneous microsphere measurements, the noninvasive flow estimates correlated linearly to invasively measured microsphere MBFs over a range of flows from about 0.5 ml · min^{-1} · g^{-1} up to 5 ml · min^{-1} · g^{-1}.[47,48] Further, intra-dog comparisons of the 2- and the 3-compartment models confirmed that both approaches yield equally accurate estimates of MBF.[49]

Initial applications in humans demonstrated a close correlation of ^{13}N-ammonia-based flow estimates with cardiac work as defined by the rate pressure product (RPP)[50] and, in a second study, an average 4.8-fold increase in MBF with intravenous dipyridamole[45] that was comparable to that observed with intracoronary flow velocity probes.[51] Finally, global and regional MBF rates determined with ^{13}N-ammonia in humans were recently found to correlate closely with flow estimates determined with the inert argon gas washout technique.[52] Intra-subject comparisons studies further report a close linear correlation between flow estimates by the ^{15}O-labeled water (i.v. bolus) and the ^{13}N-ammonia technique over a range of flows from 0.5 ml to 5.0 ml · min^{-1} · g^{-1}. In that study, the slope of the regression line also approached unity.[53]

^{82}Rubidium chloride

GENERAL CONSIDERATIONS

The cation ^{82}Rb^{+} substitutes for potassium on the sodium-potassium-dependent transmembranous ion exchange system and is actively transported across the sarcolemmal membranes into the cell. In arterially perfused isolated hearts, ^{82}Rb cations were found to rapidly exchange across the capillary membranes.[54] Active transport across the sarcolemmal membrane then competes with backdiffusion of tracer from the interstitial to the vascular space. Because the rate of back-diffusion is a function of MBF, first-pass retention fractions decline in a nonlinear fashion with increasing MBFs (Figure 6-8). Comparable relationships between MBF and the retention fractions have been observed in canine myocardium with the use of either external scintillation detectors or dynamic imaging with PET.[55–57] For the permeability surface (PS) product, values of 0.9 min^{-1} have been reported for canine[58] and of 0.82 ± 0.09 min^{-1} for human myocardium.[59] When entered into the Renkin–Crone equation, the first-pass extraction fraction to the MBF relationship with a flow-dependent PS product and, further, the net uptake to blood flow relationship can be derived (Table 6-1 and Figure 6-8).

Theoretically, the energy-requiring active transport of tracer into the cell potentially renders myocardial tracer uptake susceptible to metabolic alterations. However, in canine myocardium, hyperglycemia, insulin, digoxin, and propranolol remained without significant effects on the first-pass extraction fraction.[55] Increased plasma pH levels similarly did not alter on the extraction fraction, whereas acidosis reduced it. The latter effect was attributed to hyperkalemia and competition from K^{+} for uptake of ^{82}Rb^{+}. The first-pass extraction fraction in acutely ischemic and postischemic myocardium did not significantly deviate from the flow extraction fraction relationship.[60,61] However, ^{82}Rb^{+} subsequently leaked from irreversibly injured [nontriphenyltetrazolium chloride (TTC)-staining] myocardium but was retained or continued to accumulate in only reversibly injured (TTC-staining) myocardium.

A major advantage of ^{82}Rb is its availability through an ion exchange generator-based infusion system. The parent isotope, Strontium-82, has a 23-day physical half-life, and permits the use of the generator system for about 4 weeks to 5 weeks. The short 78-second physical half-life of ^{82}Rb affords repeat studies of MBF at short time intervals, for example, every 8 minutes to 10 minutes. Largely automated infusion systems are pushbutton operated and deliver a preselected dose of activity at a preselected rate of infusion. Typically, 1480 MBq to 2220 MBq of ^{82}Rb are administered intravenously and 60 seconds to 90 seconds are allowed for clearance of tracer from blood before imaging for 5 minutes to 7 minutes begins.

QUANTIFICATION OF MYOCARDIAL BLOOD FLOW

The physical properties of ^{82}Rb, in particular the short physical half-life of 78 seconds, complicate measurements of MBF with this tracer because very high activity boluses are required so that, after more than 1 half-life, myocardial images of acceptable count densities are obtained. This activity, in turn, causes considerable deadtime losses during the initial tracer transit through the central circulation when the arterial input function is determined. Conversely, if lower activity doses are injected in order to reduce deadtime-related losses of counts during the arterial input function, the subsequent myocardial images are of poor diagnostic quality and suffer from considerable image noise. Nevertheless, an early study in dogs, using a 2-compartment tracer kinetic model (a freely diffusible and metabolically trapped compartment) yielded accurate values of flow at baseline but underestimated hyperemic MBFs.[62] The recently introduced wavelet-based noise reduction protocol appears to overcome some of these limitations and improves the signal-to-noise ratio of the myocardial and especially, of the blood pool time activity curves.[63,64] For this approach, an average dose of 0.01 MBq $\cdot$ kg^{-1} of ^{82}Rb, selected to keep the system's dead time below 30%, is injected intravenously and serial images are acquired for 7 minutes (thirty 6-sec frames, eight 15-sec frames, and four 30-sec frames). The wavelet noise reduction protocol is then applied to the regional myocardial and blood pool time-activity curves. Estimates of MBF with this approach in 11 normal volunteers were compared to near simultaneously MBFs measured with ^{15}O-labeled water. At baseline, MBF measured with ^{82}Rb averaged 0.80 $\pm$ 0.26 ml $\cdot$ min^{-1} $\cdot$ g^{-1}and with ^{15}O-labeled water 0.92 $\pm$ 0.19 ml $\cdot$ min^{-1} $\cdot$ g^{-1}. During dipyridamole hyperemia, ^{82}Rb flows averaged 1.85 $\pm$ 0.56 ml $\cdot$ min^{-1} $\cdot$ g^{-1} as compared to 1.89 $\pm$ 0.50 ml $\cdot$ min^{-1} $\cdot$ g^{-1} for the ^{15}O-labeled water technique. Further, regional MBFs by the two approaches correlated linearly and closely over a flow range of 0.45 ml $\cdot$ min^{-1} $\cdot$ g^{-1} to 2.75 ml $\cdot$ min^{-1} $\cdot$ g^{-1} with a slope of the regression line of 1.03 (r = 0.94; p < 0.001).

Copper-62-labeled PTSM

GENERAL CONSIDERATIONS

The lipophilic copper (II) complex, pyruvaldehyde bis(N4-methylthiosemicarbazonato)-copper(II), referred to as PTSM and labeled with ^{62}Cu, has been proposed as a potentially useful tracer of flow.[65] In tumors, these complexes diffuse across the cell membrane and are reduced by sulfhydryl groups with the liberation of copper, which binds nonspecifically to intracellular macromolecules.

If the same redox process does, in fact, occur in myocardium, it explains the retention of radioactive copper in the hearts of rats, monkeys, and gerbils.[65] Of the total administered dose of ^{62}Cu-PTSM, 4.0% and 2.2% were retained in the hearts of monkeys and rats, respectively. In isolated arterially perfused rabbit hearts, the first-pass extraction fraction of ^{62}Cu-labeled PTSM averaged 0.45 ± 0.07 at flows of 1.5 ml · min^{-1} · g^{-1} and declined with higher flows (see also Figure 6-8 and Table 6-1).[66,67] Hypoxia and ischemia failed to significantly alter the extraction fraction of ^{62}Cu-PTSM. Importantly, the radiolabel becomes fixed in myocardium, as evidenced by clearance half-times greater than 3600 minutes but rapidly clears from blood, as demonstrated in dog studies.[66] MBF images recorded with PET are of good diagnostic quality and reflect accurately the regional distribution of MBF, as confirmed by the close correlation between tracer and microsphere concentrations in myocardial tissue samples by in vitro counting.

Images in humans have been of equally good quality.[68] Myocardial clearance half-times average 105 ± 49 minutes at rest and 101 ± 65 minutes after adenosine administration. The myocardial retention as an index of the net uptake was 0.41 ± 0.10 at rest and increased to 0.79 ± 0.24 (arbitrary units) during adenosine-induced hyperemia. Rest and stress MBF imaging with ^{62}Cu-PTSM (740 MBq i.v.) has been shown in preliminary investigations to accurately detect CAD in humans.[69] Accordingly, the compound appears particularly attractive as a tracer of MBF with PET because it does not require an on-site cyclotron. The half-life of the parent isotope of the zinc-62/copper-62 generator is 9.2 h, so that one generator system could be used clinically for 1 day to 2 days. The short physical half-life of ^{62}Cu of 9.7 minutes allows repeat imaging studies at time intervals similar to those for ^{13}N-ammonia (40–50 minutes).

The tracer also promises to be useful for measurements of MBF. A 2-compartment tracer kinetic model has been developed in animal experiments and has been tested in humans.[70] While flows of approximately 1.5 ml · min^{-1} · g^{-1} correlated well with those determined with near simultaneous measurements with ^{15}O-labeled water, the accuracy of the PTSM approach remained unsatisfactory for measurements of hyperemic MBFs, although its clinical utility for detecting CAD remains important.

Other tracers of myocardial blood flow

^{38}POTASSIUM CHLORIDE

Some laboratories use the cation ^{38}K$^+$ as a tracer of MBF.[71] Analogous to ^{82}Rb$^+$, it is transported actively into and retained in the myocardium in proportion to MBF. For canine myocardium, a first-pass extraction fraction of 71% at rest of MBF has been reported.[72] Relatively low temporal sampling rates in this study probably resulted in an underestimation of the intracoronary tracer input function so that the first-pass tracer extraction fraction is probably lower. The physical half-life of ^{38}K$^+$ is 7.7 minutes and thus similar to that of ^{13}N-ammonia so that repeated evaluations of MBF are possible within one study session.

[C-11] ACETATE

Several studies in patients with CAD have demonstrated that the initial net uptake of [C-11] acetate (at approximately 3 to 4 min after tracer administration) correlates linearly with the distribution of MBF as, for example, determined with ^{13}N-ammonia.[73] Some investigations have, therefore, used [C-11] acetate for imaging the relative distribution of MBF.[74] Subsequent studies, using tracer kinetic models, have shown that MBF can indeed be measured in absolute units.[75] More recently, a 2-compartment tracer kinetic model was applied to the initial 3-minute imaging data.[76] In normal volunteers, MBF at rest averaged with the [C-11] acetate method 0.93 ± 0.17 ml · min^{-1} · g^{-1} as compared to 0.96 ± 0.12 ml · min^{-1} · g^{-1} with the ^{15}O-labled water technique. In 13 patients with concentric LV hypertrophy, the corresponding flow values were 1.12 ± 0.18 ml · min^{-1} · g^{-1} with [C-11] acetate and 1.06 ± 0.22 ml · min^{-1} · g^{-1} with ^{15}O-labeled water. Overall, regional MBFs estimated with [C-11] acetate correlated with those by ^{15}O-labeled water by y = 0.21 + 0.81x (r = 0.80; p < 0.0001). With these properties, [C-11] acetate represents an interesting compound where the initial uptake serves as a measure of MBF and the subsequent clearance as a measure of oxidative metabolism (see Myocardial Oxygen Consumption and Oxidative Metabolism, p. 414).

TC-94M SESTAMIBI AND TC-94M TEBOROXIME

Initial reports indicate the feasibility of labeling technetium-based MBF-imaging agents used in single-photon emission computed tomography (SPECT), with the positron-emitting isotope technetium-94m. However, both tracers have thus far remained relatively unexplored.[77,78]

Reproducibility of blood flow measurements

Estimates of MBF both at rest and during adenosine or dipyridamole hyperemia are reproducible. With the ^{13}N-ammonia approach, repeat measurements at rest during the same study session or several days or weeks apart demonstrated nearly identical average values.[79] Interstudy differences for MBF estimates at rest were randomly distributed and averaged 16% ± 16%. Differences in cardiac work between studies accounted to some extent for this variability. Once normalized for the RPP, repeat measurements differed by only 10% ± 11%. Flow measurements during hyperemia were similarly reproducible as indicated by an only 12% ± 9% randomly distributed difference between studies. Interstudy differences for regional MBFs in, for example, the three coronary vascular territories of the LV myocardium were, as expected, somewhat greater both at rest and during hyperemia. The ^{15}O-labeled water technique offers a similar degree of reproducibility.[80] Measurements of global MBFs within 1 h differed by an average of 13% ± 11% at rest and by about 10% ± 14% during adenosine induced hyperemia. Finally, as initial multicenter trials have shown,[81] estimates of MBF obtained at different institutions are comparable, provide identical data analysis, and use comparable PET imaging equipment.

The observed homogeneity of MBF serves as another indicator of the reliability of estimates of reaching a MBF rate with the various flow tracer approaches. As determined with the microsphere technique in nonhuman primates, MBF per se is heterogeneous.[82,83] The observed heterogeneity in MBF, also referred to as relative dispersion (RD), depends on several factors and can be described by:

$$RD^2_{observed} = RD^2_{temporal} + RD^2_{spatial} + RD^2_{method} \qquad (6\text{-}7)$$

Based on well-counting of myocardial tissue samples with an average weight of 0.17 g for determining tissue activity concentrations of microspheres (15 ± 3 μ in diameter), the observed relative dispersion averaged 0.283 ± 0.066 in awake baboons.[83] The temporal RD averaged 0.114 and the spatial RD 0.26. The observed RD depends further on the size of the tissue sample that is being interrogated. The RD for different sample sizes can be adjusted by the square root of the ratio of the different sample sizes.[14] If, in fact, the temporal and spatial RDs are the same in human as in nonhuman normal myocardium, it is then possible to assess the method-related RD which then offers a means for assessing and comparing the accuracy of regional estimates of MBF as obtained with the different PET approaches.

Choice of tracer of myocardial blood flow

Use of a specific positron-emitting tracer often depends on practical and logistical considerations. For a stand-alone (satellite) PET facility without a cyclotron, generator-produced tracers like ^{82}Rb or, when available, ^{62}Cu-PTSM will be an obvious choice. For facilities with PET systems and a cyclotron, either ^{15}O-labeled water or ^{13}N-ammonia can be used. If only the relative distribution of MBF is to be evaluated, the longer lived ^{13}N-ammonia that is also metabolically retained in the myocardium yield images of a diagnostic quality that exceeds that obtained with the shorter lived ^{15}O-labeled water. On the other hand, ^{82}Rb and ^{13}N-ammonia yield images of comparable diagnostic quality as suggested by clinical trials where both tracers were found to be equally accurate in identifying the presence of CAD.[84,85]

Comparisons of ^{13}N-ammonia and ^{15}O-labeled water for measurements of MBF in the same normal human volunteers yield essentially identical values over a wide range of flows.[53] Use of either tracer, therefore, depends often on logistical and practical reasons, that is, at what time intervals responses to physiological or pharmacological interventions need to be measured and further, coordination of the cyclotron schedule and combination with studies in other organs as, for example, measurements of cerebral blood flow.

It is important, however, to keep in mind that regional MBF estimates made with ^{13}N-ammonia and the ^{15}O-labeled water in patients with CAD and previous myocardial infarctions may markedly differ. This difference is because the ^{13}N-ammonia approach yields values of the average transmural MBF, whereas the ^{15}O-labeled water technique generally excludes scar tissue or fibrosis from the analysis. Therefore, MBF estimates with this approach are confined to viable or myocardium that exchanges water rapidly and, thus, do not reflect transmural MBFs. This reason is why studies in patients with prior myocardial infarctions report substantial differences in regional MBFs measured by the ^{13}N-ammonia and the ^{15}O-labeled water technique.[86] While the transmural MBF estimates with ^{13}N-ammonia are reduced in previously infarcted myocardium, MBFs in the same regions assessed by the ^{15}O-labeled water approach may be normal or near normal.

MYOCARDIAL SUBSTRATE METABOLISM

General considerations

According to the highly simplified depiction of myocardial substrate metabolism in Figure 6-13, the myocardium chooses between various substrates; foremost are FFAs, glucose, lactate, and ketone bodies. Selection of a given fuel

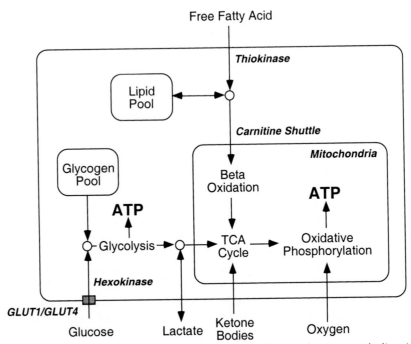

FIGURE 6-13. Schematic representation of the myocardium's substrate metabolism (see text). Abbreviations: ATP, adenosine triphosphate; GLUT1/GLUT4, glucose transporters one and two; TCA, tricarboxylic acid.

substrate depends largely on its concentration in plasma and the hormonal milieu.[87,88] These, in turn, are governed by the dietary state and physical activity but also depend on plasma concentrations of, for example, catecholamines, insulin, and glucagon. In the fasting state, circulating FFA levels are high and insulin levels are low so that as much as 70% to 80% of the myocardium's oxygen consumption can be accounted for by oxidation of FFA.[89]

Conversely, oral glucose intake raises plasma glucose and, in response, insulin levels while FFA plasma concentrations decline so that myocardium shifts its fuel selection to glucose.[88] Strenuous physical exercise increases the release of lactate from skeletal muscle so that their concentrations in plasma rise. Lactate then becomes the major fuel substrate.[90,91] In fact, as much as 60% of the oxygen consumption can be accounted for by oxidation of lactate during high level exercise. On the other hand, increases in catecholamines accelerate lipolysis so that circulating FFA levels increase, shifting the heart's substrate selection to FFA. The interrelation between glucose and FFA as myocardial substrates has also been referred to as the cycle of Randle et al.[92]

Glucose enters the cell via facilitated transport systems, the largely insulin-independent glucose transporter GLUT 1 and the largely insulin-dependent glucose transporter GLUT 4. Hexokinase phosphorylates glucose to glucose-6-phosphate that is synthesized to glycogen and/or enters glycolysis with pyruvate as its end product. Converted to lactate, it may leave the myocardium or, if activated to acetyl-CoA, enter the tricarboxylic acid (TCA) cycle as the final oxidative pathway shared by most fuel substrates. Exogenous lactate can be converted via NAD^+ to pyruvate which then again, after esterification to acyl-CoA, enters the TCA cycle. FFA like glucose may enter two different metabolic pathways (Figure 6-13). Upon entering the cells, it is esterified by the thiokinase reaction to acyl-CoA which then enters an endogenous lipid pool, consisting mostly of glycerides and phospholipids, and/or proceeds via the carnitine shuttle to the inner mitochondrial membrane. It is there where β-oxidation cleaves the long chain acyl-CoA units 2-carbon fragments that then engage in the TCA cycle. The TCA cycle metabolizes the 2-carbon units into CO2 and H2O. The rate of flux through the TCA cycle is coupled closely to oxidative phosphorylation where the energy resulting from the synthesis of oxygen and hydrogen ions is stored in the high-energy phosphate bonds of adenosine triphosphate (ATP). The latter is shuttled into the cytosol with transfer of energy to the high-energy phosphate bond of creatine phosphate as a readily available source of energy.

Bing's pioneering studies using the coronary sinus catheter technique provided initial insights into the substrate consumption of the human myocardium.[89] Differences in substrate concentrations between arterial and coronary sinus blood could be measured and, when multiplied by coronary blood flow or MBF, yielded values of substrate uptakes in absolute units. Table 6-2 lists blood concentrations and arterial-coronary sinus differences for glucose, lactate, FFA, and oxygen.[91,93,94] Extraction fractions in this table represent the ratio of arterial to coronary sinus concentration differences over the concentrations in arterial blood. They increase in proportion to the concentration in blood. The term oxygen extraction ratio refers to the fraction of each substrate that, if completely oxidized, contributes to the total myocardial oxygen consumption. Table 6-3 lists the amount of oxygen required for oxidation of glucose, lactate, and FFA and the amount of ATP generated. In his Harvey Lecture in 1954, Bing emphasized the dependency of the human myocardium's selection of substrates on their availability and thus, on their concentrations in blood.[89] In that report, the sum of the relative contributions of carbohydrates and FFA to the total oxygen consumption (that is, the oxygen extraction ratios) exceeds the actual oxygen consumption by as much as 90%. This percentage implies that with the exception of lactate, glucose and FFA are oxidized only partially. Using stable isotopes, subsequent studies in humans demonstrated that only about 20% of the glucose extracted undergoes immediate oxidation and another 13% is metabolized to lactic acid and then released from the myocardium.[94] For FFA, the fraction extracted by the myocardium and rapidly oxidized is markedly higher and averages about 85%.[29] However, the fraction of substrate that is oxidized depends on circulating substrate concentrations. For both, glucose and FFA, this fraction increases as their concentrations in blood increase.

TABLE 6-2. Substrates, Adenosine Triphosphate (ATP) Yields, and Oxygen Equivalents

Substrate	ATP yield (moles)	Oxygen (moles)
Glucose, 1 mol	36	6.0
Lactate, 1 mol	18	3.0
Free Fatty Acid, 1 mol[a]	131	23.4

[a]For free fatty acid, an average molecular weight (MW) of 256.4 has been assumed. MW for D-glucose is 180.16 and for lactate 90.08. The values for oxygen are the amounts required for complete oxidation of 1 mol of each substrate.

TABLE 6-3. Concentrations of Substrates in Arterial Blood and Arterial-Coronary Sinus Concentration Differences

Substrate	Arterial blood concentration ($\mu mol \cdot ml^{-1}$)	Art-Cor sinus difference ($\mu mol \cdot ml^{-1}$)	Extraction ratio (%)	Investigation[b]
Glucose	5.22 ± 0.37	0.23 ± 0.16	4.23 ± 3.0	Wisneski et al[94]
	3.94 ± 0.36	0.23 ± 0.11	≈ 6.0	Keul et al[91]
Lactate	0.66 ± 0.17	0.18 ± 0.14	26.0 ± 16.4	Wisneski et al[94]
	0.92 ± 0.30	0.35 ± 0.28	≈ 37	Keul et al[91]
Free Fatty Acid	0.67 ± 0.26	0.20 ± 0.7	0.20 ± 0.07	Wisneski et al[94]
	0.86 ± 0.39^a	0.15 ± 0.10^a	0.15 ± 0.10^a	Keul et al[91]
Oxygen	8.01 ± 0.69	5.01 ± 0.62	62.7 ± 7.4	Holmberg et al[93]

[a]Concentrations per milliliter of plasma; values for oxygen concentrations were converted from milliliters of $O_2 \cdot L^{-1}$ blood to $\mu mol \cdot ml^{-1}$ blood for 1.4290 g O_2 per liter of gas at 760 torr and 0°C.

[b]Wisneski et al[94] studied normal volunteers after an overnight fast and Keul et al[91] after a light breakfast. Values for O_2 were calculated for 6 normal volunteers studied at rest by Holmberg et al.[93]

Source: Data used with permission from Wisneski et al,[94] Keul et al,[90] and Holmberg et al.[93]

Myocardial oxygen consumption and oxidative metabolism

Positron-emitting tracers validated in animal experiments and used for the evaluation of myocardial substrate metabolism in humans are listed in Table 6-4. For assessments of myocardial oxidative metabolism, two tracer approaches are available: One uses molecular oxygen and yields estimates of myocardial oxygen consumption (MVO_2) in absolute units while the second approach uses [C-11] acetate and offers an index of the myocardium's oxidative metabolism.

Molecular oxygen-15

This approach expands on the ^{15}O-labeled water based measurements of MBF. In addition to the acquisition of an image of photon attenuation (transmission image), of the ^{15}O-carbon monoxide-labeled blood pool and of ^{15}O-labeled water MBF, images are recorded during the administration of $^{15}O_2$ by continuous inhalation. From these images, the myocardial oxygen extraction is determined. Multiplied by MBF and the invasively measured arterial O_2 content, estimates of the MVO_2 in $ml \cdot min^{-1} \cdot g^{-1}$ are obtained. Validated in dog experiments,[95] studies with this approach in normal volunteers report an average O_2 extraction fraction of 60% $\pm$ 11% at an MBF of 0.88% $\pm$ 0.18 $ml \cdot min^{-1} \cdot g^{-1}$ and an average MVO_2 of 0.097 $\pm$ 0.022 $ml \cdot min^{-1} \cdot g^{-1}$ (see Table 6-5).[96] These values are comparable to those measured invasively with the Fick principle (for example, 0.0973 $\pm$ 0.0063 $ml \cdot min^{-1} \cdot g^{-1}$ at a MBF of 0.88 $\pm$ 0.63 $ml \cdot min^{-1} \cdot g^{-1}$) in normal volunteers.[93] The approach has also been used for estimating MVO_2 in patients with hypertension with and without

TABLE 6-4. Tracers of Substrate Metabolism

Abbreviation	Generic name	Function
$^{15}O_2$		Oxygen consumption
[C-11] Acetate	[1-^{11}C]acetate	Tricarboxylic acid cycle activity, oxidative metabolism
^{11}C-palmitate	1-[^{11}C]-palmitate	Fatty acid metabolism
FTHA	14(R,S)-[^{18}F]fluoro-6-thia-heptadecanoic acid	Fatty acid uptake, β-oxidation
^{11}C-Glucose	[1-^{11}C]glucose	Glucose metabolism
FDG	FDG	Exogenous glucose uptake

TABLE 6-5. Normal Values of Myocardial Oxygen Consumption Estimated with $^{15}O_2$

Number of normal volunteers	MBF $(ml \cdot min^{-1} \cdot g^{-1})$	MVO_2 $(ml \cdot min^{-1} \cdot ^{-1})$	Extraction (%)	Investigation
6	0.88 ± 0.18	0.097 ± 0.022	0.60 ± 0.11	Iida et al, 1996[96]
10	0.84 ± 0.16	0.09 ± 0.02	0.59 ± 0.02	Laine et al, 1997[97]

Abbreviations: MBF, myocardial blood flow; MVO, myocardial oxygen consumption.

Source: Data used with permission from Iida et al[96] and Laine et al.[97]

LV hypertrophy and in endurance athletes.[97,98] Per mass of myocardium, MVO_2 was reduced in endurance athletes, it was found to be normal in patients with hypertension and LV hypertrophy, but it was increased in hypertensive patients without LV hypertrophy.

[C-11] acetate

GENERAL CONSIDERATIONS

This tracer evaluates the flux rate of substrates through the tricarboxylic acid (TCA) cycle. Because the TCA cycle activity is linked closely to oxidative phosphorylation, the tracer approach yields estimates of MVO_2. Myocardium extracts acetate avidly. First-pass extraction fractions of [C-11] acetate in canine myocardium average 63% at flows of $1 \ ml \cdot min^{-1} \cdot g^{-1}$ but are inversely related to MBF. In cytosol, the tracer is activated to acetyl-CoA, which is oxidized in mitochondria by the TCA cycle to ^{11}C-carbon dioxide and water. Following an intravenous bolus injection, [C-11] acetate rapidly clears from blood into myocardium. Serial images and the derived myocardial time-activity curves demonstrate the biexponential clearance of [C-11] activity from the myocardium (Figure 6-14). The biexponential clearance pattern implies distribution of tracer between at least two metabolic pools of different sizes and turnover rates. The rapid clearance phase corresponds to the release of ^{11}C-carbon dioxide from myocardium and thus to the rate of oxidation of [C-11] acetate to ^{11}C-carbon dioxide in the TCA cycle and its release from the myocardium.[99–104] In *in vitro* experimental systems and in intact dogs, the rate of efflux of carbon dioxide correlates closely and linearly with the externally measured rate of ^{11}C-activity clearance from myocardium or with consumption of oxygen. Furthermore, the clearance rate is independent of MBF and thus appears to depend almost exclusively on the rate of oxygen consumption and flux through the TCA cycle. Although nonmetabolized [C-11] acetate clears together with ^{11}C-carbon dioxide from myocardium, it represents only about 5% to 10% of the total activity released.[103,104] This fraction remains relatively constant, even during markedly abnormal states, such as ischemia, hypoxia, and hyperemia, so that the tissue clearance slope of ^{11}C activity reliably and accurately reflects the rate of oxidative turnover of [C-11] acetate and, consequently, of oxidative metabolism. Finally, changes in dietary state associated with changes in circulating plasma substrate and hormone levels do not significantly affect the myocardial clearance curve morphology or the myocardial clearance rates in normal volunteers.[105]

STUDY PROTOCOL

A 30-second bolus of [C-11] acetate (550 to 925 MBq) is injected intravenously while acquisition of serial imaging commences. Acquisition sequences consist, for example, of twelve 10-second images, five 60-second images, three 120-second images, two 300-second images, and one 600-second image amount-

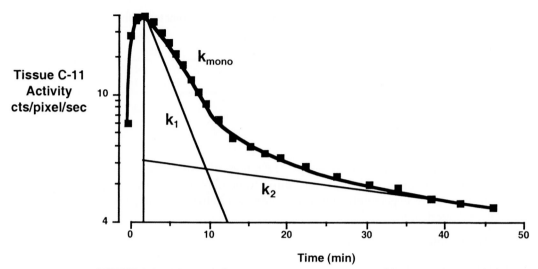

FIGURE 6-14. Myocardial time-activity curve in a normal human volunteer following the intravenous injection of [C-11] acetate. Serial images were acquired over a total period of 50 minutes. Notice the initial steep increase in tissue activity concentrations followed by exponential clearance of ^{11}C activity from the myocardium. Least-square fitting of the biexponential portion of the time-activity curves indicates the slopes of the two clearance curve components, k_1 and k_2. An index of the clearance rate can also be obtained by fitting only the linear portion of the initial rapid clearance phase, commonly referred to as k_{mono}.

ing to a total imaging time of 33 minutes. Myocardial time activity curves are then derived from the reoriented short axis images. Tissue activity clearance curves of [C-11] acetate are analyzed by biexponential or monoexponential least-square fitting routines (Figure 6-14).[103,105,106] On biexponential fitting, the relative size and slope of the slow clearance phase (k_2) have been found to remain relatively constant over a wide range of oxygen consumption. In contrast, the slope of the rapid clearance-curve component (k_1) correlates linearly in intact dogs with MVO$_2$ and in normal human volunteers with the RPP as an index of cardiac work and oxygen consumption.[103,105,106]

Because the slow clearance phase is not always adequately visualized on the tissue time-activity curves, especially when tissue clearance rates are slow, as, for example, at rest, biexponential clearance curve fitting often proves to be difficult or impossible. Slopes are then obtained by least-square fitting of only the early monoexponential portion of the clearance curve (k_{mono}). These monoexponential slopes are less sensitive to fitting errors because of low count rates and thus statistical noise toward the end of the clearance curve. Slopes by monoexponential fitting correlate well with oxygen consumption in dogs and with the heart rate-blood pressure product in humans (Tables 6-6 and 6-7).[103,105,106] In intact dogs and normal human volunteers, MVO$_2$ measured by the Fick method correlated linearly with k_{mono}.[75,103]

TRACER COMPARTMENT MODEL

In isolated, arterially perfused rabbit hearts, a 6-compartment tracer kinetic model for [C-11] acetate has been established through biochemical assays.[107] These studies demonstrated that release of the tracer label from the myocardium

TABLE 6-6. Correlations Between Cardiac Work and [C-11] Acetate Clearance Rates

	Correlation	Investigation
k_{mono}	$k_{mono} = 0.014 + 5.8908 \cdot 10^{-6}$ RPP (supine exercise)	Armbrecht et al, 1989[105]
k_1	$k_1 = -0.25 + 1.25 \cdot 10^{-5}$ RPP (dobutamine)	Henes et al, 1989[106]
	$k_{mono} = 0.0197 + 0.0027$ MVO$_2$ (ml $\cdot$ min^{-1} $\cdot$ 100 g^{-1})	Sun et al, 1998[75]
	$k_1 = 0.0393 + 0.0156$ MVO$_2$ (ml $\cdot$ min^{-1} g^{-1})	Buxton et al, 1992[440]

Abbreviations: k_1, the slope of the rapid clearance curve; k_{mono}, the linear portion of the initial rapid clearance phase; MVO$_2$, myocardial oxygen consumption; RPP, rate pressure product.

Source: Data from Armbrecht et al,[105] Henes et al,[106] Sun et al,[75] and Buxton et al[440]; the regression equation reported by Buxton et al[440] was derived from canine myocardium.

occurs during the second turn of the tracer label through the TCA cycle. Further, in myocardium, the major fraction of the ^{11}C label resides in a relatively large pool of glutamate and glutamine that primarily accounts for the slow clearance curve component. The rapid clearance curve component depends largely on the rate of oxidative flux through the TCA cycle but also on the size of the pool of TCA cycle intermediates. Subsequent studies reduced the initial 6-compartment model to a 2-compartment model configuration in order to reduce the error sensitivity of the model.[108] After exploring the validity of the simplified tracer kinetic model in canine myocardium, estimates of MVO$_2$ with this approach were validated against invasively measured values for MVO$_2$, again using the Fick principle.[75] Model-based estimates of MVO$_2$ in that study correlated well with invasively measured MVO$_2$ over a range of 0.049 ml $\cdot$ g^{-1} $\cdot$ min^{-1} to 0.097 ml $\cdot$ g^{-1} $\cdot$ min^{-1} (y = -0.019 + 1.008x; r = 0.74).

Comparison of the $^{15}O_2$ and the [C-11] acetate approach

The two approaches for estimating regional MVO$_2$ have been compared in patients with CAD.[109] In that study, the monoexponential fit of the early portion of the [C-11] acetate myocardial clearance curve was used as an index of oxygen consumption. In myocardial regions with normal or moderately decreased MBF, estimates by both approaches correlated well. In myocardial regions with greater than 50% flow reductions, however, the [C-11] acetate approach overestimated metabolic rates of oxygen by as much as 30% to 40% relative to the $^{15}O_2$ inhalation approach. One possible explanation is that the $^{15}O_2$ approach but not the [C-11] acetate approach excludes the nonwater exchanging tissue fraction from

TABLE 6-7. Normal Values for [C-11] Acetate Clearance Rates

Condition	RPP		k_{mono} (min^{-1})	Investigation
Rest	6516 ± 1553	LV	0.048 ± 0.004	Armbrecht et al, 1989[105]
	7328 ± 1445	LV	0.054 ± 0.014[a]	Henes et al, 1989[106]
	8140 ± 1370	LV	0.065 ± 0.015	Tamaki et al, 1993[174]
Supine exercise	17198 ± 4121	LV	0.121 ± 0.025	Armbrecht et al, 1989[105]
Dobutamine	14150 ± 2960	LV	0.112 ± 0.020	Tamaki et al, 1993[174]
	17493 ± 3582	LV	0.198 ± 0.043[a]	Henes et al, 1989[106]
Rest	8140 ± 1370	RV	0.034 ± 0.016	Tamaki et al, 1993[174]
Dobutamine	14150 ± 2960	RV	0.080 ± 0.018	Tamaki et al, 1993[174]

Abbreviations: k_{mono}, linear portion of the initial rapid clearance phase; LV and RV, clearance rates from the left and the right ventricular myocardium, [a]k_1; RPP, rate pressure product.

Source: Data from Armbrecht et al,[105] Henes et al,[106] and Tamaki et al.[174]

the analysis. It is also possible that [C-11]-acetate clearance is weighted towards normal myocardium with higher MBFs and hence, greater ^{11}C-acetate supply to such myocardium which then would dominate the clearance curve. Further, if hypoperfused myocardial regions are also ischemic, ischemia-related reductions in the pool size of TCA cycle intermediates could lead to a more rapid clearance of ^{11}C label from the myocardium.

Metabolism of free fatty acid

Besides ^{11}C palmitate as the very first positron-emitting radiopharmaceutical applied with PET to the study of the heart, a free fatty acid analog, [18]FHTA has recently become available for measurements of myocardial FFA metabolism.

C-11 LABELED PALMITATE

General considerations For ^{11}C-palmitate, the ^{11}C label is attached to palmitate in the one position of the 16-carbon FFA chain (1-[^{11}C]-palmitate). The tracer is suspended in 6% albumin and continues to be reversibly bound to albumin in blood. Because of first-pass extraction fractions of about 0.67 at flows of 1 ml · min^{-1} · g^{-1} (as observed in dog experiments),[27,110] the initial uptake and regional distribution of tracer in the myocardium are determined largely by regional MBF. Transmembranous exchange occurs presumably via passive diffusion along a concentration gradient, although other mechanisms, including a facilitated transport system, have been proposed. In cytosol, the radiotracer becomes esterified to ^{11}C-acyl-CoA. The thiokinase-mediated and energy-dependent reaction is largely unidirectional and is, therefore, thought of as the effective step of tracer sequestration into the myocardium. Esterification of tracer competes with back-diffusion of nonmetabolized ^{11}C-palmitate into the vascular space.[27,110,111] Once activated to acyl-CoA, the metabolic fate of ^{11}C-palmitate branches (see Figure 6-13). One fraction moves via the carnitine shuttle to the inner mitochondrial membrane, where β-oxidation cleaves two carbon fragments from the long carbon chain, which enter the tricarboxylic acid (TCA) cycle and are oxidized to carbon dioxide and water. Another fraction of acyl-CoA becomes esterified and the tracer label is deposited mostly in the form of triglycerides and phospholipids in the endogenous lipid pool.

[11]C-palmitate characteristically clears from the myocardium in a biexponential fashion (Figure 6-15). Animal experimental data support the notion that the rapid clearance curve component reflects oxidation of ^{11}C-palmitate and thus corresponds to FFA oxidation.[27,110,112] Its slope and relative size correlate with cardiac work and oxygen consumption as well as with production and release of ^{11}C-carbon dioxide as the oxidative end product of ^{11}C-palmitate. Further, the clearance-curve morphology appropriately changes in response to physiologic interventions and, thus, correctly tracks known changes in FFA metabolism. For example, increases in glucose and lactate and decreases in FFA plasma concentrations induce changes in myocardial substrate selection and oxidation. The resultant decrease in FFA oxidation in favor of increased carbohydrate oxidation is associated with a proportionate decline in the relative size and slope of the rapid clearance-curve component (Figure 6-16). Changes in the clearance-curve morphology in response to the inhibition of specific steps in the FFA metabolic pathway have substantiated further the nature of the rapid clearance-curve component. For example, impairment of FFA oxidation by inhibiting the trans-

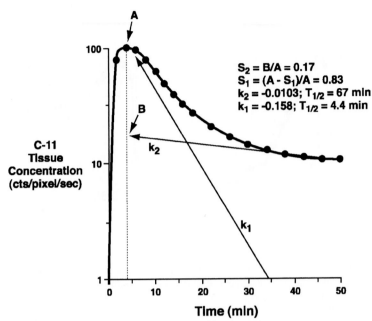

A

$S_2 = B/A = 0.17$
$S_1 = (A - S_1)/A = 0.83$
$k_2 = -0.0103; T_{1/2} = 67$ min
$k_1 = -0.158; T_{1/2} = 4.4$ min

C-11
Tissue
Concentration
(cts/pixel/sec)

B

k_2

k_1

Time (min)

FIGURE 6-15. Myocardial uptake and subsequent clearance of ^{11}C-palmitate in a normal volunteer derived from serially acquired images. Following the initial uptake of tracer into the myocardium, ^{11}C activity clears in a characteristic biexponential fashion, indicating distribution of radiotracer between at least two different metabolic pools with different turnover rates. The relative size and the clearance rate of the two clearance-curve components can be determined by least-square biexponential fitting of the time-activity curves. They provide information on the relative distribution of ^{11}C-palmitate between immediate oxidation and initial storage of tracer in larger lipid pools (see text). Abbreviations: A, peak activity; B, intercept of slow clearance phase at time of peak activity; k_1, slope of the rapid clearance-curve component; k_2, slope of the slow clearance phase; S_1, relative size of the rapid clearance phase; S_2, relative size of the slow clearance phase.

fer of acyl-CoA units into mitochondria with 2-tetradecylglycidic acid, an inhibitor of the carnitine acyltransferase I, resulted in a marked decline or even an absence of the rapid clearance-curve component.[113]

Biochemical tissue assays are important for adequate interpretation of the tissue time-activity curves. They confirm that the slow clearance-curve component corresponds to incorporation of ^{11}C label into the endogenous lipid pool (Figure 6-17).[112] The rapid clearance-curve component reflects oxidation of ^{11}C-palmitate and the rate of release of metabolic end products from myocardium. Biochemical tissue assays further point out limitations of the slope of the early clearance-curve component as an index of FFA oxidation. First, the slope may be contaminated by increased back-diffusion of nonmetabolized ^{11}C-palmitate. Indeed, the rate of back-diffusion may exceed the rate of release of ^{11}C-carbon dioxide from myocardium, especially during ischemia.[110,111] Second, the rate of activity clearance from the myocardium depends not only on substrate flux through the oxidative pathway but also on the volume of distribution of metabolites. For example, the increase in the fraction of tracer label found in the aqueous phase, reflecting ^{11}C bound to carbon dioxide, acyl-CoA, and acetyl

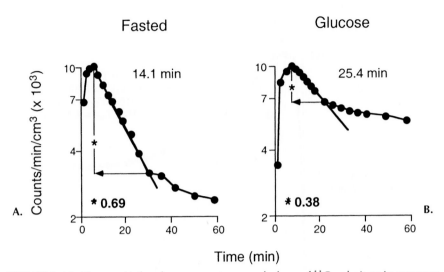

FIGURE 6-16. Changes in the clearance curve morphology of ^{11}C-palmitate in response to changes in substrate availability. A (left) demonstrates the clearance curve obtained in a normal volunteer studied after an overnight fast and B (right) was obtained following oral administration of glucose. Notice the marked decrease in the relative size of the rapid clearance curve component from fasted to glucose indicating that less FFA immediately proceeds to β-oxidation following increases in glucose blood concentrations and a shift in the myocardium's substrate selection from predominantly FFA to glucose. The relative size of the rapid clearance curve component was derived from the inflexion point on the clearance curve. The slopes defined by clearance halftimes were obtained by monoexponentially fitting the initial downslope of the clearance curve.

CoA, may delay the tissue tracer clearance rate and, thus, cause an underestimation of the true flux rate through oxidative pathways.

Study protocol For studies in humans, a 30-second bolus of 555 MBq to 740 MBq of ^{11}C-palmitate is injected intravenously. Acquisition of serial images commences at the time of tracer injection and continues for 60 minutes. A typical image acquisition may be as follows: ten 2-minute frames, five 3-minute frames followed by three 5-minute frames. The serially acquired image sets are reoriented into short axis slices and time-activity curves derived for the LV myocardium and the blood pool. Analysis of the myocardial time activity curve by biexponential least-square fitting renders the slopes (k_1 and k_2) and the relative sizes of the two clearance curve components.

Tissue time-activity curves characteristic for different dietary states, exercise, and ischemia are depicted in Figure 6-16. Under conditions of preferential FFA utilization as, for example, after an overnight fast, the major fraction of tracer enters the rapid turnover pool and is rapidly oxidized, as indicated by the large relative size and steep slope of the rapid clearance-curve component. Under conditions of low FFA and high glucose plasma concentrations, disproportionately more glucose is oxidized, which on the tissue time-activity curve is reflected by a decrease in both the relative size and slope of the rapid clearance-curve component. Impairment of FFA oxidation during ischemia causes a similar decline in both curve parameters but occurs characteristically in a well-defined myo-

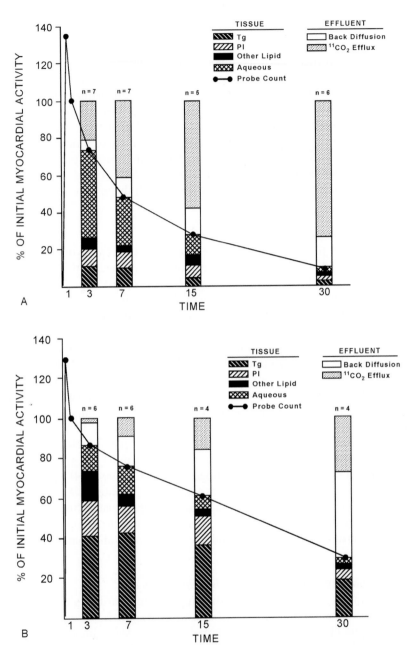

FIGURE 6-17. Metabolic fate of ^{11}C-palmitate in myocardium and coronary sinus effluent following intracoronary bolus administration of ^{11}C-palmitate in open-chest dog experiments at control (A) and low flow ischemia (B). The solid lines depict the tissue residue function and represent the average percentage of initially extracted tracer at each biopsy time point. The values above the curve at each time point indicate the cumulative contributions of ^{11}C-carbon dioxide and ^{11}C-palmitate efflux to tracer clearance from myocardium. The values below the curve depict the fractional distribution of the radiolabel between various pools of fatty acid metabolites in the myocardium as determined by tissue assays. As shown in B, ischemia causes an increase in the efflux of the nonmetabolized ^{11}C-palmitate and a disproportionate increase in the fraction of ^{11}C label deposited in tissue as triglycerides (Tg) and phospholipids (Pl). (Reproduced from Rosamond et al [112] with permission of the Society of Nuclear Medicine.)

cardial region and strikingly differs from the normal appearance of the clearance curve in normally perfused myocardial regions.

Animal experimental studies suggest the possibility of measuring myocardial FFA metabolism in absolute units.[114] Using a 4-compartment tracer kinetic model and measuring arterial FFA plasma concentrations, ^{11}C-palmitate provided estimates of the myocardial utilization of palmitate and total FFA in absolute units and, based on the myocardial clearance curve morphology, of the fraction of FFA undergoing immediate oxidation. In normal human volunteers, the model yielded estimates of the myocardial free fatty acid utilization that are in agreement with those determined earlier through the invasive coronary sinus catheter technique (see Table 6-2).[115]

^{18}F-FLUORO-6-THIA-HEPTADECANOIC ACID

14(R,S)-[18F]fluoro-6-thia-heptadecanoic acid (FTHA), a fluorinated, long carbon chain FFA analog, becomes metabolically trapped in the myocardium. The rate of metabolic trapping is thought to be proportional to the rate of β-oxidation of long chain FFA. Inhibition of the carnitine palmitoyl-transferase I and, in response, of β-oxidation in the myocardium of mice was observed to be associated with an 87% reduction in tracer uptake and retention.[116,117] Further, in extracorporally perfused pig hearts, the tracer extraction fraction correlated directly with the rate of palmitate oxidation.[117,118] These studies also found minimal back-diffusion of the tracer from the myocardium into blood so that analogous to FDG, a unidirectional transport model can be used for quantifying regional myocardial FFA uptake. Initial investigations with this compound in humans are promising. In patients with CAD, for example, estimates of the FFA uptake in normal myocardium by this approach averaged 5.8 ± 1.7 μmol $\cdot$ 100 g^{-1} $\cdot$ min^{-1} in the fasted state and declined as expected to 1.4 ± 0.5 μmol $\cdot$ 100 g^{-1} $\cdot$ min^{-1} during an insulin clamp.[119] Further, in congestive heart failure (CHF) patients with low LVEFs, myocardial FFA uptake was found to be elevated (19.3 ± 2.3 μmol $\cdot$ 100 g^{-1} $\cdot$ min^{-1}).[120] Thus, FTHA appears to appropriately trace directional changes in myocardial substrate selection in response to compensatory alterations in cardiovascular disease and in response to pharmacological interventions.

Exogenous utilization and metabolism of glucose

Two tracers are available for studying the myocardial glucose metabolism. One is the natural D-glucose labeled with ^{11}C and the second one the glucose analogue FDG, subsequently referred to as ^{18}F-deoxyglucose.

C-11-LABELED GLUCOSE

Glucose can readily be labeled with ^{11}C while fully maintaining its biochemical properties. Accordingly, the radiolabeled ^{11}C glucose has been used in animal experimental and in human investigations. However, there are several limitations to the utility of this tracer. One is the complexity of the glucose metabolism. The tracer label, therefore, distributes into multiple metabolic pools with loss of label from the myocardium during the transit of metabolic intermediates through the glycolytic and the final oxidative pathway which complicate the interpretation of the uptake and clearance data of the tracer. The second one is the low extraction of glucose by myocardium and, hence, little tracer accumulation in the myocardium so that the resulting myocardial images suffer from poor signal-to-noise ratios.

Nonetheless, some of these limitations can be overcome. Different from the earlier photosynthetic method for labeling glucose where the radiolabel becomes distributed among the six carbon atoms of glucose and which precludes accurate tracking of the metabolic fate of the tracer label, more recent synthesis approaches have succeeded in specifically labeling the carbon-1 atom of the glucose molecule.[121–123] The metabolic fate of the 1-[^{11}C]-glucose is described by a 4-compartment model. Compartment 1 describes the nonmetabolized tracer in tissue (interstitial and intracellular space), compartment 2 the phosphorylated glucose, compartment 3 the radiolabel in the glycogen pool, and compartment 4 the flux of radiotracer through the anaerobic pathway and oxidation. The approach entails the determination of the myocardial glucose extraction fraction from time-activity curves derived from serially acquired images following the intravenous administration of ^{11}C-glucose and measurements of MBF with ^{15}O-labeled water.[124] Estimates of the myocardial metabolic rate of glucose (MMR-Glc) derived noninvasively with this approach from the arterial glucose concentration, the myocardial glucose extraction, and MBF correlated with those obtained from the invasively determined arterial coronary sinus difference for glucose and PET-measured MBFs. Used in humans, the approach yielded estimates of MMRGlc of 125 ± 64 nmol · g^{-1} · min^{-1}.[115] These values obtained in 12 young healthy individuals after a 12-h overnight fast agree with estimates derived through the invasive coronary sinus catheter technique.[29]

F-18-LABELED 2-FLUORO-2-DEOXYGLUCOSE

General considerations 2-deoxy-2-[F-18]fluoro-D-glucose (FDG) (^{18}F-deoxyglucose) is transported across the capillary and sarcolemmal membranes in proportion to glucose. In cytosol, FDG competes with glucose for hexokinase and is phosphorylated to FDG-6-phosphate (see also Figure 6-13). Unlike natural glucose-6-phosphate, the phosphorylated glucose analog is a poor substrate for glycogen synthesis, glycolysis, and the fructose-phosphate shunt. It is also relatively impermeable to the sarcolemmal membrane. Because the activity of phosphatase, the enzyme that reverses the initial phosphorylation of glucose, is low in normal myocardium, the reaction product FDG-6-phosphate is trapped in cells, so that images of the myocardial ^{18}F tissue concentrations reflect the relative distribution of exogenous glucose utilization in myocardium.[125]

Following intravenous administration, ^{18}F-deoxyglucose crosses the capillary and cellular membranes. Concentrations of ^{18}F initially rise rapidly in the myocardium. Back transport of FDG then competes with its phosphorylation and effective sequestration as FDG-6-phosphate into myocardium. The rate of rise of myocardial ^{18}F activity concentrations progressively declines and may finally reach a plateau. This leveling off occurs at about 50 minutes to 60 minutes after tracer injection, when tracer concentrations in arterial blood have declined and a relative steady state between phosphorylated tracer, tracer in tissue, and tracer in arterial blood has been attained. At that time, more than 80% of the ^{18}F-label in myocardium is contained as FDG-6-phosphate.[126] In normal myocardium, the rate of effective sequestration of FDG (e.g., transmembranous transport and phosphorylation minus loss due to back-diffusion of tracer) relative to phosphorylation of glucose has been found to be relatively constant. In vitro studies suggest that this constancy is also maintained during abnormal states, for example, hypoxia and ischemia.[126]

Because ^{18}F-deoxyglucose traces only the initial metabolic steps of exogenous glucose in myocardium, it provides limited information on the metabolic fate of glucose beyond the major branch point between glycolysis and glycogen formation (see Figure 6-13). Therefore, the fraction of glucose that is subsequently synthesized to glycogen or the fraction that is directly catabolized through glycolysis remains unknown. This is also true for the contribution of endogenous glucose from the breakdown of glycogen to the overall glycolytic flux. However, when the radiotracer is used under strict steady-state conditions and when rates of exogenous glucose utilization can be assumed to be at equilibrium with rates of glycogen formation and breakdown, some inferences on overall glycolytic flux are possible. Furthermore, under extreme conditions, as, for example, during ischemia, when glycogen stores are depleted, the rate of exogenous glucose utilization determined with FDG is likely to approach the rate of glycolytic flux.

Study protocol The qualitative evaluation of the relative distribution of myocardial glucose utilization requires acquisition of a single image set at about 30 minutes to 50 minutes after intravenous injection of approximately 185 MBq to 370 MBq of FDG. On these images, regional activity concentrations represent relative rates of regional glucose utilization. If exogenous glucose utilization is to be quantified, acquisition of serial images commences at the time of tracer injection and continues for about 60 minutes. Through ROIs assigned to the myocardium and arterial blood, tissue time-activity curves are obtained for estimating rates of MMRGlc.

Quantitative studies of myocardial glucose utilization Measurements of regional MMRGlc in millimoles of glucose per minute per gram of myocardium use a 3-compartment tracer kinetic model proposed initially for autoradiographic measurements of regional cerebral glucose metabolism in the rat.[127] A 3-compartment model describes the tissue kinetics of FDG. As seen in Figure 6-18, compartment 1 represents tracer concentrations in blood, compartment 2 the tracer concentration in tissue, and compartment 3 the concentration of the phosphorylated compound FDG-6-phosphate in myocardium. The linear rate constants k_1 and k_2 describe the forward and reverse transport, respectively, of tracer between blood and tissue (transmembranous exchange); k_3 the hexokinase-mediated rate of phosphorylation; and k_4 the rate of phosphatase-mediated dephosphorylation. Although the activity of phosphatase is very low in myocardium, modifications of Sokoloff 's initial tracer kinetic model now accommodate dephosphorylation rates.

The model relates the MMRGlc to the measured rate constants for ^{18}F-deoxyglucose by

$$MMRGlc = \frac{C_p}{LC} \cdot \frac{k_1 k_3}{k_2 + k_3} \tag{6-8}$$

where $k_1 \cdot k_3/k_2 + k_3$ (also referred to as K) reflects the rate of effective metabolic sequestration or clearance of FDG from plasma into myo-cardium. The term C_p is the concentration of glucose in plasma. The lumped constant (LC)

FIGURE 6-18. Three-compartment tracer kinetic model for FDG (see text).

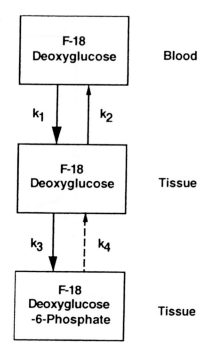

adjusts for differences in transport and phosphorylation rates between glucose and FDG as both compete for the same transport sites and are competitive substrates for hexokinase.

For measurements of rates of myocardial glucose utilization of exogenous glucose, the regional myocardial tissue time-activity curves derived from serially acquired images for 60 minutes to 90 minutes after injection of FDG are fitted with the operational equation (Figure 6-19). Individual rate constants k_1 to k_4 are obtained and are entered together with the arterial plasma glucose concentrations into Equation 8. For the LC, a fixed value of 0.67 is used, as determined in canine myocardium.[128] Estimates of glucose utilization by this approach were found to correlate in dog experiments with glucose consumption rates, as determined by the Fick principle (Figure 6-20). They predicted glucose utilization rates in normal human subjects that were similar to those reported previously in the literature.[129]

At present, most studies use a simplified approach for estimating rates of glucose utilization. The approach takes advantage of the trapping of FDG-6-phosphate and is commonly referred to as the Patlak and Blasberg graphical analysis.[130] Tracer concentrations at time t in myocardium (A_m) over tracer concentrations in plasma are plotted against the integral of the arterial tracer input function divided by the arterial tracer concentration at time t.[129] The slope corresponds to $k_1 \cdot k_3/(k_2 + k_3)$, and, thus, K, that reflects the fraction of FDG in plasma that is phosphorylated and metabolically sequestered into myocardium. The approach also includes corrections for bidirectional spillover of activity between myocardium and blood. The activity of phosphatase is assumed to be neglible so that k_4 is set to 0. In normal volunteers, estimates of glucose metabolism with this approach closely agree with those obtained by the traditional derivation of individual rate

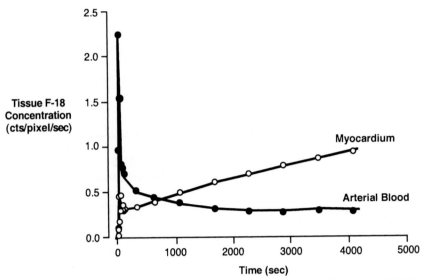

FIGURE 6-19. ^{18}F activity concentrations as determined from serially acquired PET images in arterial blood and in myocardium following intravenous FDG.

FIGURE 6-20. Comparison of noninvasively measured rates of myocardial glucose utilization using FDG and serial imaging with simultaneous measurements of myocardial glucose uptake using the Fick principle. Notice the linear correlation (LC) between both approaches over a wide range of glucose metabolic rates. (Reproduced from Ratib et al [128] with permission of the Society of Nuclear Medicine.)

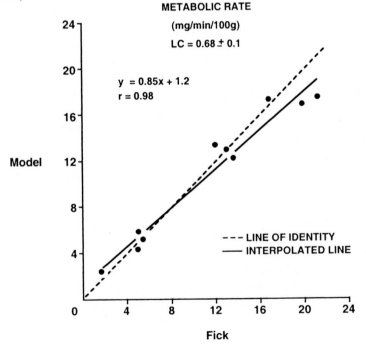

constants by least-square fitting of the time-activity curve.[129] The graphical approach offers several advantages: It is computationally fast, corrects for activity spillover, and can be performed from only 3 tissue time points. Further, the approach is suitable for generating parametric images with pixel-by-pixel display of regional glucose utilization rates.[17]

Despite the success of the FDG approach, several issues remain unresolved. Foremost is the fixed value for linear correlation (LC). Although found relatively constant in isolated heart preparations and in canine myo-cardium,[126,128] subsequent studies in isolated working heart preparations observed no effects of fasting or feeding or postischemia on the LC but report lower LCs for perfusates with pharmacological concentrations of insulin and higher LCs for physiological insulin concentrations.[131–135] Further, perturbations of steady-state conditions in isolated arterially perfused hearts affected the LC and thus emphasized the importance of steady-state conditions during measurements as one of the fundamental requirements of tracer kinetic principles.[136] It thus seems possible that the LC is, in fact, not constant but related to the metabolic study conditions. A possible solution to such variability of the LC, the intercept of K on the Patlak and Blasberg graphical plot may represent an estimated LC specific for each study or measurement.[135]

STANDARDIZATION OF STUDY CONDITIONS

Activation of rate-limiting enzyme systems along the glycolytic pathway together with translocation and increased expression of the relatively insulin-independent glucose transporter GLUT 1 are believed to be flux-generating steps for glycolysis. Hence, they are likely to account for the selective regional increase in glucose utilization and, thus, in FDG uptake in reversibly dysfunctional myocardium. Therefore, when glucose utilization in normal myocardium is suppressed by high circulating FFA and low insulin levels as, for example, after 5 h to 24 h of fasting, myocardium that selectively accumulates FDG should be considered ischemic or reversibly dysfunctional. Indeed, some laboratories utilize this approach, for example, administration of FDG after 5 h to 6 h of fasting for identifying ischemia-related alterations in regional myocardial glucose metabolism. Other laboratories again refer to serious shortcomings with the fasting approach, for example, slow tracer clearance from the blood pool and poor uptake into the myocardium and, hence, low signal-to-noise ratios with suboptimal or diagnostically unacceptable images. Most laboratories, therefore, standardize dietary conditions by raising glucose utilization in normal myocardium and accelerating tracer clearance from blood in order to optimize the myocardial FDG images.

Several approaches for standardization are currently in use:

1. *Glucose loading.* Following a light standardized breakfast several hours prior to the study, glucose plasma concentrations are determined 1 h prior to injecting FDG. Oral administration of 50 g to 70 g glucose stimulates insulin secretion and lowers plasma FFA levels—factors that enhance myocardial glucose uptake and usually produce images of good diagnostic quality.

2. *Hyperinsulinemic-euglycemic clamp.* The clamp involves continuous infusion of insulin (for example, $1 \text{ mU} \cdot \text{kg}^{-1} \cdot \text{min}^{-1}$ in one study) while normo-

glycemia is maintained through simultaneous infusion of 20% dextrose in water.[137–139] One study, for example, described an initial infusion rate of 0.16 U min^{-1} · kg^{-1} for the first 4 minutes, followed for the next 3 minutes with a lower rate of 0.08 U min^{-1} · kg^{-1} after which the infusion rate was maintained at 0.04 U min^{-1} · kg^{-1}.[140] The infusion rate of glucose is titrated in order to maintain the plasma glucose level within the range of normal. Repeated measurements of blood glucose levels are required, performed best at 10- to 15-minute time intervals. Once the target glucose level has been achieved, the rate of infusion is maintained throughout the imaging study, that is, during the initial uptake and image acquisition period. Again, this standardization approach produces high-quality myocardial FDG images.[140,141] Myocardium-to-blood ^{18}F activity ratios with this approach usually exceed those achievable with oral glucose loading, although rates of exogenous glucose utilization, in units of micromoles of glucose per minute per gram of myocardium are comparable for both. Finally, in a survey of 131 patients, glucose clamping for 2 h was found to be safe, and no serious adverse effects occurred.[141]

3. *Pharmacological lowering of FFA plasma levels.* A third standardization approach is intravenous administration of nicotinic acid or one of its derivatives.[142–144] These agents lower circulating FFA levels, shifting the competition between FFA and glucose for myocardial substrate selection in favor of glucose, thereby augmenting myocardial FDG uptake. Again, images of high diagnostic quality can be achieved with this pharmacological approach.

4. *Patients with abnormal glucose handling or with type 1 or type 2 diabetes.* In numerous patients, however, diabetes or insulin resistance may have remained undiagnosed or, if diagnosed, may not have not been communicated to the nuclear medicine physician. Therefore, it is important to determine blood glucose levels in all patients 1 h prior to the FDG injection. Guidelines provided by the American Diabetes Association (Table 6-8) are useful for determining the presence of insulin-resistant or type 2 diabetes. These guidelines also aid in standardizing study conditions and in optimizing the diagnostic quality of the myocardial ^{18}F-deoxyglucose images.

If oral glucose is used for optimizing myocardial FDG uptake, then, according to guidelines established by the American Diabetes Association (Table 6-8), glucose should be given orally only if fasting blood glucose levels are less than 110 mg%. Determination of blood glucose levels should be repeated 1 h after glucose loading in order to ascertain the absence of insulin-resistant or type 2 diabetes. At that time, blood glucose levels should be less than 160 mg%.

For fasting blood glucose levels ranging from 110 mg% to 126 mg%, no oral

TABLE 6-8. American Diabetes Association Criteria for Diabetes[a]

	Fasting glucose levels (mg · dL^{-1})	*2-h Post glucose levels (mg · dL^{-1})*
Normal	< 110	< 140
Abnormal glucose handling	> 100 and < 126	< 200
Diabetes	> 126	≥ 200

[a]Glucose levels are given in milligrams per deciliter of plasma; fasting is overnight and 2 h post glucose values are after 75 g of glucose orally.

TABLE 6-9. Use of Oral Glucose and Intravenous Regular Insulin in Type 2 Diabetes

Plasma glucose (fasting)		Oral glucose	Insulin
< 7 mmol/L	< 126 mg · dL⁻¹	25 g	None
7–11 mmol/L	126 mg − 200 mg · dL⁻¹	None	5 IU iv
> 11 mmol/L	< 200 mg · dL⁻¹	None	10 IU iv
Repeat plasma glucose levels after 15 min			
< 8 mmol/L	< 126 mg · dL⁻¹	None	None
8–11 mmol/L	126 − 200 mg · dL⁻¹	None	5 IU iv
> 11 mmol/L	< 200 mg · dL⁻¹	None	10 IU iv

Source: Schedule reprinted with permission from Vitale et al.[144]

glucose should be administered because insulin resistance may exist. One might even consider intravenous administration of 3 IU to 5 IU of regular, short-acting insulin about 15 minutes to 20 minutes prior to injecting FDG, in order to promote its uptake and retention by the myocardium. Essential is repeat monitoring of blood glucose levels so that, should hypoglycemia occur, blood glucose concentrations can be restored by oral or, if necessary, intravenous glucose administration.

For blood glucose levels of greater than 126 mg%, again, no glucose should be administered if these levels suggest the presence of type 2 diabetes. Rather, regular short-acting insulin might be administered intravenously. In most instances, insulin doses of 3 IU to 5 IU should be administered about 20 minutes prior to the FDG injection with the aim of lowering glucose concentrations by 10% to 20%. It might be advantageous to inject ^{18}F-deoxyglucose at the time of declining blood glucose levels in order to optimize clearance of the radiotracer into the myocardium. If the initial insulin administration remains, however, without effect on blood glucose concentration, repeat insulin injections may be necessary in order to lower blood glucose concentrations by at least 10% to 20%. Some laboratories have developed and report more detailed standardization protocols with doses of intravenous insulin adjusted to the initially measured plasma glucose levels. One such protocol designed specifically for type 2 diabetes patients is listed in Table 6-9.[144]

As mentioned above, for patients with modestly increased fasting blood glucose levels, continued monitoring of blood glucose concentrations for identifying hypoglycemia is important. Patients should also be familiarized with symptoms of hypoglycemia and its management, as for example, ingestion of orange juice. Further, in patients with severely impaired LV function and potentially unstable hemodynamic conditions, consultation with the referring clinician prior to administration of insulin is advisable.

STUDIES IN THE NORMAL HUMAN HEART

Myocardial blood flow and its determinants

Myocardial blood flow at rest

Numerous laboratories have published extensive information on MBF in the normal human myocardium, both at rest and during physical and pharmacologically induced stress. Regardless of the methodological approach used, that is, either the ^{15}O-labeled water or the ^{13}N-ammonia approach, considerable interindividual differences in MBF at rest with the volunteer in the supine position have been described. MBF rates at rest range from 0.4 ml · min^{-1} · g^{-1} to 1.6 ml · min^{-1} · g^{-1}. Whether MBFs at rest depend also on gender has remained uncertain. One study reports no such difference[50] while a second one reports higher resting MBF in women than in men (1.18 ± 0.75 versus 0.93 ± 0.19 ml · min^{-1} · g^{-1}; p < 0.001).[145] It is now clear that interindividual differences in cardiac work as estimated by the RPP frequently account for these variations in MBF. This explanation is consistent with findings from invasive approaches.[93] It is also consistent with changes in MBF that occur in proportion to changes in cardiac work in response to physical stress during supine exercise or to inotropic stimulation. With supine bicycle exercise, MBF increased in 13 healthy volunteers from 0.75 ± 0.43 ml · min^{-1} · g^{-1} at rest to 1.50 ± 0.74 ml · min^{-1} · g^{-1}.[44] The average 2.2-fold increase in MBF was accompanied by a comparable increase in RPP. Similar changes are reported for intravenous dobutamine. In 21 healthy individuals, infusion of 40 μg of dobutamine per minute per kilogram raised MBF from 0.77 ± 0.14 ml · min^{-1} · g^{-1} to 2.25 ± 0.28 ml · min^{-1} · g^{-1}.[146] This flow increase again was associated with a commensurate increase in the RPP. This dependency of MBF on cardiac work as depicted in Figure 6-21 has, therefore, prompted investigators to normalize flows to the RPP as follows:[50]

$$\text{MBF}_{\text{corr}} = \text{MBF} / \text{RPP}(10^{-4}) \tag{6-9}$$

It is, therefore, important to monitor heart rate and blood pressure during the MBF measurements so that resting flows can be appropriately corrected for. MBF at rest was also found to be related to age.[50,147,148] One study in 40 normal volunteers reported average flows of 0.76 ± 0.17 ml · min^{-1} · g^{-1} for individuals less than 50 years of age (n = 18; 31 ± 9 years) as compared to 0.92 ±

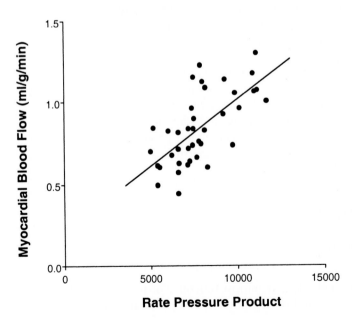

FIGURE 6-21. Dependency of myocardial blood flow as determined noninvasively with ^{13}N-ammonia and dynamic PET imaging on cardiac work as determined from the product of heart rate and systolic blood pressure (RPP) in 40 normal volunteers (closed circles) (Data used with permission from Czernin et al.[50])

0.25 ml · min^{-1} · g^{-1} (p $<$ 0.05) for normal volunteers older than 50 years of age (n = 22; 64 $\pm$ 9 years).[50] This age dependency was associated with progressive, age-dependent increases in the RPP. Based on the regression equation between age and MBFs at rest (MBF = 0.56 + 0.005 years), MBF at rest increases linearly with age. Such age dependency of MBF at rest is important because many studies compare findings in cardiac patients who usually are older to findings in normal control subjects who often are younger. Lifestyle and physical activity do not appear to independently modify MBF at rest. Endurance athletes were found to have 33% lower MBF than sedentary males although the lower flows are most likely explained by lower RPP in the endurance athletes.[98,149] Elite rowing athletes similarly revealed normal resting MBFs.[150]

Responses of myocardial blood flow to stress

Various forms of stress are used. One is supine bicycle exercise; a second one is the use of predominantly vascular smooth muscle dilating agents, for example, dipyridamole, adenosine or, more recently, ATP, and a third one, pharmacological stimulation with inotropic agents like dobutamine. Specific examples of stress acting on MBF are:

1. *For exercise stress,* a bicycle ergometer is mounted to the end of the imaging table while the subjects chest is positioned in the field of view of the imaging gantry.[44] While the patient bicycles at a constant work load, the flow tracer is injected intravenously while bicycle exercise is maintained for another 1 to 2 minutes in order to assure trapping of the radiotracer in the myocardium.

2. *Dipyridamole* (0.56 mg · kg^{-1}) is infused intravenously over a 4-minute period. Because the agent inhibits the catabolism of adenosine, tissue concentrations of adenosine progressively increase so that the maximum hyperemic response occurs at about 3 minutes to 5 minutes after completion of the dipyridamole infusion.[151] At that time, the flow tracer is administered. Raising the dipyridamole dose by 50% failed to produce higher MBFs, so that the standard dipyridamole dose appears to be adequate for achieving maximum hyperemic MBFs.[152]

3. *Adenosine* is infused at a rate of 140 μg · min^{-1} · kg^{-1}. As invasive studies have shown, coronary flow velocities rapidly reach maximum levels.[51] The standardized approach entails a total infusion time of 6 minutes. The tracer is administered at 3 minutes with the additional 3 minutes needed for trapping tracer in the myocardium. Both adenosine and dipyridamole induce comparable levels of hyperemia as determined with quantitative measurements of MBF.[153] The standard dose schedule of adenosine of 140 μg · min^{-1} · kg^{-1} appears to produce maximum flows, at least according to dosing studies in longterm smokers.[154] Conversely, lower doses, for example, of only 70 μg · min · g, produce disproportionately lower flow responses that in one study averaged only about 60% of MBFs induced by standard dose adenosine.[155]

4. *Adenosine triphosphate (ATP)* has also been used as a coronary vasodilator agent.[156] Infused at a rate of 0.16 mg · kg^{-1} · min^{-1} for 9 minutes, it increases MBF rates in young normal volunteers from 0.80 $\pm$ 0.17 ml · min · $^{-1}$ · g^{-1} at rest to 3.69 $\pm$ 0.76 ml · min · $^{-1}$ · g^{-1} during hyperemia, resulting in a myocardial flow reserve of 4.03 $\pm$ 0.68.

5. *Dobutamine* stress is primarily used when adenosine or dipyridamole are contraindicated, for example, because of bronchial asthma. Typically, intravenous dobutamine infusions begin at low doses such as $5\,\mu g \cdot min^{-1} \cdot kg^{-1}$, or $10\,\mu g \cdot min^{-1} \cdot kg^{-1}$ and, according to patient tolerance, are subsequently increased to $30\,\mu g \cdot min^{-1} \cdot kg^{-1}$ or $40\,\mu g \cdot min^{-1} \cdot kg^{-1}$.[146] Because the agent is a predominantly β_2 adrenoreceptor agonist, heart rates may not markedly increase so that some laboratories supplement the dobutamine stress with intravenous atropine (typically, 0.5 mg).[157]

6. *Cold pressor testing (CPT)* as another form of stress has been used in invasive studies of the coronary circulation for probing flow-dependent and mostly endothelial-mediated coronary vasodilator responses.[158–161] Immersion of a hand into a slush of ice-cold water is followed by a rapid rise in heart rate and in systolic blood pressure and, thus, in cardiac work. This increase in cardiac work, as estimated from the change in the RPP, normally averages about 50% to 60% and, in the normal coronary circulation, is associated with a proportionate, probably metabolism-dependent increase in MBF. Local norepinephrine release modulates the flow response.[161,162] The predominantly α-adrenergic effect of norepinephrine leads to α-adrenoreceptor-mediated vascular smooth muscle constriction which in the normal coronary circulation is opposed by nitric oxide released by the endothelium in response to increased sheer stress and to direct norephinephrine stimulation of endothelial α-adrenergic receptors. If release of nitric oxide or its bioavailability is diminished because of an impairment of endothelial function, the opposing vasodilator effect is diminished or even absent so that the vasoconstrictor action of norepinephrine prevails. Consequently, the increase in MBF relative to that of cardiac work becomes attenuated, may be absent or, conversely, MBF may actually decline.

For CPT, the participant immerses one hand in a slush of ice water. Heart rate and systemic blood pressure promptly rise within 10 seconds to 15 seconds and usually reach a maximum at about 30 seconds when the flow tracer is administered intravenously. The CPT is maintained for an additional 90 seconds required for trapping the flow tracer in the myocardium. The normal average of an approximate 50% increase in RPP provoked by CPT is paralleled by a proportionate approximate 50% increase in MBF.[163,164] This increase is markedly diminished or even absent in asymptomatic longterm smokers, in insulin-resistant diabetes and diabetes but also in postmenopausal women with risk factors for CAD.[156,163,164]

RESPONSES TO DIPYRIDAMOLE AND ADENOSINE

Hyperemic MBFs of $3.5\,ml \cdot min^{-1} \cdot g^{-1}$ to $6.0\,ml \cdot min^{-1} \cdot g^{-1}$ in response to pharmacologically induced vascular smooth muscle relaxation have been observed in young normal volunteers (Table 6-10). Adenosine and dipyridamole produce comparable levels of hyperemic MBFs. In 20 normal volunteers, for example, MBF averaged $4.4 \pm 0.9\ ml \cdot min^{-1} \cdot g^{-1}$ during adenosine infusion which was virtually identical to the average of $4.3 \pm 1.3\ ml \cdot min^{-1} \cdot g^{-1}$ after dipyridamole.[153] Importantly, hyperemic MBFs due to vascular smooth muscle relaxants, may vary considerably between normal individuals as has also been reported with intracoronary flow velocity measurements.[51] These normal interindividual differences in pharmacologically induced hyperemic blood flows

TABLE 6-10. Estimates of Myocardial Blood Flow at Rest and During Stress

Investigation	N	Age (years)	Technique	Stress	MBF Rest (ml · min⁻¹ · g⁻¹)	MBF Stress (ml · min⁻¹ · g⁻¹)	MF reserve
Bergmann et al, 1989[31]	11	25.5	¹⁵O-water	Dipyr	0.90 ± 0.22	3.55 ± 1.15	4.1 ± 1.2
Araujo et al, 1991[34]	11	26–67	¹⁵O-water	Dipyr	0.84 ± 0.09	3.52 ± 1.12	4.2 ± 1.3
Pitkänen et al, 1996[214]	20	31 ± 8	¹⁵O-water	Dipyr	0.83 ± 0.13	4.49 ± 1.27	5.4 ± 15
Yokoyama et al, 1998[220]	13	56 ± 7	¹⁵O-water	Dipyr	0.80 ± 0.39	2.92 ± 1.66	3.7 ± 1.4
Kaufmann et al, 1999[80]	21	45 ± 8	¹⁵O-water	Adenosine	0.89 ± 0.15	3.51 ± 0.45	NA
Tadamura et al, 2001[157]	20	23 ± 3	¹⁵O-water	Dipyr	0.67 ± 0.16	4.33 ± 1.23	NA
			¹⁵O-water	Dob + Atr	NA	5.89 ± 1.58	NA
Iwado et al, 2002[156]	12		¹⁵O-water	ATP	0.80 ± 0.17	3.69 ± 0.76	4.03 ± 0.68
Krivokapich et al, 1989[44]	13	24 ± 8	¹³N-ammonia	Exercise	0.75 ± 0.43	1.50 ± 0.74	2.2 ± 0.7
Hutchins et al, 1990[45]	7	24 ± 4	¹³N-ammonia	Dipyr	0.88 ± 0.17	4.17 ± 1.12	4.8 ± 1.3
Chan et al, 1992[153]	20	35 ± 16	¹³N-ammonia	Dipyr	1.1 ± 0.2	4.3 ± 1.3	4.0 ± 1.3
			¹³N-ammonia	Adenosine	NA	4.4 ± 0.9	4.3 ± 1.6
Senneff et al, 1991[147]	11	25 ± 4	¹⁵O-water	Dipyr	1.16 ± 0.32	4.25 ± 1.54	3.9 ± 1.5
	15	55 ± 9	¹⁵O-water	Dipyr	1.17 ± 0.33	3.12 ± 1.09	3.0 ± 1.4
Czernin et al, 1993[50]	18	31 ± 9	¹³N-ammonia	Dipyr	0.76 ± 0.25	3.0 ± 0.8	4.1 ± 0.9
	22	64 ± 9	¹³N-ammonia	Dipyr	0.92 ± 0.25	2.7 ± 0.25	3.0 ± 0.7

Abbreviations: Dipyr, dipyridamole; Dob + Atr, dobutamine and atropine; MBF, myocardial blood flow; MF, myocardial flow; N, number of patients; NA, not available.

Source: Data tabulated with permission from: Bergmann et al,[31] Araujo et al,[34] Pitkänen et al,[214] Yokoyama et al,[220] Kaufmann et al,[80] Tadamura et al,[157] Iwado et al,[156] Krivokapich et al,[44] Hutchins et al,[45] Chan et al,[153] Senneff et al,[147] and Czernin et al.[50]

and flow reserves appear, however, unrelated to exercise capacity.[165] Both adenosine and dipyridamole act directly on the vascular smooth muscle of the coronary resistance vessels. More recent experimental evidence suggests, however, an additional, endothelial-mediated effect of adenosine that appears to augment the total hyperemic flow. This effect of adenosine may be direct by stimulation of adenosine receptors of endothelial cells or indirect by a flow-dependent, probably sheer stress-mediated vasodilation.[166,167]

The hyperemia produced by adenosine or dipyridamole is independent of cardiac work and, hence, no longer correlates with the RPP. Antagonists of both agents, for example, caffeine or theophylline-containing substances, attenuate or even abolish the hyperemic response and, therefore, should be withheld for at least 24 h.[168] Although adenosine- or dipyridamole-induced hyperemia depends on coronary driving pressure and, thus, on the mean arterial blood pressure, increases in blood pressure induced by handgrip or by physical exercise lowered maximum hyperemic MBFs, possibly because of an associated increase in extravascular resistance.[152,169] Hyperemic MBFs may also depend on the adrenergic control of the coronary vessels as demonstrated by effects of β-adrenergic blockers on hyperemic MBFs, although it remains uncertain whether the observed augmentation of hyperemic MBF results directly from an effect on the adrenergic coronary control or indirectly from, for example, a decline in extravascular resistant forces.[170] There also appears to be no effect of α_1-adrenergic activity on hyperemic MBFs in normal subjects as demonstrated with dexamethasone.[171] Intravenous insulin, however, has been shown to augment hyperemic flow responses. In young, healthy men, hyperisulinemic-euglycemic clamping produced a 20% increase in adenosine hyperemic MBFs (from 0.38 ± 0.97 to 4.28 ± 1.57 ml $\cdot$ min^{-1} $\cdot$ g^{-1}).[171] This increase is dose dependant. For example, at plasma insulin concentrations of 65 mU/L, adenosine-stimulated flows increased from 3.92 ± 1.17 ml $\cdot$ min^{-1} $\cdot$ g^{-1} to 4.72 ± 0.96 ml $\cdot$ min^{-1} $\cdot$ g^{-1} ($p < 0.05$) and further to 5.61 ± 1.03 ml $\cdot$ min^{-1} $\cdot$ g^{-1} at supraphysiological plasma insulin concentrations of 460 mU/L.[172]

Whether hyperemic MBF truly declines with age has remained controversial, even though some reports point to somewhat lower hyperemic MBFs in normal volunteers older than 50 years of age when compared to young normal volunteers.[147] For example, one study reports hyperemic MBFs of 4.25 ± 1.54 ml $\cdot$ min^{-1} $\cdot$ g^{-1} in 11 normal subjects with an average age of 25 ± 4 years as compared to average MBFs of 3.12 ± 1.09 ml $\cdot$ min^{-1} $\cdot$ g^{-1} in 15 normal subjects with an average age of 55 ± 9 years. In contrast, another study finds in 22 normal subjects with an average age of 64 ± 9 years average hyperemic MBFs that are nearly identical to those in a comparison group of 18 younger normal subjects (31 ± 9 years), although the minimum myocardial MBF resistance (see below) was modestly, though significantly higher in older than in younger normal subjects.[50]

DOBUTAMINE

Different from dipyridamole or adenosine hyperemia, MBF increases in response to inotropic agents, for example, dobutamine in proportion to increases in cardiac work or the RPP.[146] Supplementation of the maximum 40 μg $\cdot$ kg^{-1} $\cdot$ min^{-1} dose of dobutamine by intravenous atropine (at split doses of

0.5 mg at 1-min intervals of up to 1 mg) in order to increase heart rates produced levels of hyperemic flows that exceeded those achieved with standard dose dipyridamole (5.89 ± 1.58 ml $\cdot$ min^{-1} $\cdot$ g^{-1} versus 4.33 ± 1.23 ml $\cdot$ min^{-1} $\cdot$ g^{-1}).[157]

Myocardial flow reserve and resistance

Several other parameters of the coronary circulation can be derived from the MBF estimates. One is the MBF reserve as the ratio of hyperemic to rest MBFs. A second one is the coronary resistance as the ratio of the mean arterial blood pressure over MBF,[173] and a third one is the coronary conductance as the ratio of MBF over mean arterial blood pressure. The latter two indices relate or normalize MBF during hyperemia to the coronary driving pressure.

Myocardial substrate metabolism and substrate selection

Oxygen consumption and oxidative metabolism

Estimates of MVO_2, of the myocardial oxygen extraction and of the corresponding MBFs obtained with the ^{15}O-labeled water and the ^{15}O-oxygen approach are listed in Table 6-5.[96,97] They are comparable to those determined invasively with the coronary sinus catheter technique and as listed in Table 6-2.[93]

Average values reported for the myocardial clearance rates of [C-11] acetate and thus for rates of oxidative metabolism in normal volunteers are listed in Table 6-7.[105,106,174] Generally, the tissue clearance rates were obtained in these studies by monoexponential fitting of the early portion of the LV myocardial clearance time-activity curve. Oxidative metabolism can be estimated also in the thin-walled myocardium of the right ventricle.[175] Clearance rates in 9 normal volunteers indicated that oxidative metabolism in the right ventricular myocardium was $42\% \pm 10\%$ lower than in the interventricular septum. This difference is comparable to that observed with invasive techniques. In the same study, clearance rates in the right ventricular myocardium in patients with aortic valve disease but normal right ventricular pressures averaged 0.037 ± 0.007 min^{-1} compared with 0.065 ± 0.11 min^{-1} in the interventricular septum. These values are comparable to those reported in another investigation in 14 normal volunteers, in whom k_{mono} averaged 0.065 ± 0.015 min^{-1} for the left and 0.034 ± 0.016 min^{-1} for the right ventricular myocardium.[174]

Similar to MBF, rates of myocardial oxidative metabolism as determined with [C-11] acetate markedly differ between normal individuals, primarily as a function of cardiac work and, hence, oxygen demand. Supine bicycle exercise accelerates the myocardial clearance of [C-11] acetate and, thus, k_{mono}.[105] Similar, increases in cardiac work induced by inotropic stimulation as, for example, with dobutamine produced corresponding increases in the myocardial [C-11] acetate clearance.[106] In these studies, the RPP as an index of cardiac work generally correlated linearly with k_{mono} as shown in Table 6-6. The same table also includes regression equations for converting tissue clearance rates of [C-11] acetate into values of MVO_2. As an example, one study describes a correlation of $k_{mono} = 0.014 + 5.8908 \cdot 10^{-6}$ RPP in normal volunteers submitted to bicycle exercise and the second one of $k_1 = -0.25 + 1.25 \cdot 10^{-5}$ RPP in normal volunteers submitted to dobutamine stimulation (the greater steepness of the slope of the regression line in the latter study is probably because the curves during dobutamine were analyzed with a biexponential fit while the first study used only k_{mono}.

Myocardial free fatty acid metabolism

Rates of myocardial FFA utilization and of β-oxidation depend on substrate availability and, thus, on the dietary state. As listed in Table 6-11, they may increase by more than four times from the preferential glucose to the preferential FFA utilization state. Different from studies with [18]FTHA, the use of ^{11}C-palmitate offers more information on the metabolic fate of FFA in the myocardium. The radiotracer clears from myocardium in a characteristic biexponential fashion (Figure 6-16). The pattern of substrate selection, for example, between FFA, glucose, and lactate as well as cardiac work, determine the relative sizes and clearance rates of the two clearance components. In the fasting state when FFA serves as the major substrate fuel, the relative size of the rapid clearance curve component averages approximately 40%.[176] The corresponding clearance halftimes average about 11 minutes. When glucose is administered in order to shift myocardial substrate selection from FFA to glucose, the relative size of the rapid clearance phase decreases to 10% while the clearance halftime increases to 20 minutes, reflecting the anticipated decline in the fraction of FFA undergoing immediate oxidation. Increases in FFA oxidation in response to increases in cardiac work, for example, induced by atrial pacing, further accentuate the rapid clearance-curve component; when depending on the magnitude of the increase in cardiac work, its relative size increases in proportion and its slope becomes steeper (for example, from 46% to 64% for the relative size and from 22 min to 13.4 min for the halftime of the rapid clearance phase).[177] Using a 4-compartment tracer kinetic model for ^{11}C-palmitate,[114] estimates of myocardial FFA utilization in normal volunteers averaged 2.13 ± 4.9 nmol $\cdot$ min^{-1} $\cdot$ g^{-1}.[115]

Myocardial glucose utilization

The glucose analogue FDG distributes homogeneously throughout the normal LV myocardium with the exception of a regional increase in the posterolateral wall.[178] This increase is especially prominent when studies are performed in the fasted state and myocardial FDG uptake is low (about 25%

TABLE 6-11. Estimates of Myocardial Glucose and Free Fatty Acid (FFA) Utilization by FDG, ^{11}C-Glucose, ^{11}C-Palmitate, and [18]FTHA[a]

	Dietary state	Glucose (mmol $\cdot$ L^{-1})	FFA (mmol $\cdot$ L^{-1})	Utilization (μmol $\cdot$ min^{-} $\cdot$ 1 g^{-1})	Investigation
Glucose	Fasting	4.8 ± 0.3	0.30 ± 0.25	0.24 ± 0.17	Choi et al, 1993[179]
		5.7 ± 0.05	1.07 ± 0.46	0.13 ± 0.09	Ohtaki et al, 1995[441]
		4.9 ± 0.4	0.67 ± 0.17	0.13 ± 0.06	Davila-Roman et al, 2002[115]
	Post glucose	8.6 ± 1.8	0.19 ± 0.14	0.69 ± 0.11	Choi et al, 1993[179]
		10.2 ± 0.4	N/A	0.69 ± 0.03	Knuuti et al, 1992[180]
		7.0 ± 0.13	0.31 ± 0.20	0.52 ± 0.05	Ohtaki et al, 1995[441]
	Clamp	5.1 ± 0.2	N/A	0.74 ± 0.02	Knuuti et al, 1992[180]
		5.4 ± 0.13	0.34 ± 0.20	0.54 ± 0.11	Ohtaki et al, 1993[441]
FFA	Fasting	5.3 ± 0.4	0.560 ± 0.080	5.8 ± 1.7	Mäki et al, 1998[119]
		4.9 ± 0.4	0.67 ± 0.17	0.21 ± 0.05	Davila-Roman et al, 2002[115]
	Clamp	5.4 ± 0.8	0.110 ± 0.030	1.4 ± 0.5	Mäki et al, 1998[119]

[a]Fasting studies performed after an overnight fast; post glucose, 1 h after 75 g glucose orally; and clamp study performed during hyperinsulinemic-euglycemic glucose clamping; N/A, data not reported; values for FFA uptake are given in μmol $\cdot$ min^{-1} $\cdot$ 100 g^{-1}.

Source: Data taken with permission from Choi et al,[179] Knuuti et al,[180] Ohtake et al,[441] Mäki et al,[119] and Davila-Roman et al.[115]

higher in the posterolateral than in the anterior wall).[179] Under conditions of glucose loading and, thus, optimization of myocardial FDG uptake, this regional increase in tracer uptake in the posterolateral wall is less prominent. The mechanism accounting for this observation has remained uncertain but may be related to regional variations in the LC and, thus, to the affinity of FDG or, more likely, reflects a true variation in regional myocardial glucose metabolism.

Estimates of MMRGlc depend on circulating substrate and hormone levels. After oral glucose loading when myocardial glucose utilization is optimized, most investigations report a MMRGlc in normal volunteers of about 0.7 μmol $\cdot$ min^{-1} $\cdot$ g^{-1} (see Tables 6-2 and 6-11).[129,179] Similar values are achieved in normal myocardium with the hyperinsulinemic-euglycemic glucose clamp (see Table 6-11),[179,180] although differences exist between the two approaches. During the hyperinsulinemic-euglycemic clamp, a higher k_3 or phosphorylation rate constant accounts for the high MMRGlc whereas higher plasma glucose concentrations rather than k_3 are responsible for the higher MMRGlc after oral glucose loading.[180] Estimates of MMRGlc derived noninvasively with PET match estimates reported in the literature as determined invasively with the coronary sinus catheter technique. For example, for the blood levels and the myocardial extraction fraction for glucose listed in Table 6-2, when one assumes a resting MBF of 0.7 ml $\cdot$ min^{-1} $\cdot$ g^{-1}, the MMRGlc is about 0.8 μmol $\cdot$ min^{-1} $\cdot$ g^{-1}. This value is consistent with the PET derived estimates of the MMRGlc as listed for fasting normal volunteers in Table 6-11. Comparable estimates of MMRGlc have also been obtained with ^{11}C-labeled glucose.[115] They averaged 0.125 μmol $\cdot$ min^{-1} $\cdot$ g^{-1} in normal volunteers in the fasting state.

Despite careful standardization of study conditions with the aim of achieving rates of glucose metabolism that are comparable between study participants, considerable interindividual variations in MMRGlc exist. For example, the coefficient variation averages 0.26 for normal individuals after glucose loading, which is not significantly different from the coefficient variation of 0.26 observed for normal volunteers when studied using the hyperinsulinemic-euglycemic clamp.[180]

Substrate regulation and competition

Preferential utilization of a given fuel substrate, for example, glucose, lactate, or FFA, depends on its concentration in arterial blood which, in turn, depends on the dietary state, serum levels of insulin, or on physical stress.[181] A change in the myocardium's preferential substrate utilization from FFA to glucose, also referred to as Randle's cycle, can be demonstrated with either ^{11}C-palmitate and FDG or both.[119,179,181,182] When plasma levels of FFA are high and glucose and insulin are low, the use of FFA as the preferred substrate is reflected on the ^{11}C-palmitate curve by the large relative size of the rapid clearance phase and its steep slope (both corresponding to increased FFA oxidation) and the low or even undetectable FDG uptake. MMRGlc in this condition may be only 0.24 $\pm$ 0.17 μmol $\cdot$ min^{-1} $\cdot$ g^{-1} or 0.33 $\pm$ 0.24 μmol $\cdot$ min^{-1} $\cdot$ g^{-1},[182,179], which is only about 30% to 40% of the MMRGlc under conditions when glucose is the primary fuel (Table 6-11). Ingestion of carbohydrates raises glucose plasma concentrations and stimulates insulin secretion but reduces FFA plasma levels. Similar effects are achieved by the hyperinsulinemic-euglycemic clamp and, conversely, by raising FFA plasma concentrations with intravenous heparin and intralipid.[182] The corresponding shift to myocardial glucose utilization and oxidation is then reflected by a decline in the size and slope of the rapid clearance phase of ^{11}C-palmitate. Simultaneous measurements of myocardial and skeletal muscle glucose uptake with FDG together with total body glucose disposal rates demonstrated the operation of the cycle of Randle et al.[92] in humans.[182]

STUDIES OF CARDIOVASCULAR DISEASE AND CLINICAL IMPLICATIONS

Detection of clinical coronary artery disease

Qualitative studies of myocardial blood flow

Numerous clinical investigations confirmed PET's high diagnostic performance for the detection of CAD (Table 6-12 and Figure 6-22).[85,183–190] Sensitivities range from 87% to 97% and specificities from 78% to 100%. Most of these studies compared rest or stress-induced flow defects to arteriographic findings by visual analysis and most defined a 50% to 70% diameter luminal narrowing as significant stenoses sufficient to produce detectable reductions in MBF. Given the limitation of visual analysis, two investigations graded severity of stenosis based on estimates of the coronary flow reserve by quantitative arteriography.[84,85] Coronary arteries were classified as follows: moderately to severely stenosed if the predicted coronary flow reserve was less than 3, intermediate if the coronary flow reserve ranged from 3 to 4, and minimal for coronary flow reserve values of greater than 4. According to this classification, 94% of vessels with moderate to severe, 49% of vessels with intermediate, and 5% of vessels with minimal stenosis were accurately identified with PET and pharmacological vasodilator stress.[85]

COMPARISON OF PET TO CONVENTIONAL TECHNIQUES

While impressive, the diagnostic accuracy of PET must, however, be directly compared to that by more conventional approaches in order to more clearly define the diagnostic gain. One study indirectly compared the findings on PET with those made in another laboratory using ^{201}Tl single-photon emission computed tomography (SPECT) but using an identical angiographic approach for

TABLE 6-12. Detection of Coronary Artery Disease by PET Stress/Rest Perfusion Imaging

Investigation	N	Stenosis	Tracer	Stress	Sensitivity (%)	Specificity (%)	Accuracy (%)
Schelbert et al, 1982[85a]	45	> 50%	NH₃	DIp	97	100	98
Demer et al, 1989[85]	193	SFR 3< 3	NH₃, Rb	DIP	94	95	94
Yonekura et al, 1987[85b]	50	≥ 50%	NH₃	EX	93	100	94
Stewart et al, 1991[188]	81	≥ 50%	Rb	DIP	84	88	85
Go et al, 1990[187]	202	≥ 50%	Rb	DIp	93	78	90
Williams et al, 1994[190]	287	≥ 67%	Rb	DIP	87	88	88
Simone et al, 1992[189]	225	≥ 67%	Rb	DIP	82	91	89

Abbreviations: DIP, dipyridamole; EX, exercise; N, number of patients; NH₃, ^{13}N-ammonia; Rb, rubidium-82; Stenosis, percent of luminal narrowing considered significant; SFR, coronary flow reserve estimated by quantitative angiography.

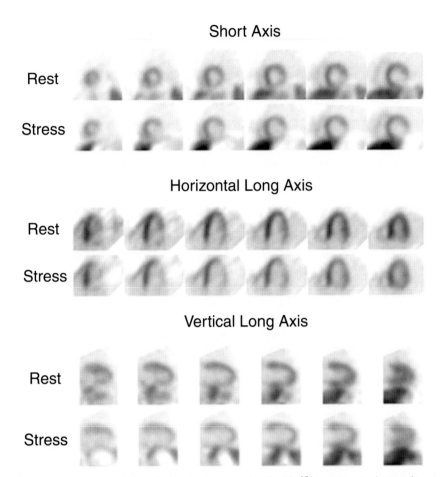

FIGURE 6-22. Myocardial perfusion images obtained with ^{13}N-ammonia during dipyridamole-induced hyperemia and at rest in a patient with angiographically documented coronary artery disease. Notice the decreased tracer activity and, thus, perfusion defect, in the antero-lateral and the lateral wall during pharmacological stress and the normal homogeneous tracer distribution on the rest study.

defining stenosis severity.[85,191] PET outperformed SPECT. Both studies defined stenosis severity by the angiographically predicted coronary flow reserve. Moderate-to-severe coronary stenoses were detected with a 95% sensitivity with PET and a 72% sensitivity with SPECT; intermediate stenoses were detected with a 49% sensitivity with PET while none was detected by SPECT.

Other studies compared the PET to the more conventional SPECT approach in the same patients (Table 6-13). An early study used supine bicycle stress and ^{13}N-ammonia in 48 patients with CAD and reported comparable diagnostic performances for PET and SPECT.[186] Another investigation examined the relative merits of PET and SPECT in 202 patients during the same pharmacological stress.[187] MBF was evaluated with ^{82}Rb at rest and again 4 minutes after dipyridamole infusion. About 8 minutes to 9 minutes later, or a total of 12 minutes to 13 minutes after the end of the dipyridamole infusion, ^{201}Tl was injected and

TABLE 6-13. Comparative Accuracies for SPECT and PET Perfusion Imaging

Investigation	No. of patients	Stenosis (%0	Sensitivity PET (%)	Sensitivity SPECT (%)	Specificity PET (%)	Specificity SPECT (%)	Accuracy PET (%)	Accuracy SPECT (%)
Tamaki et al, 1988[186]	48	≥ 50	98	96	N/A	N/A	N/A	N/A
Go et al, 1990[187]	202	≥ 50	93[a]	76	78	80	90[a]	77
Stewart et al, 1991[188]	81	≥ 50	84	84	88[a]	53	85[a]	79

[a]Statistically significant difference to SPECT.

Source: Data used with permission from Tamaki et al,[186] Go et al,[187] and Stewart et al[188]; Tamaki et al[186] used treadmill exercise and Go et al[187] and Stewart et al[188] intravenous dipyridamole.

SPECT imaging performed within 10 minutes. PET and SPECT exhibited comparable specificities while PET demonstrated a significantly higher sensitivity than SPECT. The results were similar when only 132 of the 202 patients without prior cardiac events such as percutaneous transdermal coronary angioplasty (PTCA) or bypass grafting were analyzed. A third study reported somewhat different findings in 81 patients.[188] Again, all patients underwent rest and dipyridamole stress imaging with ^{82}Rb and PET; for the ^{201}Tl SPECT study, 38 (47%) of the patients underwent treadmill stress and the remaining 43 (53%) pharmacological stress with dipyridamole. In that study, PET and SPECT exhibited comparable sensitivities; however, the specificity was higher for PET than for SPECT. The diagnostic accuracies were similar for patients submitted to treadmill stress testing and patients with pharmacologically induced hyperemia for ^{201}Tl SPECT imaging.

Thus, the two patient comparison studies performed with pharmacological stress confirm the high diagnostic accuracy of PET. However, the studies differ in terms of higher sensitivities and specificities. While it might be argued that in the study with ^{82}Rb and ^{201}Tl injected during the same dipyridamole induced a hyperemic episode, the hyperemic effects of dipyridamole had dissipated at the time of the ^{201}Tl injection, thus, accounting for the lower sensitivity of SPECT; continuous coronary sinus flow measurements have demonstrated an average decay half-time of 33 minutes for the hyperemic response. This amounts to only a 10% decline in the hyperemic response over a 4-minute period[151] which is unlikely to fully explain the lower sensitivity of ^{201}Tl SPECT imaging. More plausible is the gain in specificity in the second study which compared both imaging modalities in a different study session. The higher specificity of PET likely resulted from the adequate correction of photon attenuation and thus a reduction of falsely positive findings. Although the reasons for the observed differences between both studies remain unclear, image analysis at different points of the receiver operating curve (ROC) might be one explanation. Further, the absence of a significant difference between PET and SPECT findings in the first study[186] might be attributed to the use of first generation PET imaging instrumentation.

On balance, the reported studies demonstrate a statistically significant gain in diagnostic accuracy for the detection of CAD by PET. Although larger clinical trials, especially in previously undiagnosed patients with normal MBF and normal wall motion at baseline, are needed for defining more clearly the diagnostic gain, current information nevertheless indicates an improved diagnostic accuracy that might eliminate additional diagnostic procedures like coronary arteriography. This seems confirmed by recent reports that compared the effect of PET and of SPECT on subsequent referral to coronary angiography in 1490 and 102 patients, respectively.[189,190] Pretest likelihoods for CAD were similar for patient groups evaluated with SPECT and with PET. The rate of angiography was, however, significantly less (16.7%) after PET than after SPECT (31.4%) which produced an approximate 23% cost saving per patient.

PROGNOSTIC IMPLICATIONS FOR REST/STRESS *PET* PERFUSION IMAGING

Only few investigations have explored the prognostic value of PET stress and rest MBF imaging. One preliminary survey of 108 patients with a relatively low pretest likelihood of CAD found a zero cardiac morbidity or mortality for 2 years after a normal PET study.[192] When PET was used in a population with strongly suspected or known CAD, the prognostic value of PET was maintained.[193] By following 685 patients for an average period of 41 months, a normal PET study was associated with a 0.9% annual cardiac mortality rate as compared to a 4.3% annual mortality rate in patients with rest and/or stress-induced MBF defects.

PET's value for assessing the preoperative risk in patients scheduled for aortic, carotid, and femoral artery surgery has also been explored.[194] A normal PET study had a 92% negative predictive accuracy for a cardiac event. Conversely, extensive ischemic defects involving at least 5 of 24 myocardial segments were 64% accurate in predicting a perioperative cardiac event. While these values are similar to those reported for SPECT, the use of PET would seem justified especially in patients with inferior image quality on SPECT, for example, for obesity.

STRESS AND REST MYOCARDIAL PERFUSION IMAGING WITH *PET* IN ASYMPTOMATIC PATIENTS

To our knowledge, no information or investigational support on the use of PET myocardial perfusion imaging for screening for CAD is available. However, in asymptomatic but high-risk individuals, PET imaging may prove useful for uncovering subclinical or early coronary atherosclerosis. For example, in 32 asymptomatic first-degree relatives of patients with CAD, quantitative analysis of dipyridamole and rest PET myocardial perfusion images revealed myocardial perfusion defects in 50% of patients.[195] These defects were independent of other risk factors, appeared to be associated with a family trait of CAD and were attributed to structural or functional abnormalities of the coronary circulation probably reflecting preclinical coronary atherosclerosis. If, in fact, such association between flow defects and preclinical disease can be demonstrated, PET imaging in high-risk individuals could provide a rationale for initiating therapeutic measures for primary prevention.

LIFESTYLE MODIFICATION AND MYOCARDIAL PERFUSION ON *PET*

Beneficial effects of risk factor modification on myocardial perfusion in patients with CAD can be demonstrated noninvasively by evaluating the relative distribution of MBF at rest and during pharmacological stress with PET. For example, one clinical investigation randomized patients with CAD into two groups.[196] In one group, 20 patients were assigned to risk factor modification consisting of a very low fat vegetarian diet, stress management, group support and mild-to-moderate exercise. In the second group, 15 patients remained under the care of their private physician with treatment consisting mainly of antianginal treatment. Five years after randomization, repeat imaging with PET revealed that the extent of stress-induced flow defects had slightly but significantly declined by 5.1% ± 4.8% in the (first aggressive treatment) group whereas importantly, the defect size had increased by 10.3% ± 5.6% in the control group patients. The findings on perfusion images parallel those on quantitative angiography so that progression and regression of coronary artery stenosis can be accurately identified noninvasively with PET MBF imaging.

Measurements of myocardial blood flow in CAD

Evaluations of the relative distribution of MBF for the detection of CAD by any radionuclide test are inherently limited. Relative reductions in regional tracer uptake are equated with hemodynamically significant coronary stenosis whereas myocardium with the highest tracer concentration is considered to be supplied by normal coronary vessels. Such myocardium may, however, also be supplied by vessels with hemodynamically significant disease, though less severe. This is where measurements of MBF can uncover additional disease. For example, one study in patients with single vessel disease observed in remote myocardium normal MBF at rest but a severely reduced myocardial flow reserve.[197]

This observation, attributed to microcirculatory abnormalities, is at variance with findings from other investigations of markedly higher flows in such myocardial regions although the hyperemic responses were usually attenuated relative to those in normal volunteers.[198,199] A consistent finding has been that hyperemic MBF in myocardium supplied by vessels with greater than 50% to 70% diameter stenosis is significantly reduced.[198,200–202] Most studies failed to find a correlation between stenosis severity and the degree of attenuation of hyperemic flows, possibly because of vessels with stenosis-in-series and or with the subtended myocardium supplied by collaterals. Only one study described a curvilinear relationship between cross-sectional luminal narrowing and hyperemic MBFs as well as myocardial flow reserves (Figure 6-23).[198] The finding of such curvilinear correlation, resembling the results of Gould, Lipscomb, and Hamilton[203] now considered a classic relationship between anatomical and functional stenosis severity in canine experiments, was attributed to careful selection of vessels without stenoses-in-series and without collaterals. Nevertheless, the considerable scatter of the data about the regression line in this study suggested, in addition to methodological noise disparities between anatomical alterations and their functional, fluid dynamic consequences. Use of the fractional flow reserve as an invasively derived measure of the functional or fluid dynamic effects of a coronary stenosis uncovered similar disparities between the anatomic severity and its effect on coronary blood flow.[204] The approach determines with intracoronary pressure wires the pressure gradient across a coronary stenosis at rest and during pharmacologically induced hyperemia; it relates the pressure gradients to the coronary pressures in a normal, nondiseased coronary artery in the same patient. In 22 patients with isolated stenoses of the left anterior descending coronary artery, the fractional coronary flow reserve correlated poorly with the anatomical stenosis severity with quantitative angiography but, importantly, correlated closely and linearly with the noninvasively measured regional myocardial perfusion reserve measured with ^{15}O-labeled water and PET (relative MBF by PET = 1.12 fractional flow reserve − 0.17; r = 0.89; SEE = 0.13).[204]

Responses of regional MBF to dobutamine stimulation in patients with CAD are similar. For example, in myocardium supplied by less than 50% diameter

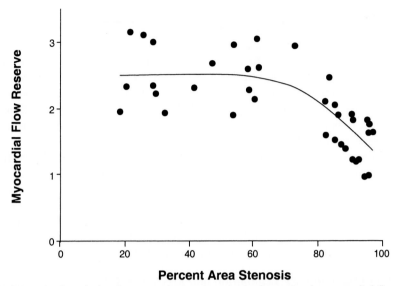

FIGURE 6-23. Correlation between the noninvasively determined myocardial flow reserve as the ratio of hyperemic to resting myocardial blood flow obtained with ^{13}N-ammonia and the severity of coronary artery stenosis as determined by quantitative angiography. (Reproduced with permission from DiCarli et al.[198])

stenoses, MBF increased 2.4 times the baseline with dobutamine. This MBF increase was markedly attenuated in myocardium subtended by greater than 50% diameter stenoses. Importantly, the increase in regional MBF was inversely correlated with the stenosis severity on quantitative coronary angiography.[205]

MBF responses to pharmacological stress have also been used to explore entirely collateral-dependent myocardium. For example, among 26 patients with complete proximal occlusion of the left anterior descending coronary artery, hyperemic MBF was normal in 9.[206] These patients also revealed normal motion of the anterior wall. In contrast, the remaining patients demonstrated severely diminished hyperemic MBFs and, consequently, markedly diminished flow reserves. Of notice, wall motion in the collateral-dependent myocardium was consistently diminished. A more recent and detailed analysis found MBFs at rest in collateral-dependent myocardium to be normal when compared to flows in a normal control population.[207] Only 25% of all collateral-dependent myocardial regions exhibited normal function. MBF in these normally contracting regions increased in response to adenosine by about 80%, markedly less than the 260% increase in the normal control group. Flow responses were even more diminished in dysfunctional collateral-dependent myocardium regions. In nearly 50% of such regions, MBF did increase but by only a modest 30% whereas in the other 50% of regions MBF actually declined by about 35%, supporting the notion of a true coronary steal in collateral-dependent myocardium. The wall motion abnormalities did not differ in severity between the two latter types of collateral-dependent myocardium. In another study, decreases rather than increases in regional MBF during dipyridamole-induced hyperemia in 8 of 18 patients with multivessel CAD were similarly attributed to a true coronary steal.[208] Because of a statistically significant association between these flow reductions and the occurrence of electrocardiographic sinus tachycardia (ST)-segment elevations or the combination of angina and ST-segment depression, these dipyridamole-induced flow reductions were considered to cause true myocardial ischemia.

Responses of regional MBF at rest and, especially, during stress to interventional revascularization has also been examined quantitatively. As observed by evaluating the relative distribution of MBF following mechanical interventions like coronary artery bypass grafting (CABG) or PTCA, stress-induced flow defects improve or resolve entirely. PTCA combined with stent placement promptly normalized regional hyperemic MBFs when measured after 1.6 ± 0.6 days.[209] Flow values in such revascularized territories thus no longer differed from those in myocardium subtended by angiographically normal coronary arteries. Other studies again suggest that such normalization of hyperemic flows does not occur immediately but may be delayed. One study reports full restoration of the vasodilator capacity at only 3 months following PTCA, whereas in early post PTCA (at day 7) the hyperemic response remained unchanged,[210] raising the possibility of vascular stunning immediately after PTCA.

Abnormal coronary vasomotion and preclinical CAD

GENERAL CONSIDERATIONS

Studies with intracoronary Doppler flow velocity probes and quantitative angiography have characterized the effect of coronary risk factors on the function of the large epicardial conduit and on the coronary resistance vessels. First was the observation of a paradoxical flow-dependent constriction of the epicardial conduit vessels in patients with CAD.[158] The constriction occurred when papaverine or adenosine was injected directly into the coronary artery in order to increase coronary flow velocities. In the normal coronary artery, such increases cause a flow-dependent or endothelium-mediated dilation of the epicardial conduit vessels. Second, intracoronary injections of acetylcholine, an agonist of endothelial muscarinic receptors was used to test the vasomotion-related function of the endothelium. Intracoronary acetylcholine produces in normal coronary vessels marked increases in coronary flow that are either diminished or absent in patients with risk factors for CAD.[162,211] Frequently, acetylcholine injections in such patients may even reduce coronary flow. Of interest, the majority of these studies demonstrating abnormal flow responses to intracoronary acetylcholine report normal or near normal flow responses to intracoronary direct vascular smooth muscle relaxants like adenosine or papaverine.[162,211]

CORONARY RISK FACTORS AND MYOCARDIAL BLOOD FLOW

Initial studies with noninvasive MBF measurements by PET in hypercholesteremia patients without CAD demonstrated for the first time a significant attenuation of hyperemic MBFs and thus, of the myocardial MBF reserve (Figure 6-24).[212] Hyperemic MBFs averaged 2.17 ± 0.56 ml $\cdot$ min^{-1} $\cdot$ g^{-1} as compared to 2.64 ± 0.39 ml $\cdot$ min^{-1} $\cdot$ g^{-1} in age-matched control subjects. The myocardial MBF reserve in these hypercholesteremic patients was reduced by 32%. In fact, there was an inverse correlation between the ratio of total to high-density lipoprotein (HDL) cholesterol and the myocardial MBF reserve. Specific lipid abnormalities may also affect hyperemic MBFs, at least according to studies reporting gender-related differences in MBF at rest and during stress-induced hyperemia.[213] Higher flows at rest and during hyperemia in hypercholesteremic

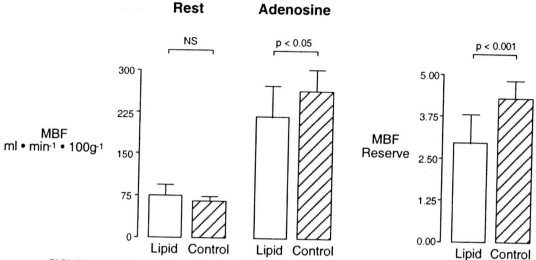

FIGURE 6-24. Comparison of myocardial blood flow at rest and during adenosine-induced hyperemia in normal volunteers (control) and in patients with hypercholesterolemia (lipid) and the corresponding myocardial blood flow reserves (right). Notice the significantly lower hyperemic blood flows and the lower flow reserves in the hypercholesterolemia patients when compared to the normal controls. (Data used with permission from Dayanikli et al.[212])

postmenopausal women than in age-matched men were ascribed to distinctly different lipid profiles.

Subsequent studies in hypercholesteremia patients reported even more severe reductions in hyperemic MBFs in patients with familial hypercholesterolemia (Table 6-14).[214–219] Some of these studies describe significant correlations between the reduced hyperemic response and total plasma cholesterol while others again indicate that such correlation exists only for low-density lipoprotein (LDL) and not for total plasma cholesterol.[219] Elevated plasma triglyceride levels apparently are also associated with a diminished vasodilator capacity.[220] Of interest, different laboratories report comparable reductions in the total vasodilator capacity, all in the range of 20% to 35% (Table 6-14). This reduction is comparable to the decline of the total adenosine stimulated vasodilator capacity observed after pharmacological inhibition of nitric oxide synthase (NOS).[167] It is, therefore, tempting to ascribe the hypercholesterolemia-related impairment to reduced nitric oxide (NO) bioavailability or to endothelial dysfunction. A series of investigations in young asymptomatic men but with a family history of premature CAD or with borderline hypertension but without LV hypertrophy further report attenuated hyperemic MBFs.[221,222]

Of interest are investigations in types 2 and 1 diabetic patients demonstrating attenuated hyperemic MBFs and, thus, a diminished total vasodilator capacity.[223–226] It is questioned whether such attenuation results directly from hyperglycemia as indicated by studies comparing patients with elevated and with normal plasma glucose levels but with comparable glucose disposal rates and, hence, insulin resistance.[225,226] Also, hyperinsulinemia in type 2 diabetes has been shown to augment hyperemic flows.[171]

TABLE 6-14. Coronary Risk Factors and Myocardial Blood Flow

Investigation	Patients MBF ($ml \cdot min^{-1} \cdot g^{-1}$)			Controls MBF ($ml \cdot min^{-1} \cdot g^{-1}$)			$Diff^c$	P^c
	N	Rest	Hyperemia	N	Rest	Hyperemia		
Hypercholesteremia								
Dayanikli et al, 1994[212]	16	0.76 ± 0.19	2.18 ± 0.56	11	0.66 ± 0.09	2.64 ± 0.39	−17%	< 0.001
Pitkänen et al, 1996[214]	15	0.92 ± 0.24	3.19 ± 1.59	20	0.83 ± 0.13	4.49 ± 1.27	−29%	< 0.011
Yokoyama et al, 1996[216]	11	0.70 ± 0.21	2.10 ± 0.71	11	0.75 ± 0.35	3.22 ± 1.74	−35%	< 0.01
	11	0.81 ± 0.31	1.29 ± 0.19				−60%	< 0.01
Pitkänen et al, 1999[218]	21	0.79 ± 0.19	3.54 ± 1.59	21	0.88 ± 0.20	4.54 ± 1.17	−22%	< 0.025
Hypertriglyceridemia								
Yokoyama et al, 1998[220]	15	0.74 ± 0.24	1.98 ± 1.06	13	0.81 ± 0.37	2.62 ± 1.20	−30%	< 0.01
Diabetes								
Pitkänen et al, 1998[224]	12	0.84 ± 0.18	3.17 ± 1.57	12	0.88 ± 0.25	4.45 ± 1.37	−29%	< 0.05
Di Carli et al, 1999[230]	15[a]	0.96 ± 0.17	2.53 ± 0.61	11	0.90 ± 0.17	3.18 ± 0.49	−20%	< 0.001
	13[b]	0.91 ± 0.16	2.48 ± 0.43				−22%	< 0.001
Yokoyama et al, 1997[223]	25	0.74 ± 0.24	1.84 ± 0.99	12	0.73 ± 0.17	2.62 ± 1.20	−30%	< 0.01
Hypertension								
Laine et al, 1998[222]	16	0.83 ± 0.21	2.85 ± 1.20	19	0.80 ± 0.22	3.80 ± 1.44	−25%	

[a,b]Yokoyama et al[216] studied patients with secondary (a) and familial (b) hypercholesteremia; Di Carli et al[230] studied patients without (a) and with (b) diabetic sympathetic neuropathy.

[c]Diff and P represent percentage difference and statistical significance, respectively, between hyperemic myocardial blood flow in patients with risk factors and normal control subjects.

Abbreviations: MBF, myocardial blood flow; N, number of patients or control subjects.

Source: Data used with permission from: Dayanikli et al,[212] Pitkänen et al,[214] Yokoyama et al,[216] Pitkänen et al,[218] Yokoyama et al,[220] Pitkänen et al,[224] DiCarli et al,[230] Yokoyama et al,[223] and Laine et al.[222]

Because invasive studies with intracoronary papaverine or adenosine found the flow response to direct vascular smooth muscle relaxation to be preserved in the presence of coronary risk factors,[159,162,211] hyperemic flow responses to intravenous dipyridamole or adenosine and measured noninvasively with PET most probably reflect the total integrated coronary vasomotor function. They include vascular smooth muscle dilation, flow-dependent or endothelium-mediated dilation of the large conduit and of the prearteriolar vessels combined with decreases in the downstream resistance. Consistent with this possibility is the approximate 30% decrease in adenosine-stimulated forearm blood flow after inhibition of the NO synthase with L-N^G–monomethyl arginine (L-NMMA)[166] and the approximate 21% reduction in adenosine MBF after inhibition with N^G-nitro-L-arginine methyl ester (L-NAME).[167] Also, a flow-dependent dilation of the 400-μ diameter prearterioles might contribute to a reduction in peripheral resistance and, thus, potentiate the effect of direct vascular smooth muscle relaxation.[227] Under abnormal conditions of associated endothelial dysfunction and reduced NO bioactivity, such augmentation will be diminished or even absent so that the total hyperemic MBF response is reduced.

Myocardial flow response to adrenergic stimulation Early in the course of invasive explorations of the coronary vasomotor function, responses of the lumen of the coronary conduit and, subsequently, of the coronary resistance vessels to CPT were found to be abnormal in the presence of coronary risk factors.[158,159] Moreover, the degree of the abnormal response of the coronary resistance vessels to adrenergic stimulation, elicited by CPT, was found to be correlated with the abnormal resistance responses to intracoronary acetylcholine.[158,159,162] These observations suggested that an α-adrenergically mediated vasoconstrictor effect was, under normal conditions, opposed by an α-adrenergically mediated endothelial-dependent NO release so that the vasodilator effect prevailed. Hence, the adrenergically mediated cold pressor test may reveal information on endothelial function.

That efferent adrenergic neurons are indeed intimately involved in mediating flow responses to CPT was confirmed by recent findings with PET. In addition to noninvasive measurements of regional MBF, these studies also evaluated regional adrenergic neuronal function, using a carbon-11-labeled analogue of epinephrine. The agent, ^{11}C-hydroxy-ephedrine (HED), accumulates via the uptake II mechanism in adrenergic nerve terminals.[228] Its uptake is diminished in neuronal dysfunction or in states of de-innervation, for example, in cardiac allografts but also in patients with diabetic neuropathy.[229,230] Regional reductions in the myocardial retention of ^{11}C-hydroxy-ephedrine (HED) in cardiac allografts and in patients with diabetic neuropathy were associated with diminished MBF responses to CPT. Moreover, in autonomic diabetic neuropathy, hyperemic MBF responses were preserved best in myocardial regions with normal ^{11}C-HED uptake.[231] These observations again suggest that sympathetic activity and endothelial function modulate the total coronary vasodilator capacity and implicate cardiac sympathetic innervation as an important signaling pathway for mediating coronary vasomotor responses to CPT. It also appears from these findings that, under normal conditions, the endothelial-dependent vasodilator effect supersedes the α-adrenergically mediated vasoconstrictor effect on the vascular smooth muscle.

Mental stress, also proposed as a test of endothelial function, might more realistically reflect MBF responses to activities during daily life. Mental stress provoked by anxiety to solve algebraic tasks of increasing difficulty raised cardiac work as reflected by higher RPPs. This increase was associated with a commensurate increase in MBF in normal volunteers[232] but not in patients with CAD in whom flow responses were attenuated or even absent despite comparable increases in RPP.[233] While endothelial factors and the cardiac sympathetic innervation appear to be involved in these flow responses, their determinants appear to be more complex. The longer duration of the test raises circulating norepinephrine and, especially, epinephrine levels implicating a systemic response by the adrenal medulla [232] so that the predominantly α-adrenergic effect of norepinephrine may, therefore, be mixed with the more β-adrenergic effect of epinephrine. Therefore, the flow response may be less specific to the endothelium.

It might be argued that forearm blood flow measurements are a more readily available means of assessing endothelial function. Again, this approach evaluates both the endothelial-dependent responsiveness of the large conduit and the resistance vessels. Inherent in many of these studies using this approach is the assumption that vasomotor abnormalities in the brachial artery system can be equated with those in the coronary circulation. This assumption, however, awaits verification. One argument against this assumption is that forearm, unlike coronary, vessels are rarely affected by clinically significant atherosclerotic disease. Further, some studies evaluate the reactivity of both the coronary and forearm vessels but demonstrate disparate findings. For example, PET-based measurements of MBF failed to observe correlations between vasomotor abnormalities in the coronary and the forearm circulation.[230,234]

Graded, longitudinal, base-to-apex reductions in myocardial perfusion Finally, there is a more subtle but conceptually intriguing observation of a longitudinal, base-to-apex perfusion gradient that has only recently been observed with quantitative analysis of images of the relative distribution of MBF in patients with clinical CAD.[235] This longitudinal perfusion gradient was attributed to diffuse luminal narrowing of the epicardial vessels, causing a decline in intracoronary pressure along the conduit vessels with diminished perfusion of the distal vascular territory. Such gradient was also observed in asymptomatic individuals with coronary risk factors.[236] The gradient was, however, not apparent on semiquantitative image analysis but only when MBF was measured during dipyridamole hyperemia. Though small in magnitude, this hyperemic perfusion gradient between the mid and the apical portions of the LV myocardium was statistically significant and was absent in age-matched normal subjects or young volunteers without coronary risk factors. Dipyridamole hyperemia in these at-risk patients did not induce regional flow defects nor was the magnitude of the hyperemic MBF diminished.

The mechanism underlying this observation may be related to an abnormality in coronary vasomotor function. If endothelial dysfunction precludes a flow-dependent dilation of the large conduit vessels in response to higher flow velocities and shear stresses, then the resistance to high-velocity flows along the large epicardial vessels markedly increases as a function of the fourth power of the radius and thus causes a decline of the coronary pressure along the coronary vascular tree.

Analogous to diffuse anatomical narrowing, this then leads to a longitudinal gradient in myocardial perfusion. Indeed, intracoronary pressure measurements confirmed the existence of a proximal to distal pressure gradient and thus lend support to this concept.[237] In coronary vessels free of stenoses in patients with CAD, the coronary pressure declined from proximal to distal by about 5 mm Hg at rest and by 10 mm Hg during hyperemia. In 8% of such coronary vessels the pressure declined by more than 25% and thus, reached ischemic levels.

Integrated approach to the study of abnormal coronary vasomotion Based on observations with PET measurements of MBF in patients with CAD or in patients with only coronary risk factors, a hierarchy of functional abnormalities emerges. In this scenario, a stress-induced regional flow defect as a consequence of anatomical narrowing of fluid dynamic significance represents the most severe state. A globally diminished vasodilator capacity as evidenced by attenuated hyperemic MBFs in response to adenosine or dipyridamole and exemplified by findings in patients with hypercholesteremia or diabetes follows. A more subtle, somewhat lesser functional abnormality is present when such attenuation occurs only at the more distal portion of the coronary vascular tree as evidenced by the longitudinal, base-to-apex perfusion gradient in patients with coronary risk factors but with a still normally preserved global hyperemic myocardial flow response. Finally, an abnormal flow response to CPT, as seen as the only abnormality in longterm smokers or in insulin resistance, may represent the mildest and perhaps earliest form of a functional abnormality of the coronary circulation.

TRANSPLANT VASCULOPATHY

Disease of the coronary arteries represents the most common complication of cardiac allografts. Its diffuseness frequently precludes detection with noninvasive techniques, for example, myocardial perfusion imaging or even with invasive coronary angiography.[238] It is detected most reliably with intracoronary ultrasound but may be identifiable with noninvasive measurements of MBF.[239] Early following cardiac transplantation, MBFs both at rest and during pharmacological stress as well as the myocardial flow reserve are normal.[240] Several months after transplantation, the myocardial flow reserve declines. While hyperemic MBFs remain normal, resting MBF is commonly increased accounting for the decline of the ratio of hyperemic to resting MBFs, that is, the myocardial flow reserve.[240,241] Renal toxicity of immunosuppressive treatment associated with hypertension most commonly accounts for the increase in resting MBFs that occur in proportion to an increase in the RPP. When studied after 2 to 3 years, hyperemic MBFs have usually declined.[242] Also, responses of MBF to CPT become markedly attenuated or are absent, suggesting the presence of endothelial dysfunction. The attenuation of the hyperemic MBF response to dipyridamole correlated inversely with the degree of intimal thickening as determined by intracoronary ultrasound. Thus, endothelial-dependent and -independent factors including increased arterial wall stiffness and microcirculatory abnormalities are, therefore, likely causes of the observed abnormalities in MBF in transplant vasculopathy.

MONITORING RESPONSES TO PHARMACOLOGICAL INTERVENTIONS

Measurements of MBF can characterize functional responses of the coronary circulation to therapeutic interventions. Cardiovascular conditioning has been advocated as a means of improving cardiovascular health, although its effect on the function of the coronary vasculature remains largely unexplored. In 13 individuals, 5 with clinical evidence of CAD or coronary risk factors, MBF was measured at baseline and after a 6-week course of cardiovascular conditioning, consisting of daily physical exercise, dietary changes and lifestyle modification.[243] Total and LDL cholesterol plasma levels declined by 16% ± 10% and 18% ± 10%, respectively. Heart rate and systolic blood pressure were significantly lower at followup then at baseline. As anticipated from the 16% decrease in cardiac work, as defined by the RPP, MBF at rest had declined in proportion and averaged 0.69 ± 0.14 ml $\cdot$ min^{-1} $\cdot$ g^{-1} at followup as compared to 0.78 ± 0.18 ml $\cdot$ min^{-1} $\cdot$ g^{-1} at baseline (p < 0.05). This alone produced a significant increase in the myocardial MBF reserve. However, hyperemic MBFs had also increased by 9% indicating a beneficial effect of cardiovascular conditioning on the integrated total vasodilator capacity (Table 6-15). Although the mechanisms underlying such improvement in vasodilator capacity may be several ones, including decreases in extravascular resistive forces, changes in blood viscosity and reductions in plasma cholesterol levels, they may also entail an exercise-related improvement in endothelial function as recently demonstrated.[244]

Multicenter trials present convincing evidence for primary and secondary prevention of cardiac events by chronic 3-hydroxy-3-methylglutaryl Coenzyme A (HMG–CoA) reductase inhibitor treatment.[245] This beneficial effect in the secondary prevention trials occurred despite minimal, if any, effects on the anatomical severity of coronary stenoses. The protective effects of HMG–CoA reductase inhibitors were attributed, therefore, to an improvement in endothelial function and stabilization of coronary plaques. There are now several studies, though in only small patient populations, that have explored noninvasive measurements of MBF responses to cholesterol lowering and/or treatment with HMG–CoA reductase inhibitors (Table 6-15).

In one study, for example, repeat measurements of MBF in 51 asymptomatic, young men with moderately elevated plasma cholesterol levels failed to demonstrate a significant effect of 6 months of pravastatin (4 mg/day) on adenosine hyperemic blood flows or on the myocardial flow reserve (Table 6-15).[246] Importantly, however, the mean hyperemic blood flows as well as if the flow reserve were normal at baseline. A posthoc analysis of the 15 study participants with diminished hyperemic MBFs at baseline (less than 4 ml $\cdot$ min^{-1} $\cdot$ g^{-1}) did demonstrate a significant (27%) increase in hyperemic MBFs and a similar increase in the myocardial flow reserve (Table 6-15). Similar improvements are reported for asymptomatic patients with familial hypercholesterolemia following 9 to 15 months of treatment with simvastatin (5 to 10 mg/day)[247] as well as for patients who were either normal or only minimally diseased (less than 30% diameter narrowing or irregular luminal surface) on coronary angiography after 6 months of treatment with simvastatin (20 mg/day).[248]

Total and LDL cholesterol plasma concentrations declined by approximately 20% to 30% and approximately 30% to 40%, respectively, in these studies in asymptomatic patients (Table 6-15). Whether the improvement in the coronary vasodilator capacity relates directly and quantitatively to the reductions in total or LDL cholesterol plasma concentrations has remained uncertain. The improvement in dipyridamole hyperemic MBF within 18 h to 20 h after plasma LDL-apheresis might suggest such direct effect.[249] Plasma LDL concentrations

TABLE 6-15. Effect of Cholesterol-Lowering Treatment of Myocardial Blood Flow

Investigation	N	MBF at Baseline $(ml \cdot min^{-1} \cdot g^{-1})$		MBF at Followup $(ml \cdot min^{-1} \cdot g^{-1})$		Change (%)	P
		Rest	Stress	Rest	Stress		
Cardiovascular conditioning							
Czernin et al, 1995[243]	13	0.78 ± 0.18	2.06 ± 0.35	0.69 ± 0.14	2.25 ± 0.40	+9.2	< 0.05
HMG-CoA reductase inhibitors							
Huggins et al, 1998[155]	12	0.95 ± 0.35	2.63 ± 0.41	0.83 ± 0.16	2.35 ± 0.64	−10.6[a]	NS
Guethlin et al, 1999[199]	15	0.73 ± 0.19	1.29 ± 0.33	0.74 ± 0.18	1.89 ± 0.79	+46.5[b]	< 0.01
Yokoyama et al, 1999[254]	27	0.70 ± 0.20	1.70 ± 0.50	0.70 ± 0.20	2.30 ± 0.90	+35.3	< 0.01
Baller et al, 1999[248]	23	0.89 ± 0.15	1.89 ± 0.75	0.83 ± 0.12	2.26 ± 0.85	+19.6	< 0.01
Yokoyama et al, 2001[247]	16	0.87 ± 0.20	1.82 ± 0.36	0.92 ± 0.19	2.38 ± 0.58	+30.8	< 0.001
Janatuinen et al, 2001[a][246]	23	0.77 ± 0.12	1.89 ± 0.75	0.75 ± 0.96	2.26 ± 0.85	+19.6	< 0.05
Janatuinen et al, 2001[b][246]	15	0.85 ± 0.27	3.61 ± 1.04	0.86 ± 0.23	3.79 ± 1.31	+5	NS
		0.82 ± 0.20	3.06 ± 0.47	0.81 ± 0.17	3.88 ± 1.34	+26.8	< 0.05

Abbreviations: Change, change in hyperemic blood flows; HMG-CoA, 3-hydroxy-3-methylglutaryl Coenzyme A; MBF, myocardial blood flow; N, number of patients; P, significance.

[a,b]Czernin et al[243] enrolled normal subjects and patients with CAD for a 6-week course of exercise, cholesterol-lowering diet and counseling; Huggins et al[155] found in patients with CAD no significant effect of a 4-month treatment with simvastatin on blood flow in remote myocardium (a) but a significant effect on blood flow in myocardium supplied by stenosed coronary arteries (b), whereas Guethlin et al[199] reported improvements in myocardium supplied by normal and diseased coronary arteries. Yokoyama et al[254] studied patients treated with different statins, and Baller et al[248] examined patients with hypercholesteremia but without angiographically significant CAD. Janatuinen et al[246] studied asymptomatic young men with borderline elevated cholesterol levels. Only for 15 participants with hyperemic blood flows at baseline of less than 4.0 ml · min⁻¹ · g⁻¹ was there a significant improvement at followup.

Source: Data from Czernin et al,[243] Huggins et al,[155] Guethlin et al,[199] Yokoyama et al,[248] Baller et al,[254] Yokoyama et al,[247] and Janatuinen et al.[246]

in this study were high at baseline (194 ± 38 mg $\cdot$ dl^{-1}) and had decreased by 58% while hyperemic MBFs had increased by 31%. This observation of a significant improvement in coronary vasodilator capacity differs from findings of a delayed improvement in coronary vasoreactivity in hypercholesterolemia patients submitted to 6 months of treatment with fluvastatin (Figure 6-25).[199] After 2 months of treatment, total and LDL cholesterol plasma concentrations had declined by 28% and 37%, respectively, while hyperemic MBFs remained unchanged. When restudied at 6 months, no further changes in plasma lipids were noted but hyperemic MBFs had improved by 35%. Different from the investigation with LDL-plasma apheresis, the delayed increase in coronary vasodilator capacity in the fluvastatin study argues against a direct effect of plasma cholesterol being lower and suggests that the beneficial vasomotor effects of HMG-CoA reductase inhibitors may be independent of plasma cholesterol concentrations or, further, the effects of reductions in plasma cholesterol levels are mediated by other structural and functional mechanisms. Because of the striking reductions in plasma LDL cholesterol concentrations in the LDL-apheresis study, it is, therefore, possible that rheologic factors rather than a direct effect on coronary vasomotor function accounted for the higher postapheresis hyperemic MBFs.[249] Consistent with this possibility is a statistically significant (6.3%) decrease in plasma viscosity that would reduce resistance to flow and, thus, result in higher hyperemic blood flows. It is further possible that the delay in improvement in the Fluvastatin study was associated with structural improvements of the coronary vessels that required time, for example, a decrease in the intima media thickness as well as with an improvement in the bioactivity of NO or, as postulated by others, a down regulation of the angiotension II receptors on the endothelial cells.[250–253]

Measurements of MBF in other studies have also demonstrated improvements in hyperemic flows and the flow reserve in patients with clinically and angiographically documented CAD.[155,199,254] These studies generally have demonstrated a beneficial effect on blood flow in myocardium subtended by normal and diseased coronary arteries confirmed with angiography. In only one study was the beneficial effect of HMG-CoA reductase inhibitors confined to myocardial territory supplied by normal vessels confirmed with angiography.[155] Possible explanations for the lack of improvement in remote myocardial territories include the shorter duration of the treatment with HMG-CoA reductase inhibitors (only 4 months as compared to 6 months or more in the other studies) or, as is listed in Table 6-15, hyperemic MBFs and myocardial flow reserves that were essentially normal in the remote myocardium at baseline.

Effects of therapy on coronary vasomotion in type 2 diabetes have also been studied but yielded more equivocal findings. Effective diabetes control with normal fasting blood glucose levels appeared to enhance the total coronary vasodilator capacity.[225,226] Hyperemic MBFs were higher than in untreated or poorly controlled patients. Hyperemic MBF correlated best with fasting plasma glucose concentrations. This might also imply a direct effect of glucose-mediated function or, alternatively, of abnormal glucose disposal rates and, hence, the degree of insulin resistance on coronary vasomotion and, as discussed below, on endothelium-dependent coronary vasomotor function.

Endothelial dysfunction has now become a major target for pharmacological interventions. As mentioned above, longterm smoking per se causes an abnormal flow response to CPT despite normal hyperemic MBFs (Figure 6-26).[163]

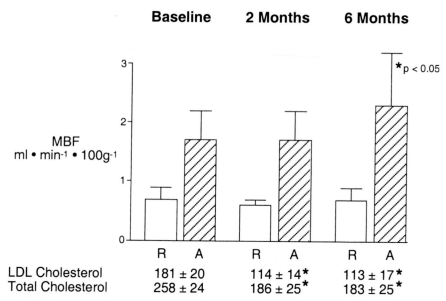

	Baseline		2 Months		6 Months	
	R	A	R	A	R	A
LDL Cholesterol	181 ± 20		114 ± 14*		113 ± 17*	
Total Cholesterol	258 ± 24		186 ± 25*		183 ± 25*	

FIGURE 6-25. Effect of 6-months of treatment with simvastatin on myocardial blood flow at rest and during adenosine-induced hyperemia and on plasma cholesterol levels. The patients with CAD were studied with PET at baseline and again at 2 and 6 months of treatment. Notice the significant decrease in plasma LDL cholesterol and total cholesterol at 2 months while hyperemic MBF remains unchanged from baseline. At 6 months however, a significant improvement in the hyperemic flow response is observed. (Data used with permission from Guethlin et al.[199]) Abbreviations: CAD, coronary artery disease; LDL, low density lipoprotein; MBF, myocardial blood flow; PET, positron emission tomography; R and A, MBF at rest and during adenosine, respectively.

If this abnormality is related to endothelial dysfunction, then administration of L-arginine as the substrate for NOS might modify the response to CPT. This, in fact, occurred in studies in longterm smokers who otherwise were healthy.[164] Acute intravenous administration of L-arginine had no effect on baseline hemodynamics and baseline MBFs. Importantly, the diminished or even absent MBF response to CPT normalized after L-arginine (Figure 6-27). The 47% increase in the RPP, unchanged from baseline, was accompanied by a commensurate 48% increase (as compared to an 11% increase at baseline) in MBF.

Although the above observation supports the notion that flow responses to CPT provide a measure of endothelial function, the mechanism(s) explaining the improvement of L-arginine remain uncertain. One mechanism might involve increased production and, thus, increased bioactivity of NO by driving the L-arginine and citrulline reaction. However, the low K_m of the nitric oxide synthase (NOS)-mediated reaction argues against low L-arginine levels as rate limiting.[255] A second explanation includes competition with asymmetric dimethylarginine (ADMA) as an endogenous inhibitor of NOS.[256] Elevated cholesterol levels interfere with the degradation of ADMA so that its concentrations in plasma increases as has been observed in young hypercholesteremia patients.[257] Finally, L-arginine's effect may also be mediated by insulin. Infusion of L-arginine produced a 4.5-fold increase in plasma insulin concentrations in the

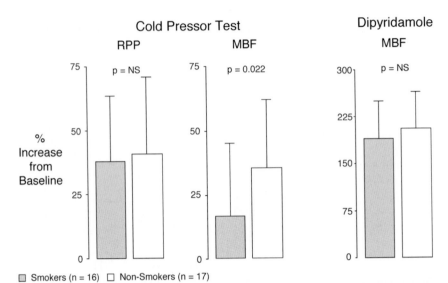

FIGURE 6-26. Responses of the rate pressure product (RPP) and of myocardial blood flow (MBF) to cold pressor testing in 16 smokers and 17 nonsmokers and hyperemic blood flows induced by intravenous dipyridamole. Responses to cold pressor testing are depicted as percent increases from baseline values. Notice the similar responses in the RPP but the attenuated response of MBF in the smokers when compared to that in the nonsmokers. Hyperemic blood flows achieved by smokers and nonsmokers were similar. (Data used with permission from Campisi et al.[163])

healthy longterm smokers. An insulin mediated effect on NOS or the bioactivity of NO could thus serve as a third explanation.

An insulin-mediated effect could be consistent with the reported increase in MBF during the euglycemic-hyperinsulinemic clamp.[171] It is also consistent with recent findings in patients with insulin resistance but without clinical diabetes.[258] As mentioned above, the total vasodilator capacity as tested with dipyridamole was normal in insulin resistance, but flow responses to CPT were attenuated or insignificant, most likely as the result of an impairment of insulin-mediated bioactivity of NO. However, 3 months of treatment with a new class of insulin sensitizers, thiazolidinediones, had no effect on MBF at rest but normalized the flow response to CPT. This observation supports the notion that by improving its access to the endothelial cell, insulin enhances production and or/release of NO and, thus, its bioactivity. The exact mechanism of action of these novel insulin sensitizers still remains incompletely understood, although their effect appears to be mediated by the phosphatidylinositol 3-kinase pathway that is important for glucose transport into skeletal muscle cells and also for endothelial NO production and insulin-mediated vasodilation.[259]

Measurements of MBF with PET have also been used for examining the effects of hormone replacement therapy (HRT) in postmenopausal women. These studies found no effect of short-term HRT on MBF at rest or during pharmacological vasodilation.[260,261] In contrast, longterm estrogen replacement appears to beneficially affect endothelial function in postmenopausal women.[262] Different from postmenopausal women without longterm hormone replacement therapy, women on hormone replacement either with estrogen alone or in combi-

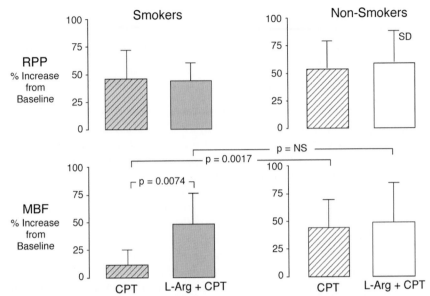

FIGURE 6-27. Responses of the rate pressure product (RPP; upper panel) and the my-ocardial blood flow (MBF; lower panel) to cold pressor testing (CPT). The panel on the left depicts the responses in smokers and the panel on the right depicts those in non-smokers. For each pair of bars, the left bars represent the responses at baseline and the bars on the right indicate those following intravenous infusion of L-arginine. Notice the comparable responses in RPP at baseline and following intravenous L-arginine in both smokers and nonsmokers. At baseline, the flow response to CPT in the smokers was markedly attenuated but normalized following intravenous L-arginine; this flow response no longer differs from that observed in nonsmokers. (Data used with permission from Campisi et al.[164])

nation with progestogens revealed MBF responses to CPT identical to those in young women with normal plasma estrogen concentrations. Of notice, such nor-malization was not observed in postmenopausal women with coronary risk fac-tors including hypercholesteremia, obesity, hypertension, or a family history of premature CAD.

The responses to pharmacological interventions are consistent with those observed with invasive techniques using quantitative angiography and intra-coronary flow velocity probes.[263] This particularly applies to studies on the ef-fects of HMG–CoA reductase inhibitors and, to some extent, the treatment of diabetes. Further, the improvement of the integrated coronary vasomotor func-tion or vasodilator capacity might be consistent with the primary and second-ary preventive effects of longterm HMG–CoA reductase inhibitor treatment. This will especially be true if an improvement in endothelial function significantly contributes to the total coronary vasodilator capacity. This then might imply that MBF responses, either to CPT and/or to direct vascular smooth muscle dila-tors, could serve as a surrogate endpoint for longterm beneficial effects of phar-macological agents. Obviously, longterm followup studies are needed for ex-ploring this possibility, especially whether a correlation between improvements in coronary vasomotion and a longterm reduction in cardiac events can be doc-umented. Recent observations on the predictive value of endothelial dysfunction for cardiac events support such possible correlation and, hence, the value of noninvasive assessments of coronary vasomotor motor function and, thus, importance for evaluating the efficacy of current and emerging pharmacological agents.[264,265]

Myocardial substrate metabolism

LEFT VENTRICULAR HYPERTROPHY AND HYPERTROPHIC CARDIOMYOPATHY

Secondary LV hypertrophy commonly results from arterial hypertension. Most studies in arterial hypertension and secondary LV hypertrophy have explored MBF and its response to pharmacological vasodilation. Even borderline hypertension without an increase in myocardial mass has been reported to be associated with an attenuated hyperemic MBF response while MBF at rest remained normal.[222] In addition to a diminished hyperemic blood flow response, clinically manifested arterial hypertension without LV hypertrophy is accompanied by elevated resting MBFs, most likely because of the increased RPP and, thus, cardiac work.[266] As LV hypertrophy develops, MBF per unit mass of myocardium returns to normal, although hyperemic blood flows remain attenuated. At the same time, myocardial efficiency as determined by a disproportionate increase in MVO_2 relative to the increase in myocardial mass was found to be reduced while MMRGlc remained normal.[97]

Findings by PET are more complex in patients with hypertrophic cardiomyopathy as a more heterogeneous disease entity. MBFs averaged over the entire LV myocardium are within the range of normal while dipyridamole hyperemia is markedly reduced.[267] Dipyridamole flows averaged 1.64 ± 0.44 ml/min/g in one study in 12 hypertrophic cardiomyopathy patients as compared to 3.50 ± 0.95 ml/min/g in 40 normal control subjects.[266] Flow measurements in the thickened interventricular septum (25.4 ± 5.8 mm) revealed moderately reduced subendocardial flows during dipyridamole hyperemia suggestive of possible subendocardial ischemia.[268] The same investigators found the myocardial flow reserves markedly diminished in both the thickened interventricular septum and the normally thick lateral wall.[267] Hypertrophic cardiomyopathy most likely represents a rather heterogeneous disease entity, which may explain the often-disparate findings on PET. For example, in one study, measurements of MBF with the ^{15}O-labeled water approach revealed comparable flows in the hypertrophic septum and the normal lateral wall but relatively increased FDG concentrations (by approximately 40%) in those patients with greater systolic thickening of the lateral wall.[269] While attributed to greater regional myocardial work, the observation may also have been associated with partial volume-related differences because the calculation of flows with the ^{15}O-labeled water technique is independent of partial volume effects while wall thickness of the lateral wall, averaged over the entire cardiac circle for the FDG uptake, might have resulted in apparently higher tracer activity concentrations. Other investigations into the substrate metabolism of hypertrophic cardiomyopathy report diminished FDG concentrations in the interventricular septum but rendered normal MBFs and ^{11}C-palmitate uptake and clearance rates at rest, thus arguing against the presence of resting myocardial ischemia.[11,12] Of interest, MBF failed to increase with supine bicycle exercise[12] or, in another study in adolescents, with hypertrophic cardiomyopathy with intravenous dipyridamole.[270]

STUDIES IN IDIOPATHIC-DILATED CARDIOMYOPATHY

A dominant feature of the markedly enlarged left and right ventricular myocardium in idiopathic-dilated cardiomyopathy is the homogeneously distributed MBF. In general, MBF at rest has been found to be normal or comparable to that in normal volunteers, although the MBF reserve is diminished.[271–274] Some investigators ascribe the attenuated flow reserve to microvascular disease but increased extravascular resistant forces due to increased myocardial wall tension may also serve as an explanation. High extravascular resistant forces due to the greater left ventricular diameter and the associated increase in wall tension might be responsible for the attenuation of hyperemic MBFs. Microvascular disease appears to be an additional explanation. For example, the mostly endothelium-dependent flow response to CPT was markedly diminished in patients with idiopathic-dilated cardiomyopathy.[275] Despite comparable cold-induced approximate 50% increases in the RPP, flow increased by 52% in normal subjects but by only 20% (p < 0.008) in idiopathic-dilated cardiomyopathy patients. Importantly, the dipyridamole-stimulated MBFs appear to offer predictive information. In a study in 64 patients with idiopathic-dilated cardiomyopathy and an average left ventricular ejection fraction of only 34% ± 10%, only 35.8% of patients with a hyperemic MBF of less then 1.36 ml $\cdot$ min^{-1} $\cdot$ g^{-1} survived the 5-year followup period free of a cardiac event (including worsening on congestive heart failure systems, cardiac transplantation, or cardiac death).[274] In contrast, 79% of patients with dipyridamole-stimulated flows of greater than 1.36 ml $\cdot$ min^{-1} $\cdot$ g-$^{-1}$ remained event free over the same time period.

Similarly, rates of myocardial oxidative metabolism as determined with [C-11] acetate have also been found to be normal while higher wall stresses as a result of the LV enlargement would predict an increase.[276] Whether this is due to the intrinsic myopathic process or a diminished contractile state remains uncertain at present. Nevertheless, several studies using ^{11}C-acetate and estimates of cardiac work from measurements of LV chamber dimensions and systolic blood pressure report a diminished mechanical efficiency.[276–278]

Observations on myocardial metabolism of FFA have been of particular interest. Early investigations reported a heterogeneous myocardial uptake of ^{11}C-palmitate.[279,280] Regional reductions in tracer uptake were scattered throughout the LV myocardium and were in locations unrelated to the coronary vascular territories. Of even greater interest were paradoxical responses in the clearance of ^{11}C-palmitate to changes in substrate utilization.[281] In patients with idiopathic-dilated cardiomyopathy, the relative size of the rapid clearance curve component and its slope revealed the normal decline from the fasted to the glucose-loaded state. In contrast, approximately 50% of patients demonstrated a paradoxical response with an increase in the relative size of the rapid clearance curve component and increase in clearance rate from the fasted to the postglucose state. While this observation might imply an improvement in myocardial FFA oxidation in response to greater glucose availability with replenishment of TCA cycle intermediates, it also could reflect diminished metabolic sequestration of ^{11}C-palmitate into the myocardium and, hence, back-diffusion of unmetabolized tracer.

The myocardial uptake of FDG in idiopathic-dilated cardiomyopathy is characteristically homogeneous (Figure 6-28),[282] although a recent study refers to some relatively small regions of diminished perfusion and enhanced FDG uptake as evidence of regional ischemia attributed to the increased wall stress in

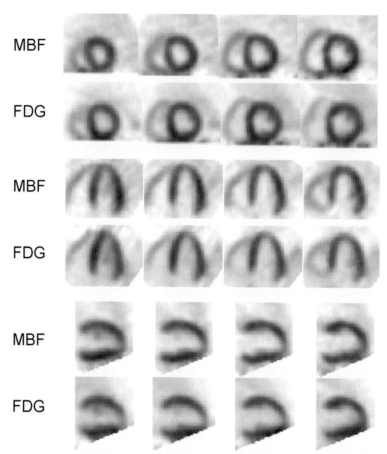

FIGURE 6-28. Examples of myocardial perfusion with ^{13}N-ammonia (MBF) and FDG uptake images in a patient with idiopathic-dilated cardiomyopathy. Notice the markedly enlarged LV cavity. Myocardial perfusion and glucose uptake are characteristically homogeneous. The upper row represents the short axis, the middle row the horizontal long axis, and the lower row the vertical long access images.

the presence of a diminished flow reserve.[273] Nevertheless, homogenous uptake of FDG in a relatively thin-walled but enlarged left ventricle is a dominant feature of idiopathic-dilated cardiomyopathy, and together with the homogeneously distributed MBF, allows the differentiation of idiopathic-dilated from ischemic cardiomyopathy. In addition to heart failure symptoms, ischemic cardiomyopathy shares several other features with idiopathic-dilated cardiomyopathy, for example, the LV enlargement, diffuse hypokinesis, low LVEF and, frequently, mitral regurgitation. Biventricular enlargement has been considered a feature characteristic of idiopathic-dilated cardiomyopathy but can also be present in ischemic cardiomyopathy. Conduction abnormalities often limit the accuracy of ECG criteria to distinguish between both entities. Additionally, an intrinsic myopathic process including LV remodeling may also exist in patients with CAD so that the major cause of the poor LV function may remain unknown or difficult to elucidate. Distinction between both disease types is important because of strikingly different therapeutic approaches. Combined imaging of MBF and glucose metabolism distinguished between both disease entities with an overall accuracy of 85%.[282] This value exceeded the diagnostic accuracy of ECG criteria, regional wall motion abnormalities, or right ventricular enlargement.

ISCHEMIC CARDIOMYOPATHY

General considerations Findings in experimental animals provided the base for the study of ischemic cardiomyopathy as well as for the detection of myocardial viability. These early studies indicated that known alterations in substrate metabolism during acute myocardial ischemia could, indeed, be demonstrated noninvasively with tracers of myocardial substrate metabolism.[283] Consistent with an impaired FFA oxidation was the diminished initial uptake of ^{11}C-palmitate and its delayed clearance rate from the myocardium. Additionally, the known increase in glucose extraction and glucose utilization was reflected by a regional increase in FDG uptake.[110,181,284] Initial studies in patients with clinical evidence of acute myocardial ischemia had revealed MBF and glucose metabolism patterns that were virtually identical to those in animals, for example, enhanced FDG uptake in hypoperfused dysfunctional myocardial regions.[285,286] Unexpected was the existence of the same pattern in patients with chronic CAD but without clinical signs of acute ischemia (Figure 6-29). This then raised the question as to whether the MBF metabolism

FIGURE 6-29. Blood flow metabolism mismatch in a patient with subtotal occlusion of the proximal left anterior descending coronary artery. On the images on the left are shown the markedly decreased perfusion in the anterior wall (top image, arrows) but the enhanced [1]FDG uptake (bottom). The center and right panels depict followup studies in the same patient after percutaneous transdermal angioplasty (PTCA). Notice the marked improvement in perfusion to the anterior wall and the normalization of FDG uptake. At baseline, there was akinesis of the anterior wall. Following restoration of resting myocardial blood flow (MBF) after angioplasty, wall motion normalized while myocardial blood flow and glucose utilization became normal.

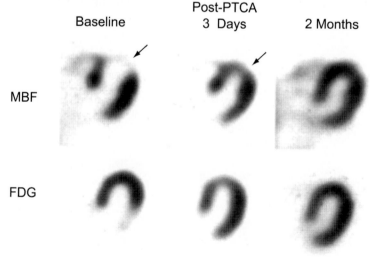

Post-PTCA

| Baseline | 3 Days | 2 Months |

pattern as observed on PET was indeed unique to acute ischemia or whether it represented a more general metabolic pattern in chronically dysfunctional and hypoperfused myocardium.

Study protocol and image analysis The evaluation of ischemic cardiomyopathy characteristically entails a 2-step approach, that is, the evaluation of regional myocardial MBF with ^{13}N-ammonia or [82]Rb and PET or, more recently, with ^{201}Tl or ^{99m}Tc-labeled sestamibi or tetrofosmin and SPECT. In the second step, the distribution of myocardial glucose utilization is evaluated with FDG. The MBF and FDG images are then analyzed for regional perfusion defects and further, whether the distribution of FDG follows that of MBF. This is most often accomplished by visual analysis but is frequently aided by a more quantitative image analysis. The short axis slices of both the MBF and the FDG images are assembled into polar maps. The MBF polar maps are then compared against a database of normal values for determining presence, location, and extent of MBF defects. Regional reductions in flow tracer concentrations by more than 2 standard deviations (SD) below the normal mean are considered as flow defects. The polar maps of myocardial FDG uptake are then normalized to those of MBF, which is accomplished by adjusting the FDG polar map to the myocardial region with the highest MBF. The MBF polar map is then subtracted from the FDG polar map. Again, regional differences (rather than ratios) of greater than 2 SDs of the normal mean are considered as regional increases in glucose uptake.

Three distinct patterns of regional MBF and glucose utilization are observed:

1. Normal MBF, normal or enhanced glucose uptake (Figure 6-30).
2. Reduced MBF, normal or enhanced glucose uptake, or reduced glucose uptake but markedly in excess of MBF (mismatch; Figure 6-31).
3. Reduced MBF and proportionately reduced glucose uptake (match; Figure 6-32).[285,286]

While these terms are purely operational, they infer, at least to some extent, the underlying pathophysiology accounting for the contractile dysfunction. Normal flow and/or metabolism might represent stunned while the classic mismatch might be consistent with hibernating myocardium. Both patterns predict a

FIGURE 6-30. Myocardial blood flow (MBF) and FDG images in a normal volunteer. Short axis together with horizontal and vertical long axis images are shown. Notice the homogeneous distribution of both tracers in the left ventricular myo-cardium. Abbreviations: FDG, 2-deoxy-2-[F-18]fluoro-D-glucose; HLA, horizontal long axis; MBF, myo-cardial blood flow; VLA, vertical long axis.

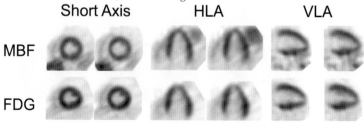

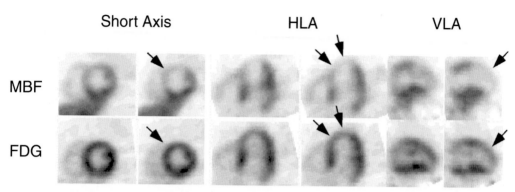

FIGURE 6-31. Images of myocardial perfusion with ^{13}N-ammonia and myocardial glucose utilization with FDG in a patient with ischemic cardiomyopathy, demonstrating a mismatch. Again, short axis and vertical and horizontal long axis images of the LV myocardium are shown. Notice the decreased perfusion in the anteroseptal anterior and anterolateral wall but the preserved FDG uptake in these regions. Abbreviations: FDG, 2-deoxy-2-[F-18]fluoro-D-glucose; HLA, horizontal long axis; MBF, myocardial blood flow; VLA, vertical long axis.

postrevascularization improvement in contractile function, whereas concordant reductions in MBF and metabolism predict that function will not improve. It should be emphasized that the severity of the regional flow reduction in both matches and mismatches may considerably differ between patients. Modest concordant reductions in both MBF and FDG uptake reflect a prior nontransmural infarction as compared to severe reductions or even near absence of MBF consistent with transmural infarctions.[287]

Evaluation of MBF alone Because of an inverse correlation between tissue fibrosis and relative flow tracer uptake, as, for example, observed for ^{13}N-ammo-

FIGURE 6-32. Images of myocardial blood flow and glucose metabolism in a patient with ischemic cardiomyopathy, showing a match. Short axis and horizontal and vertical long axis images are shown. Notice the severely decreased perfusion in the anterior, anterolateral, and lateral walls that is associated with a proportionate reduction in FDG uptake. Abbreviations: FDG, 2-deoxy-2-[F-18]fluoro-D-glucose; HLA, horizontal long axis; MBF, myocardial blood flow; VLA, vertical long axis.

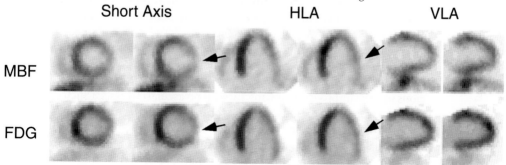

nia,[288,289] the evaluation of regional MBF alone can provide information on the presence of reversible contractile dysfunction.[290] Severely reduced (less than 25% of normal) or near absent MBF reflects complete or nearly complete transmural scar tissue formation and, hence, nonreversibility. According to another study, flow reductions greater than 60% were highly accurate in predicting nonreversibility of contractile dysfunction.[291] Conversely, completely normal or only mild reductions (less than 20%) of MBF in dysfunctional myocardium argue against the presence of significant amounts of fibrosis; it possibly reflects myocardial stunning and thus indicates functional reversibility. However, moderate MBF reductions are less reliable discriminators; for example, a nontransmural infarction may result in a mild flow reduction. If the remainder of the myocardial wall consists of normal myocardium, then revascularization would be unlikely to improve contractile function. If combined with a metabolic study, the FDG uptake in this case would be reduced in proportion to MBF.[292] Conversely, an increase in glucose metabolism would indicate the coexistence of reversibly dysfunctional myocardium with scar tissue and predict an improvement in contractile function.

Assessment of FDG uptake alone This approach derives from comparative studies with gated MRI and PET and assumes that regional reductions in FDG of greater than 50% relative to remote myocardium represent irreversible contractile dysfunction, whereas mildly reduced or normal uptake indicates the presence of reversible dysfunction.[293,294] Used for some time as a benchmark measure for defining the accuracy of ^{201}Tl-based techniques for assessing myocardial viability,[293] only recent studies have tested the validity of this particular approach against the postrevascularization outcome in regional contractile function.[295] ECG-gated image acquisition affords simultaneous evaluation of regional function and metabolism and, thus, can further augment the predictive accuracy of the FDG stand-alone approach.[296,297] A more recent report emphasizes the utility of measurements of exogenous glucose utilization. Using a threshold value of 0.25 μmol $\cdot$ min^{-1} $\cdot$ g^{-1} provided a 93% positive and a 95% negative predictive accuracy for the improvement of contractile dysfunction.[298] Similarly, as evidenced by findings in a multicenter trial in 157 patients, relative regional FDG utilization rates of greater than 45% of those in normal remote myocardium appear to accurately identify dysfunctional myocardium as viable.[140] Nevertheless, limitations with this approach remain, especially when glucose utilization and FDG uptake cannot be sufficiently and consistently standardized. In such instances, it may be difficult to distinguish between scar tissue, normal myocardium, and reversibly contractile dysfunction, which then could readily be clarified by evaluating the distribution of regional MBF.[299]

A clinically more difficult issue is the pattern of normal regional MBF and glucose metabolism associated with mild-to-severe hypokinesis in severely dysfunctional LVs. One study reports that of 32 such myocardial regions, only 8 regions or 25% improved following surgical revascularization.[300] Such regions may, therefore, represent remodeled LV myocardium. On the other hand, a postrevascularization improvement in wall motion may have been consistent with prior myocardial stunning. If suspected, careful evaluation of the coronary anatomy, or, if unavailable, the addition of a pharmacological stress study can aid in distinguishing between stunned and remodeled LV myocardium (Figure 6-33).

FIGURE 6-33. Three contiguous cross-sectional images of myocardial blood flow (MBF) at rest (upper panel), during dipyridamole stress (middle panel) and of FDG uptake (bottom panel). On the resting images, myocardial perfusion is relatively homogenous. During hyperemia, there is a stress-induced flow defect in the lateral wall (arrows) that is on the FDG image associated with regionally enhanced glucose utilization. This pattern is most likely consistent with myocardial stunning.

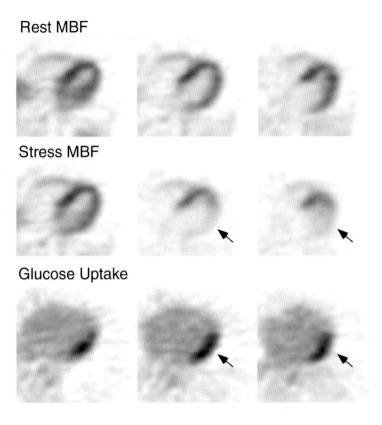

Rest MBF

Stress MBF

Glucose Uptake

SPECT imaging of MBF and FDG uptake More recent approaches rely on the use of multipurpose SPECT-like systems, either equipped with ultra-high photon energy general purpose collimators or with coincidence detection systems. Little information, thus far, has become available on the clinical performance of coincidence detection systems[301–304] whereas systematic studies with ultra-high photon energy general purpose collimator SPECT systems, using ^{201}Tl or ^{99m}Tc-labeled flow tracers and FDG, report predictive accuracies that are comparable to those reported with dedicated PET systems.[305,306]

Alternative metabolic approaches for assessing myocardial viability One approach evaluates regional myocardial oxidative metabolism with [C-11] acetate in dysfunctional myocardium.[307] The approach has been reported to predict with an 85% accuracy an improvement and with an 87% accuracy irreversibility of regional contractile dysfunction following revascularization in patients with chronic CAD.[307–309] More recent reports, however, found lower predictive accuracies for the [C-11] acetate approach.[74,310] In these studies, the degree of regional flow reduction discriminated more accurately between reversibly and irreversibly dysfunctional myocardium than the regional myocardial clearance rates of [C-11] acetate.

Possible mechanisms of the blood flow metabolism pattern The mechanisms underlying the MBF-FDG mismatch remain uncertain. Patients with CAD undergoing supine bicycle exercise revealed in stress-induced flow defects an augmented FDG uptake when the radiotracer was administered 20 minutes to 30 minutes after exercise and after the stress-induced flow defect had resolved.[311] This then implied that the enhanced tracer uptake might indeed represent stunned myocardium, a possibility supported by observations in animal experiments and more recently in patients with either collaterized myo-cardium or unstable angina.[206,312,313] These studies had demonstrated the evolution of an MBF metabolism pattern in chronically reperfused myocardium: an immediate postreperfusion decrease in glucose metabolism was followed by an increase that subsequently declined to normal as contractile function returned.[312] The enhanced FDG uptake was attributed to increased lactate release and, thus, anaerobic glycolysis that persisted even after full restoration of MBF.[312] The evolution of such a metabolic pattern might pertain also to early postinfarction patients[314] but does not fully explain the flow metabolism observations in patients with chronic CAD. Another possibility is repetitive stunning.[315] An impairment in contractile function associated with enhanced glucose metabolism was noted in collateral-dependent myocardium only if the flow reserve was markedly restricted.[206] It limits the coronary circulation's ability to appropriately respond to transient and frequent increases in oxygen demand during daily life leading to transient ischemic episodes, each followed by stunning and preventing contractile function to recover. Contractile dysfunction due to stunning can be induced in coronary artery disease patients with dobutamine stress.[316–318] The degree of dysfunction induced by dobutamine stress correlates with the stenosis severity of the supplying coronary artery and the attenuation of the flow response to dobutamine.

Myocardial hibernation serves as another explanation.[319] The postulated downregulation of contractile function in response to diminished supply is thought to be associated with an alteration of the myocardium's substrate metabolism with a dominant role for the more oxygen-efficient glucose. Hibernation in its truest sense then implies that the downregulated energy requirements match the diminished energy supply. A new supply and demand imbalance is established but at a lower level. Such new balance would, however, be precarious because even moderate increases in demand or decreases in supply could disturb this balance and cause ischemia. It is, thus, possible and likely that both, hibernation and stunning coexist to varying extents in many patients. Observations in experimental animals suggest that sustained reductions in both MBF and contractile function can be maintained for some time without significant necrosis, but, with development of structural alterations that resemble those in patients with chronic CAD. These findings provide an animal experimental underpinning for the concept of hibernation.[320–322] Both concepts, repetitive stunning and hibernation, may, in their purest form, represent the two ends of a spectrum. This spectrum begins with a reduction in MBF reserve where increased demand can no longer be matched by an appropriate increase in supply and ends with a complete loss of the MBF reserve and a reduction in regional MBF at rest, associated with a downregulation of contractile function and adaptation of substrate metabolism. Such spectrum could represent a temporal progression in coronary stenosis severity. Recent findings in chronically instrumented animals with a progressive decline and ultimately loss of regional flow reserve associated with a decrease in rest MBF support such a scenario.[321–324] On the other hand, MBF reductions may also occur suddenly in view of the high incidence of MBF metabolism mismatches in early postinfarction patients.[285,325,326] As acute animal experimental studies have demonstrated, sudden but moderate regional MBF reductions that are initially associated with signs of acute ischemia, for example, produce release of lactate and enhanced glucose uptake. An apparent resetting or adjustment of demand occurs thereafter when lactate release converts to uptake, high energy phosphate stores are replenished, and a new supply and demand balance seems to have returned.[320,327] Some debate has focused on the issue whether MBF at rest can indeed be chronically reduced.[328] This was because hibernating myocardium no longer demonstrated the postulated perfusion contraction match. To some extent, this may be because of a coexistence of scar tissue or replacement fibrosis but also because of ultrastructural changes of myocytes with loss of contractile proteins that is neither specific to repetitive stunning nor to myocardial hibernation.

Technical differences in the measurement approaches contribute to the controversy on the levels of MBF in reversibly dysfunctional myocardium. The flow tracers ^{13}N-ammonia and ^{82}Rb depict and estimate the total transmural MBF. Interstitial fibrosis and scar tissue, commonly present in dysfunctional myocardium, result in regional reductions in transmural blood flow. The regional myocardial ^{13}N-ammonia uptake, for example, declines as the tissue fraction of fibrosis increases as observed through histological analysis of biopsy samples removed from dysfunctional myocardium during CABG (Figure 6-34).[288,289] Despite this linear correlation between the fractional tissue fibrosis and transmural MBFs, it is difficult to determine whether the reduction in blood flow can be attributed to fibrotic tissue alone or to a combination of fibrosis and abnormal dysfunctional and hypoperfused myocytes. In contrast, the ^{15}O-labeled water approach measures blood flow only in the fraction of the myocardium capable of rapidly exchanging water so that in most reports using this technique, regional MBFs are found to be normal or only slightly reduced. Again, if the tissue fraction of hibernating myocardium is, in fact, hypoperfused and unable to exchange water, the ^{15}O-labeled water technique would examine primarily normal myocardium. This might account for the normal or only mildly reduced flow estimates in reversibly dysfunctional myocardial regions. Arguments in favor of a

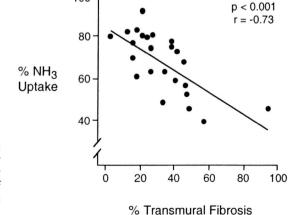

FIGURE 6-34. Relationship between the fraction of transmural fibrosis as determined from biopsy samples in patients undergoing coronary artery bypass grafting (CABG) and the relative uptake of ^{13}N-ammonia. (Data used with permission from Depré et al.[289])

true hypoperfusion of chronically hibernating myocardium include regional flow reductions in an animal experimental model of longterm hibernation free of necrosis and scar tissue formation[321] and increases in regional MBF following revascularization of reversibly dysfunctional myocardium.[74,329,330]

If myocardial hibernation represents an adaptive process to a limitation in substrate supply, and thus, regional MBF, it should preclude increases in MBF, for example, in response to increased demand. Consistent with this notion are preliminary observations of an absent myocardial flow reserve in dysfunctional myocardium,[331] although more recent investigations with the ^{15}O-labeled water technique report a residual flow reserve, although markedly diminished and ranging from about 1.2 to 1.5.[332,333] Increases in regional flow in dysfunctional myocardium in response to inotropic stimulation with intravenous dobutamine are similarly consistent with some residual flow reserve.[334]

A preserved contractile reserve is another key feature of reversible dysfunction and, thus, viable myocardium. This reserve has been used advantageously with low dose dobutamine stress echocardiography for identifying the presence of viable myocardium. Most comparison studies implicate the contractile reserve as a less sensitive but more specific index of myocardial viability.[335–337] Other investigations again refer to the increased FDG uptake in dysfunctional myocardium as a more accurate predictor of the postrevascularization outcome in segmental function as compared to dobutamine stress echocardi-ography.[338] This is because the absence of FDG rather than the segmental inotropic response predicts more accurately that function will not improve following revascularization. Conversely, in these studies, the increased ^{18}F-deoxyglucose uptake rather than the loss of contractile reserve predicted a postrevascularization and improvement in segmental wall motion.

Dysfunctional myocardial regions that do not improve function in response to revascularization generally exhibit a greater amount of interstitial fibrosis (20% vs. only 2.7% in reversibly dysfunctional segments), associated with more severely reduced blood flow, absent systolic wall thickening (0% vs. 18%), and essentially no increase in systolic wall thickening in response to low dose dobutamine stimulation (3% vs. 28%).[339] However, as many as 30% of dysfunctional myocardial regions with preserved or enhanced FDG uptake and, thus, with sustained metabolic activity may no longer respond to inotropic stimulation. They are then associated with a loss in contractile reserve.[334,340] Despite comparable reductions in blood flow and levels of FDG uptake, morphological changes including the fraction of abnormal myocytes or the fraction of fibrosis may vary considerably between dysfunctional segments and patients.[341,342] Histological and ultrastructural assays of transmural biopsies from dysfunctional myocardium identified loss of contractile proteins as the only independent predictor of the inotropic reserve[342] which then might explain the disparity between a loss of inotropic reserve and sustained metabolic activity.

Ultrastructural and histochemical observations Other attempts to gain mechanistic insights into the enhanced FDG uptake include morphometric and histochemical analysis of biopsy specimens harvested from dysfunctional human myocardium during surgical revascularization (Figure 6-35). What had been known from prior autopsy studies was the existence of a general correlation between the degree of regional myocardial fibrosis and the severity of the impairment of

FIGURE 6-35. Electron micrograph of myocardium obtained during coronary artery bypass grafting (CABG) from the dysfunctional myocardium in a patient with ischemic cardiomyopathy. Notice the irregularly shaped nucleus, the perinuclear loss of myofibrils and the replacement by glycogen granules. (Courtesy of Marcel Borgers.)

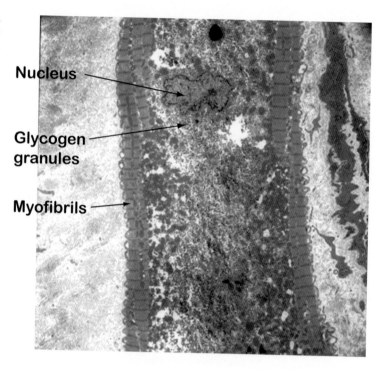

regional contractile function. Yet, there were exceptions.[343] In some instances, dyskinetically moving myocardium was free of fibrosis on autopsy or, conversely, some normally contracting myocardium contained as much as 40% fibrosis.[344] It was also known that abnormal myocytes existed in chronically dysfunctional myocardium.[345] Recent investigations noted correlations between the externally determined relative MBFs and relative FDG concentrations on the one hand and the morphometrically determined fractions of fibrosis, abnormal myocytes, and normal myocardium on the other hand.[206,288,289] Several studies agree on a general correlation between relative MBF and the fraction of tissue fibrosis[206,288,289] but differ in regards to the fraction of abnormal myocytes. In one study, this fraction is virtually the same in reversibly and irreversibly dysfunctional myocardium[288] while a second study notes a significantly greater fraction in reversibly than in irreversibly dysfunctional myocardium.[289] Because of centrally located glycogen granules as one of the key features of such abnormal myocytes and a statistically significant correlation between the fraction of such abnormal myocytes and the relative FDG uptake, these abnormal myocytes have been thought of as the ultrastructural correlate of the enhanced FDG uptake in chronically dysfunctional myocardium.

Other observations argue against such explanation. Again, electron microscopy and histochemistry of biopsy samples retrieved during surgical bypass grafting from the center of the dysfunctional myocardial wall demonstrate highly different degrees in the severity of morphologic alterations in myocardial regions with comparable MBF metabolism mismatches.[346] Despite identical flow metabolism findings on PET imaging, nearly half of the patients in this study exhibited minimal if any significant morphologic changes while the other half demonstrated the structural abnormalities as described above. Such variability in morphologic alterations argues against the structurally abnormal myocyte and, especially, the glycogen granules as an explanation of the enhanced FDG uptake. More likely explanations include: 1) translocation and possibly upregulation of the relatively insulin-independent glucose transporter GLUT1[347–349] as the flux-generating step; 2) multisite mostly passive modulation of the glycolytic flux along the anaerobic pathway with active control by glucose phosphate isomerase (GPiso) and PGM/eno (phosphoglycerate mutase to enolase)[350]; 3) uncoupling of glycolysis from glucose oxidation, probably effected by malonyl-CoA and carnitine palmitate transferase I[351]; and, thus, 4) increased tissue accumulation of lactate. An additional contributing factor may be an ischemia-related loss of adrenergic innervation or function[352] shown to be associated with increased exogenous glucose utilization, as recently demonstrated in partially reinnervated cardiac allografts where glucose utilization in denervated myocardium was about 7% higher than in reinnervated myocardium.[353] The increase in anaerobic ATP production with higher rates of glycolysis has been viewed to be critical for protecting or preserving membrane function. Yet, as oxidative metabolism appears to persist in chronic dysfunctional myocardium, high-energy phosphate tissue contents have been found to be normal.[354]

Abnormal myocytes in chronically dysfunctional myocardium Whether abnormal myocytes found in biopsy material from mismatched myocardium point specifically in the direction of or are ingredients unique to any particular pathophysiological mechanism underlying the chronic, though potentially reversible, impairment of contractile function remains uncertain. Two schools of thought exist: One holds that the morphologic alterations result from (1) contractile unloading, (2) increased wall stress (stretch), and (3) a substrate switch to preferential glucose utilization.[355] In fact, contractile unloading has recently been demonstrated to lead to virtually identical structural changes.[356,357] The expression and distribution patterns of other features such as of α-smooth muscle actin, cardiotin, and titin[355] as well as increased expression of glucose transporter 1 (GLUT1) mRNA,[347] with features that resemble those in embryonic and/or neonatal myocytes, suggested that the changes of abnormal myocytes may represent dedifferentiation.[355] Histochemical analysis further uncovered alterations in the extracellular matrix with increased amounts of collagen and fibronectin surrounding the abnormal myocytes.[355] Finally, similar to neonatal myocytes, these abnormal myocytes have been found to be more resistant to ischemia.[358] The absence of true degenerative changes has further been involved in support of this possibility and argues in favor of a reexpression of the fetal gene program or suppression of the adult relative to the fetal gene program.[359,360]

The other school of thought emphasizes a progressive deterioration of the cell's morphology and, therefore, refers to hibernation as incomplete adaptation to ischemia.[361] The process begins with few if any structural changes but a switch in substrate selection to glucose, either because of its greater oxygen efficiency or, alternatively, loss of enzymes essential for FFA oxidation, followed by loss of contractile protein and accumulation of glycogen and mitochondrial and nuclear alterations, ultimately leading to cell death and scar tissue formation.[341]

Other studies again report reduced expression of contractile and cytoskeletal proteins associated with increased expression of extracellular matrix proteins,[361] implying a progressive loss of contractile protein and deterioration of the cell structure that is paralleled by accelerated formation of tissue fibrosis and, hence, a progressive loss of viability found to be associated with apoptosis and replacement fibrosis.

Clinical observations lend support to such a downhill course. Biopsies from patients with preoperatively viable myocardium but without a postrevascularization improvement in contractile dysfunction demonstrated an approximate 3-fold increase in mRNA of Caspase-3, a promoter of apoptosis, together with an approximate 50% reduction in the expression of the antideath genes Bcl-2 and p53, again consistent with continued cell death and replacement fibrosis.[362] Chronic animal experimental studies similarly demonstrate increases in apoptotic myocytes in hibernating myocardium with reduced rest MBF and critically reduced or absent flow reserve.[323] The observation that myocyte apoptosis in these studies occurred scattered and not in clusters raises the question of whether apoptosis is, indeed, the endpoint of the progressively deteriorating abnormal myocyte or whether such apoptosis represents a parallel process.

A progressive deterioration of reversibly dysfunctional myocardium is also consistent with clinical observations. Studies point to the high prevalence of mismatch patterns in patients with prior myocardial infarctions[285,363] but note a declining incidence of MBF metabolism mismatches as a function of time after an acute myocardial infarction.[326] Moreover, the loss of the potential to improve LVEF if revascularization is delayed by more than 6 months,[364] or an increase in fibrosis and loss of functional recovery after revascularization as a function of the duration of clinical symptoms,[365] seems to support such progression and raise the question whether a new supply and demand balance at rest at a lower level can, in fact, be sustained permanently. If not, then the MBF metabolism mismatch represents a more transient rather than permanent state of reversibly dysfunctional myocardium.

In the clinical setting, prompt restoration of adequate tissue perfusion through interventional revascularization will, therefore, be essential. As it remains uncertain at what stage the structural alterations become irreversible, it would seem that ultimately the return of contractile function will depend upon the amount of connective tissue. Once fibrosis and scar tissue occupy more than 35% to 40% of the myocardium, dysfunction has been shown to be irreversible.[37,38] As another clinical implication, the presence of structural changes in viable myocardium as demonstrated with MBF metabolism imaging implies that if the contractile machinery in abnormal or dedifferentiated myocytes can be restored, the recovery of contractile function will not be immediate but slow as clinical investigations demonstrated.[366,367] The time required for repair of the structural alterations of myocytes is also likely to account for the persistence of the increased FDG uptake following surgical revascularization,[368] especially because the time to resumption or to a measurable improvement of contractile function is longest in those myocardial regions with the greatest number of structurally altered or hibernating myocytes. Indeed, the rate of recovery of contractile function was shown to be correlated with the fraction of abnormal myocytes.[367]

Clinical implications of MBF and FDG uptake patterns

GENERAL CONSIDERATIONS

Viability assessment with PET can decisively affect therapeutic strategies in patients with advanced CAD and ischemic cardiomyopathy. Therapeutic options in these patients range from aggressive medical management to surgical revascularization and cardiac transplantation. While conservative, pharmacological approaches have markedly improved over the past decade, the longterm survival of medically treated patients remains poor.[369] Cardiac transplantation as another approach offers better longterm survival and an improvement in the quality of life but supply of donor hearts has not kept pace with the increasing demand so that this therapeutic option remains limited. The number of cardiac transplantations in the United States has declined over the past several years; it was 2,198 in the year 2002, while the incidence of cardiomyopathy and congestive heart failure (CHF) is on the rise (2002 Heart and Stroke Statistical Update, American Heart Association).

At present, the prevalence of ischemic cardiomyopathy in the United States alone amounts to about 2.5 million cases, thus affecting roughly 1% of the U.S. population. The same statistics indicate an annual incidence of ischemic cardiomyopathy of about 400,000 with 200,000 deaths resulting from ischemic cardiomyopathy each year. Interventional revascularization by PTCA or, more commonly, CABG, often remains the third choice. The Coronary Artery Surgery Study (CASS) clearly demonstrates a significant 5-year survival benefit of surgery as compared to medical management and improvement or relief of anginal symptoms.[370,371] However, the CASS registry found no significant benefit of CABG for CHF-related symptoms which are most often the leading and most disabling complication in patients with ischemic cardiomyopathy. At the same time, it remains difficult and often impossible to predict with conventional clinical criteria the postrevascularization outcome in CHF-related symptoms and in global left ventricular function. Moreover, patients with ischemic cardiomyopathy face a high perioperative risk.

There is also compelling evidence for the clinical impact of viability assessment, especially for evaluating the risk of cardiac death and the benefits of interventional revascularization. For example, data were collected from 24 investigations that reported patient survival relative to the presence or absence of myocardial viability and relative to treatment. In a total of 3,088 patients with ischemic cardiomyopathy and an average left ventricular ejection fraction of only 32% $\pm$ 8%, viability was assessed with ^{201}Tl-myocardial perfusion imaging, FDG, or dobutamine stress echocardiography.[372] Patients without viability had intermediate mortality rates; the annual mortality rate averaged 6.2% on medical and 7.7% on revascularization treatment. Importantly, patients with viability and on medical treatment had a 16% annual mortality rate that significantly declined to 3.2% (chi-square; p < 0.0001) for patients on revascularization treatment. This then indicates a particularly high risk of cardiac deaths for patients with viability on medical treatment and, importantly, a 79.6% reduction of the annual mortality rate achieved through revascularization.

Perioperative morbidity and mortality MBF and glucose metabolism studies with PET can contribute to predicting the surgical risk. Two investigations have explored the contribution of PET to the surgical risk assessment.[373,374] Both studies combined include a total of 317 patients with ischemic cardiomyopathy and an LVEF of less than 35%. The patients were categorized into two groups. Group one (35 and 88 patients, respectively in each study) underwent CABG based on standard clinical criteria, including LV size or LVEF, the suitability of the coronary anatomy for surgical revascularization, and the presence of comorbidities. The same criteria were also applied to the second group (41 and 153 patients per study) which, however, also underwent MBF metabolism imaging with PET. Thirty-four (83%) of 41 patients in one and 110 (72%) of 153 patients in the other group demonstrated evidence of reversibly dysfunctional myocardium involving at least 20% to 30% of the LV and subsequently underwent bypass grafting. Both studies demonstrated lower perioperative mortality rates in patients with PET-demonstrated viability (30-day mortality rates of 0% and 0.9%) as compared to mortalities of 11.4% and 19.8% in the patients not evaluated by PET. Additionally, 1-year cardiac mortalities were lower for the PET-selected (3% and 10%, respectively) than for those not evaluated with PET (21% and 30%, respectively.). Patients with viability by PET required less inotropic support or intra-aortic balloon pumping, had higher cardiac output and shorter stays in the intensive care unit. Further confirmation of such short-term benefits seems warranted. If confirmed, PET evaluations of patients with ischemic cardiomyopathies would then offer important and possibly critical prognostic information on the immediate and longterm risks of cardiovascular surgery in this group of patients.

Left ventricular function Numerous clinical investigations have reported the high accuracy of FDG imaging with PET in predicting the post-revascularization outcome in regional LV wall motion.[286,294,375–381] Even though some of these investigations used permutations of the initially described MBF metabolism approach or relied only on the evaluation of only regional FDG uptake in dysfunctional myocardium,[294,381] the predictive accuracy both positive and negative, remains high. Such studies have been important because they prove the concept of MBF metabolism patterns as accurate predictors of the outcome of regional wall motion after restoration of MBF. More relevant in the clinical setting is, however, whether MBF metabolism patterns predict the postrevascularization outcome in LVEF.

Early studies demonstrated a correlation between the extent of the MBF metabolism mismatch and the postrevascularization gain in LVEF.[286] Patients with MBF metabolism mismatches that occupied at least 2 or more of a total of 7 myocardial segments revealed a significant increase in LVEF following CABG.[286] No such improvement was observed in patients with only one mismatch segment or with only matches. Subsequent studies confirmed these initial observations and reported significant gains in LV function in patients with MBF metabolism mismatches as compared to no improvement in those patients without metabolic evidence of viability. Table 6-16 summarizes the findings in 19 investigations including a total of 570 patients.[286–289,300,310,329,338,341,364,373,377,378,382–388,400,406] Further, the gain in LVEF is more prominent in patients with LV ejection fractions of less than 35%. There was an average 34% postsurgical increase in the LV ejection fraction in patients with more severely depressed LV function (LVEF < 35%) as compared to a 19% (p < 0.02) improvement in patients with with less severely reduced LV function (LVEF > 35%). Additionally, recent stud-

TABLE 6-16. Changes in Left Ventricular Ejection Fraction after Surgical Revascularization in Patients

Investigation	MBF/FDG[a]	Nt	Mismatch				Match			
				LVEF				LVEF		
			N	Pre	Post	P	N	Pre	Post	P
Tillisch et al, 1986[286]	PETn/PET	17	11	30 ± 11	45 ± 14	0.005	6	30 ± 11	31 ± 12	NS
Carrel et al, 1992[377]	PETr/PET	21	21	34 ± 14	52 ± 11	0.001				
Lucignani et al, 1992[378]	SPECTs/PET	14	14	38 ± 5	48 ± 9	0.001				
Marwick et al, 1992[382] b	PETr/PET	24	9	37 ± 11	40 ± 9	NS	6	38 ± 13	13 ± 18	NS
Maes et al, 1994[288]	PETn/PET	33	12	51 ± 11	60 ± 10	0.05	15	46 ± 11	48 ± 10	NS
Dreyfus et al, 1994[406]	PETw/PET	40	40	23 ± 6	39 ± 13	0.05				
vom Dahl et al, 1994[384]	PETn/PET	37	37	34 ± 10	36 ± 10	0.001				
Paolini et al, 1994[383]	PET/PET	17	9	28 ± 5	43 ± 8	0.001				
Depré et al, 1995[289]	PETn/PET	23	16	43 ± 18	51 ± 15	0.05	7	35 ± 9	23 ± 9	NS
Maes et al, 1995[329]	PETn/PET	30	15	51 ± 11	61 ± 6	0.001	15	46 ± 11	48 ± 10	NS
Schwarz et al, 1996[341]	SPECTs/PET	24	20	44 ± 12	54 ± 9	0.01				
vom Dahl et al, 1996[287]	SPECTs/PET	43	23	47 ± 10	54 ± 10	0.001				
Hata et al, 1996[310]	PETn/PET	28	13	45 ± 4	62 ± 6	0.001	15	43 ± 5	44 ± 6	NS
Wolpers et al, 1996[310a]	PETa/PET	30	17	40 ± 10	43	0.003	13	46 ± 13	48	NS
Haas et al, 1997[373]	PETn/PET	44	22	26 ± 4	35 ± 12	0.01	22	30 ± 4	34 ± 12	NS
Bax et al, 1997[385]	SPECTt/SPECT	55	19	28 ± 8	35 ± 9	0.001	36	45 ± 14	44 ± 14	NS
Fath–Ordoubadi et al, 1998[387]	PETn/PET	47	27	22 ± 6	31 ± 10	0.001	21	43 ± 9	43 ± 12	NS
Pagano et al, 1998[338]	PETn/PET	35	18	22 ± 5	38 ± 10	0.001	11	29 ± 8	31 ± 8	NS
Beanlands et al, 1998[364]	PETr/PET	12	12	24 ± 7	29 ± 8	0.001				
Flameng et al, 1997[386]	PETn/PET	59	23	47 ± 15	56 ± 15	0.005	20	49 ± 15	50 ± 16	NS
Schöder et al, 1999[300]	PETn/PET	40	40	30 ± 6	37 ± 8	0.01				
Zhang et al, 2001[400]	SPECTs/PET	42	42	36 ± 5	51 ± 9					

Abbreviations and Terms: FDG, 2-deoxy-2-[F-18]fluoro-D-glucose; LVEF, left ventricular ejection fraction; MBF, myocardial blood flow; MBF/FDG, imaging of MBF and FDG; Mismatch and Match, patients with mismatch and patients without mismatches or only small mismatches; N, number of patients; P, P value; PET, positron emission tomography; Pre and Post, prior to and after coronary artery bypass grafting; SPECT, single-photon emission computed tomography.

[a]MBF evaluated with PET and ^{13}N-ammonia (PETn), ^{82}Rb (PETr), ^{15}O-labeled water (PETw) or [C-11] acetate (PETa) or with SPECT and ^{99m}Tc-sestamibi (SPECTs) or ^{201}Tl (SPECTt).

[b]Marwick et al[382] determined viability from stress myocardial blood flow images and rest ^{18}F-deoxyglucose uptake.

Source: Data from Tillisch et al,[286] Carrel et al,[377] Lucignani et al,[378] Marwick et al,[382] Maes et al,[288] Dreyfus et al,[406] vom Dahl et al,[384] Paolini et al,[383] Depré et al,[289] Maes et al,[329] Schwarz et al,[341] vom Dahl et al,[287] Hata et al,[310] Wolpers et al,[310a] Haas et al,[373] Bax et al,[385] Fath–Ordoubadi et al,[387] Pagano et al,[338] Beanlands et al,[364] Flameng et al,[386] Schöder et al,[300] and Zhang et al.[400]

ies report statistically significant correlations between the percentage of the LV with a MBF metabolism mismatch and the postrevascularization increase in the LVEF.[300,389] This then implies that the extent of a MBF metabolism mismatch is of predictive value on the postsurgical gain in global LV performance (Figure 6-36).

Most clinical investigations invariably report significant postrevascularization improvements in LV function at rest in patients with large MBF glucose metabolism mismatches. One laboratory finds no such improvement in resting LV function.[390] MBF in these studies was evaluated with [82]Rb at rest and during pharmacological stress. However, distribution of MBF during stress was compared to the myocardial glucose metabolism at rest. The approach, therefore, identifies both stress-induced ischemia and viable myocardium at rest. Hence, MBF and, possibly, wall motion at rest may be normal in some patients so that revascularization predominantly improves the capacity of the LV to more appropriately respond to exercise rather than left ventricular function at rest.[390,391]

The improvement in regional and especially global LV function may not occur immediately but rather slowly and progressively following revascularization. Again, in a highly selected patient group, MBF was shown to recover promptly following revascularization by PTCA while contractile function remained initially unchanged.[366] On reexamination 67 days ± 19 days later, no further improvements in regional MBF had occurred, but systolic wall motion had significantly improved. The disparity between recovery of MBF and contractile function might be attributed to stunning, but may also be related to rebuilding of the contractile machinery in hibernating myocytes. The more rapid functional

FIGURE 6-36. Extent of blood flow metabolism mismatch and postrevascularization improvement in the left ventricular ejection fraction. The figure compares the number of myocardial segments with blood flow-metabolism mismatches to the postsurgical improvement in the left ventricular ejection fraction. (Reproduced from Pagano et al., with permission from Elsevier.[389]) Abbreviations: Delta-EF, left ventricular ejection fraction; PET, positron emission tomography.

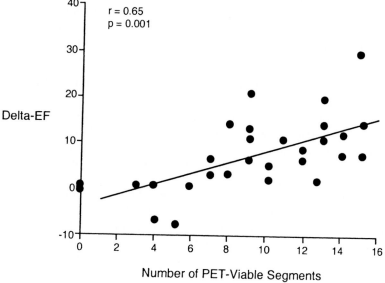

recovery of myocardial regions with relatively well-preserved MBF as compared to a more delayed improvement in regions with more severely reduced flows appears to support this possibility.[392]

Congestive heart failure symptoms A related clinical question is whether such improvement is also associated with relief or amelioration of LVEF symptoms. Several retrospective studies do, in fact, indicate such possible symptomatic improvement. For example, two investigations conclude that patients with MBF metabolism mismatches undergoing surgical revascularization demonstrated a significantly higher incidence of an improvement in functional class (NYHA Congestive Heart Failure Class) than patients without mismatches or patients with matches also submitted to surgical revascularization.[393,394] Among the 52 patients with mismatches and CHF Class III or IV, 81% of the 26 patients undergoing revascularization revealed a significant improvement in CHF class (by at least one grade) as compared to only 23% of 26 patients treated conservatively.[394] While a causal relationship is still lacking, it nevertheless appears that improvements in CHF symptoms are associated with an improvement in global left ventricular function.[395]

The amount of viable myocardium contains information on the magnitude of the postrevascularization improvement in CHF symptoms.[396] The level of physical activity patients performed prior to and 24 months ± 14 months following CABG was graded on a specific activity scale and expressed in metabolic equivalents (METs).[397] Among the 36 patients in this study with an average LVEF of only 28% ± 6% prior to revascularization, the extent of the MBF metabolism mismatch ranged from 0 to 74% (mean, 23% ± 22%) on polar map analysis. When patients were grouped according to the extent of the mismatch, 11 patients with a mismatch occupying less than 5% of the LV myocardium revealed a statistically significant but only mild improvement in functional status (34% increase in METs). Intermediate-sized mismatches (5% to 17%) in 8 patients were associated with a 42% increase in METs whereas large mismatches, that is greater than 18%, in 17 patients were followed after revascularization by an average increase of 107% in METS. Furthermore, as seen in Figure 6-37, there was a statistically significant correlation between the improvement in functional status and the anatomic extent of the MBF metabolism mismatch. Lastly, MBF metabolism mismatches equal to or greater than 18% were 70% sensitive and 78% specific in predicting an improvement in physical activity or functional status following successful surgical revascularization.

Longterm survival Several studies examined the longterm fate of patients after being evaluated for MBF and metabolism with PET.[393,394,398–400] These studies presented compelling evidence for the notion of an increased incidence of cardiac events in patients with MBF metabolism mismatches not submitted to interventional revascularization (Table 6-17). They also imply that revascularization of MBF metabolism mismatch segments might avert future nonfatal and fatal cardiac events.

Despite this general agreement, important differences emerge from these studies. One study in 129 chronic CAD patients followed clinically for an average of 17 months ± 19 months found the presence of mismatches in the absence of revascularization to be independent predictors of the 17 nonfatal ischemic events.[399] Nevertheless, the LVEF and the patient's age contained the highest predictive values for the 13 cardiac deaths in this patient group. Given a wide

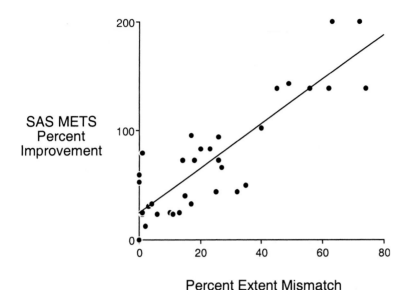

FIGURE 6-37. Comparison between the percent improvement in physical activity and the extent of the blood flow metabolism mismatch prior to bypass grafting. The improvement in physical activity was measured by a specific activity score and expressed in metabolic units (METs). (Data used with permission from DiCarli et al.[396])

range of functional compromise of the LV in the patients of this study, the high predictive value of the LVEF is not surprising. In patient groups with more homogeneously depressed LV function, the predictive value of a low LVEF applied equally to all groups. This then affords an analysis of other factors as prognosticators of cardiac mortality. As shown in Figure 6-38, the cumulative longterm survival was lowest in the patient subgroup with MBF metabolism mismatches that was on medical treatment. Of notice, all four subgroups were similar in regards to age and clinical and hemodynamic findings. There were no significant intergroup differences in the LVEF, which for the whole patient group averaged 25% ± 7%. In addition, patients with mismatches undergoing revascularization revealed a significantly better cumulative survival which no longer differed significantly from that of the groups without mismatches. In this study, the LVEF was without significant predictive value while with Cox model analysis the extent of a mismatch had a significant ($p < 0.02$) negative effect on survival and revascularization of mismatch patients a significant ($p < 0.04$) positive effect on survival.[394] While submitted to a less rigorous statistical analysis, a second study in patients with a similar uniform depression of LVEFs reached similar conclusions.[393,400] Among the patient groups with and without mismatches, the subgroup of patients with mismatches demonstrated markedly higher incidences of cardiac deaths during the 12-month followup period as compared to a very low mortality rate in patients with mismatches undergoing revascularization.

Alternate imaging approaches for the identification of myocardial viability

These alternate approaches include myocardial perfusion imaging with ^{201}Tl, dobutamine stress echocardiography, and, more recently, late contrast enhancement on magnetic resonance imaging (MRI).

TABLE 6-17. Flow Metabolism Patterns and Cardiac Mortality[a]

Investigation	Pts	Months	LVEF	Mismatch Surgical No	Deaths N(%)	Mismatch Medical No	Deaths N(%)	Match Surgical No	Deaths N(%)	Match Medical No	Deaths N(%)
Eitzman et al, 1992[393]	82	12	34 ± 13	26	1 (4%)	18	6 (33%)	14	0 (0%)	24	2 (8%)
Di Carli et al, 1994[394]	93	13.6	25 ± 6	26	3 (12%)	17	8 (47%)	17	1 (6%)	33	3 (9%)
Tamaki N et al, 1993[174]	84	23 ± 13	N/G			48	3 (6%)			36	0 (0%)
Rohatgi R et al, 2001[394a]	99	25 ± 9	22 ± 6	29	0 (0%)	29	10 (34%)	8	0 (0%)	33	5 (15%)
Zhang X et al, 2001[400]	123	26 ± 10	35 ± 6	42	0 (0%)	30	8 (27%)	25	2 (8%)	26	1 (4%)
Lee et al, 1994[399]	129	17 ± 9	38 ± 16	49	4 (8%)	21	3 (14%)	19	1 (5%)	40	5 (12%)
	610			172	4.8%	163	26.8%	83	3.8%	192	8.0%

Abbreviations: LVEF, left ventricular ejection fraction; N, number of patients involved in mismatches or matches; N/G, not given; Pts, total number of patients in each study cited.

[a]Incidents of cardiac deaths according to blood flow metabolism patterns on positron emission tomography (PET) and according to treatment as reported in 6 investigations. For each investigation, the number of patients, the average followup period (months) and the average LVEF are given. Patients are then grouped according to presence of mismatch (left) and match (right) and further according to treatment (revascularization or surgical and medical). For each subgroup, the number of patients and the number of cardiac deaths (expressed in percent in parentheses) are listed.

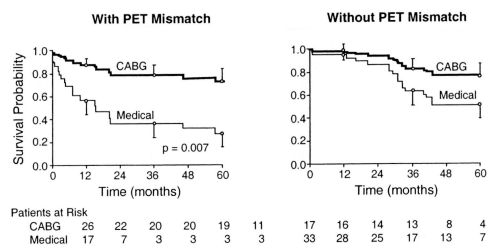

FIGURE 6-38. Five-year survival according to the findings on blood flow metabolism imaging with PET and according to treatment. Abbreviations: CABG, coronary artery bypass grafting; medical, medical treatment. (Reproduced with permission from Di Carli et al., with permission from Elsevier.[439])

THALLIUM-201 SPECT IMAGING

The concept inherent to the use of ^{201}Tl is that early after administered to the patient when at rest, the radiotracer delineates myocardial perfusion and, thus, identifies myocardial regions that are hypoperfused at rest. As a potassium analogue, the tracer subsequently equilibrates between blood and myocardium so that images recorded between 4 h and 24 h after ^{201}Tl administration reflect the myocardial potassium pool. Accordingly, hypoperfused myocardium that on delayed imaging demonstrates an increase in ^{201}Tl uptake is considered viable. In contrast, persistence of a defect on late imaging is attributed to scar tissue and is, hence, considered nonviable.

Generally found to be highly sensitive and specific,[335,401–405] the accuracy of the ^{201}Tl rest-redistribution approach may be limited in patients with ischemic cardiomyopathy and severely reduced left ventricular function. In one study, for example, myocardial perfusion-metabolism imaging with PET identified myocardial viability in 18 of 20 patients with fixed defects on SPECT ^{201}Tl imaging.[406] Another investigation reported metabolic evidence of viability in 17 of 33 patients with fixed defects or equivocal findings on ^{201}Tl rest redistribution SPECT imaging.[388] Revascularization in the patients of both studies led to substantial improvements in left ventricular function. The reported prevalence of metabolic evidence of myocardial viability in patients with fixed ^{201}Tl defects in both studies is comparable to the prevalence of mismatches reported for myocardial segments with fixed defects on 4 h and 24 h delayed ^{201}Tl imaging.[363,407,408] Some investigators have attributed the failure of ^{201}Tl to redistribute into hypoperfused though viable myocardial regions to diminished tracer availability, mostly because of clearance of ^{201}Tl and, thus, loss of tracer from blood. Reinjection of ^{201}Tl has been advocated to overcome this limitation. It would seem that the resulting reinjection images again primarily reflect the distribution of MBF rather than the true potassium pool. Indeed, in instances of redistribution or in resolving defects on late images, reinjection may produce new defects in regions with diminished blood flow at rest. Rather than limitations of tracer kinetics, methodological shortcomings may likely explain the limited accuracy of ^{201}Tl rest-redistribution imaging in patients with severely depressed left ventricular function. Poor signal-to-noise ratios lower the diagnostic accuracy of identifying regional reductions in myocardial tracer activity and their time-dependent changes.

Dobutamine stress echocardiography This approach identifies the presence of contractile reserve as another indicator of myocardial viability or potentially reversible contractile dysfunction. Responses of dysfunctional myocardial regions to intravenous administration of dobutamine are monitored with 2-D echocardiography. An improvement in wall motion and/or in wall thickening indicates the presence of viability whereas an absent response signifies irreversible contractile dysfunction. Findings in clinical investigations support the high predictive accuracy of stress echocardiography for the identification of myocardial viability.[409–414] Further, comparison studies between stress-echocardiography and PET myocardial perfusion and metabolism imaging report comparable overall diagnostic accuracies, although the PET approach appears to be less specific but more sensitive than stress echocardiography,[338] possibly for two reasons: First, metabolic imaging with PET possibly identifies small fractions of metabolically abnormal but viable myocardium, which are of little, if any, significance for regional myocardial wall motion and its response to revascularization. Conversely, metabolism imaging may identify viable myocardium that has remained metabolically active and may recover contractile function, although contractile proteins have been largely lost, precluding a functional response to inotropic stimulation.

Contrast-enhanced magnetic resonance imaging The approach with contrast-enhanced MRI represents the most recent addition to the diagnostic tools for distinguishing between reversible and irreversible contractile dysfunction. Retention of gadolinium contrast and, thus, hyperenhancement of myocardium on MR images has been observed to be correlated with an acute but also chronic irreversible injury.[415–417] Although the mechanism of such contrast retention awaits further clarification, abnormal membrane permeability after an acute injury and distribution of gadolinium-contrast into the interstitial space of scar tissue have been invoked as possible explanations.[415]

The transmural extent of the hyperenhancement, therefore, reflects the transmural extent of irreversibly injured myocardium or scar tissue. Accordingly, contractile function failed to improve following revascularization in nearly 100% of all dysfunctional segments with greater than 75% and in 90% of segments with greater than 51% of transmural hyperenhancement.[416] Conversely, contractile function improved following coronary revascularization in 78% of all dysfunctional segments without hyperenhancement. Thus, MRI offers an addition to information on global and regional contractile function, regional wall thickness, and systolic wall thickening predictive of information on the potential reversibility of contractile dysfunction.

Different from both the ^{201}Tl redistribution and the ^{1}FDG approaches with ischemically compromised but viable myocardium as the diagnostic target, the MRI hyperenhancement approach delineates the transmural amount of scar tissue and, thus, irreversibly injured myocardium. Both targets are critical features of potentially irreversible contractile dysfunction. Regional wall motion will improve only if 1) the transmural fraction of irreversible tissue injury remains small, and 2) the transmural fraction of reversibly dysfunctional myocardium is sufficiently large to support a possible improvement in contractile function. While the size of this transmural fraction remains to be determined, there is relatively good agreement on the transmural fraction of irreversibly injured tissue. The MRI hyperenhancement approach as well as the perfusable tissue index as an analogous approach for assessing the fraction amount of scar tissue indicate that wall motion becomes impaired irreversibly once the transmural fraction of fibrosis exceeds 35% to 40%.[37,38]

Similar estimates have been forthcoming from studies of regional myocardial perfusion. Relative reductions in the myocardial uptake of radiotracers of blood flow, for example, ^{13}N-ammonia, ^{201}Tl, or ^{99m}Tc-labeled agents, have been found to be correlated inversely with the fractional amounts of fibrosis and scar tissue in the myocardium of patients with coronary artery disease.[206,288] This is why the evaluation of MBF alone can provide prognostic information on irreversible contractile dysfunction. Severe reductions in resting MBF generally correspond to substantial amounts of scar tissue and, thus, nonreversibility, whereas normal or near normal MBFs predict reversibility. This also explains the general agreement between findings on MRI hyperenhancement and on PET where regional MBF inversely correlates to the transmural hyperenhancement.[418] Further, if patients are studied in the glucose-loaded state, then there is likely to be a general inverse correlation between the hyperenhancing tissue fraction and the regional FDG uptake, a correlation that, however, may no longer apply to mismatched myocardium. Regional FDG concentrations then no longer depend solely on the hyperenhancing myocardial (scar) tissue fraction or, conversely, on the fraction of normal myocardium, but to varying degrees on the amount of coexisting ischemically injured and viable myocardium.

These considerations entail several implications for the assessment of myocardium viability. If, as demonstrated, perfusion depends on the fractional amount of scar tissue, then the relative regional MBF contains predictive information on myocardium viability.[206,288,289] The predictive value of regional flows would appear to be especially high at both ends of the spectrum of regional MBFs, that is, either for normal or near normal flows and for severely reduced regional flows but is likely to be lower for intermediate flow reductions. Similar arguments can be made for the predictive value of regional myocardial FDG concentrations. In the glucose-loaded state, absent or conversely normal FDG uptake would depend on the fractional amount of scar tissue and, thus, predict reversible and reversible contractile dysfunction.[419] However, the predictive accuracy for intermediate uptake reductions will be markedly lower (i.e., by 40% to 60%). Similar considerations seem to apply to the MRI hyperenhancement, where intermediate transmural hyperenhancing tissue fractions may discriminate less accurately between reversibility and irreversibilty of contractile dysfunction. Finally, the same considerations might also apply to the perfusable tissue index. Based on a direct comparison study, delineation of the nonperfusable tissue fraction or scar tissue alone predicted somewhat less accurately than the assessment of the myocardial metabolic activity with FDG and, by inference, of both normal and of coexisting ischemically injured myocardium the postrevascularization outcome in left ventricular function.[420]

Acute myocardial infarction

Relatively few investigations have been performed in patients with acute myocardial infarctions, either during the very acute phase or the periinfarction period.[325,421] The dominant finding in these patients, especially during the prethrombolysis era was the reduction in regional MBF corresponding in location to that of the impaired wall motion and, in many instances, to that of electrocardiographic criteria. Nearly half of the acute infarct patients studied within 3 days after onset of symptoms exhibited absolute or relative (to MBF) increases in FDG uptake, thus signifying persistent myocardial viability. Such mismatches are frequently associated with a longterm improvement of regional wall motion while patients with proportionate reductions in MBF and glucose utilization usually do not recover contractile function. Marked improvements or even normalization of wall motion impairments have, however, been noted in some patients exhibiting even initially severe reductions in both regional MBF and glucose utilization (Schelbert et al, unpublished observations).

Studies on myocardial FFA metabolism in subacute myocardial infarctions reveal regional reductions in ^{11}C-palmitate uptake in the infarcted myocardium.[325,421] Generally, these reductions parallel the reductions in MBF because of the flow-dependent uptake of ^{11}C-palmitate in myocardium. Regional clearance rates of ^{11}C-palmitate from infarcted myocardium are, however, markedly delayed with a decrease in the size and slope of the rapid clearance-curve component indicating that most of the tracer label becomes incorporated into the endogenous lipid pool. This is because of the sensitivity of FFA oxidation to ischemia so that most of the FFA extracted and retained by infarcted myocardium is shifted away from β-oxidation and esterified to triglycerides and lipids. Consistent with the regional decrease in oxidative metabolism is the delayed clearance of [C-11] acetate.[422] Again, its initial uptake largely follows the distribution of MBF and, thus, is diminished in the infarcted myocardium.

Comparison studies of MBF and oxidative metabolism, assessed with ^{13}N-ammonia and [C-11] acetate, demonstrate that oxidative metabolism declines with decreasing MBFs in a biphasic rather than linear fashion.[422,423] As shown in Figure 6-39, oxidative metabolism is relatively well preserved with mild-to-modest reductions in MBF. However, once regional MBF declines to less that $0.5 \text{ ml} \cdot \text{min}^{-1} \cdot \text{g}^{-1}$, oxidative metabolism, as demonstrated by k_{mono} on the [C-11] acetate clearance curves, sharply decreases. The observed biphasic relationship between blood flow and oxidative metabolism is consistent with that modeled from animal experimental data[423] and suggests the operation of compensatory mechanisms where the O_2 extraction increases initially with decreasing flows so that O_2 supply to tissue is relatively well preserved. Once the O_2 extraction reaches a maximum, further flow reductions produce a steep decline in oxygen delivery and, hence, oxidative metabolism.

Thrombolysis in acute myocardial infarction results in the majority of patients in a partial or complete restoration of MBF when evaluated for 24 with ^{13}N-ammonia. In one study in 30 patients, regional MBF remained severely reduced by more than 50% relative to that in remote myocardium.[424] Regional wall motion failed to recover in such segments when reexamined at 3 months. In 23% of patients with entirely normal MBFs at 24 h, regional wall motion recovered in all, whereas in the remaining patients with persistent but only intermediate reductions in MBF and relative increases in regional FDG uptake at 5

FIGURE 6-39. Regional myocardial blood flow and oxygen consumption (determined with [C-11] acetate) in early postinfarction patients (● remote, □ match and ▲ mismatch myocardial region). With modest reduction in blood flow, oxygen consumption declines disproportionately less as the extraction of oxygen increases but declines steeply with more severe flow reduction (see text).

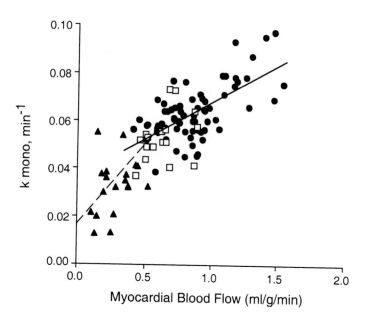

days post myocardial infarction, contractile function improved after additional angioplasty. In a subsequent review of 62 acute myocardial infarct patients, the same investigators concluded that contractile function in infarcted myocardium recovers only if MBF is greater than Thrombolysis in Myocardiac Infarction (TIMI) grade III or if a MBF metabolism mismatch is present and additional angioplasty is performed.[330]

Clinical indications

The following section describes clinical indications of cardiac PET. It emphasizes those that are generally accepted as clinically useful and effective but also addresses indications that are in the future likely to be of value for the clinical decision-making process or, at least, contribute to it. Finally, this section discusses the potential value of cardiac PET for assessing the efficacy of new pharmaceuticals

Assessment of myocardial viability

The evaluation of MBF and FDG uptake for identifying the presence of potentially reversible wall-motion abnormalities has become the clinically most widely recognized and accepted PET procedure. It is part of the practice guidelines of the American College of Cardiology and is considered a class I procedure (usually appropriate and considered useful). These guidelines are on the internet at http://www.acc.org/clinical/guidelines/radio/dirIndex.htm. Further, the Health Care Finance Administration (HCFA) now includes metabolic imaging of the heart with FDG as clinically indicated and thus reimbursable by MediCare for the assessment of myocardial viability if findings on conventional SPECT are equivocal or if SPECT demonstrates only a fixed defect (HCFAL memorandum December 15, 2001). PET assessments of myocardial viability are clinically most useful in patients with ischemic cardiomyopathy and those with acute myocardial infarction.

ISCHEMIC CARDIOMYOPATHY

The diagnostic algorithm used by the University of California, Los Angeles Heart Failure Program for stratifying patients to specific treatment approaches is depicted in Figure 6-40. According to this diagram, the LV function and LV dimensions are determined first by echocardiography. Patients with an end-diastolic diameter of less than 70 mm are referred for a myocardial viability study that might, in addition to the MBF and FDG study at rest, also include a pharmacological stress study. The latter uncovers fluid dynamically significant coronary stenosis in myocardial territories with normal blood flow and wall motion at rest and, thus, contributes to estimating the extent and severity of CAD. If viability is present and involves more than 25% of the LV myocardium (previously referred to as involving at least two segments[425]), patients proceed to coronary angiography for assessing the suitability of the coronary anatomy for bypass grafting. If adequate, patients are then considered for surgical revascularization. Patients with an end-diastolic LV dimension of greater than 70 mm generally do not benefit from revascularization; they are assigned to aggressive medical management. If this management remains without hemodynamic and clinical benefits, patients are then considered for cardiac transplantation. Furthermore, if the viability study fails to identify the presence of adequate amounts of potentially dysfunctional myocardium, or, the coronary anatomy proves unsuitable for bypass grafting, patients are similarly assigned to aggressive medical management. Additional criteria entering this algorithm include comorbidities that may alter the stratification of patients to a specific treatment approach and the decision for revascularization or even cardiac transplantation. Further, the algorithm must take into account existing diagnostic information obtained by the referring clinician or institution. A survey of the outcome of this algorithm reported in preliminary form has determined its cost-effectiveness.[426,427] Of 112 patients evaluated by this algorithm and considered initially for cardiac trans-

FIGURE 6-40. Algorithm in use at University of California, Los Angeles for stratifying patients with ischemic cardiomyopathy to treatment (see text). Abbreviations: ANGIO, cardioangiography; Cor, coronary; CABG, coronary artery bypass grafting; ECHO, echocardiography; LVEDD, left ventricular end-diastolic diameter; PET, positron emission tomography; Rx, treatment.

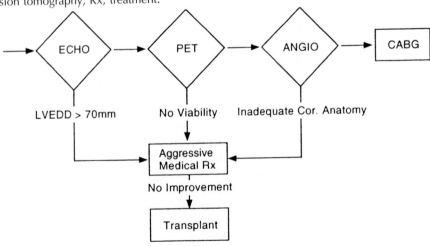

plantation, 38 had PET myocardial viability; of these, 8 refused surgery or had poor vascular targets. Thus, 30 were assigned to CABG. Importantly, their 71.4% actuarial 5-year survival rate of patients was similar (80.1%) to that of patients with cardiac transplantation and significantly exceeded that (42.4%; $p < 0.05$) of patients assigned to aggressive medical management or on the waiting list for cardiac transplantation.

COMPLETENESS OF REVASCULARIZATION

Revascularization by either angioplasty or bypass grafting in patients with advanced CAD and poor LV function remains technically difficult. Persistence or recurrence of symptoms may suggest incomplete revascularization or restenosis. If regional perfusion has not improved, assessment of viability with ^{18}F-deoxyglucose may aid in deciding on further invasive interventions for improving regional MBF.

ACUTE MYOCARDIAL INFARCTION

Despite thrombolysis, a residual, fluid dynamically significant coronary stenosis may impair regional MBF at rest. Normal regional perfusion at rest, and, especially during stress, even in the presence of abnormal wall motion, argues in favor of a complete patency of the infarct vessel. Conversely, a persistent flow defect may result from irreversibly injured myocardium but also from a hemodynamically high-grade coronary stenosis. (Figure 6-41). Sustained metabolic activity in such myocardium as evidenced by increased FDG uptake provides objective evidence of residual myocardial viability and hence, establishes the need for additional interventions, for example, angioplasty.[329,330,428]

Assessment and characterization of coronary artery disease

DIAGNOSIS OF CORONARY ARTERY DISEASE

Conventional SPECT approaches identify the presence of CAD and its extent with a high degree of accuracy. In addition, they contain considerable prognostic information. Shortcomings include the propensity for false positive studies, most

FIGURE 6-41. Example of myocardial perfusion and metabolism images in a patient with acute myocardial infarction. Notice the reduced perfusion of the anterior wall and anterior-lateral wall (arrows) which on the FDG images is associated with enhanced glucose utilization; the patient, therefore, exhibits a blood flow metabolism mismatch that is likely to benefit from additional revascularization. Abbreviations: FDG, 2-deoxy-2-[F-18]-fluoro-D-glucose; MBF, myocardial blood flow.

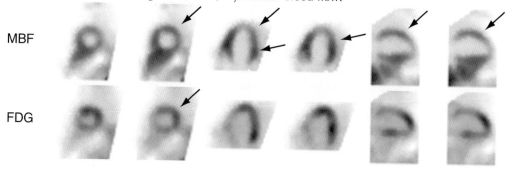

MBF

FDG

frequently related to technical limitations as, for example, photon attenuation due to the liver and the hemidiaphragm or in women to breast tissue. New correction techniques for photon attenuation together with gated SPECT image acquisition and wall-motion assessment have largely overcome these limitations. More difficult to resolve are limitations of the ^{99m}Tc-labeled flow tracers because of the relatively poor uptake response to hyperemic blood flows. Accordingly, mild stenoses may remain undetected. The superior flow to myocardial uptake response of most positron-emitting flow tracers together with the higher spatial and contrast resolution of PET should, therefore, enable detection of less severe coronary stenosis.[84,85] Additionally, because the PET MBF images are free of photon attenuation-related artifacts, PET myocardial perfusion imaging is specifically suited for the detection of CAD for obese patients and women.

This clinical indication appears also indicated for patients at risk for CAD. As demonstrated in siblings of patients with premature CAD, conventional SPECT imaging uncovered in 29% of men and 9% of women asymptomatic siblings of patients with premature CAD (< 60 years of age) mild, stress-induced perfusion defects and, thus, asymptomatic or clinically silent CAD.[429,430] Again, given its superior performance characteristics, PET myocardial rest and stress imaging represents a more sensitive technique for uncovering clinically silent disease and, thus, would be indicated in patients at high risk for CAD. Similar observations have been reported for PET studies in first-degree relatives of patients with CAD.[195] Fifty percent of these patients with a sibling or parent with CAD demonstrated a flow defect.

MONITORING CORONARY ARTERY DISEASE

The high spatial and contrast resolution of the photon attenuation-free PET images together with superior properties of flow tracers renders PET ideal for monitoring progression and regression of CAD. Reports on the effect of strict dietary and lifestyle changes on the extent and severity of perfusion defects on PET MBF images serves as an example for this particular clinical indication of PET.[196,431]

IDENTIFICATION OF PATIENTS AT HIGH RISK FOR CORONARY EVENTS

Numerous trials with especially HMG-CoA reductase inhibitors have conclusively demonstrated their effectiveness for secondary and primary prevention of coronary events. This then raises the question of how to identify patients who are likely to benefit from such treatment for primary prevention. Pivotal to its success and cost effectiveness remains the identification of patients with the highest risk of a future cardiac event. Evaluation of the relative distribution and, in particular, measurement of MBF and of the myocardial flow reserve would seem to be an appropriate and noninvasive component of such risk assessment. Patients at risk, as shown in several studies in patients with abnormal lipid profiles, with diabetes, insulin resistance, or with a family trait of CAD, have demonstrated reduced hyperemic blood flows and flow reserves (see also Table 6-14). Beyond the initial assessment, measurements of MBF in absolute units could also prove useful as means for monitoring beneficial therapeutic effects.

Pediatric cardiovascular diseases

Congenital cardiovascular diseases, for example, cardiomyopathies or anomalous coronary arteries or, following surgical corrections of, for example, transposition of the great vessels, but also acquired disorders such as Kawasaki's disease, can be associated with diminished LV function.[270,432,433] The functional impairment may result from abnormal myocardial perfusion that is amenable to treatment with angioplasty or surgical repair of stenotic coronary reimplantation sites. Use of SPECT for delineating myocardial perfusion patterns in such patients may be limited because of its relatively poor spatial resolution. Therefore, PET with its markedly higher spatial resolution capability can offer especially in small children images of MBF and substrate metabolism of diagnostically meaningful and accurate information. As shown in Figure 6-42, MBF at rest and in response to pharmacological vasodilation as well as myocardial FDG uptake can be evaluated in even very young children (or as in this patient, a 2-month-old infant) and provide diagnostically useful information.

Opportunities for the evaluation of new pharmaceuticals

Besides established clinical indications and those of clinical potential value, cardiac PET further seems ideally suited for evaluating the efficacy of new pharmaceuticals. For example, studies in relatively small patient populations have allowed demonstration of beneficial effects of new antiatherosclerotic or lipid-lowering agents or of insulin sensitizers on the function of the human coronary circulation (Table 6-15). Efficacy studies of many of these agents require demonstration of beneficial effects on structural as well as functional alterations of the coronary circulation. Clearly, PET measurements can provide the functional component to structural changes. Effects of other agents, for example, anti-ischemic compounds, can similarly be evaluated and documented by probing the metabolism of ischemic myocardium with positron-emitting tracers.

FUTURE DEVELOPMENTS

This chapter attempted to provide an account of the current state of cardiac PET. It focused on well-established and, to a lesser extent, on currently emerging techniques used for probing noninvasively cardiovascular function in humans and

FIGURE 6-42. Example of a myocardial blood flow (MBF) and glucose uptake study in an infant following surgical correction of the great vessels. Short axis, vertical long axis, and horizontal long access cuts are shown from left to right. Notice on the myocardial perfusion images at rest the moderate decrease in perfusion in the anterior, the anterior-lateral wall, and the antereceptum. With dipyridamole stress, these defects become more severe. The FDG images do show, however, enhanced glucose utilization in the anterior interventricular septum and the right ventricular myocardium.

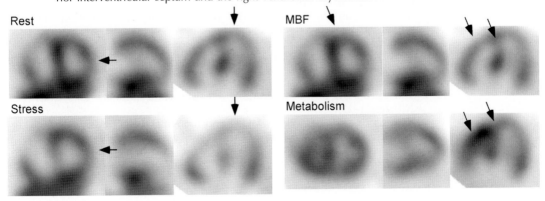

for identifying abnormal processes and cardiovascular disease. Admittedly, some aspects of the current PET technology in cardiology that include a large body of experimental and clinical investigations, for example, studies on the neuronal activity and control, have not been included in this chapter, simply for reasons of brevity. Nevertheless, it must be emphasized that such studies on neuronal control have provided novel and exciting insights in the reinnervation of the deinnervated transplant heart, on functional aspects of neuronal control of the coronary circulation and on the possible interaction between neuronal activity and substrate metabolism.[353,434,435] No less important have been studies demonstrating with PET phenotypic consequences of genetically determined cardiovascular disorders, for example, in myotonic dystrophy.[436,437] These studies found significant correlations between the severity of the genetic alteration (for example, the number of triplet repeats) and abnormalities in myocardial flow reserve and glucose phosphorylation.[436,437]

These areas of research promise even more comprehensive insights into the function of the cardiovascular system. Other developments include the transfer of the PET technology into small animals thereby offering the unique opportunity to define, for example, phenotypic expressions of genetic modifications. PET imaging techniques have also been used for monitoring myocardial repair through, for example, myoblast transplantation into human myocardium.[438] They hold promise for imaging expression of a specifically targeted gene and, thus, are likely to serve as vehicles for designing, validating, and implementing gene therapy approaches.

REFERENCES

1. Hoffman EJ, Phelps ME, Wisenberg G, Schelbert HR, Kuhl DE. Electrocardiographic gating in positron emission computed tomography. *J Comp Assist Tomogr.* 1979;3:733–739.
2. Yamashita K, Tamaki N, Yonekura Y, et al. Quantitative analysis of regional wall motion by gated myocardial positron emission tomography: Validation and comparison with left ventriculography. *J Nucl Med.* 1989;30:1775–1786.
3. Yamashita K, Tamaki N, Yonekura Y, et al. Regional wall thickening of left ventricle evaluated by gated positron emission tomography in relation to myocardial perfusion and glucose metabolism. *J Nucl Med.* 1991;32:679–685.
4. Porenta G, Kuhle W, Sinha S, et al. Parameter estimation of cardiac geometry by ECG-gated PET imaging: validation using magnetic resonance imaging and echocardiography. *J Nucl Med.* 1995;36:1123–1129.
5. Boyd HL, Gunn RN, Marinho NV, et al. Non-invasive measurement of left ventricular volumes and function by gated positron emission tomography. *Eur J Nucl Med.* 1996;23:1594–1602.
6. Boyd HL, Rosen SD, Rimoldi O, Cunningham VJ, Camici PG. Normal values for left ventricular volumes obtained using gated PET. *Gior Ital Cardiol.* 1998;28:1207–1214.
7. Hattori N, Bengel FM, Mehilli J, et al. Global and regional functional measurements with gated FDG PET in comparison with left ventriculography. *Eur J Nucl Med.* 2001;28:221–229.
8. Hoffman EJ, Huang SC, Phelps ME. Quantitation in positron emission computed tomography: 1. Effect of object size. *J Comp Assist Tomogr.* 1979;3:299–308.
9. Henze E, Huang SC, Ratib O, Hoffman E, Phelps ME, Schelbert HR. Measurements of regional tissue and blood-pool radiotracer concentrations from serial tomographic images of the heart. *J Nucl Med.* 1983;24:987–996.
10. Sinha S, Sinha U, Czernin J, Porenta G, Schelbert HR. Noninvasive assessment of myo-

cardial perfusion and metabolism: feasibility of registering gated MR and PET images. *Am J Roentgen.* 1995;164:301–307.

11. Grover-McKay M, Schwaiger M, Krivokapich J, Perloff JK, Phelps ME, Schelbert HR. Regional myocardial blood flow and metabolism at rest in mildly symptomatic patients with hypertrophic cardiomyopathy [see comments]. *J Am Coll Cardiol.* 1989;13:317–324.

12. Nienaber CA, Gambhir SS, Mody FV, et al. Regional myocardial blood flow and glucose utilization in symptomatic patients with hypertrophic cardiomyopathy. *Circulation.* 1993;87:1580–1590.

13. Parodi O, Schelbert HR, Schwaiger M, Hansen H, Selin C, Hoffman EJ. Cardiac emission computed tomography: underestimation of regional tracer concentrations due to wall motion abnormalities. *J Comp Assist Tomogr.* 1984;8:1083–1092.

14. Kuhle WG, Porenta G, Huang SC, et al. Quantification of regional myocardial blood flow using 13N-ammonia and reoriented dynamic positron emission tomographic imaging. *Circulation.* 1992;86:1004–1107.

15. Porenta G, Kuhle W, Czernin J, et al. Semiquantitative assessment of myocardial blood flow and viability using polar map displays of cardiac PET images. *J Nucl Med.* 1992;33:1628–1636.

16. Nekolla SG, Miethaner C, Nguyen N, Ziegler SI, Schwaiger M. Reproducibility of polar map generation and assessment of defect severity and extent assessment in myocardial perfusion imaging using positron emission tomography. *Eur J Nucl Med.* 1998;25:1313–1321.

17. Choi Y, Hawkins RA, Huang SC, et al. Parametric images of myocardial metabolic rate of glucose generated from dynamic cardiac PET and 2-[18F]fluoro-2-deoxy-d-glucose studies. *J Nucl Med.* 1991;32:733–738.

18. Blanksma PK, Willemsen AT, Meeder JG, et al. Quantitative myocardial mapping of perfusion and metabolism using parametric polar map displays in cardiac PET. *J Nucl Med.* 1995;36:153–158.

19. Hicks K, Ganti G, Mullani N, Gould KL. Automated quantitation of three-dimensional cardiac positron emission tomography for routine clinical use. *J Nucl Med.* 1989;30:1787–1797.

20. Laubenbacher C, Rothley J, Sitomer J, et al. An automated analysis program for the evaluation of cardiac PET studies: Initial results in the detection and localization of coronary artery disease using nitrogen-13-ammonia. *J Nucl Med.* 1993;34:968–978.

21. Gould KL. Myocardial perfusion after cholesterol lowering. *J Atheroscler Thromb.* 1996;3:59–61.

22. Wu HM, Hoh CK, Buxton DB, et al. Quantification of myocardial blood flow using dynamic nitrogen-13-ammonia PET studies and factor analysis of dynamic structures. *J Nucl Med.* 1995;36:2087–2093.

23. Wu HM, Hoh CK, Choi Y, et al. Factor analysis for extraction of blood time-activity curves in dynamic FDG-PET studies. *J Nucl Med.* 1995;36:1714–1722.

24. Hermansen F, Ashburner J, Spinks TJ, Kooner JS, Camici PG, Lammertsma AA. Generation of myocardial factor images directly from the dynamic oxygen-15-water scan without use of an oxygen-15-carbon monoxide blood-pool scan. *J Nucl Med.* 1998;39:1696–1702.

25. Renkin EM. Transport of potassium-42 from blood tissue in isolated mammalian skeletal muscles. *Am J Physiol.* 1959;197:1205–1210.

26. Crone C. Permeability of capillaries in various organs as determined by use of the indicator diffusion method. *Acta Physiol Scand.* 1963;58:292–305.

27. Schön HR, Schelbert HR, Robinson G, et al. C-11 labeled palmitic acid for the noninvasive evaluation of regional myocardial fatty acid metabolism with positron-computed tomography. I. Kinetics of C-11 palmitic acid in normal myocardium. *Am Heart J.* 1982;103:532–547.

28. Schelbert HR, Henze E, Schon HR, et al. C-11 palmitate for the noninvasive evaluation of regional myocardial fatty acid metabolism with positron computed tomography. III. In vivo demonstration of the effects of substrate availability on myocardial metabolism. *Am Heart J.* 1983;105:492–504.

29. Wisneski JA, Gertz EW, Neese RA, Mayr M. Myocardial metabolism of free fatty acids. Studies with 14C-labeled substrates in humans. *J Clin Invest.* 1987;79:359–366.

30. Bergmann SR, Fox KA, Rand AL, et al. Quantification of regional myocardial blood flow in vivo with H215O. *Circulation.* 1984;70:724–733.

31. Bergmann SR, Herrero P, Markham J, Weinheimer CJ, Walsh MN. Noninvasive quantitation of myocardial blood flow in human subjects with oxygen-15-labeled water and positron emission tomography. *J Am Coll Cardiol.* 1989;14:639–652.

32. Iida H, Takahashi A, Tamura Y, Ono Y, Lammertsma AA. Myocardial blood flow: comparison of oxygen-15-water bolus injection, slow infusion and oxygen-15-carbon dioxide slow inhalation. *J Nucl Med.* 1995;36:78–85.

33. Hermansen F, Rosen SD, Fath-Ordoubadi F, et al. Measurement of myocardial blood flow with oxygen-15 labelled water: comparison of different administration protocols. *Eur J Nucl Med.* 1998;25:751–759.

34. Araujo L, Lammertsma A, Rhodes C, et al. Noninvasive quantification of regional myocardial blood flow in coronary artery disease with oxygen-15-labeled carbon dioxide inhalation and positron emission tomography. *Circulation.* 1991;83:875–885.

35. Iida H, Rhodes C, de Silva R, et al. Myocardial tissue fraction-correction for partial volume effects and measure of tissue viability. *J Nucl Med.* 1991;32:2169–2175.

36. Iida H, Tamura Y, Kitamura K, Bloomfield PM, Eberl S, Ono Y. Histochemical correlates of (15)O-water-perfusable tissue fraction in experimental canine studies of old myocardial infarction. *J Nucl Med.* 2000;41:1737–1745.

37. de Silva R, Yamamoto Y, Rhodes CG, et al. Preoperative prediction of the outcome of coronary revascularization using positron emission tomography. *Circulation.* 1992;86: 1738–1742.

38. Yamamoto Y, De Silva R, Rhodes C, et al. A new strategy for the assessment of viable myocardium and regional myocardial blood flow using ^{15}O-water and dynamic positron emission tomography. *Circulation.* 1992;86:167–178.

39. Phelps ME, Hoffman EJ, Raybaud C. Factors which affect cerebral uptake and retention of 13NH3. *Stroke.* 1977;8:694–702.

40. Post RL, Jolly PC. The linkage of sodium, potassium and ammonium active transport across the human erythrocyte membrane. *Biochim Biophys Acta.* 1957;25:118–128.

41. Schelbert HR, Phelps ME, Huang SC, et al. N-13 ammonia as an indicator of myocardial blood flow. *Circulation.* 1981;63:1259–1272.

42. Bergmann SR, Hack S, Tewson T, Welch MJ, Sobel BE. The dependence of accumulation of 13NH3 by myocardium on metabolic factors and its implications for quantitative assessment of perfusion. *Circulation.* 1980;61:34–43.

43. Krivokapich J, Keen RE, Phelps ME, Shine KI, Barrio JR. Effects of anoxia on kinetics of [13N] glutamate and 13NH3 metabolism in rabbit myocardium. *Circulat Res.* 1987;60: 505–516.

44. Krivokapich J, Smith GT, Huang SC, et al. 13N ammonia myocardial imaging at rest and with exercise in normal volunteers. Quantification of absolute myocardial perfusion with dynamic positron emission tomography [see comments]. *Circulation.* 1989;80: 1328–1337.

45. Hutchins GD, Schwaiger M, Rosenspire KC, Krivokapich J, Schelbert H, Kuhl DE. Noninvasive quantification of regional blood flow in the human heart using N-13 ammonia and dynamic positron emission tomographic imaging. *J Am Coll Cardiol.* 1990;15: 1032–1042.

46. Bellina CR, Parodi O, Camici P, et al. Simultaneous in vitro and in vivo validation of nitrogen-13-ammonia for the assessment of regional myocardial blood flow. *J Nucl Med.* 1990;31:1335–1343.

47. Bol A, Melin JA, Vanoverschelde JL, et al. Direct comparison of [13N]ammonia and [15O]water estimates of perfusion with quantification of regional myocardial blood flow by microspheres. *Circulation.* 1993;87:512–525.

48. Muzik O, Beanlands RS, Hutchins GD, Mangner TJ, Nguyen N, Schwaiger M. Validation of nitrogen-13-ammonia tracer kinetic model for quantification of myocardial blood flow using PET. *J Nucl Med.* 1993;34:83–91.

49. Choi Y, Huang SC, Hawkins RA, et al. Quantification of myocardial blood flow using 13N-ammonia and PET: comparison of tracer models. *J Nucl Med.* 1999;40:1045–1055.

50. Czernin J, Müller P, Chan S, et al. Influence of age and hemodynamics on myocardial blood flow and flow reserve. *Circulation.* 1993;88:62–69.

51. Wilson R, Laughlin D, Ackell P. Transluminal subselective measurement of coronary artery blood flow velocity and vasodilator reserve in man. *Circulation.* 1985;72:82–89.

52. Kotzerke J, Glatting G, van den Hoff J, et al. Validation of myocardial blood flow estimation with nitrogen-13 ammonia PET by the argon inert gas technique in humans. *Eur J Nucl Med.* 2001;28:340–345.

53. Nitzsche EU, Choi Y, Czernin J, Hoh CK, Huang SC, Schelbert HR. Noninvasive quantification of myocardial blood flow in humans. A direct comparison of the [13N]ammonia and the [15O]water techniques. *Circulation.* 1996;93:2000–2006.

54. Huang SC, Williams BA, Krivokapich J, Araujo L, Phelps ME, Schelbert HR. Rabbit myocardial 82Rb kinetics and a compartmental model for blood flow estimation. *Am J Physiol.* 1989;256:H1156–H1164.

55. Goldstein RA, Mullani NA, Marani SK, Fisher DJ, Gould KL, O'Brien HA Jr. Myocardial perfusion with rubidium-82. II. Effects of metabolic and pharmacologic interventions. *J Nucl Med.* 1983;24:907–915.

56. Mullani NA, Goldstein RA, Gould KL, et al. Myocardial perfusion with rubidium-82. I. Measurement of extraction fraction and flow with external detectors. *J Nucl Med.* 1983;24:898–906.

57. Mullani NA. Myocardial perfusion with rubidium-82: III. Theory relating severity of coronary stenosis to perfusion deficit. *J Nucl Med.* 1984;25:1190–1196.

58. Budinger TF, Yano Y, Moyer B, Twitchell J, Huesman RH. Myocardial extraction of Rb-82 vs. flow determined by positron emission tomography. *J Nucl Med.* 1983;68:III-81.

59. Glatting G, Bergmann K, Stollfub J, et al. Myocardial Rb extraction fraction: Determination in humans. *J Am Coll Cardiol.* 1995;25:364A.

60. Goldstein RA. Kinetics of rubidium-82 after coronary occlusion and reperfusion. Assessment of patency and viability in open-chested dogs. *J Clin Invest.* 1985;75:1131–1137.

61. Goldstein RA. Rubidium-82 kinetics after coronary occlusion: Temporal relation of net myocardial accumulation and viability in open-chested dogs. *J Nucl Med.* 1986;27:1456–1461.

62. Herrero P, Markham J, Shelton ME, Weinheimer CJ, Bergmann SR. Noninvasive quantification of regional myocardial perfusion with rubidium-82 and positron emission tomography. Exploration of a mathematical model. *Circulation.* 1990;82:1377–1386.

63. Lin JW, Laine AF, Akinboboye O, Bergmann SR. Use of wavelet transforms in analysis of time-activity data from cardiac PET. *J Nucl Med.* 2001;42:194–200.

64. Lin JW, Sciacca RR, Chou RL, Laine AF, Bergmann SR. Quantification of myocardial perfusion in human subjects using 82Rb and wavelet-based noise reduction. *J Nucl Med.* 2001;42:201–208.

65. Green MA, Mathias CJ, Welch MJ, et al. Copper-62-labeled pyruvaldehyde bis(N4-methylthiosemicarbazonato)copper(II): synthesis and evaluation as a positron emission tomography tracer for cerebral and myocardial perfusion. *J Nucl Med.* 1990;31:1989–1996.

66. Shelton ME, Green MA, Mathias CJ, Welch MJ, Bergmann SR. Kinetics of copper-PTSM in isolated hearts: a novel tracer for measuring blood flow with positron emission tomography. *J Nucl Med.* 1989;30:1843–1847.

67. Marshall R, Leidholdt EJ, Zhang D, Barnett C. Technetium-99m hexakis 2-methoxy-2-isobutyl isonitrile and thallium-201 extraction, washout, and retention at varying coronary flow rates in rabbit heart. *Circulation.* 1990;82:998–1007.

68. Beanlands RS, Muzik O, Mintun M, et al. The kinetics of copper-62-PTSM in the normal human heart. *J Nucl Med.* 1992;33:684–690.

69. Wallhaus TR, Lacy J, Stewart R, et al. Copper-62-pyruvaldehyde bis(N-methyl-thiosemicarbazone) PET imaging in the detection of coronary artery disease in humans. *J Nucl Cardiol.* 2001;8:67–74.

70. Herrero P, Markham J, Weinheimer CJ, et al. Quantification of regional myocardial perfusion with generator-produced 62Cu-PTSM and positron emission tomography. *Circulation.* 1993;87:173–183.

71. Mélon P, Brihaye C, Degueldre C, et al. Myocardial kinetics of potassium-38 in humans and comparison with Copper-62-PTSM. *J Nucl Med.* 1994;35:1116–1122.

72. Poe ND. Comparative myocardial uptake and clearance characteristics of potassium and cesium. *J Nucl Med.* 1972;13:557–560.

73. Chan SY, Brunken RC, Phelps ME, Schelbert HR. Use of the metabolic tracer carbon-11-acetate for evaluation of regional myocardial perfusion. *J Nucl Med.* 1991;32:665–672.

74. Wolpers HG, Burchert W, van den Hoff J, Weinhardt R, Meyer GJ, Lichtlen PR. Assessment of myocardial viability by use of 11C-acetate and positron emission tomography. Threshold criteria of reversible dysfunction. *Circulation.* 1997;95:1417–1424.

75. Sun KT, Yeatman LA, Buxton DB, et al. Simultaneous measurement of myocardial oxygen consumption and blood flow using [1-carbon-11]acetate. *J Nucl Med.* 1998;39: 272–280.

76. Sciacca RR, Akinboboye O, Chou RL, Epstein S, Bergmann SR. Measurement of myocardial blood flow with PET using 1-11C-acetate. *J Nucl Med.* 2001;42:63–70.

77. Nickles R, Nunn A, Stone C, Christian B. Technetium-94m-teboroxime: synthesis, dosimetry and initial PET imaging studies. *J Nucl Med.* 1993;34:1058–1066.

78. Stone C, Christian B, Nickles R, Perlman S. Technetium 94m-labeled methoxyisobutyl isonitrile: Dosimetry and resting cardiac imaging with positron emission tomography. *J Nucl Cardiol.* 1994;1:425–433.

79. Nagamachi S, Czernin J, Kim AS, et al. Reproducibility of measurements of regional resting and hyperemic myocardial blood flow assessed with PET. *J Nucl Med.* 1996;37:1626–1631.

80. Kaufmann PA, Gnecchi-Ruscone T, Yap JT, Rimoldi O, Camici PG. Assessment of the reproducibility of baseline and hyperemic myocardial blood flow measurements with 15O-labeled water and PET. *J Nucl Med.* 1999;40:1848–1856.

81. Iida H, Yokoyama I, Agostini D, et al. Quantitative assessment of regional myocardial blood flow using oxygen-15-labelled water and positron emission tomography: a multicentre evaluation in Japan. *Eur J Nucl Med.* 2000;27:192–201.

82. Marcus M, Kerber R, Erhardt J, Falsetti H, Davis D, Abboud F. Spatial and temporal heterogeneity of left ventricular perfusion in awake dogs. *Am Heart J.* 1977;94:748–754.

83. King R, Bassingthwaighte J, Hales J, Rowell L. Stability of heterogeneity of myocardial blood flow in normal awake baboons. 1985;57:285–295.

84. Gould KL, Goldstein RA, Mullani NA, et al. Noninvasive assessment of coronary stenoses by myocardial perfusion imaging during pharmacologic coronary vasodilation. VIII. Clinical feasibility of positron cardiac imaging without a cyclotron using generator-produced rubidium-82. *J Am Coll Cardiol.* 1986;7:775–789.

85. Demer LL, Gould KL, Goldstein RA, et al. Assessment of coronary artery disease severity by positron emission tomography. Comparison with quantitative arteriography in 193 patients. *Circulation.* 1989;79:825–835.

85a. Schelbert HR, Wisenberg G, Phelps ME, Gould KL, Henze E, Hoffman EJ, Gomes A, Kuhl DE. Noninvasive assessment of coronary stenoses by myocardial imaging during pharmacologic coronary vasodilation. VI. Detection of coronary artery disease in human beings with intravenous N-13 ammonia and positron computed tomography. *Am J Cardiol.* 1982;49:1197–1207.

85b. Yonekura Y, Tamaki N, Senda M, Nohara R, Kambara H, Konishi Y, Koide H, Kureshi SA, Saji H, Ban T, et al. Detection of coronary artery disease with 13N-ammonia and high-resolution positron-emission computed tomography. *Am Heart J.* 1987;113:645–654.

86. Gerber BL, Melin JA, Bol A, et al. Nitrogen-13- and oxygen-15-water estimates of absolute myocardial perfusion in left ventricular ischemic dysfunction. *J Nucl Med.* 1998;39: 1655–1662.

87. Opie LH. Metabolism of the heart in health and disease. I. *Am Heart J.* 1968;76:685–698.

88. Liedtke AJ. Alterations of carbohydrate and lipid metabolism in the acutely ischemic heart. *Prog Cardiovasc Dis.* 1981;23:321–336.

89. Bing RJ. The metabolism of the heart. In: Harvey Society of NY ed. *Harvey Lecture Series.* New York: Academic Press; 1954:27–70.

90. Keul J, Doll E, Steim H, Fleer U, Reindell H. Über den Stoffwechsel des menschlichen Herzens. III. Der oxidative Stoffwechsel des menschlichen Herzens unter verschiedened Arbeitsbedingungen II. *Pflugers Archiv Gesamte Physiol Menschen Tiere.* 1965;282:43–53.

91. Keul J, Doll E, Steim H, Homburger H, Kern H, Reindell H. Uber den Stoffwechsel des menschlichen Herzens. I. Substratversorgung des gesunden Herzens in Ruhe, während und nach körperlicher Arbeit. *Pflugers Archiv Gesamte Physiol Menschen Tiere.* 1965;282:1–27.

92. Randle RJ, Garland BP, Hales CN, Newsholme EA. The glucose fatty acid cycle: its role in insulin sensitivity and the metabolic disturbances in diabetes mellitus. *Lancet.* 1963;1:785–789.

93. Holmberg S, Serzysko W, Varnauskas E. Coronary circulation during heavy exercise in control subjects and patients with coronary heart disease. *Acta Med Scand.* 1971;190: 465–480.

94. Wisneski JA, Gertz EW, Neese RA, Gruenke LD, Morris DL, Craig JC. Metabolic fate of extracted glucose in normal human myocardium. *J Clin Invest.* 1985;76:1819–1827.

95. Yamamoto Y, de Silva R, Rhodes CG, et al. Noninvasive quantification of regional myocardial metabolic rate of oxygen by 15O2 inhalation and positron emission tomography. Experimental validation. *Circulation.* 1996;94:808–816.

96. Iida H, Rhodes CG, Araujo LI, et al. Noninvasive quantification of regional myocardial metabolic rate for oxygen by use of 15O2 inhalation and positron emission tomography. Theory, error analysis, and application in humans. *Circulation.* 1996;94:792–807.

97. Laine H, Katoh C, Luotolahti M, et al. Myocardial oxygen consumption is unchanged but efficiency is reduced in patients with essential hypertension and left ventricular hypertrophy. *Circulation.* 1999;100:2425–2430.

98. Takala TO, Nuutila P, Katoh C, et al. Myocardial blood flow, oxygen consumption, and fatty acid uptake in endurance athletes during insulin stimulation. *Am J Physiol.* 1999; 277:E585–E590.

99. Brown M, Marshall DR, Sobel BE, Bergmann SR. Delineation of myocardial oxygen utilization with carbon-11-labeled acetate. *Circulation.* 1987;76:687–696.

100. Brown MA, Myears DW, Bergmann SR. Noninvasive assessment of canine myocardial oxidative metabolism with carbon-11 acetate and positron emission tomography. *J Am Coll Cardiol.* 1988;12:1054–1063.

101. Buxton DB, Schwaiger M, Nguyen A, Phelps ME, Schelbert HR. Radiolabeled acetate as a tracer of myocardial tricarboxylic acid cycle flux. *Circulat Res.* 1988;63:628–634.

102. Brown MA, Myears DW, Bergmann SR. Validity of estimates of myocardial oxidative metabolism with carbon-11 acetate and positron emission tomography despite altered patterns of substrate utilization. *J Nucl Med.* 1989;30:187–193.

103. Buxton DB, Nienaber CA, Luxen A, et al. Noninvasive quantitation of regional myocardial oxygen consumption in vivo with [1-11C]acetate and dynamic positron emission tomography. *Circulation.* 1989;79:134–142.

104. Armbrecht JJ, Buxton DB, Schelbert HR. Validation of [1–11C]acetate as a tracer for noninvasive assessment of oxidative metabolism with positron emission tomography in normal, ischemic, postischemic, and hyperemic canine myocardium. *Circulation.* 1990; 81:1594–1605.

105. Armbrecht JJ, Buxton DB, Brunken RC, Phelps ME, Schelbert HR. Regional myocardial oxygen consumption determined noninvasively in humans with [1–11C]acetate and dynamic positron tomography. *Circulation.* 1989;80:863–872.

106. Henes CG, Bergmann SR, Walsh MN, Sobel BE, Geltman EM. Assessment of myocardial oxidative metabolic reserve with positron emission tomography and carbon-11 acetate. *J Nucl Med.* 1989;30:1489–1499.

107. Ng CK, Huang SC, Schelbert HR, Buxton DB. Validation of a model for [1–11C]acetate as a tracer of cardiac oxidative metabolism. *Am J Physiol.* 1994;266:H1304–H1315.

108. Sun KT, Chen K, Huang SC, et al. Compartment model for measuring myocardial oxygen consumption using [1–11C]acetate. *J Nucl Med.* 1997;38:459–466.

109. Ukkonen H, Knuuti J, Katoh C, et al. Use of [11C]acetate and [15O]O2 PET for the assessment of myocardial oxygen utilization in patients with chronic myocardial infarction. *Eur J Nucl Med.* 2001;28:334–339.

110. Schön HR, Schelbert HR, Najafi A, et al. C-11 labeled palmitic acid for the noninvasive evaluation of regional myocardial fatty acid metabolism with positron-computed tomography. II. Kinetics of C-11 palmitic acid in acutely ischemic myocardium. *Am Heart J.* 1982;103:548–561.

111. Fox KA, Abendschein DR, Ambos HD, Sobel BE, Bergmann SR. Efflux of metabolized and nonmetabolized fatty acid from canine myocardium. Implications for quantifying myocardial metabolism tomographically. *Circulat Res.* 1985;57:232–243.

112. Rosamond TL, Abendschein DR, Sobel BE, Bergmann SR, Fox KA. Metabolic fate of radiolabeled palmitate in ischemic canine myocardium: implications for positron emission tomography. *J Nucl Med.* 1987;28:1322–1329.

113. Wyns W, Schwaiger M, Huang SC, et al. Effects of inhibition of fatty acid oxidation on myocardial kinetics of 11C-labeled palmitate. *Circulat Res.* 1989;65:1787–1797.

114. Bergmann SR, Weinheimer CJ, Markham J, Herrero P. Quantitation of myocardial fatty acid metabolism using PET. *J Nucl Med.* 1996;37:1723–1730.

115. Davila-Roman VG, Vedala G, Herrero P, et al. Altered myocardial fatty acid and glu-

cose metabolism in idiopathic dilated cardiomyopathy. *J Am Coll Cardiol.* 2002;40: 271–277.

116. Stone CK, Pooley RA, DeGrado TR, et al. Myocardial uptake of the fatty acid analog 14-fluorine-18-fluoro-6-thia-heptadecanoic acid in comparison to beta-oxidation rates by tritiated palmitate. *J Nucl Med.* 1998;39:1690–1696.

117. DeGrado TR, Wang S, Holden JE, Nickles RJ, Taylor M, Stone CK. Synthesis and preliminary evaluation of (18)F-labeled 4-thia palmitate as a PET tracer of myocardial fatty acid oxidation. *Nucl Med Biol.* 2000;27:221–231.

118. Renstrom B, Rommelfanger S, Stone CK, et al. Comparison of fatty acid tracers FTHA and BMIPP during myocardial ischemia and hypoxia. *J Nucl Med.* 1998;39:1684–1689.

119. Mäki MT, Haaparanta M, Nuutila P, et al. Free fatty acid uptake in the myocardium and skeletal muscle using fluorine-18-fluoro-6-thia-heptadecanoic acid. *J Nucl Med.* 1998;39:1320–1327.

120. Taylor M, Wallhaus TR, Degrado TR, et al. An evaluation of myocardial fatty acid and glucose uptake using PET with [18F]fluoro-6-thia-heptadecanoic acid. *J Nucl Med.* 2001;42:55–62.

121. Hawkins RA, Mans AM, Davis DW, Vina JR, Hibbard LS. Cerebral glucose use measured with [14C]glucose labeled in the 1, 2, or 6 position. *Am J Physiol.* 1985;248: C170–C176.

122. Stone-Elander S, Halldin C, Langstrom B, et al. Production method for [11C]-D-glucose labeled in carbon-1 for positron emission tomography of glucose metabolism. *Acta Radiol Suppl.* 1991;376:102–103.

123. Dence CS, Powers WJ, Welch MJ. Improved synthesis of 1-[11C]D-glucose. *Appl Radiat Isot.* 1993;44:971–980.

124. Herrero P, Weinheimer CJ, Dence C, Oellerich WF, Gropler RJ. Quantification of myocardial glucose utilization by PET and 1-carbon-11-glucose. *J Nucl Cardiol.* 2002;9:5–14.

125. Phelps ME, Hoffman EJ, Selin C, et al. Investigation of [18F]2-fluoro-2-deoxyglucose for the measure of myocardial glucose metabolism. *J Nucl Med.* 1978;19:1311–1319.

126. Krivokapich J, Huang SC, Selin CE, Phelps ME. Fluorodeoxyglucose rate constants, lumped constant, and glucose metabolic rate in rabbit heart. *Am J Physiol.* 1987;252:H777–H787.

127. Sokoloff L, Reivich M, Kennedy C, et al. The [14C]-deoxyglucose method for the measurement of local cerebral glucose utilization: Theory, procedure and normal values in the conscious and anesthetized albino rat. *J Neurochem.* 1977;28:897–916.

128. Ratib O, Phelps ME, Huang SC, Henze E, Selin CE, Schelbert HR. Positron tomography with deoxyglucose for estimating local myocardial glucose metabolism. *J Nucl Med.* 1982;23:577–586.

129. Gambhir SS, Schwaiger M, Huang SC, et al. Simple noninvasive quantification method for measuring myocardial glucose utilization in humans employing positron emission tomography and fluorine-18 deoxyglucose. *J Nucl Med.* 1989;30:359–366.

130. Patlak CS, Blasberg RG. Graphical evaluation of blood-to-brain transfer constants from multiple-time uptake data. *J Cereb Blood Flow Metab.* 1985;5:584–590.

131. Schneider CA, Nguyen VT, Taegtmeyer H. Feeding and fasting determine postischemic glucose utilization in isolated working rat hearts. *Am J Physiol.* 1991;260:H542–H548.

132. Russell RR III, Nguyen VT, Mrus JM, Taegtmeyer H. Fasting and lactate unmask insulin responsiveness in the isolated working rat heart. *Am J Physiol.* 1992;263:E556–E561.

133. Russell RR III, Cline GW, Guthrie PH, Goodwin GW, Shulman GI, Taegtmeyer H. Regulation of exogenous and endogenous glucose metabolism by insulin and acetoacetate in the isolated working rat heart. A three tracer study of glycolysis, glycogen metabolism, and glucose oxidation. *J Clin Invest.* 1997;100:2892–2899.

134. Doenst T, Taegtmeyer H. Complexities underlying the quantitative determination of myocardial glucose uptake with 2-deoxyglucose. *J Molec Cell Cardiol.* 1998;V30:1595–1604.

135. Botker HE, Goodwin GW, Holden JE, Doenst T, Gjedde A, Taegtmeyer H. Myocardial glucose uptake measured with fluorodeoxyglucose: A prospect method to account for variable lumped constants. *J Nucl Med.* 1999;40:1186–1196.

136. Hariharan R, Bray M, Ganim R, Doenst T, Goodwin GW, Taegtmeyer H. Fundamental limitations of [F-18]2-deoxy-2-fluoro-D-glucose for assessing myocardial glucose uptake. *Circulation.* 1995;91:2435–2444.

137. DeFronzo RA, Tobin JD, Andres R. Glucose clamp technique: a method for quantifying insulin secretion and resistance. *Am J Physiol.* 1979;237:E214–E223.

138. Hicks R, von Dahl J, Lee K, Herman W, Kalff V, Schwaiger M. Insulin-glucose clamp for standardization of metabolic conditions during F-18 fluoro-deoxyglucose PET imaging. *J Am Coll Cardiol.* 1991;17:381A.

139. Meaki M, Luotolahti M, Nuutila P, et al. Glucose uptake in the chronically dysfunctional but viable myocardium. *Circulation.* 1996;93:1658–1666.

140. Gerber BL, Ordoubadi FF, Wijns W, et al. Positron emission tomography using(18)F-fluoro-deoxyglucose and euglycaemic hyperinsulinaemic glucose clamp: optimal criteria for the prediction of recovery of post-ischaemic left ventricular dysfunction. Results from the European Community Concerted Action Multicenter Study on Use of (18)F-fluoro-deoxyglucose Positron Emission Tomography for the Detection of Myocardial Viability. *Eur Heart J.* 2001;22:1691–1701.

141. Bax JJ, Visser FC, Poldermans D, et al. Feasibility, safety and image quality of cardiac FDG studies during hyperinsulinaemic-euglycaemic clamping. *Eur J Nucl Med.* 2002;29:452–457.

142. Nuutila P, Knuuti M, Raitakari M, et al. Effect of antilipolysis on heart and skeletal muscle glucose uptake in overnight fasted humans. *Am J Physiol.* 1994;267:E941–E946.

143. Stone C, Holden J, Stanley W, Perlman S. Effect of nicotinic acid on exogenous myocardial glucose utilization. *J Nucl Med.* 1995;36:996–1002.

144. Vitale GD, deKemp RA, Ruddy TD, Williams K, Beanlands RSB. Myocardial glucose utilization and optimization of ^{18}F-FDG PET imaging in patients with non-insulin-dependent diabetes mellitus, coronary artery disease, and left ventricular dysfunction. *J Nucl Med.* 2001;42:1730–1736.

145. Chareonthaitawee P, Kaufmann PA, Rimoldi O, Camici PG. Heterogeneity of resting and hyperemic myocardial blood flow in healthy humans. *Cardiovasc Res.* 2001;50:151–161.

146. Krivokapich J, Huang SC, Schelbert HR. Assessment of the effects of dobutamine on myocardial blood flow and oxidative metabolism in normal human subjects using nitrogen-13 ammonia and carbon-11 acetate. *Am J Cardiol.* 1993;71:1351–1356.

147. Senneff MJ, Geltman EM, Bergmann SR. Noninvasive delineation of the effects of moderate aging on myocardial perfusion [published erratum appears in *J Nucl Med* 1992; 33(2):201] [see comments]. *J Nucl Med.* 1991;32:2037–2042.

148. Uren NG, Camici PG, Melin JA, et al. Effect of aging on myocardial perfusion reserve. *J Nucl Med.* 1995;36:2032–2036.

149. Kalliokoski KK, Nuutila P, Laine H, et al. Myocardial perfusion and perfusion reserve in endurance-trained men. *Med Sci Sports Exerc.* 2002;34:948–953.

150. Radvan J, Choudhury L, Sheridan DJ, Camici PG. Comparison of coronary vasodilator reserve in elite rowing athletes versus hypertrophic cardiomyopathy. *Am J Cardiol.* 1997;80:1621–1623.

151. Brown BG, Josephson MA, Peterson RB, et al. Intravenous dipyridamole combined with isometric handgrip for near maximal acute increase in coronary flow in patients with coronary artery disease. *Am J Cardiol.* 1981;48:1077–1085.

152. Czernin J, Auerbach M, Sun KT, Phelps M, Schelbert HR. Effects of modified pharmacologic stress approaches on hyperemic myocardial blood flow. *J Nucl Med.* 1995;36:575–580.

153. Chan SY, Brunken RC, Czernin J, et al. Comparison of maximal myocardial blood flow during adenosine infusion with that of intravenous dipyridamole in normal men. *J Am Coll Cardiol.* 1992;20:979–985.

154. Kaufmann PA, Gnecchi-Ruscone T, di Terlizzi M, Schäfers KP, Lüscher TF, Camici PG. Coronary heart disease in smokers: vitamin C restores coronary microcirculatory function. *Circulation.* 2000;102:1233–1238.

155. Huggins GS, Pasternak RC, Alpert NM, Fischman AJ, Gewirtz H. Effects of short-term treatment of hyperlipidemia on coronary vasodilator function and myocardial perfusion in regions having substantial impairment of baseline dilator reserve. *Circulation.* 1998;98:1291–1296.

156. Iwado Y, Yoshinaga K, Furayama H, et al. Decreased endothelium-dependent coronary vosmotion in healthy young smokers. *Eur J Nucl Med.* 2002;29:984–990.

157. Tadamura E, Iida H, Matsumoto K, et al. Comparison of myocardial blood flow during dobutamine-atropine infusion with that after dipyridamole administration in normal men. *J Am Coll Cardiol.* 2001;37:130–136.

158. Nabel EG, Ganz P, Gordon JB, Alexander RW, Selwyn AP. Dilation of normal and constriction of atherosclerotic coronary arteries caused by the cold pressor test. *Circulation.* 1988;77:43–52.

159. Zeiher AM, Drexler H, Wollschlaeger H, Saurbier B, Just H. Coronary vasomotion in response to sympathetic stimulation in humans: importance of the functional integrity of the endothelium [see comments]. *J Am Coll Cardiol.* 1989;14:1181–1190.

160. Zeiher AM, Drexler H. Coronary hemodynamic determinants of epicardial artery vasomotor responses during sympathetic stimulation in humans. *Basic Res Cardiol.* 1991; 86:203–213.

161. Zeiher AM, Schachlinger V, Hohnloser SH, Saurbier B, Just H. Coronary atherosclerotic wall thickening and vascular reactivity in humans. Elevated high-density lipoprotein levels ameliorate abnormal vasoconstriction in early atherosclerosis. *Circulation.* 1994;89: 2525–2532.

162. Zeiher AM, Drexler H, Wollschlager H, Just H. Endothelial dysfunction of the coronary microvasculature is associated with coronary blood flow regulation in patients with early atherosclerosis. *Circulation.* 1991;84:1984–1992.

163. Campisi R, Czernin J, Schöder H, et al. Effects of long-term smoking on myocardial blood flow, coronary vasomotion, and vasodilator capacity. *Circulation.* 1998;98:119–125.

164. Campisi R, Czernin J, Schöder H, Sayre JW, Schelbert HR. L-Arginine normalizes coronary vasomotion in long-term smokers. *Circulation.* 1999;99:491–497.

165. Raitakari OT, Toikka J, Laine H, Viikari J, Knuuti J, Hartiala J. Reduced myocardial flow reserve does not impair exercise capacity in asymptomatic men. *Am J Cardiol.* 1999;84: 1253–1255, A8.

166. Smits P, Williams S, Lipson D, Banitt P, Rongen G, Creager M. Endothelial release of nitric oxide contributes to the vasodilator effect of adenosine in humans. *Circulation.* 1995;92:2135–2141.

167. Buus NH, Bottcher M, Hermansen F, Sander M, Nielsen TT, Mulvany MJ. Influence of nitric oxide synthase and adrenergic inhibition on adenosine-induced myocardial hyperemia. *Circulation.* 2001;104:2305–2310.

168. Böttcher M, Czernin J, Sun KT, Phelps ME, Schelbert HR. Effect of caffeine on myocardial blood flow at rest and during pharmacological vasodilation. *J Nucl Med.* 1995;36:2016–2021.

169. Müller P, Czernin J, Choi Y, et al. Effect of exercise supplementation during adenosine infusion on hyperemic blood flow and flow reserve. *Am Heart J.* 1994;128:52–60.

170. Böttcher M, Czernin J, Sun K, Phelps ME, Schelbert HR. Effect of beta 1 adrenergic receptor blockade on myocardial blood flow and vasodilatory capacity. *J Nucl Med.* 1997; 38:442–446.

171. Laine H, Nuutila P, Luotolahti M, Meyer C, Ronnemaa T, Knuuti J. Insulin-induced increment of coronary flow reserve is not abolished by dexamethasone in healthy young men. *J Am Coll Cardiol.* 2000;35:419A.

172. Sundell J, Nuutila P, Laine H, et al. Dose-dependent vasodilating effects of insulin on adenosine-stimulated myocardial blood flow. *Diabetes.* 2002;51:1125–1130.

173. Marcus M. Methods of calculating coronary vascular resistance. *The Coronary Circulation in Health and Disease.* New York: McGraw-Hill; 1983:107–109.

174. Tamaki N, Magata Y, Takahashi N, et al. Oxidative metabolism in the myocardium in normal subjects during dobutamine infusion. *Eur J Nucl Med.* 1993;20:231–237.

175. Hicks R, Kalff V, Savas V, Starling M, Schwaiger M. Assessment of right ventricular oxidative metabolism by positron emission tomography with C-11 acetate in aortic valve disease. *Am J Cardiol.* 1991;67:753–757.

176. Schelbert HR, Henze E, Sochor H, et al. Effects of substrate availability on myocardial C-11 palmitate kinetics by positron emission tomography in normal subjects and patients with ventricular dysfunction. *Am Heart J.* 1986;111:1055–1064.

177. Grover-McKay M, Schelbert HR, Schwaiger M, et al. Identification of impaired metabolic reserve by atrial pacing in patients with significant coronary artery stenosis. *Circulation.* 1986;74:281–292.

178. Gropler RJ, Siegel BA, Lee KJ, et al. Nonuniformity in myocardial accumulation of fluorine-18-fluorodeoxyglucose in normal fasted humans [see comments]. *J Nucl Med.* 1990;31:1749–1756.

179. Choi Y, Brunken RC, Hawkins RA, et al. Factors affecting myocardial 2-[F-18]fluoro-2-deoxy-D-glucose uptake in positron emission tomography studies of normal humans. *Eur J Nucl Med.* 1993;20:308–318.

180. Knuuti M, Nuutila P, Ruotsalainen U, et al. Euglycemic hyperinsulinemic clamp and oral glucose load in stimulating myocardial glucose utilization during Positron Emission Tomography. *J Nucl Med.* 1992;33:1255–1262.
181. Schelbert HR, Henze E, Keen R, et al. C-11 palmitate for the noninvasive evaluation of regional myocardial fatty acid metabolism with positron-computed tomography. IV. In vivo evaluation of acute demand-induced ischemia in dogs. *Am Heart J.* 1983;106:736–750.
182. Nuutila P, Koivisto VA, Knuuti J, et al. Glucose-free fatty acid cycle operates in human heart and skeletal muscle in vivo. *J Clin Invest.* 1992;89:1767–1774.
183. Gould KL, Schelbert HR, Phelps ME, Hoffman EJ. Noninvasive assessment of coronary stenoses with myocardial perfusion imaging during pharmacologic coronary vasodilatation. V. Detection of 47 percent diameter coronary stenosis with intravenous nitrogen-13 ammonia and emission-computed tomography in intact dogs. *Am J Cardiol.* 1979;43:200–208.
184. Schelbert HR, Phelps ME, Hoffman EJ, Huang SC, Selin CE, Kuhl DE. Regional myocardial perfusion assessed with N-13 labeled ammonia and positron emission computerized axial tomography. *Am J Cardiol.* 1979;43:209–219.
185. Tamaki N, Yonekura Y, Senda M, et al. Myocardial positron computed tomography with 13N ammonia at rest and during exercise. *Eur J Nucl Med.* 1985;11:246–251.
186. Tamaki N, Yonekura Y, Senda M, et al. Value and limitation of stress thallium-201 single photon emission computed tomography: comparison with nitrogen-13 ammonia positron tomography. *J Nucl Med.* 1988;29:1181–1188.
187. Go RT, Marwick TH, MacIntyre WJ, et al. A prospective comparison of rubidium-82 PET and thallium-201 SPECT myocardial perfusion imaging utilizing a single dipyridamole stress in the diagnosis of coronary artery disease [see comments]. *J Nucl Med.* 1990;31:1899–1905.
188. Stewart R, Schwaiger M, Molina E, et al. Comparison of rubidium-82 Positron Emission Tomography and thallium-201 SPECT imaging for detection of coronary artery disease. *Am J Cardiol.* 1991;67:1303–1310.
189. Simone G, Mullani N, Page D, Anderson B Sr. Utilization statistics and diagnostic accuracy of a nonhospital-based positron emission tomography center for the detection of coronary artery disease using rubidium-82. *Am J Physiol Imag.* 1992;7:203–209.
190. Williams B, Millani N, Jansen D, Anderson B. A retrospective study of the diagnostic accuracy of a community hospital-based PET center for the detection of coronary artery disease using rubidium-82. *J Nucl Med.* 1994;35:1586–1592.
191. Zijlstra F, Fioretti P, Reiber JH, Serruys PW. Which cineangiographically assessed anatomic variable correlates best with functional measurements of stenosis severity? A comparison of quantitative analysis of the coronary cineangiogram with measured coronary flow reserve and exercise/redistribution thallium-201 scintigraphy. *J Am Coll Cardiol.* 1988;12:686–691.
192. Flamm SD, Khanna S, Dicarli M, Phelps M, Schelbert HR, Maddahi J. Prognostic significance of normal adenosine stress myocardial perfusion PET study in patients presenting with chest pain. *J Nucl Med.* 1994;35:60P.
193. Marwick TH, Shan K, Patel S, Go RT, Lauer MS. Incremental value of rubidium-82 positron emission tomography for prognostic assessment of known or suspected coronary artery disease. *Am J Cardiol.* 1997;80:865–870.
194. Marwick TH, Shan K, Go RT, MacIntyre WJ, Lauer MS. Use of positron emission tomography for prediction of perioperative and late cardiac events before vascular surgery. *Am Heart J.* 1995;130:1196–1202.
195. Sdringola S, Patel D, Gould KL. High prevalence of myocardial perfusion abnormalities on positron emission tomography in asymptomatic persons with a parent or sibling with coronary artery disease. *Circulation.* 2001;103:496–501.
196. Gould KL, Ornish D, Scherwitz L, et al. Changes in myocardial perfusion abnormalities by positron emission tomography after long-term, intense risk factor modification [see comments]. *JAMA.* 1995;274:894–901.
197. Sambuceti G, Parodi O, Marcassa C, et al. Alteration in regulation of myocardial blood flow in one-vessel coronary artery disease determined by positron emission tomography. *Am J Cardiol.* 1993;72:538–543.

198. Di Carli M, Czernin J, Hoh CK, et al. Relation among stenosis severity, myocardial blood flow, and flow reserve in patients with coronary artery disease. *Circulation*. 1995;91: 1944–1951.

199. Guethlin M, Kasel AM, Coppenrath K, Ziegler S, Delius W, Schwaiger M. Delayed response of myocardial flow reserve to lipid-lowering therapy with fluvastatin. *Circulation*. 1999;99:475–481.

200. Uren NG, Melin JA, De Bruyne B, Wijns W, Baudhuin T, Camici PG. Relation between myocardial blood flow and the severity of coronary-artery stenosis. *N Engl J Med*. 1994; 330:1782–1788.

201. Beanlands RS, Muzik O, Melon P, et al. Noninvasive quantification of regional myocardial flow reserve in patients with coronary atherosclerosis using nitrogen-13 ammonia positron emission tomography. Determination of extent of altered vascular reactivity. *J Am Coll Cardiol*. 1995;26:1465–1475.

202. Muzik O, Duvernoy C, Beanlands RS, et al. Assessment of diagnostic performance of quantitative flow measurements in normal subjects and patients with angiographically documented coronary artery disease by means of nitrogen-13 ammonia and positron emission tomography. *J Am Coll Cardiol*. 1998;31:534–540.

203. Gould KL, Lipscomb K, Hamilton GW. Physiologic basis for assessing critical coronary stenosis. Instantaneous flow response and regional distribution during coronary hyperemia as measures of coronary flow reserve. *Am J Cardiol*. 1974;33:87–94.

204. De Bruyne B, Baudhuin T, Melin J, et al. Coronary flow reserve calculated from pressure measurements in humans. Validation with positron emission tomography. *Circulation*. 1994;89:1013–1022.

205. Krivokapich J, Czernin J, Schelbert HR. Dobutamine positron emission tomography: absolute quantitation of rest and dobutamine myocardial blood flow and correlation with cardiac work and percent diameter stenosis in patients with and without coronary artery disease. *J Am Coll Cardiol*. 1996;28:565–572.

206. Vanoverschelde JL, Wijns W, Depré C, et al. Mechanisms of chronic regional postischemic dysfunction in humans. New insights from the study of noninfarcted collateral-dependent myocardium [see comments]. *Circulation*. 1993;87:1513–1523.

207. Holmvang G, Fry S, Skopicki HA, et al. Relation between coronary "steal" and contractile function at rest in collateral-dependent myocardium of humans with ischemic heart disease. *Circulation*. 1999;99:2510–2516.

208. Akinboboye OO, Idris O, Chou RL, Sciacca RR, Cannon PJ, Bergmann SR. Absolute quantitation of coronary steal induced by intravenous dipyridamole. *J Am Coll Cardiol*. 2001;37:109–116.

209. Kosa I, Blasini R, Schneider-Eicke J, et al. Early recovery of coronary flow reserve after stent implantation as assessed by positron emission tomography. *J Am Coll Cardiol*. 1999;34:1036–1041.

210. Uren NG, Crake T, Lefroy DC, DeSilva R, Davies GJ, Maseri A. Delayed recovery of coronary resistive vessel function after coronary angioplasty. *J Am Coll Cardiol*. 1993;21: 612–621.

211. Egashira K, Inou T, Hirooka Y, Yamada A, Urabe Y, Takeshita A. Evidence of impaired endothelium-dependent coronary vasodilatation in patients with angina pectoris and normal coronary angiograms [see comments]. *N Engl J Med*. 1993;328:1659–1664.

212. Dayanikli F, Grambow D, Muzik O, Mosca L, Rubenfire M, Schwaiger M. Early detection of abnormal coronary flow reserve in asymptomatic men at high risk for coronary artery disease using positron emission tomography. *Circulation*. 1994;90:808–817.

213. Duvernoy CS, Meyer C, Seifert-Klauss V, et al. Gender differences in myocardial blood flow dynamics: lipid profile and hemodynamic effects. *J Am Coll Cardiol*. 1999;33: 463–470.

214. Pitkänen OP, Raitakari OT, Niinikoski H, et al. Coronary flow reserve is impaired in young men with familial hypercholesterolemia. *J Am Coll Cardiol*. 1996;28:1705–1711.

215. Yokoyama I, Murakami T, Ohtake T, Momomura S, Nishikawa J, Sasaki Y, Omata M. Reduced coronary flow reserve in familial hypercholesterolemia. *J Nucl Med*. 1996;37: 1937–42.

216. Yokoyama I, Ohtake T, Momomura S, Nishikawa J, Sasaki Y, Omata M. Reduced coronary flow reserve in hypercholesterolemic patients without overt coronary stenosis. *Circulation*. 1996;94:3232–3238.

217. Yokoyama I, Ohtake T, Momomura S, et al. Impaired myocardial vasodilation during hyperemic stress with dipyridamole in hypertriglyceridemia. *J Am Coll Cardiol.* 1998;31: 1568–1574.

218. Pitkänen OP, Nuutila P, Raitakari OT, et al. Coronary flow reserve in young men with familial combined hyperlipidemia. *Circulation.* 1999;99:1678–1684.

219. Kaufmann PA, Gnecchi-Ruscone T, Schäfers KP, Lüscher TF, Camici PG. Low density lipoprotein cholesterol and coronary microvascular dysfunction in hypercholesterolemia. *J Am Coll Cardiol.* 2000;36:103–109.

220. Yokoyama I, Ohtake T, Momomura S, et al. Altered myocardial vasodilatation in patients with hypertriglyceridemia in anatomically normal coronary arteries. *Arterioscler Thromb Vasc Biol.* 1998;18:294–299.

221. Pitkanen OP, Raitakari OT, Ronnemaa T, et al. Influence of cardiovascular risk status on coronary flow reserve in healthy young men. *Am J Cardiol.* 1997;79:1690–1692.

222. Laine H, Raitakari OT, Niinikoski H, et al. Early impairment of coronary flow reserve in young men with borderline hypertension. *J Am Coll Cardiol.* 1998;32:147–153.

223. Yokoyama I, Momomura S, Ohtake T, et al. Reduced myocardial flow reserve in non-insulin-dependent diabetes mellitus [see comments]. *J Am Coll Cardiol.* 1997;30:1472–1477.

224. Pitkänen OP, Nuutila P, Raitakari OT, et al. Coronary flow reserve is reduced in young men with IDDM. *Diabetes.* 1998;47:248–254.

225. Yokoyama I, Ohtake T, Momomura S, et al. Hyperglycemia rather than insulin resistance is related to reduced coronary flow reserve in NIDDM. *Diabetes.* 1998;47:119–124.

226. Yokoyama I, Yonekura K, Ohtake T, et al. Coronary microangiopathy in type 2 diabetic patients: relation to glycemic control, sex, and microvascular angina rather than to coronary artery disease. *J Nucl Med.* 2000;41:978–985.

227. Bache RJ. Vasodilator reserve: a functional assessment of coronary health [editorial; comment]. *Circulation.* 1998;98:1257–1260.

228. Schwaiger M, Kalff V, Rosenspire K, et al. Noninvasive evaluation of sympathetic nervous system in human heart by positron emission tomography [see comments]. *Circulation.* 1990;82:457–464.

229. Di Carli MF, Tobes MC, Mangner T, et al. Effects of cardiac sympathetic innervation on coronary blood flow. *N Engl J Med.* 1997;336:1208–1215.

230. Di Carli MF, Bianco-Batlles D, Landa ME, et al. Effects of autonomic neuropathy on coronary blood flow in patients with diabetes mellitus. *Circulation.* 1999;100:813–819.

231. Stevens MJ, Raffel DM, Allman KC, et al. Cardiac sympathetic dysinnervation in diabetes: implications for enhanced cardiovascular risk. *Circulation.* 1998;98:961–968.

232. Schöder H, Silverman DH, Campisi R, et al. Regulation of myocardial blood flow response to mental stress in healthy individuals. *Am J Physiol Heart Circ Physiol.* 2000;278: H360–H366.

233. Schöder H, Silverman DH, Campisi R, et al. Effect of mental stress on myocardial blood flow and vasomotion in patients with coronary artery disease. *J Nucl Med.* 2000;41:11–16.

234. Bottcher M, Madsen MM, Refsgaard J, et al. Peripheral flow response to transient arterial forearm occlusion does not reflect myocardial perfusion reserve. *Circulation.* 2001; 103:1109–1114.

235. Gould KL, Nakagawa Y, Nakagawa K, et al. Frequency and clinical implications of fluid dynamically significant diffuse coronary artery disease manifest as graded, longitudinal, base-to-apex myocardial perfusion abnormalities by noninvasive positron emission tomography. *Circulation.* 2000;101:1931–1939.

236. Hernandez-Pampaloni M, Keng FYY, Kudo T, Sayre JS, Schelbert HR. Abnormal longitudinal base to apex myocardial perfusion gradient by quantitative blood flow measurements in patients with coronary risk factors. *Circulation.* 2001;104:527–532.

237. De Bruyne B, Hersbach F, Pijls NH, et al. Abnormal epicardial coronary resistance in patients with diffuse atherosclerosis but "Normal" coronary angiography. *Circulation.* 2001;104:2401–2406.

238. Smart FW, Ballantyne CM, Cocanougher B, et al. Insensitivity of noninvasive tests to detect coronary artery vasculopathy after heart transplant. *Am J Cardiol.* 1991;67:243–247.

239. Hosenpud JD. Noninvasive diagnosis of cardiac allograft rejection. Another of many searches for the grail [editorial; comment]. *Circulation.* 1992;85:368–371.

240. Chan SY, Kobashigawa J, Stevenson LW, Brownfield E, Brunken RC, Schelbert HR. Myocardial blood flow at rest and during pharmacological vasodilation in cardiac transplants during and after successful treatment of rejection. *Circulation.* 1994;90:204–212.

241. Senneff MJ, Hartman J, Sobel BE, Geltman EM, Bergmann SR. Persistence of coronary vasodilator responsivity after cardiac transplantation. *Am J Cardiol.* 1993;71:333–338.

242. Kofoed KF, Czernin J, Johnson J, et al. Effects of cardiac allograft vasculopathy on myocardial blood flow, vasodilatory capacity, and coronary vasomotion. *Circulation.* 1997; 95:600–606.

243. Czernin J, Barnard RJ, Sun KT, et al. Effect of short-term cardiovascular conditioning and low-fat diet on myocardial blood flow and flow reserve. *Circulation.* 1995;92:197–204.

244. Hambrecht R, Wolf A, Gielen S, et al. Effect of exercise on coronary endothelial function in patients with coronary artery disease [see comments]. *N Engl J Med.* 2000;342:454–460.

245. Smith SC, Jr. Risk-reduction therapy: the challenge to change. Presented at the 68th Scientific Sessions of the American Heart Association, November 13, 1995, Anaheim, California. *Circulation.* 1996;93:2205–2211.

246. Janatuinen T, Laaksonen R, Vesalainen R, et al. Effect of lipid-lowering therapy with pravastatin on myocardial blood flow in young mildly hypercholesterolemic adults. *J Cardiovasc Pharmacol.* 2001;38:561–568.

247. Yokoyama I, Yonekura K, Inoue Y, Ohtomo K, Nagai R. Long-term effect of simvastatin on the improvement of impaired myocardial flow reserve in patients with familial hypercholesterolemia without gender variance. *J Nucl Cardiol.* 2001;8:445–451.

248. Baller D, Notohamiprodjo G, Gleichmann U, Holzinger J, Weise R, Lehmann J. Improvement in coronary flow reserve determined by positron emission tomography after 6 months of cholesterol-lowering therapy in patients with early stages of coronary atherosclerosis. *Circulation.* 1999;99:2871–2875.

249. Mellwig KP, Baller D, Gleichmann U, et al. Improvement of coronary vasodilatation capacity through single LDL apheresis. *Atherosclerosis.* 1998;139:173–178.

250. John S, Schlaich M, Langenfeld M, et al. Increased bioavailability of nitric oxide after lipid-lowering therapy in hypercholesterolemic patients: a randomized, placebo-controlled, double-blind study. *Circulation.* 1998;98:211–216.

251. Laufs U, La Fata V, Plutzky J, Liao JK. Upregulation of endothelial nitric oxide synthase by HMG CoA reductase inhibitors. *Circulation.* 1998;97:1129–1135.

252. Kaesemeyer WH, Caldwell RB, Huang J, Caldwell RW. Pravastatin sodium activates endothelial nitric oxide synthase independent of its cholesterol-lowering actions. *J Am Coll Cardiol.* 1999;33:234–241.

253. Nickenig G, Baumer AT, Temur Y, Kebben D, Jockenhovel F, Bohm M. Statin-sensitive dysregulated AT1 receptor function and density in hypercholesterolemic men. *Circulation.* 1999;100:2131–2134.

254. Yokoyama I, Momomura S, Ohtake T, et al. Improvement of impaired myocardial vasodilatation due to diffuse coronary atherosclerosis in hypercholesterolemics after lipid-lowering therapy. *Circulation.* 1999;100:117–122.

255. Kurz S, Harrison DG. Insulin and the arginine paradox [editorial]. *J Clin Invest.* 1997;99:369–370.

256. Boger RH, Bode-Boger SM, Szuba A, et al. Asymmetric dimethylarginine (ADMA): a novel risk factor for endothelial dysfunction: its role in hypercholesterolemia. *Circulation.* 1998;98:1842–1847.

257. Boger RH, Bode-Boger SM, Sydow K, Heistad DD, Lentz SR. Plasma concentration of asymmetric dimethylarginine, an endogenous inhibitor of nitric oxide synthase, is elevated in monkeys with hyperhomocyst(e)inemia or hypercholesterolemia. *Arterioscler Thromb Vasc Biol.* 2000;20:1557–1564.

258. Pampaloni MH, Hsueh WA, Quinones M, Sayre JS, Schelbert HR. PET determined myocardial blood flow demonstrates abnormal coronary vasomotion in insulin resistance without diabetes. *J Nucl Med.* 2000;41:44P.

259. Hsueh WA, Law RE. Insulin signaling in the arterial wall. *Am J Cardiol.* 1999;84:21J–24J.

260. Duvernoy CS, Rattenhuber J, Seifert-Klauss V, Bengel F, Meyer C, Schwaiger M. Myocardial blood flow and flow reserve in response to short-term cyclical hormone replacement therapy in postmenopausal women. *J Gend Specif Med.* 2001;4:21–27.

261. Peterson LR, Eyster D, Davila-Roman VG, et al. Short-term oral estrogen replacement therapy does not augment endothelium-independent myocardial perfusion in postmenopausal women. *Am Heart J.* 2001;142:641–647.

262. Campisi R, Nathan L, Pampaloni MH, Schoder H, Sayre JW, Chaudhuri G, Schelbert HR. Noninvasive assessment of coronary microcirculatory function in postmenopausal women and effects of short-term and long-term estrogen administration. *Circulation.* 2002;105:425–430.

263. Vita JA, Yeung AC, Winniford M, et al. Effect of cholesterol-lowering therapy on coronary endothelial vasomotor function in patients with coronary artery disease. *Circulation.* 2000;102:846–851.

264. Schachinger V, Britten MB, Zeiher AM. Prognostic impact of coronary vasodilator dysfunction on adverse long-term outcome of coronary heart disease. *Circulation.* 2000;101: 1899–906.

265. Suwaidi JA, Hamasaki S, Higano ST, Nishimura RA, Holmes DR Jr, Lerman A. Long-term follow-up of patients with mild coronary artery disease and endothelial dysfunction. *Circulation.* 2000;101:948–954.

266. Choudhury L, Rosen SD, Patel D, Nihoyannopoulos P, Camici PG. Coronary vasodilator reserve in primary and secondary left ventricular hypertrophy. A study with positron emission tomography. *Eur Heart J.* 1997;18:108–116.

267. Camici P, Chiriatti G, Lorenzoni R, et al. Coronary vasodilation is impaired in both hypertrophied and nonhypertrophied myocardium of patients with hypertrophic cardiomyopathy: a study with nitrogen-13 ammonia and positron emission tomography. *J Am Coll Cardiol.* 1991;17:879–886.

268. Choudhury L, Elliott P, Rimoldi O, et al. Transmural myocardial blood flow distribution in hypertrophic cardiomyopathy and effect of treatment. *Bas Res Cardiol.* 1999;94:49–59.

269. Perrone-Filardi P, Bacharach SL, Dilsizian V, Panza JA, Maurea S, Bonow RO. Regional systolic function, myocardial blood flow and glucose uptake at rest in hypertrophic cardiomyopathy. *Am J Cardiol.* 1993;72:199–204.

270. Tadamura E, Yoshibayashi M, Yonemura T, et al. Significant regional heterogeneity of coronary flow reserve in paediatric hypertrophic cardiomyopathy. *Eur J Nucl Med.* 2000; 27:1340–1348.

271. Drzezga A, Blasini R, Ziegler S, et al. Quantitative flow measurement using N-13 ammonia positron emission tomography during rest and stress by cold pressor test in normal subjects and patients with dilated cardiomyopathy. *J Nucl Med.* 1995;36:3P.

272. Weismueller S, Czernin J, Sun KT, Fung C, Phelps ME, Schelbert HR. Reduced coronary vasodilator capacity in idiopathic dilated cardiomyopathy. *J Nucl Med.* 1996;37:82P–83P.

273. van den Heuvel AF, van Veldhuisen DJ, van der Wall EE, et al. Regional myocardial blood flow reserve impairment and metabolic changes suggesting myocardial ischemia in patients with idiopathic dilated cardiomyopathy. *J Am Coll Cardiol.* 2000;35:19–28.

274. Neglia D, Michelassi C, Trivieri MG, et al. Prognostic role of myocardial blood flow impairment in idiopathic left ventricular dysfunction. *Circulation.* 2002;105:186–193.

275. Drzezga AE, Blasini R, Ziegler SI, Bengel FM, Picker W, Schwaiger M. Coronary microvascular reactivity to sympathetic stimulation in patients with idiopathic dilated cardiomyopathy. *J Nucl Med.* 2000;41:837–844.

276. Bengel FM, Permanetter B, Ungerer M, Nekolla S, Schwaiger M. Non-invasive estimation of myocardial efficiency using positron emission tomography and carbon-11 acetate—comparison between the normal and failing human heart. *Eur J Nucl Med.* 2000;27:319–326.

277. Wolpers HG, Buck A, Nguyen N, et al. An approach to ventricular efficiency by use of carbon 11-labeled acetate and positron emission tomography. *J Nucl Cardiol.* 1994;1:262–269.

278. Beanlands RS, Nahmias C, Gordon E, et al. The effects of beta(1)-blockade on oxidative metabolism and the metabolic cost of ventricular work in patients with left ventricular dysfunction: A double-blind, placebo-controlled, positron-emission tomography study. *Circulation.* 2000;102:2070–2075.

279. Geltman EM, Smith JL, Beecher D, Ludbrook PA, Ter-Pogossian MM, Sobel BE. Altered regional myocardial metabolism in congestive cardiomyopathy detected by positron tomography. *Am J Med.* 1983;74:773–785.

280. Eisenberg JD, Sobel BE, Geltman ED. Differentiation of ischemic from nonischemic cardiomyopathy with positron emission tomography. *Am J Cardiol.* 1987;59:1410–1414.

281. Sochor H, Schelbert H, Schwaiger M, Henze E, Phelps M. Studies of fatty acid metabolism with positron emission tomography in patients with cardiomyopathy. *Eur J Nucl Med.* 1986;12:S66–S69.

282. Vaghaiwalla Mody F, Brunken R, Warner-Stevenson L, Nienaber C, Phelps M, Schelbert H. Differentiating cardiomyopathy of coronary artery disease from non-ischemic dilated cardiomyopathy utilizing positron tomography. *J Am Coll Cardiol.* 1991;17:373–383.

283. Opie LH, Owen P, Riemersma RA. Relative rates of oxidation of glucose and free fatty acids by ischemic and non-ischemic myocardium after coronary artery ligation in the dog. *Eur J Clin Invest.* 1973;3:419–435.

284. Schelbert HR, Phelps ME, Selin C, Marshall RC, Hoffman EJ, Kuhl DE. Regional myocardial ischemia assessed by [18]Fluoro-2-deoxyglucose and positron emission computed tomography. In: Kreuzer H, Parmley WW, Rentrop P, Heiss HW, eds. *Quantification of Myocardial Ischemia.* New York: Gehard Witzstrock Publishing House; 1980:437–447.

285. Marshall RC, Tillisch JH, Phelps ME, Huang SC, Carson R, Henze E, Schelbert HR. Identification and differentiation of resting myocardial ischemia and infarction in man with positron computed tomography, 18F-labeled fluorodeoxyglucose and N-13 ammonia. *Circulation.* 1983;67:766–78.

286. Tillisch J, Brunken R, Marshall R, et al. Reversibility of cardiac wall-motion abnormalities predicted by positron tomography. *N Engl J Med.* 1986;314:884–888.

287. vom Dahl J, Altehoefer C, Sheehan F, et al. Recovery of regional left ventricular dysfunction after coronary revascularization: Impact of myocardial viability assessed by nuclear imaging and vessel patency at follow-up angiography. *J Am Coll Cardiol.* 1996;28:948–958.

288. Maes A, Flameng W, Nuyts J, et al. Histological alterations in chronically hypoperfused myocardium. Correlation with PET findings. *Circulation.* 1994;90:735–745.

289. Depré C, Vanoverschelde JL, Melin JA, et al. Structural and metabolic correlates of the reversibility of chronic left ventricular ischemic dysfunction in humans. *Am J Physiol.* 1995;268:H1265–H1275.

290. Gewirtz H, Fischman A, Abraham S, Gilson M, Strauss H, Alpert N. Positron emission tomographic measurements of absolute regional myocardial blood flow permits identification of nonviable myocardium in patients with chronic myocardial infarction. *J Am Coll Cardiol.* 1994;23:851–859.

291. Duvernoy CS, vom Dahl J, Laubenbacher C, Schwaiger M. The role of nitrogen 13 ammonia positron emission tomography in predicting functional outcome after coronary revascularization. *J Nucl Cardiol.* 1995;2:499–506.

292. Bax JJ, Poldermans D, Elhendy A, et al. Improvement of left ventricular ejection fraction, heart failure symptoms and prognosis after revascularization in patients with chronic coronary artery disease and viable myocardium detected by dobutamine stress echocardiography. *J Am Coll Cardiol.* 1999;34:163–169.

293. Bonow RO, Dilsizian V, Cuocolo A, Bacharach SL. Identification of viable myocardium in patients with chronic coronary artery disease and left ventricular dysfunction. Comparison of thallium scintigraphy with reinjection and PET imaging with 18F-fluorodeoxyglucose [see comments]. *Circulation.* 1991;83:26–37.

294. Knuuti M, Saraste M, Nuutila P, Härkönen R, Wegelius U, Haapanen A. Myocardial viability: fluorine-18-deoxyglucose positron emission tomography in prediction of wall motion recovery after revascularization. *Am Heart J.* 1994;127:785–796.

295. Baer FM, Voth E, Deutsch HJ, Schneider CA, Schicha H, Sechtem U. Assessment of viable myocardium by dobutamine transesophageal echocardiography and comparison with fluorine-18 fluorodeoxyglucose positron emission tomography. *J Am Coll Cardiol.* 1994;24:343–353.

296. Buvat I, Bartlett M, Srinivasan G, et al. Can gated FDG PET assess LV function as well as gated bloodpool SPECT? *J Nucl Med.* 1996;37:39P.

297. Buvat I, Kitsiou A, Srinivasan G, Dilsizian V, Bacharach S. Relationship between metabolism and function in CAD patients using gated FDG PET. *J Nucl Med.* 1996;37:161P.

298. Fath-Ordoubadi F, Beatt KJ, Spyrou N, Camici PG. Efficacy of coronary angioplasty for the treatment of hibernating myocardium. *Heart.* 1999;82:210–216.

299. DePuey EG, Ghesani M, Schwartz M, Friedman M, Nichols K, Salensky H. Comparative performance of gated perfusion SPECT wall thickening, delayed thallium uptake, and F-18 fluorodeoxyglucose SPECT in detecting myocardial viability. *J Nucl Cardiol.* 1999;6:418–428.

300. Schöder H, Campisi R, Ohtake T, et al. Blood flow-metabolism imaging with positron emission tomography in patients with diabetes mellitus for the assessment of reversible left ventricular contractile dysfunction. *J Am Coll Cardiol.* 1999;33:1328–1337.

301. Erler H, Zaknun J, Donnemiller E, et al. One year's clinical experience of 18F-FDG PET with a modified SPECT camera using molecular coincidence detection. *Nucl Med Commun.* 1999;20:1009–1015.

302. Fukuchi K, Sago M, Nitta K, et al. Attenuation correction for cardiac dual-head gamma camera coincidence imaging using segmented myocardial perfusion SPECT. *J Nucl Med.* 2000;41:919–925.

303. Nowak B, Zimny M, Schwarz ER, et al. Diagnosis of myocardial viability by dual-head co-incidence gamma camera fluorine-18 fluorodeoxyglucose positron emission tomography with and without non-uniform attenuation correction. *Eur J Nucl Med.* 2000;27:1501–1508.

304. Di Bella EV, Kadrmas DJ, Christian PE. Feasibility of dual-isotope coincidence/single-photon imaging of the myocardium. *J Nucl Med.* 2001;42:944–950.

305. Bax JJ, Cornel JH, Visser FC, et al. F18-fluorodeoxyglucose single-photon emission computed tomography predicts functional outcome of dyssynergic myocardium after surgical revascularization. *J Nucl Cardiol.* 1997;4:302–308.

306. Bax JJ, Visser FC, Elhendy A, et al. Prediction of improvement of regional left ventricular function after revascularization using different perfusion-metabolism criteria. *J Nucl Med.* 1999;40:1866–1873.

307. Gropler RJ, Geltman EM, Sampathkumaran K, et al. Functional recovery after coronary revascularization for chronic coronary artery disease is dependent on maintenance of oxidative metabolism. *J Am Coll Cardiol.* 1992;20:569–577.

308. Gropler RJ, Siegel BA, Sampathkumaran K, et al. Dependence of recovery of contractile function on maintenance of oxidative metabolism after myocardial infarction. *J Am Coll Cardiol.* 1992;19:989–997.

309. Rubin PJ, Lee DS, Dávila-Román VG, et al. Superiority of C-11 acetate compared with F-18 fluorodeoxyglucose in predicting myocardial functional recovery by positron emission tomography in patients with acute myocardial infarction. *Am J Cardiol.* 1996;78:1230–1235.

310. Hata T, Nohara R, Fujita M, et al. Noninvasive assessment of myocardial viability by positron emission tomography with 11C acetate in patients with old myocardial infarction. Usefulness of low-dose dobutamine infusion. *Circulation.* 1996;94:1834–1841.

310a. Wolpers HG, Burchert W, van den Hoff J, Weinhardt R, Meyer GJ, Lichtlen PR. Assessment of myocardial viability by use of 11C-acetate and positron emission tomography. Threshold criteria of reversible dysfunction. *Circulation.* 1997;95:1417–1424.

311. Camici P, Araujo LI, Spinks T, et al. Increased uptake of ^{18}F-fluorodeoxyglucose in postischemic myocardium of patients with exercise-induced angina. *Circulation.* 1986; 74:81–88.

312. Schwaiger M, Schelbert HR, Ellison D, et al. Sustained regional abnormalities in cardiac metabolism after transient ischemia in the chronic dog model. *J Am Coll Cardiol.* 1985;6:336–347.

313. Gerber BL, Wijns W, Vanoverschelde JL, et al. Myocardial perfusion and oxygen consumption in reperfused noninfarcted dysfunctional myocardium after unstable angina: direct evidence for myocardial stunning in humans. *J Am Coll Cardiol.* 1999;34:1939–1946.

314. Schwaiger M. Time course of metabolic findings in coronary occlusion and reperfusion and their role for assessing myocardial salvage. *Eur J Nucl Med.* 1986;12 Suppl: S54–S58.

315. Bolli R. Myocardial 'stunning' in man. *Circulation.* 1992;86:1671–1691.

316. Barnes E, Baker CS, Dutka DP, et al. Prolonged left ventricular dysfunction occurs in patients with coronary artery disease after both dobutamine and exercise induced myocardial ischaemia. *Heart.* 2000;83:283–289.

317. Barnes E, Dutka DP, Khan M, Camici PG, Hall RJ. Effect of repeated episodes of reversible myocardial ischemia on myocardial blood flow and function in humans. *Am J Physiol Heart Circ Physiol.* 2002;282:H1603–H1608.

318. Barnes E, Hall RJ, Dutka DP, Camici PG. Absolute blood flow and oxygen consumption in stunned myocardium in patients with coronary artery disease. *J Am Coll Cardiol.* 2002;39:420–427.

319. Rahimtoola SH. The hibernating myocardium. *Am Heart J.* 1989;117:211–221.

320. Schulz R, Rose J, Martin C, Brodde O-E, Heusch G. Development of short-term myocardial hibernation-Its limitation by the severity of ischemia and inotropic stimulation. *Circulation.* 1993;88:684–695.

321. Fallavollita J, Bryan P, Cantry J. ^{18}F-2-deoxyglucose deposition and regional flow in pigs with chronically dysfunctional myocardium: evidence for transmural variations in chronic hibernating myocardium. *Circulation.* 1997;95:1900–1909.

322. Fallavollita JA, Canty JM Jr. Differential 18F-2-deoxyglucose uptake in viable dysfunctional myocardium with normal resting perfusion: evidence for chronic stunning in pigs. *Circulation.* 1999;99:2798–2805.

323. Lim H, Fallavollita JA, Hard R, Kerr CW, Canty JM Jr. Profound apoptosis-mediated regional myocyte loss and compensatory hypertrophy in pigs with hibernating myocardium. *Circulation.* 1999;100:2380–2386.

324. Shivalkar B, Flameng W, Szilard M, Pislaru S, Borgers M, Vanhaecke J. Repeated stunning precedes myocardial hibernation in progressive multiple coronary artery obstruction. *J Am Coll Cardiol.* 1999;V34:2126–2136.

325. Schwaiger M, Brunken R, Grover-McKay M, et al. Regional myocardial metabolism in patients with acute myocardial infarction assessed by positron emission tomography. *J Am Coll Cardiol.* 1986;8:800–808.

326. Fragasso G, Chierchia S, Lucignani G, et al. Time dependence of residual tissue viability after myocardial infarction assessed by [18F] fluorodeoxyglucose and positron emission tomography. *Am J Cardiol.* 1993;72:131G–139G.

327. Fedele FA, Gewortz J, Capone RJ, Sharaf B, Most AS. Metabolic response to prolonged reduction of myocardial blood flow distal to a severe coronary artery stenosis. *Circulation.* 1988;78:729–735.

328. Camici PG, Wijns W, Borgers M, et al. Pathophysiological mechanisms of chronic reversible left ventricular dysfunction due to coronary artery disease (hibernating myocardium). *Circulation.* 1997;96:3205–3214.

329. Maes A, Flameng W, Borgers M, et al. Regional myocardial blood flow, glucose utilization and contractile function before and after revascularization and ultrastructural findings in patients with chronic coronary artery disease. *Eur J Nucl Med.* 1995;22:1299–1305.

330. Maes A, Mortelmans L, Nuyts J, et al. Importance of flow/metabolism studies in predicting late recovery of function following reperfusion in patients with acute myocardial infarction. *Eur Heart J.* 1997;18:954–962.

331. Czernin J, Porenta G, Rosenquist G, et al. Loss of coronary perfusion reserve in PET ischemia. *Circulation.* 1991;84:II-47.

332. Pagano D, Bonser RS, Camici PG. Myocardial revascularization for the treatment of post-ischemic heart failure. *Curr Opin Cardiol.* 1999;14:506–509.

333. Pagano D, Fath-Ordoubadi F, Beatt KJ, Townend JN, Bonser RS, Camici PG. Effects of coronary revascularisation on myocardial blood flow and coronary vasodilator reserve in hibernating myocardium. *Heart.* 2001;85:208–212.

334. Sun KT, Czernin J, Krivokapich J, et al. Effects of dobutamine stimulation on myocardial blood flow, glucose metabolism, and wall motion in normal and dysfunctional myocardium [see comments]. *Circulation.* 1996;94:3146–3154.

335. Pasquet A, Robert A, D'Hondt AM, Dion R, Melin JA, Vanoverschelde JL. Prognostic value of myocardial ischemia and viability in patients with chronic left ventricular ischemic dysfunction. *Circulation.* 1999;100:141–148.

336. Pasquet A, Williams MJ, Secknus MA, Zuchowski C, Lytle BW, Marwick TH. Correlation of preoperative myocardial function, perfusion, and metabolism with postoperative function at rest and stress after bypass surgery in severe left ventricular dysfunction. *Am J Cardiol.* 1999;84:58–64.

337. Pasquet A, Lauer MS, Williams MJ, Secknus MA, Lytle B, Marwick TH. Prediction of global left ventricular function after bypass surgery in patients with severe left ventricular dysfunction. Impact of pre-operative myocardial function, perfusion, and metabolism [see comments]. *Eur Heart J.* 2000;21:125–136.

338. Pagano D, Bonser RS, Townend JN, Ordoubadi F, Lorenzoni R, Camici PG. Predictive value of dobutamine echocardiography and positron emission tomography in identifying hibernating myocardium in patients with postischaemic heart failure. *Heart.* 1998;79:281–288.

339. Nagueh SF, Mikati I, Weilbaecher D, et al. Relation of the contractile reserve of hibernating myocardium to myocardial struture in humans. *Circulation.* 1999;100:490–496.
340. Bax JJ, Poldermans D, Visser FC, et al. Delayed recovery of hibernating myocardium after surgical revascularization: implications for discrepancy between metabolic imaging and dobutamine echocardiography for assessment of myocardial viability. *J Nucl Cardiol.* 1999;6:685–687.
341. Schwarz ER, Schaper J, vom Dahl J, et al. Myocyte degeneration and cell death in hibernating human myocardium. *J Am Coll Cardiol.* 1996;27:1577–1585.
342. Pagano D, Camici PG. Relation of contractile reserve of hibernating myocardium to myo-cardial structure in humans. *Circulation.* 2000;102:E189–E190.
343. Stinson E, Billingham M. Correlative study of regional left ventricular histology and contractile function. *Am J Cardiol.* 1977;39:378–383.
344. Cabin HS, Clubbs KS, Vita N, Zaret BL. Regional dysfunction by equilibrium radionuclide angiography: A clinicopathologic study evaluating the relation of degree of dysfunction to the presence and extent of myocardial infarction. *J Am Coll Cardiol.* 1987; 10:743–747.
345. Flameng W, Suy R, Schwarz F, et al. Ultrastructural correlates of left ventricular contraction abnormalities in patients with chronic ischemic heart disease: determinants of reversible segmental asynergy post-revascularization surgery. *Am Heart J.* 1981;102:846–857.
346. Schwarz E, Schaper J, vom Dahl J, et al. Myocardial hibernation is not sufficient to prevent morphological disarrangements with ischemic cell alterations and increased fibrosis. *Circulation.* 1994;90:I-378.
347. Schwaiger M, Sun D, Deeb G, et al. Expression of myocardial glucose transporter (GLUT) mRNAs in patients with advanced coronary artery disease (CAD). *Circulation.* 1994;90: I-113.
348. Brosius FC, III, Liu Y, Nguyen N, Sun D, Bartlett J, Schwaiger M. Persistent myocardial ischemia increases GLUT1 glucose transporter expression in both ischemic and non-ischemic heart regions. *J Molec Cell Cardiol.* 1997;29:1675–1685.
349. Brosius FC, III, Nguyen N, Egert S, et al. Increased sarcolemmal glucose transporter abundance in myocardial ischemia. *Am J Cardiol.* 1997;80:77A–84A.
350. Vogt AM, Nef H, Schaper J, et al. Metabolic control analysis of anaerobic glycolysis in human hibernating myocardium replaces traditional concepts of flux control. *FEBS Lett.* 2002;517:245–250.
351. Lopaschuk G, Stanley W. Glucose metabolism in the ischemic heart. *Circulation.* 1997; 95:313–315.
352. Allman K, Wieland D, Muzik O, Degrado T, Wolfe E, Schwaiger M. Carbon-11 hydroxyephedrine with positron emission tomography for serial assessment of cardiac adrenergic neuronal function after acute myocardial infarction in humans. *J Am Coll Cardiol.* 1993;22:368–375.
353. Bengel F, Ueberfuhr P, Ziegler SI, et al. Effect of cardiac sympathetic innervation on metabolism of the human heart determined by positron emission tomography. *Circulation.* 1999;110:I.201.
354. Wiggers H, Noreng M, Paulsen PK, et al. Energy stores and metabolites in chronic reversibly and irreversibly dysfunctional myocardium in humans. *J Am Coll Cardiol.* 2001; 37:100–108.
355. Borgers M, Ausma J. Structural aspects of the chronic hibernating myocardium in man. *Basic Res Cardiol.* 1995;90:44–46.
356. Ausma J, Wijffels M, van Eys G, et al. Dedifferentiation of atrial cardiomyocytes as a result of chronic atrial fibrillation. *Am J Pathol.* 1997;151:985–997.
357. Depré C, Havaux X, Dion R, Vanoverschelde JL. Morphologic alterations of myocardium under conditions of left ventricular assistance. *J Thorac Cardiovasc Surg.* 1998;115: 478–479.
358. Ausma J, Thonae F, Dispersyn GD, et al. Dedifferentiated cardiomyocytes from chronic hibernating myocardium are ischemia-tolerant. *Molec Cell Biochem.* 1998;186:159–168.
359. Depré C, Vanoverschelde JL, Taegtmeyer H. Glucose for the heart. *Circulation.* 1999; 99:578–588.
360. Razeghi PW, Young ME, Alcorn JL, Moravec CS, Frazier OH, Taegtmeyer H. Metabolic gene expression in fetal and failing human heart. *Circulation.* 2001;104:2923–2931.

361. Elsässer A, Schlepper M, Kleovekorn WP, et al. Hibernating myocardium: an incomplete adaptation to ischemia. *Circulation*. 1997;96:2920–2931.

362. Elsaesser A, Greiber S, Hein S, et al. Hibernating myocardium: Upregulation of the caspase-3 gene and reduction of bcl-2. *Circulation*. 1999;110:I.758.

363. Brunken RC, Mody FV, Hawkins RA, Nienaber C, Phelps ME, Schelbert HR. Positron emission tomography detects metabolic viability in myocardium with persistent 24-hour single-photon emission computed tomography 201Tl defects. *Circulation*. 1992;86:1357–1369.

364. Beanlands RS, Hendry PJ, Masters RG, deKemp RA, Woodend K, Ruddy TD. Delay in revascularization is associated with increased mortality rate in patients with severe left ventricular dysfunction and viable myocardium on fluorine 18-fluorodeoxyglucose positron emission tomography imaging. *Circulation*. 1998;98:II51–II56.

365. Schwarz E, Schoendube F, Kostin S, et al. Prolonged myocardial hibernation exacerbates cardiomyocyte degeneration and impairs recovery of function after revascularization. *J Am Coll Cardiol*. 1998;31:1018–1026.

366. Nienaber CA, Brunken RC, Sherman CT, et al. Metabolic and functional recovery of ischemic human myocardium after coronary angioplasty [see comments]. *J Am Coll Cardiol*. 1991;18:966–978.

367. Vanoverschelde JL, Depre C, Gerber BL, et al. Time course of functional recovery after coronary artery bypass graft surgery in patients with chronic left ventricular ischemic dysfunction. *Am J Cardiol*. 2000;85:1432–1439.

368. Marwick T, MacIntyre W, Lafont A, Nemec J, Salcedo E. Metabolic responses of hibernating and infarcted myocardium to revascularization: a follow-up study of regional perfusion, function, and metabolism. *Circulation*. 1992;85:1347–1353.

369. Stevenson W, Stevenson L, Middlekauff H, et al. Improving survival for patients with advanced heart failure: A study of 737 consecutive patients. *J Am Coll Cardiol*. 1995;26:1417–1423.

370. Alderman EL, Fisher LD, Litwin P, et al. Results of coronary artery surgery in patients with poor left ventricular function (CASS). *Circulation*. 1983;68:785–795.

371. Passamani E, Davis KB, Gillespie MJ, Killip T. A randomized trial of coronary artery bypass surgery. Survival of patients with low ejection fraction. *N Engl J Med*. 1985;312:1665–1671.

372. Allman KC, Shaw LJ, Hachamovitch R, Udelson JE. Myocardial viability testing and impact of revascularization on prognosis in patients with coronary artery disease and left ventricular dysfunction: a meta-analysis. *J Am Coll Cardiol*. 2002;39:1151–1158.

373. Haas F, Haehnel CJ, Picker W, et al. Preoperative positron emission tomographic viability assessment and perioperative and postoperative risk in patients with advanced ischemic heart disease [see comments]. *J Am Coll Cardiol*. 1997;30:1693–1700.

374. Landoni C, Lucignani G, Paolini G, et al. Assessment of CABG-related risk in patients with CAD and LVD. Contribution of PET with [18F]FDG to the assessment of myocardial viability. *J Cardiovasc Surg*. 1999;40:363–372.

375. Tamaki N, Yonekura Y, Yamashita K, et al. Positron emission tomography using fluorine-18 deoxyglucose in evaluation of coronary artery bypass grafting. *Am J Cardiol*. 1989;64:860–865.

376. Tamaki N, Yonekura Y, Yamashita K, et al. Prediction of reversible ischemia after coronary artery bypass grafting by positron emission tomography. *J Cardiol*. 1991;21:193–201.

377. Carrel T, Jenni R, Haubold-Reuter S, Von Schulthess G, Pasic M, Turina M. Improvement of severely reduced left ventricular function after surgical revascularization in patients with preoperative myocardial infarction. *Eur J Cardiothorac Surg*. 1992;6:479–484.

378. Lucignani G, Paolini G, Landoni C, et al. Presurgical identification of hibernating myocardium by combined use of technetium-99m hexakis 2-methoxyisobutylisonitrile single photon emission tomography and fluorine-18 fluoro-2-deoxy-D-glucose positron emission tomography in patients with coronary artery disease. *Eur J Nucl Med*. 1992;19:874–881.

379. Marwick TH, MacIntyre WJ, Lafont A, Nemec JJ, Salcedo EE. Metabolic responses of hibernating and infarcted myocardium to revascularization. A follow-up study of regional perfusion, function, and metabolism. *Circulation*. 1992;85:1347–1353.

380. Gropler RJ, Geltman EM, Sampathkumaran K, et al. Comparison of carbon-11-acetate with fluorine-18-fluorodeoxyglucose for delineating viable myocardium by positron emission tomography. *J Am Coll Cardiol.* 1993;22:1587–1597.

381. Baer FM, Voth E, Deutsch HJ, et al. Predictive value of low dose dobutamine transesophageal echocardiography and fluorine-18 fluorodeoxyglucose positron emission tomography for recovery of regional left ventricular function after successful revascularization. *J Am Coll Cardiol.* 1996;28:60–69.

382. Marwick TH, Nemec JJ, Lafont A, Salcedo EE, MacIntyre WJ. Prediction by postexercise fluoro-18 deoxyglucose positron emission tomography of improvement in exercise capacity after revascularization. *Am J Cardiol.* 1992;69:854–859.

383. Paolini G, Lucignani G, Zuccari M, et al. Identification and revascularization of hibernating myocardium in angina-free patients with left ventricular dysfunction. *Eur J Cardio-Thorac Surg.* 1994;8:139–144.

384. vom Dahl J, Eitzman D, Al-Aouar A, et al. Relation of regional function, perfusion, and metabolism in patients with advanced coronary artery disease undergoing surgical revascularization. *Circulation.* 1994;90:2356–2366.

385. Bax JJ, Valkema R, Visser FC, et al. Detection of myocardial viability with F-18-fluorodeoxyglucose and single photon emission computed tomography [editorial]. *Giorn Ital Cardiol.* 1997;27:1181–1186.

386. Flameng WJ, Shivalkar B, Spiessens B, et al. PET scan predicts recovery of left ventricular function after coronary artery bypass operation. *Ann Thorac Surg.* 1997;64: 1694–1701.

387. Fath-Ordoubadi F, Pagano D, Marinho NV, Keogh BE, Bonser RS, Camici PG. Coronary revascularization in the treatment of moderate and severe postischemic left ventricular dysfunction. *Am J Cardiol.* 1998;82:26–31.

388. Akinboboye OO, Idris O, Cannon PJ, Bergmann SR. Usefulness of positron emission tomography in defining myocardial viability in patients referred for cardiac transplantation. *Am J Cardiol.* 1999;83:1271–1274.

389. Pagano D, Townend JN, Littler WA, Horton R, Camici PG, Bonser RS. Coronary artery bypass surgery as treatment for ischemic heart failure: the predictive value of viability assessment with quantitative positron emission tomography for symptomatic and functional outcome. *J Thorac Cardiovasc Surg.* 1998;115:791–799.

390. Marwick T, Nemec J, Lafont A, Salcedo E, MacIntyre W. Prediction by postexercise fluoro-18 deoxyglucose positron emission tomography of improvement in exercise capacity after revascularization. *Am J Cardiol.* 1992;69:854–859.

391. Marwick TH, Zuchowski C, Lauer MS, Secknus MA, Williams J, Lytle BW. Functional status and quality of life in patients with heart failure undergoing coronary bypass surgery after assessment of myocardial viability. *J Am Coll Cardiol.* 1999;33:750–758.

392. Haas F, Augustin N, Holper K, et al. Time course and extent of improvement of dysfunctioning myocardium in patients with coronary artery disease and severely depressed left ventricular function after revascularization: correlation with positron emission tomographic findings. *J Am Coll Cardiol.* 2000;36:1927–1934.

393. Eitzman D, Al-Aouar Z, Vom Dahl J, Kirsh M, Schwaiger M. Clinical outcome of patients with advanced coronary artery disease after viability studies with Positron Emission Tomography. *J Am Coll Cardiol.* 1992;20:559–565.

394. Di Carli M, Davidson M, Little R, et al. Value of metabolic imaging with Positron Emission Tomography for evaluating prognosis in patients with coronary artery disease and left ventricular dysfunction. *Am J Cardiol.* 1994;73:527–533.

394a. Rohatgi R, Epstein S, Henriquez J, Ababneh AA, Hickey KT, Pinsky D, Akinboboye O, Bergmann SR. Utility of positron emission tomography in predicting cardiac events and survival in patients with coronary artery disease and severe left ventricular dysfunction. *Am J Cardiol.* 2001;87:1096–1099, A6.

395. Bax JJ, Visser FC, Poldermans D, et al. Relationship between preoperative viability and postoperative improvement in LVEF and heart failure symptoms. *J Nucl Med.* 2001;42: 79–86.

396. Di Carli MF, Asgarzadie F, Schelbert HR, et al. Quantitative relation between myocardial viability and improvement in heart failure symptoms after revascularization in patients with ischemic cardiomyopathy. *Circulation.* 1995;92:3436–3444.

397. Goldman L, Hashimoto B, Cook E, Loscalzo A. Comparative reproducibility and validity of systems for assessing cardiovascular functional class: advantages of a new specific activity scale. *Circulation.* 1981;64:1227–1234.

398. Tamaki N, Kawamoto M, Takahashi N, et al. Prognostic value of an increase in fluorine-18 deoxyglucose uptake in patients with myocardial infarction: comparison with stress thallium imaging. *J Am Coll Cardiol.* 1993;22:1621–1627.

399. Lee KS, Marwick TH, Cook SA, et al. Prognosis of patients with left ventricular dysfunction, with and without viable myocardium after myocardial infarction. Relative efficacy of medical therapy and revascularization. *Circulation.* 1994;90:2687–2694.

400. Zhang X, Liu XJ, Wu Q, et al. Clinical outcome of patients with previous myocardial infarction and left ventricular dysfunction assessed with myocardial (99m)Tc-MIBI SPECT and (18)F-FDG PET. *J Nucl Med.* 2001;42:1166–1173.

401. Gioia G, Powers J, Heo J, Iskandrian AS. Prognostic value of rest-redistribution tomographic thallium-201 imaging in ischemic cardiomyopathy. *Am J Cardiol.* 1995;75:759–762.

402. Gioia G, Milan E, Giubbini R, DePace N, Heo J, Iskandrian AS. Prognostic value of tomographic rest-redistribution thallium 201 imaging in medically treated patients with coronary artery disease and left ventricular dysfunction. *J Nucl Cardiol.* 1996;3:150–156.

403. Pagley PR, Beller GA, Watson DD, Gimple LW, Ragosta M. Improved outcome after coronary bypass surgery in patients with ischemic cardiomyopathy and residual myocardial viability. *Circulation.* 1997;96:793–800.

404. Petretta M, Cuocolo A, Bonaduce D, et al. Incremental prognostic value of thallium reinjection after stress-redistribution imaging in patients with previous myocardial infarction and left ventricular dysfunction. *J Nucl Med.* 1997;38:195–200.

405. Cuocolo A, Petretta M, Nicolai E, et al. Successful coronary revascularization improves prognosis in patients with previous myocardial infarction and evidence of viable myocardium at thallium-201 imaging. *Eur J Nucl Med.* 1998;25:60–68.

406. Dreyfus GD, Duboc D, Blasco A, et al. Myocardial viability assessment in ischemic cardiomyopathy: benefits of coronary revascularization. *Ann Thorac Surg.* 1994;57:1402–1407; discussion 1407–1408.

407. Brunken R, Schwaiger M, Grover-McKay M, Phelps ME, Tillisch J, Schelbert HR. Positron emission tomography detects tissue metabolic activity in myocardial segments with persistent thallium perfusion defects. *J Am Coll Cardiol.* 1987;10:557–567.

408. Brunken RC, Kottou S, Nienaber CA, et al. PET detection of viable tissue in myocardial segments with persistent defects at T1-201 SPECT. *Radiology.* 1989;172:65–73.

409. Williams MJ, Odabashian J, Lauer MS, Thomas JD, Marwick TH. Prognostic value of dobutamine echocardiography in patients with left ventricular dysfunction. *J Am Coll Cardiol.* 1996;27:132–139.

410. Afridi I, Grayburn PA, Panza JA, Oh JK, Zoghbi WA, Marwick TH. Myocardial viability during dobutamine echocardiography predicts survival in patients with coronary artery disease and severe left ventricular systolic dysfunction. *J Am Coll Cardiol.* 1998;32:921–926.

411. Anselmi M, Golia G, Cicoira M, et al. Prognostic value of detection of myocardial viability using low-dose dobutamine echocardiography in infarcted patients. *Am J Cardiol.* 1998;81:21G–28G.

412. Meluzin J, Cerny J, Frelich M, et al. Prognostic value of the amount of dysfunctional but viable myocardium in revascularized patients with coronary artery disease and left ventricular dysfunction. Investigators of this Multicenter Study. *J Am Coll Cardiol.* 1998;32:912–920.

413. Senior R, Kaul S, Lahiri A. Myocardial viability on echocardiography predicts long-term survival after revascularization in patients with ischemic congestive heart failure. *J Am Coll Cardiol.* 1999;33:1848–1854.

414. Smart SC, Dionisopoulos PN, Knickelbine TA, Schuchard T, Sagar KB. Dobutamine-atropine stress echocardiography for risk stratification in patients with chronic left ventricular dysfunction. *J Am Coll Cardiol.* 1999;33:512–521.

415. Kim RJ, Fieno DS, Parrish TB, et al. Relationship of MRI delayed contrast enhancement to irreversible injury, infarct age, and contractile function. *Circulation.* 1999;100:1992–2002.

416. Kim RJ, Wu E, Rafael A, et al. The use of contrast-enhanced magnetic resonance imaging to identify reversible myocardial dysfunction. *N Engl J Med.* 2000;343:1445–1453.

417. Gerber BL, Garot J, Bluemke DA, Wu KC, Lima JAC. Accuaracy of contrast-enhanced magnetic resonance imaging in predicting improvement in regional myocardial function in patients after acute myocardial infarction. *Circulation.* 2002;101:1083–1089.

418. Klein C, Nekolla SG, Bengel FM, et al. Assessment of myocardial viability with contrast-enhanced magnetic resonance imaging: comparison with positron emission tomography. *Circulation.* 2002;105:162–167.

419. Bonow RO, Dilsizian V, Cuocolo A, Bacharach SL. Identification of viable myocardium in patients with chronic coronary artery disease and left ventricular dysfunction. Comparison of thallium scintigraphy with reinjection and PET imaging with 18F-fluorodeoxyglucose. *Circulation.* 1991;83:26–37.

420. Bax JJ, Fath-Ordoubadi F, Boersma E, Wijns W, Camici G. Accuracy of PET in predicting functional recovery after revascularisation in patients with chronic ischaemic dysfunction: head-to-head comparison between blood flow, glucose utilisation and water-perfusable tissue fraction. *Eur J Nucl Med Mol Imaging.* 2002;29:721–727.

421. Schwaiger M, Brunken RC, Krivokapich J, et al. Beneficial effect of residual anterograde flow on tissue viability as assessed by positron emission tomography in patients with myocardial infarction. *Eur Heart J.* 1987;8:981–988.

422. Czernin J, Porenta G, Brunken R, et al. Regional blood flow, oxidative metabolism, and glucose utilization in patients with recent myocardial infarction. *Circulation.* 1993;88: 884–895.

423. Feigl E, Neat G, Huang A. Interrelations between coronary artery pressure, myocardial metabolism and coronary blood flow. *J Mol Cell Cardiol.* 1990;22:375–390.

424. Maes A, Van de Werf F, Nuyts J, Bormans G, Desmet W, Mortelmans L. Impaired myocardial tissue perfusion early after successful thrombolysis. Impact on myocardial flow, metabolism, and function at late follow-up. *Circulation.* 1995;92:2072–2078.

425. Louie HW, Laks H, Milgalter E, et al. Ischemic cardiomyopathy. Criteria for coronary revascularization and cardiac transplantation. *Circulation.* 1991;84:III290–III295.

426. Duong T, Hendi P, Fonarow G, et al. Role of Positron Emission Tomographic assessment of myocardial viability in the management of patients who are referred for cardiac transplantation. *Circulation.* 1995;92:I-123.

427. Duong T, Fonarow G, Laks H, et al. Cost effectiveness of Positron Emission Tomography (PET) in the management of ischemic cardiomyopathy patients who are referred for cardiac transplantation. *J Am Coll Cardiol.* 1996;27:144A.

428. Maes AF, Van de Werf F, Mesotten LV, et al. Early assessment of regional myocardial blood flow and metabolism in thrombolysis in myocardial infarction flow grade 3 reperfused myocardial infarction using carbon-11-acetate. *J Am Coll Cardiol.* 2001;37:30–36.

429. Blumenthal RS, Becker DM, Moy TF, Coresh J, Wilder LB, Becker LC. Exercise thallium tomography predicts future clinically manifest coronary heart disease in a high-risk asymptomatic population. *Circulation.* 1996;93:915–923.

430. Becker DM, Yook RM, Moy TF, Blumenthal RS, Becker LC. Markedly high prevalence of coronary risk factors in apparently healthy African-American and white siblings of persons with premature coronary heart disease. *Am J Cardiol.* 1998;82:1046–1051.

431. Gould KL, Martucci JP, Goldberg DI, et al. Short-term cholesterol lowering decreases size and severity of perfusion abnormalities by positron emission tomography after dipyridamole in patients with coronary artery disease. A potential noninvasive marker of healing coronary endothelium. *Circulation.* 1994;89:1530–1538.

432. Furuyama H, Odagawa Y, Katoh C, et al. Assessment of coronary function in children with a history of Kawasaki disease using (15)O-water positron emission tomography. *Circulation.* 2002;105:2878–2884.

433. Hernandez-Pampaloni M, Allada V, Fishbein MC, Schelbert HR. Myocardial perfusion and viability by PET in infants and children with coronary abnormalities: correlation with echocardiography, cor angiogr histopathol. *J Am Coll Cardiol.* 2002;41:618–626.

434. Bengel FM, Ueberfuhr P, Nekolla S, Ziegler SI, Reichart B, Schwaiger M. Oxidative metabolism of the transplanted human heart assessed by positron emission tomography using C-11 acetate. *Am J Cardiol.* 1999;83:1503–1505, A8.

435. Bengel FM, Ueberfuhr P, Ziegler SI, Nekolla S, Reichart B, Schwaiger M. Serial assessment of sympathetic reinnervation after orthotopic heart transplantation. A longitudinal study using PET and C-11 hydroxyephedrine. *Circulation.* 1999;99:1866–1871.

436. Annane D, Duboc D, Mazoyer B, et al. Correlation between decreased myocardial glu-

cose phosphorylation and the DNA mutation size in myotonic dystrophy. *Circulation.* 1994;90:2629–2634.

437. Annane D, Merlet P, Radvanyi H, et al. Blunted coronary reserve in myotonic dystrophy. An early and gene-related phenomenon. *Circulation.* 1996;94:973–977.

438. Menasche P, Hagege AA, Scorsin M, et al. Myoblast transplantation for heart failure. *Lancet.* 2001;357:279–280.

439. Di Carli MF, Maddahi J, Rokhsar S, et al. Long-term survival of patients with coronary artery disease and left ventricular dysfunction: implications for the role of myocardial viability assessment in management decisions. *J Thorac Cardiovasc Surg.* 1998;116:997–1004.

CHAPTER 7

Molecular Imaging of Biological Processes with PET: Evaluating Biologic Bases of Cerebral Function

Daniel H.S. Silverman and William P. Melega

Neuroimaging studies with positron emission tomography (PET) have advanced our understanding of the human brain by noninvasively assessing several aspects of cerebral biology and biochemistry. These aspects include glucose metabolic rates, blood flow, blood-brain barrier permeability, enzyme activity, neurotransmitter synthesis and release, receptor subtype binding, and gene expression. Changes in these processes occur with normal development and aging, neurodegenerative and cerebrovascular diseases, head trauma, psychiatric disorders, and chemotoxic insults. PET can be used to study all of these aspects and also the pharmacokinetic and pharmacodynamic effects of drugs on the central nervous system. The data that are generated can be used to address questions of relevance to basic neuroscience as well as to the clinical management of patients with neuropsychiatric disorders. Accordingly, the following sections highlight both research-oriented and clinically oriented applications of brain PET, providing illustrations of how the power of this methodology to image and quantify neurobiologic parameters can impact upon the assessment of brain function and dysfunction.

STUDIES OF NORMAL HUMAN BRAIN FUNCTION

Cerebral metabolism

As with whole-body PET studies of human biology and disease, the most commonly performed PET studies of the brain are carried out with 2-deoxy-2-[F-18]fluoro-D-glucose (FDG) as the imaged radiopharmaceutical. Because the synthesis of over 95% of the adenosine triphosphate (ATP) molecules that are hydrolyzed to fuel cerebral function originate from the catabolism of glucose, PET imaging of glucose metabolism with FDG provides an excellent way to evaluate the distributed function of the brain (see Chapter 2).[1] In the clinical arena, the resulting scans are typically interpreted qualitatively with visual analysis, that is, an experienced reader examines the relative distribution of glucose metabolism throughout the brain of the patient under scrutiny and compares it to the distribution expected for a normal subject of similar age (Figure 7-1). The patient's age is especially important to the interpretation because of major changes in cerebral metabolism that are known to occur in the course of normal development and aging (see below). Other factors that can influence scans of normal subjects—either with respect to regional activity or overall count rates—include sex, handedness, sensory environment, level of alertness, mood, drug effects, serum glucose levels, and the portion of administered tracer that passes into the brain.

Visual analysis is also used in some research studies but often, the results of semiquantitative or absolute quantitative analyses are reported in addition to (or instead) of visual interpretation. In this context, *semiquantitative* refers to results that are based on regional concentrations of measured radioactiv-

FIGURE 7-1. Normal pattern of cerebral glucose metabolism measured with FDG in the brain of a 42-year-old man. Images from plane 8 to plane 49 are from the top to the base of the brain. Images can be displayed in cross-sectional, coronal, and sagittal formats. The gray scale is proportional to cerebral metabolic rate for glucose (CM-Rglc), with black being highest. In this and later figures, images are cross-sectional and are displayed with the anterior brain at the top of each image; the left side of the brain is on the right side of the images (radiologic convention).

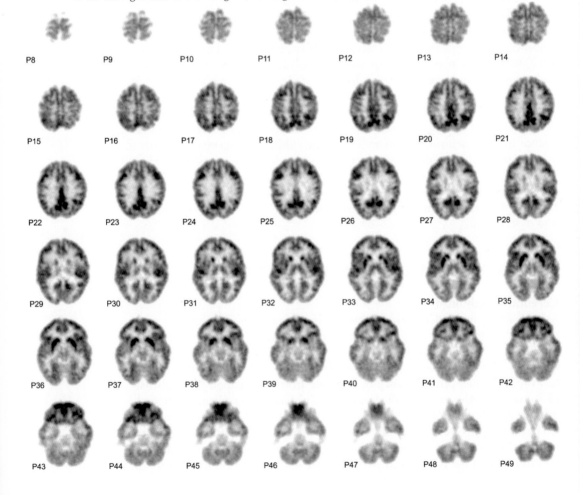

ity, normalized to some internal reference standard—for example, a reference region of the brain, the whole-brain activity, or the average whole-body concentration prior to excretion and decay-corrected to the actual time of imaging (i.e., standardized uptake value, or SUV) (see Chapter 2).[2] Those results turn out to be adequate for most clinical applications, as well as for many research applications. In contrast, *absolute quantitative* values are derived from biologically based mathematical models that reflect the partitioning of radioactivity into compartments that can reflect both physiological boundaries (e.g., the vascular space, the blood-brain barrier, and the plasma membrane of neurons) and biochemical processes (enzymatic anabolism and degradation, transport molecules, and receptor proteins). These models necessarily represent substantial simplifications of the actual biological environment but, nevertheless, have proven capable of yielding quantitative estimates in good agreement with similar measures obtained by more invasive methods (Chapter 2).

Initially, values for global human cerebral metabolic rates of glucose utilization were obtained using Kety–Schmidt methods for the combined measurement of global cerebral blood flow and the arteriovenous difference for glucose.[2–8] Kety–Schmidt techniques thus measure cerebral blood flow and arteriovenous substrate differences across the whole brain. Table 7-1 shows values for these and related biological parameters measured in this way.

In the case of FDG studies, the biological parameter that is being estimated is the rate of regional glucose utilization, based on a method described by Sokoloff and his colleagues,[12] originally developed with ^{14}C-labeled 2-deoxyglucose for use with autoradiography and subsequently validated for FDG and PET.[13–18] Early measures of regional glucose utilization rates in the human brain yielded estimates of global cerebral metabolism of approximately 5.5 mg of glucose/min/100 g, which ranged from 3.6 to 5.2 mg of glucose/min/100 g in white matter structures to 5.8 to 10.3 mg of glucose/min/100g in gray matter structures (Table 7-2). Values in the literature are also reported in units of micromoles per minutes per 100 grams to allow stoichiometric comparisons to other substrates used by the brain (e.g., oxygen, and the ketones alpha-butyrate and acetoacetate). That conversion is accomplished by

TABLE 7-1. Whole-Brain Blood Flow, Glucose, and Oxygen Utilization in Normal Adults Using the Kety–Schmidt Technique[a]

Glucose utilization (μmol/min/100g)	Glucose extraction (%)	Oxygen utilization (μmol/min/100g)	Oxygen extraction (%)	Respiratory quotient	Oxygen/ glucose molar utilization ratio	Blood flow (ml/min/100g)
30.2 ± 4.3	10.9 ± 1.8	159.7 ± 17.4	34 ± 3	$0.98 \pm .02$	5.3 ± 0.8	54.2 ± 8.4

[a]Utilization rates were determined from the product of flow and arteriovenous substrate differences. Errors are standard deviations from literature values using their reported errors as weighting factors. Compared with PET data, most reported global values refer only to the supratentorial portion of the brain, whereas values in the table are for whole brain.

Source: Data from Kety and Schmidt,[6] Kety and Schmidt,[9] Alexander et al,[10] Takeshita et al,[11] Mazziotta and Phelps[81] and from: Scheinberg P, Stead EA Jr. *J Clin Invest.* 1949;28:1161–1171; Novack P, Goluboff B, Burtin L, Soffe A, Shenkin HA. *Circulation.* 1953;7:724–731; Mangold R, Sokoloff L, Conner E, Kleinerman J, Therman P-OG, Kety SS. *J Clin Invest.* 1955;34:1092–1100; Sokoloff L, Mangold R, Wechsler RL, Kennedy C, Kety SS. *J Clin Invest.* 1955;34:1101–1108; Gottein U, Bernsmeier A, Sedlmeyer I. *Klin Wochenschr.* 1963;41:943–948; Cohen PJ, Alexander SC, Smith TC, Reivich M, Wollman H. *J Appl Physiol Physiol.* 1967;23:183–189.

TABLE 7-2. Local Metabolic Rates of Glucose Utilization Reported in the Literature (reference number in parentheses) from Both Autoradiographic and PET Studies[a]

	Rat: DG[b] (12)	Cat: DG	Monkey: DG[b]	Human: FDG–PET (17)	Human: FDG–PET (14)	Human: FDG–PET[c] (15) Left	Right
Gray matter structures							
Frontal cortex	116 ± 5	50	50 ± 2	34		43 ± 10	43 ± 10
Parietal cortex	107 ± 3		47 ± 4	38	37	43 ± 9	42 ± 10
Occipital cortex	111 ± 5		59 ± 2	57	38		
Primary visual						47 ± 11	46 ± 11
Assoc. visual						36 ± 9	37 ± 9
Inferior occipital						36 ± 6	38 ± 6
Temporal cortex	157 ± 5	32	79 ± 4	45	36	44 ± 12	43 ± 11
Cingulate cortex						43 ± 12	43 ± 11
Lenticular nuclei						45 ± 9	44 ± 8
Striatum						44 ± 10	45 ± 12
Caudate	111 ± 4	41	52 ± 3	38	32	38 ± 8	38 ± 9
Thalamus	103 ± 3	26	49 ± 2	41	32	36 ± 7	36 ± 7
Hippocampus	79 ± 1	64	39 ± 2	32			
Inferior colliculus	198 ± 7						
Superior colliculus	99 ± 3						
Medial geniculate	126 ± 5						
Lateral geniculate	92 ± 2	48	39 ± 1				
Pontine tegmentum	69 ± 3		28 ± 1				
Cerebellar cortex	66 ± 2		31 ± 2				
White matter structures							
Corpus callosum	42 ± 2		11 ± 0	20		23 ± 8	23 ± 8
Centrum semiovale						29 ± 7	28 ± 7
Frontal white		5		20	21		
Parietal white			11 ± 1	20	20		
Occipital white		5		23	20		
Cerebellar white	38 ± 2		12 ± 1				
Global value				32	29	30 ± 4	32 ± 4

Abbreviations: DG, [14C]deoxyglucose; FDG, 2-deoxy-2-[F-18]fluoro-D-glucose; PET, positron emission tomography.

[a]Units are in μmol of glucose/min/100 g.   [b]Errors are standard error of the mean.   [c]Errors are standard deviations.

Source: Data from Sokoloff et al,[12] Reivich et al,[17] Kuhl et al,[14] Mazziotta et al,[15] and Mazziotta and Phelps.[81]

dividing the grams of glucose by the molecular weight of glucose (180 g/mole). Table 7-2 includes local cerebral metabolic rate for glucose (LCMRGlc) values reported in the early literature for both autoradiographic animal studies and human PET studies. The values in humans agree well with previous global values obtained using the Kety–Schmidt[6] method (Table 7-1).

EXAMPLE 7-1

Whole-brain glucose utilization was measured to be 30 μmoles/min/100 g of brain tissue by the Kety–Schmidt technique. What is the corresponding CMRglc as measured in mg glucose/min/100 g?

ANSWER

(30 μmoles/min/100g) $\times$ (180 μgrams glucose/μmole)
$\times$ (1 mg/1000 μgrams) = 5.4 mg glucose/min/100 g

Regional values which have been more recently published[19–21] (Table 7-3), reflecting measurements using instruments and techniques with improved imaging capabilities are in substantial agreement with the initially reported values.

EXAMPLE 7-2
Succinctly describe the biochemical basis for mapping regional cerebral activity using FDG–PET images of the brain.

ANSWER
Increased cerebral activity in a brain region involves increased synaptic firing, which is energy-expensive: It requires dissipation of gradients of ions (electrically charged molecules) across neuronal membranes which are then restored through hydrolysis of the energy-rich phosphate bonds found in ATP. In fact, approximately half of all ATP consumption in the brain is to support synaptic firing. This, in turn, requires increased utilization of glucose, the primary (greater than 95%) metabolic fuel driving the synthesis of ATP in the brain, which is measured using PET with a glucose analog labeled with F-18, FDG. FDG is taken up via neuronal glucose transporters and, after being phosphorylated by hexokinase, becomes trapped intracellularly from where its radioactive emissions are detected and localized by the PET instrument.

TABLE 7-3. Rates of Regional Glucose Utilization Determined with FDG–PET in Normal Subjects[a]

Region	Minoshima et al[19] 64 ± 8 y.o. N = 22	Moeller et al.[20] <50 y.o. N = 58	Moeller et al[20] ≥50 y.o. N = 72	Ishii et al[21] 67 ± 6 y.o. N = 21
FC	7.9 (43.9)			
inf FC				7.7 (42.8)
mid FC				7.6 (42.2)
sup FC				7.2 (40.0)
ant CC				7.2 (40.0)
med FC		8.8 (48.9)	7.9 (43.9)	
lat FC		9.1 (50.6)	8.4 (46.7)	
SM	**7.7 (42.8)**	**8.7 (48.3)**	**8.0 (44.4)**	**7.6 (42.2)**
PC	**7.8 (43.3)**			
inf PC		8.9 (49.4)	8.2 (45.6)	7.7 (42.8)
sup PC				7.4 (41.1)
TC	**6.8 (37.8)**			
ant TC				6.3 (35.0)
pos TC				7.3 (40.6)
med TC		6.8 (37.8)	6.5 (36.1)	5.1 (28.3)
lat TC		6.6 (36.7)	6.1 (33.9)	
OC	**8.1 (45.0)**			
med OC		8.5 (47.2)	8.1 (45.0)	8.0 (44.4)
lat OC		8.1 (45.0)	7.9 (43.9)	7.6 (42.2)
BG		**9.7 (53.9)**	**9.2 (51.1)**	**8.4 (46.7)**
T	**8.7 (48.3)**	**8.8 (48.9)**	**8.9 (49.4)**	**7.6 (42.2)**
Crb		**5.6 (31.1)**	**6.9 (38.3)**	**6.7 (37.2)**

Abbreviations: BG, basal ganglia; Crb, cerebellum; FDG, 2-deoxy-2-[F-18]fluoro-D-glucose; FC, frontal cortex (inferior, middle, superior, anterior cingulate, medial, lateral); N, number of patients; OC, occipital cortex (medial, lateral); PC, parietal cortex (inferior, superior); PET, positron emission tomography; SM, sensorimotor strip; T, thalamus; TC, temporal cortex (anterior, posterior, medial, lateral); y.o., years old.

[a]All values are expressed in mg/min/100 g, followed by μmoles/min/100 g in parentheses; values in bold are for entire structures or lobes.

Cerebral blood flow

Cerebral blood flow (CBF) has traditionally been quantified in either of two ways: 1) as a flow rate, expressed as volume of blood flowing per unit of time (e.g., ml/min), or 2) as a rate of tissue perfusion, expressed as volume of blood flowing through a given quantity of tissue per unit of time (e.g., ml/min/100 g). By common use, CBF can refer to either blood flow or perfusion. In the healthy brain, blood flow is normally tightly coupled with local metabolic needs of brain tissue, through vasoconstrictive-vasodilatory autoregulation of blood supply. With respect to physiologic function, perfusion directly relates to the supply of nutrient delivery to tissue through the capillary beds. Within a vascular territory, measures of CBF and glucose metabolic rate covary nearly linearly. Between different vascular territories, however, different constants of proportionality can pertain. For example, because most of the lateral neocortex is supplied by the middle cerebral artery branch of the carotid circulation, the pattern of distribution of CBF imaged with the diffusible tracer $H_2^{15}O$ closely parallels that of the cerebral metabolic rate for glucose (CMRglc) throughout most of the cortical surface (Figure 7-2). In contrast, the cerebellum, despite its lower CMRglc relative to neocortex, is more richly perfused (e.g., compare planes 32 to 37 of Figure 7-2 with comparable planes 39 to 44 of Figure 7-1), being supplied by arterial branches of the vertebrobasilar circulation. Also, in certain pathologic circumstances (e.g., see section on stroke below, p. 546), the normal coupling between metabolism and CBF can be disturbed, such that a consistent relationship may not exist even within a vascular territory.

Images of regional cerebral function (rCf) can be obtained with $H_2^{15}O$ (or $^{15}O_2$), as with FDG. In the case of these former tracers, however, the short physical half-life (2 min) of the ^{15}O radionuclide makes them especially suitable for acquiring multiple data sets from the same individual over a relatively brief period. This period allows statistical analyses of changes observed in rCf (measured quantitatively or semiquantitatively, as described for FDG) during varying experimental conditions, such as resting versus motor, sensory, or cognitive activities; predrug versus postdrug and withdrawal states; waking versus various stages of sleeping; comfort versus discomfort or pain; and emotional calm versus induced sadness, anxiety, sexual arousal, fear, or anger. This paradigm for studying brain function, referred to as an activation study, has been used in thousands of investigations for the purpose of identifying cerebral correlates of normal and pathologic processes involved in mentation and behavior. It lies far beyond the scope of this chapter to provide even a superficial review of that enormous body of work. The application of the activation paradigm will, however, be examined in greater detail in a subsequent section regarding the study of visceral pain as an example of this approach because of the central importance of that perceptual experience to diverse fields of medical practice.

Efforts over the years to quantify cerebral blood flow in absolute units (generally ml/min/100 g) with PET have yielded values varying more widely than corresponding efforts to quantify glucose metabolism. Factors contributing to this variability include the tracers used, the evolving spatial resolution of scanning systems, whether and how blood volume corrections are performed, lower statistical accuracy compared to FDG studies, and whether 1-compartment or 2-compartment models are used.[22] For example, at one end of the spectrum, an early

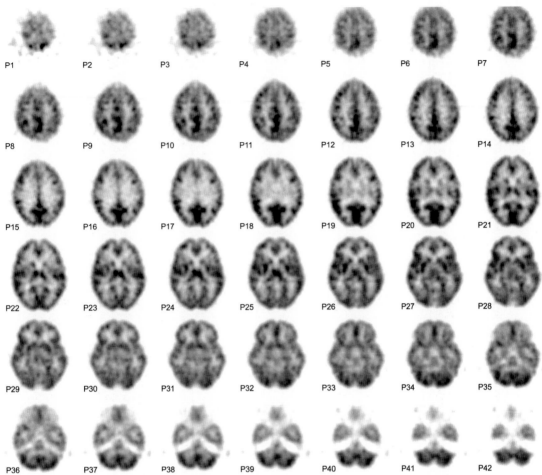

FIGURE 7-2. Baseline pattern of cerebral blood flow imaged with [O-15]water in a healthy 55-year-old woman. The display is in the same format as that of Figure 7-1 but with plane 1 through plane 42.

report of cerebral blood flow measurements[23] in 7 subjects with a mean age of 27 years, using $H_2{}^{15}O$-PET without correction for blood volume, estimated mean gray matter flow at only 39 ± 7 ml/min/100 g (Table 7-4).[23,25–28,30–33,36,37] A recent study[24] using a 1-compartment model and magnetic resonance (MR)-based, partial-volume corrections in 18 subjects with a mean age of 28 years, estimated cortical flow at 62 ± 10 ml/min/100 ml. In a systematic methodologic study,[22] 64 $H_2{}^{15}O$ scans were acquired of 8 subjects in which the investigators found a 2-compartment model to be superior to a 1-compartment model for their imaging data. Using that model with partial-volume correction yielded values of gray matter flow at 107 ± 11 ml/min/100 g (substantially higher than their estimate using the same data set, but with a 1-compartment model, which yielded values of 52 ± 7 ml/min/100 g). It should be emphasized that the above discussion includes the extremes of quantitative cerebral perfusion measurements that have been made with PET over the years. Most published studies have reported values in the range of 40 ml/min/100 g to 80 ml/min/100 g for gray mat-

TABLE 7-4. Cerebral Blood Flow, Oxygen Utilization, and Oxygen Extraction Fraction in Early PET Studies of Human Brain[a]

Reference		Frackowiak et al[30]	Avg. 43	Lenzi et al[33]	Lenzi et al[32]	18F-CH₃	Huang et al[13]
	N	14	7	14	27	13	7
	Age range (yrs)	26–74	43	49–76	50 ± [e]	32–54	Mean = 27.3
	method[b]	^{15}O-CI	^{15}O-CI	^{15}O-CI	^{15}O-CI	^{18}F-CH$_3$	^{15}O-H$_2$O
Mean gray (temporal-insula)	LCBF[c]	65.3 ± 7.2	61 ± 10		64.5 ± 17.3	55.2 ± 8.2	39.1 ± 7.2
	LCMRO$_2$	263 ± 26	109 ± 33		256 ± 50		
	LOEF	49 ± 2			47 ± 9		
Frontal cortex	LCBF			45.0	51.9 ± 5.8		
	LCMRO$_2$			185			
	LOEF			50			
Visual cortex	LCBF	63 ± 17		46.3	60.2 ± 7.9		
	LCMRO$_2$	242 ± 60		204			
	LOEF			52			
Thalamus	LCBF	49 ± 11			54.9 ± 9.6		
	LCMRO$_2$	149 ± 26					
	LOEF						
Mean white (centrum semiovale)	LCBF	21.4 ± 1.9	20 ± 7		21.2 ± 2.7	25.8 ± 5.1	18.9 ± 3.2
	LCMRO$_2$	80 ± 10	71 ± 14		82 ± 15		
	LOEF	48 ± 4			47 ± 9		
Global	LCBF	47.7[d]		39.3 ± 5.8	42.8 ± 4.2	31.1 ± 5.5	
	LCMRO$_2$	188[d]	167 ± 27				
	LOEF	49[d]		56 ± 6			

Abbreviations: CI, continuous inhalation of ^{15}O-labeled CO$_2$ and O$_2$; LCBF, cerebral blood flow (ml/min/100 g); LCBV, local cerebral blood volume; LCMRO$_2$, cerebral metabolic rate for oxygen (μmol of glucose/min/100 g); LOEF, oxygen extraction fraction (%); PET, positron emission tomography.

[a]All values are obtained with the ECAT II PET device[25]; regions of interest sizes vary; errors are standard deviations; data uncorrected for blood volume.

[b]CI, otherwise, bolus administration used; normal values for LCBF may vary significantly because of its proportional dependence on P_{aco_2}.

[c]LCBF has been measured with [^{18}F]fluoromethane, [26][^{11}C]methylglucose, [27] ^{77}Kr,[28] and both continuous and bolus administration of ^{15}O-labeled compounds (water or carbon dioxide). LCMRO$_2$, and LOEF have been measured using ^{15}O-labeled gaseous oxygen most typically with continuous inhalation.[31] As with the glucose method, PET values for LCMRO$_2$ and LCBF are in reasonably good agreement with global values for the same variable obtained with Kety–Schmidt techniques (Table 7-1). Values for LOEF and, therefore, for LCMRO$_2$, are overestimated when the effect of LCBV is not taken into consideration.[36] This overestimation is approximately 20% to 30% of the uncorrected value[37] in normal subjects compared to global values listed in Tables 7-1 and 7-2; most recent studies have measured LCBV to correct LOEF and LCMRO$_2$, values for this error.

[d]Assume 60:40 distribution of gray to white matter.

[e]N = 16, < 50 years old; N = 11, > 50 years old.

Source: Adapted with permission from Mazziotta and Phelps.[81]

ter structures. Nevertheless, given that the standard deviations for absolute flow determinations within investigations are typically 10% to 20%, but that between investigations can vary by 100% or more, the need for each study to define a baseline or control range, maintaining a consistent methodology across both experimental and control groups or conditions, is clear.

Neurotransmitter systems

PET provides a unique window through which to view neurotransmitter systems in the brain. For example, the longterm time course and regional localization of dopamine system dysfunction can be followed in motor disorders (e.g., Parkinson's disease and other Parkinsonian syndromes), psychiatric disorders (e.g., depression, obsessive-compulsive disorder, schizophrenia, and attention deficit disorder), and effects of neuroactive drugs (e.g., cocaine, methamphetamine, and alcohol). A continuing goal in PET research is to design tracers and kinetic models that can provide detailed assessments of neurotransmitter system functions in vivo. PET tracers have been synthesized for multiple components of neurotransmitter pathways, providing estimates of enzyme synthesis rates and concentrations of pre- and postsynaptic membrane-bound proteins such as uptake transporters and receptors. Novel PET methods have also been developed to assess occupancy of receptors by pharmacologic doses of drugs and the effects of drugs on neurotransmitter release. These methods provide the framework for clinical applications in normal biological and disease states. For each of several neurotransmitter systems, presynaptic activity (synthesis, storage, and release) and receptor binding will be reviewed in the context of PET tracers designed to monitor those parameters.

PET studies of the striatal dopamine system represent the most developed example of translating knowledge of neurotransmitter concepts into the design of PET studies. Because studies on other neurotransmitter systems have been largely based on the dopamine system paradigm, a detailed critique of dopaminergic PET tracers will first be presented.

Dopamine system

The potential choices for dopamine system PET tracers have been based on subcellular components that regulate major aspects of dopamine function. Those targets include the dopamine synthetic enzymes (tyrosine hydroxylase monoamineoxidase and aromatic acid decarboxylase), the dopamine transporter associated with the neuronal membrane that removes dopamine from the extracellular space, the vesicular amine transporter that sequesters dopamine from the cytoplasm into vesicles, and five receptor subtypes that bind selectively to dopamine.[38] Successful PET tracers have been more difficult to develop for some of these regulation sites, due in part to the lack of specificity for those targets, as well as limitations related to pharmacokinetic issues.[39,40] Many PET ligands, however, have been designed to study specific dopaminergic parameters in normal and disease states with markers of pre- and postsynaptic function, as well as of regional levels of the monoamine oxidase enzymes MAO-A and MAO-B (Figure 7-3).

RATE OF SYNTHESIS

Aromatic amino acid decarboxylase (AAAD) is an enzyme selective for neurotransmitter synthesis and is present in dopaminergic, noradrenergic, and sero-

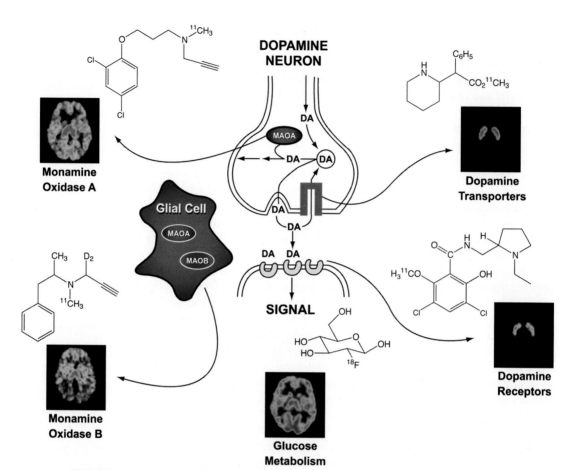

FIGURE 7-3. Overview of PET applications for molecular characterization of the dopamine system in the human brain. *Upper right:* [11C]methylphenidate binds to the dopamine transporter; the extent of its binding is used to index striatal dopamine terminal integrity. *Lower right:* [11C]raclopride binds to dopamine D_2 receptors and is used to determine receptor levels. *Lower center:* [18FDG] enters into the glycolysis metabolic pathway of all cells. After [18FDG] is metabolized by the rate-limiting enzyme, hexokinase, the [18F]FDG-6-phosphate product remains metabolically trapped, providing an index of glucose metabolic rates. [11C]d_2-deprenyl (lower left) and [11C]chlorgyline (upper left) bind irreversibly to MAO-B and MAO-A, respectively, providing selective measures of those enzyme levels. The incorporation of two deuterium atoms in the deprenyl analogue yields more favorable enzyme kinetics. (Courtesy of N.D. Volkow, MD, and J.S. Fowler, MD.)

tonergic systems. In PET studies of the striatum, uptake of the [F-18]fluorinated analog of dihydroxyphenylalanine (FDOPA) has been used to examine transport of dopamine precursor from plasma and its decarboxylation by AAAD to form fluorodopamine.[41,42] Dynamic measures of FDOPA distribution are thus used to assess AAAD-catalyzed synthesis of dopamine in neurons. These measured changes in rates of dopamine synthesis, however, cannot be used to differentiate between changes occurring in activity per neuron terminal versus changes in the total number of terminals. Without either factor being independently measured, the product of average activity per neuron and the number of terminals can be considered the dopamine synthesis capacity for the region of interest (ROI).

LABELING OF PRESYNAPTIC TRANSPORTER

Additional information can be obtained with PET tracers that bind selectively to the dopamine transporter (DAT).[43] These measurements provide an indirect assessment of dopamine terminal density, based on studies that have shown a correlation between the number of ligand binding sites and number of terminals.[44] For PET, ^{11}C and ^{18}F positron-labeled tropanes have been developed, such as the DAT ligand and a cocaine analog, [^{11}C]WIN-35,428 (WIN).[45] However, insofar as the DAT may be subject to regulation by neuronal activity and drugs, its use as a terminal density index may be compromised. In contrast, another PET ligand, $(+)$-α-[^{11}C] dihydrotetrabenazine (DTBZ), selective for the vesicular monoamine transporter (VMAT), appears to be less susceptible to regulation.[44] Hence, measurements of its binding should provide a more reliable correlate of terminal density. The VMAT is, however, not selective for dopamine and is located in norepinephrine and serotonin terminals as well. In normal subjects, PET imaging of the striatum with the tracers, FDOPA, WIN, and DTBZ show with comparable spatial resolution the corresponding presynaptic processes (Figure 7-4).

POSTSYNAPTIC TARGETS

Measurements of the equilibrium dissociation constant (K_d) and the total number of specific binding types (Bmax) individually are readily obtained from in vitro tissue studies using a range of tracer concentrations but have not often been obtained from PET studies. The necessity for multiple PET studies with the tracer at different specific activities in each subject is often a logistical problem that is compounded by the potential for changes in receptor number that may occur between studies.[46,47] Rather, most human studies have used kinetic models that yield the ratio Bmax/K_d, often referred to as binding potential, which can be obtained from a single study[48] (Chapter 2).

Among dopamine receptors in striatum, the D1 and D2 subtypes have been most systematically studied due, in part, to their relatively high abundance there[49] and because they are common therapeutic targets. In contrast, the significantly lower levels of D3 to D5 receptors in striatum and the lack of availability of selective PET tracers have not yet allowed for their quantitative characterization.

D1 and D2 PET tracers show similar spatial resolution in striatum (Figure 7-5). The majority of PET studies have measured the D2 subtype, focusing on its involvement in motor disorders, psychiatric states, and drug abuse. D2 receptor PET tracers have also been used to assess synaptic dopamine concentrations, based on the extent of displacement by pharmacological drug-induced dopamine release (Figure 7-6). Valid interpretation of these data is premised on the postulates of the receptor occupancy model.[50] Although the measurement made does not explicitly account for the presence of variable basal dopamine levels in the extracellular space, drug-induced increases in dopamine do result in greater occupancy of available receptor binding sites, thereby reducing the apparent binding potential of the PET tracer. This approach offers the possibility to determine how dopamine release may be dif-

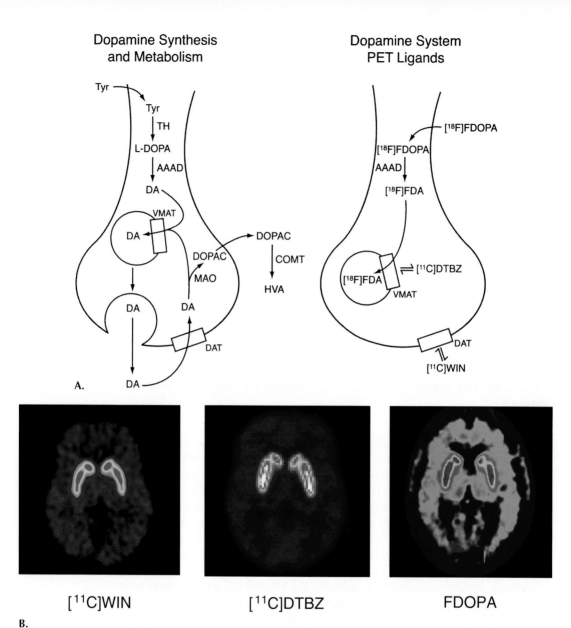

FIGURE 7-4. Imaging presynaptic parameters of striatal dopamine system integrity. A: The schematic diagrams of a presynaptic nerve terminal show the dopamine synthesis and metabolism pathway (*left*) and key proteins that are targets for PET imaging in striatum (*right*). B: The cross-sectional PET images show the striatum of human brain as generated by three differently labeled ligands that provide unique structural or functional information on dopamine system integrity. *Left:* ([^{11}C]WIN binds to the DAT which is located on dopaminergic axons. *Middle:* [^{11}C]DTBZ binds to the VMAT located on dopamine storage vesicles. *Right:* FDOPA in the striatum is a substrate for AAAD and is converted to [^{18}F]fluorodopamine which is then stored in dopamine storage vesicles. Because AAAD is contained primarily within dopaminergic neurons, the extent of [^{18}F]fluorodopamine accumulation provides an estimate of that region's dopamine synthesis capacity. Abbreviations: AAAD, aromatic acid decarboxylase; [^{11}C]DTBZ, [^{11}C](+)-dihydrotetrabenazine; [^{11}C]WIN, [^{11}C]WIN35,428]; COMT, catechol-O-methyltransferase; DA, dopamine; DAT, dopamine transporter; DOPAC, 3,4-dihydroxyphenylacetic acid; FDOPA, [F-18]fluoro-L-DOPA; [^{18}F]FDA, 6-[^{18}F]fluorodopamine; HVA, homovanillic acid; MAO, monoamine oxidase; TH, thyroid hormone; Tyr, tyrosine; VMAT, vesicular monoamine transporter. ([^{11}C]DTBZ image courtesy of K.A. Frey, MD.)

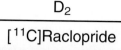

D_1	D_2
[^{11}C]NNC 112	[^{11}C]Raclopride

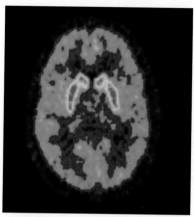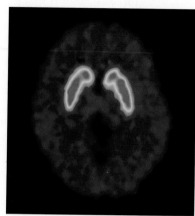

FIGURE 7-5. Imaging dopamine D_1 and D_2 receptors in striatum. Dopamine D_1 and D_2 receptors can be imaged by the binding of the labeled ligands, (+)-[^{11}C]NNC 112 and [^{11}C]raclopride which are dopamine D_1 and D_2 antagonists, respectively. The PET images show that both (+)-[^{11}C]NNC 112, *(left)*, and [^{11}C]raclopride, *(right)*, have their highest binding in striatum, the brain region with the highest concentration of D_1 and D_2 receptors. [(+)-[^{11}C]NNC 112 image reprinted with permission from Halldin et al[256]; Raclopride image reprinted from Volkow et al.,[235] with permission from the Society for Neuroscience, Copyright 2001.)]

ferentially affected in psychiatric, drug-induced changes, and motor disorders. Recent experimental data, however, show that some aspects of receptor regulation are not formally described by the receptor occupancy model. Those results indicate that ligand-receptor occupancy kinetics fail to fully account for the following: receptor internalization, receptor recycling, receptor phosphorylation, effects of G-protein-receptor interactions, and diffusion characteristics of the PET tracer across neuronal membranes. These actions on receptor dynamics remain to be incorporated into PET tracer kinetic models. The use of PET receptor binding methods for absolute quantitative assessment of drug-induced dopamine release thus awaits further validation. These and other issues related to imaging dopaminergic neurotransmission with *in vivo* competition binding methods have been comprehensively reviewed.[51]

EXAMPLE 7-3

Calculate the K_d and B_{max}, *in vivo*, for a novel labeled ligand that binds to a specific receptor subtype in brain. For this calculation, a saturation binding experiment is conducted which is based on receptor occupancy model kinetics:

$$[L] + [R] \longleftrightarrow [LR]$$
$$K_d = [L][R]/[LR]$$

Abbreviations are: L = free radioactive ligand; R = unbound receptor; R_T = total receptors; LR = bound ligand-receptor; $[R] = [R_T] - [LR]$.

Substitution and rearrangement of the above equation yields the Scatchard equation:

$$[LR] / [L] = -[LR] / K_d + [R_T] / K_d \qquad slope / K_d = -1$$

A minimum of two imaging studies is required and is often the only option for studies in humans. In the example here, four different radioligand concentrations are used to obtain more accurate values of K_d and B_{max}. For each study, the specific bound receptor concentration is determined in the region of interest at equilibrium, using an appropriate kinetic model (Chapter 1). The free ligand is estimated by using its concentration either in plasma or a ROI devoid of the receptor. Suppose the following data are obtained from an image-based binding experiment:

Study #	Specific bound in ROI ([LR])(nmol/l)	Plasma ligand concentration ([L]) (nmol/l)	Bound/free
1	0.8	0.04	20
2	24	2.4	10
3	35	5.8	6
4	52	21	2.5

Perform a linear regression (Scatchard) analysis to calculate the K_d and B_{max} (which is equivalent to $[R_T] \times$ [volume of sample])

ANSWER
Plot [LR]/[L] (bound/free) vs. [LR] (bound).

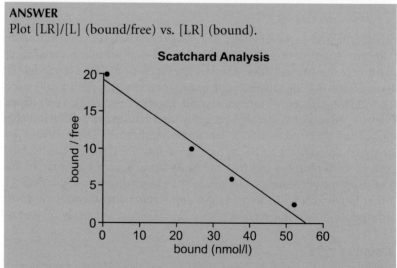

The slope can be used to calculate the K_d value and the X-intercept to obtain $[R_T]$.

$$slope = -0.35 \pm 0.04 \text{ nM}^{-1}$$
$$slope = -1 / K_d; K_d = 2.9 \text{ nM}$$
$$X\text{-intercept} = B_{max} = 55.63 \text{ nmol/L}$$

Serotonin system

The serotonin system appears to modulate activities of other neuronal systems throughout the entire brain as evidenced by its widespread projections into

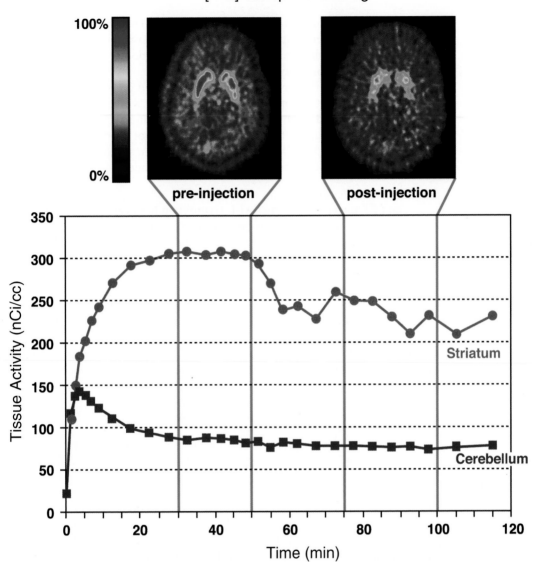

FIGURE 7-6. Imaging dopamine release in the striatum. Drugs such as d-amphetamine that release dopamine can be used in conjunction with [^{11}C]raclopride, a dopamine D$_2$ receptor antagonist that binds selectively to D$_2$ receptors, to assess the functional activity of presynaptic dopamine terminals. In this example, [^{11}C]raclopride is injected first as a bolus and then followed by constant infusion over 120 minutes. This protocol is designed to achieve steady-state levels of [^{11}C]raclopride in brain and plasma. At 50 minutes after [^{11}C]raclopride administration, amphetamine (0.2 mg/kg) is injected. The increase in extracellular dopamine concentrations caused by the drug will displace a corresponding fraction of the previously bound [^{11}C]raclopride, providing an index of dopamine release. In this example, the binding of [^{11}C]raclopride is decreased by 20% due to its displacement by the amphetamine-induced dopamine release. The effects of amphetamine are shown in the time-activity curves for striatum (red) but not for cerebellum (blue) because only the striatum contains a high concentration of dopamine terminals. The cerebellar curve is used to calculate nonspecific [^{11}C]raclopride binding. Cross-sectional PET images of [^{11}C]raclopride binding in striatum are shown before (*left*) and after (*right*) the amphetamine injection. This methodology can be used to assess alterations of dopamine terminal responsivity in normal and pathological disease states. (Reprinted with permission from Breier et al.,[257] with permission from National Academy of Sciences, U.S.A., copyright 1997.)

cortical and subcortical structures.[52] Pharmacological manipulations of the serotonin system have demonstrated its influence on behavioral states of depression, anxiety, and schizophrenia. Selective regional activation is facilitated by at least 14 serotonin receptor subtypes.

PET imaging of the serotonin system has focused on parameters analogous to those assessed in the dopamine system—namely, synthetic enzymes, the uptake transporter, and receptors. The wide distribution of serotonergic terminals and receptors throughout the brain has, however, not yielded such clear imaging resolution of ROIs as has been possible with the striatal dopamine system nor the development of comparable quantitative models.

Rate of synthesis

The PET tracer, [^{11}C]α-methyl-L-tryptophan has been synthesized in order to track serotonin synthesis through its conversion to α-methylhydroxytryptophan by the rate-limiting enzyme, tryptophan hydroxylase, and then decarboxylation to α-methylserotonin by AAAD. Unlike serotonin, this analogue is not catabolized by MAO and, therefore, the rate of its accumulation in brain was postulated to reflect the average serotonin synthesis rate. Initial studies with this tracer were thus interpreted as detecting differences in serotonin synthesis rates between groups, (e.g., sex differences[53] and increases in migraine conditions[54]). Subsequent studies in animals, however, have indicated that the extent of [^{11}C]α-methyl-L-tryptophan accumulation is limited by its rate of transport into brain, which is heavily influenced by plasma and brain concentrations of large neutral amino acids.[55] It thus remains to be clarified to what extent synthetic rates vary with age, sex, and disease states.

Labeling of presynaptic transporter

Measurements of serotonin transporter (SERT) density have been used to evaluate serotonin system integrity. Serotonin-specific reuptake inhibitors, such as the antidepressants fluoxetine and paroxetine, have relatively high affinity for SERT and have been labeled with ^{11}C or ^{18}F as potential PET tracers.[56] Investigators have found in *in vivo* studies of the pharmacology of the tracers, however, that their extensive lipophilicity results in high levels of nonspecific binding and slow clearance rates—parameters that are unfavorable for quantitative PET imaging. In contrast, studies with the SERT-ligand tracer, trans-1,2,3,5,6,10-beta-hexahydro-6-[4-(methylthio)phenyl]pyrrolo-[2,1-a]-isoquinoline ([+]-[11C]McN5652), have shown the expected regional differences in binding within the brain (e.g., greater binding in thalamus, hypothalamus, basal ganglia, and midbrain binding relative to cerebral cortex) not found with its inactive (−) enantiomer (Figure 7-7). These methods, as well as the use of kinetic models, are best suited to detecting differences in regions with a high density of specific binding sites for the ligand, due to the relatively high background contributed by nonspecific binding.[57]

Acetylcholine system

Cholinergic pharmacology has been the focus of much research on Alzheimer's disease and, to a lesser extent, Parkinson's disease and schizophrenia. Tracer development has been largely directed towards assessment of concentrations of muscarinic and nicotinic receptors and acetylcholinesterase.[58] (S)-(−)-[11C]nicotine was one of the first radioligands synthesized for the purpose of studying cholinergic systems in human brain, but its uptake appeared to reflect perfusion and extraction across the blood-brain barrier more than specific bind-

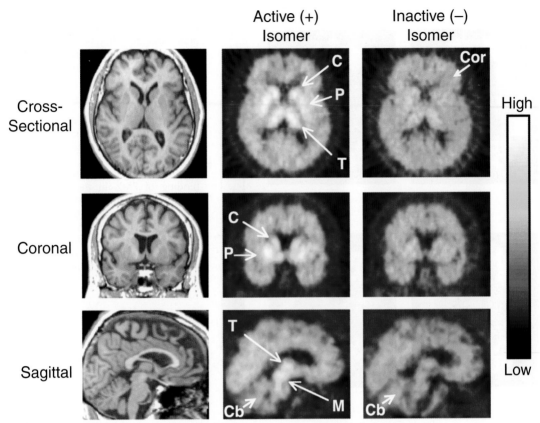

FIGURE 7-7. Imaging serotonin transporters in the brain. The labeled ligand, (+)-[^{11}C]McN 5652, binds with high affinity to the 5-HT transporter (specific binding) but also binds nonspecifically throughout the brain. Magnetic resonance (MR) images, (*left column*), are used to accurately define ROIs on the PET images. The sum of specific and nonspecific binding (total binding) is shown in the (+)-[^{11}C]McN 5652 PET images (*middle column*). The less active isomer, the labeled ligand, (−)-[^{11}C]McN 5652, binds to the 5-HT transporter with low affinity and its specific binding to the transporter is considered negligible (*right column*). It does bind to nonspecific sites, however, with an affinity similar to that of the (+)-isomer. To calculate the binding specific to the transporter, the non-specific (−)-[^{11}C]McN 5652 binding is subtracted from the (+)-[^{11}C]McN 5652 total binding. A color (heat) scale common to all PET images represents the activity in tissues and is used for visual comparison of binding differences between regions. Cross-sectional (top row), coronal (middle row), and sagittal (lower row) views are shown. Binding densities are highest in the caudate (C), putamen (P), thalamus (T), and midbrain (M). Notice that on the low affinity (−) isomer images (*right column*), the binding in cortex (Cor), a region with 5-HT transporters, is only marginally higher than that in cerebellum (Cb), a region without 5-HT transporters, indicating that the binding in both regions is predominantly nonspecific. (Reprinted with permission from Parsey et al.[258])

ing parameters.[59] More selective agents such as [18F]analogs of the nicotinic acetylcholine receptor agonist, epibatidine (exo-2-(2'-chloro-5'-pyridyl)-7-azabicyclo[2.2.1]heptane), have been proposed for human imaging, based on PET studies in baboons demonstrating thalamus and cerebellum binding ratios that reflected corresponding high and low receptor densities in those regions.[60] Tracers for muscarinic receptors such as analogues of 3-quinuclidinyl benzilate have

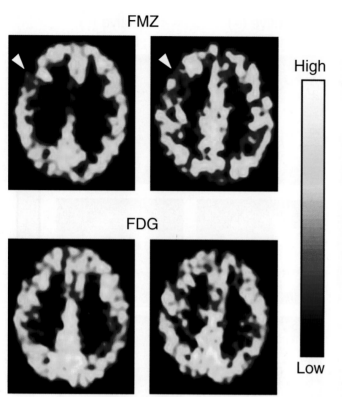

FMZ

High

FDG

Low

FIGURE 7-8. Monitoring GABA$_A$ receptor distribution in an epileptic patient. Imaging alterations in regional GABA$_A$ receptor distributions can reveal epilepsy-related pathology that is not apparent by more global assessments of brain function, such as glucose metabolic rates with FDG. *Upper:* In this study, GABA$_A$ receptors are imaged in an epileptic patient by the binding of the labeled ligand, [^{11}C]flumazenil (FMZ), a benzodiazepine antagonist. The decreased binding of FMZ in the right frontal lobe, identifies and localizes a cryptogenic epilepsy. *Lower:* In contrast, imaging with FDG shows normal glucose metabolic rates throughout the same cortical region. (Reprinted from Ryulin et al.,[259] with permission from Oxford University Press.)

also been synthesized but remain less well characterized with respect to binding kinetics and receptor selectivity.[61,62]

GABA system

As the predominant inhibitory neurotransmitter in brain, gamma-aminobutryic acid (GABA) subserves many functions by modulating neuronal firing frequency. For example, pharmacological alterations of GABA activity selectively alter states of anxiety, consciousness, sleep, and seizures.

The design of PET tracers for the GABA system has been focused on the postsynaptic benzodiazepine binding site. The most well-characterized PET tracer, the benzodiazepine antagonist, [11C]flumazenil has been used to demonstrate regions of high and low binding (Figure 7-8), particularly for the detection of asymmetries related to seizure focus localization in epilepsy.[64] Other applications include measuring GABAergic alterations in neurodegenerative disease and the effects of pharmacological drugs on the GABA system.[65,66]

Opiate system

Opiate activity both influences, and is influenced by, sensation of pain, aspects of drug addiction (Figure 7-9), and various disease processes, such as Parkinson's disease and epilepsy. PET assessment of the opiate system has been directed at mu and kappa receptor alterations as detected by binding of [18F]-cyclofoxy,[67] 11C-diprenorphine,[68] or 11C-carfentanil.[69] Possible alterations in patients with seizures or Parkinson's disease have been assessed with such tracers,[70] but the consistency with which differences between patients and control subjects can be identified has yet to be established.

Mu Opioid Receptor Binding Potential

[^{11}C]Carfentanil

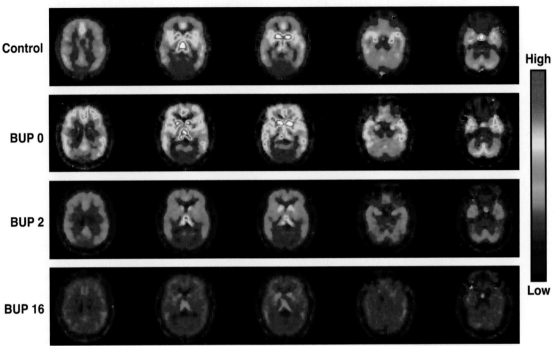

FIGURE 7-9. Monitoring dose-dependent increases in buprenorphine binding to the mu-opioid receptor. The distribution of mu-opioid receptors in a normal subject's brain (*top row*) is shown by the binding of the labeled ligand, [^{11}C]carfentanil, a selective mu-opiate receptor agonist. In a heroin-dependent subject (*row 2*), increases in [^{11}C]carfentanil binding are detected, showing an apparent upregulation of mu-opioid receptors induced by heroin drug exposure. A pharmacotherapy approach for the treatment of heroin dependence is to administer buprenorphine (BUP), a mu-opioid partial agonist. BUP would then occupy a significant fraction of mu-opioid receptors, thereby preventing heroin binding and stimulation. In this example, BUP receptor occupancy is calculated using [^{11}C]carfentanil studies obtained before and after BUP maintenance dose administration. The reduced [^{11}C]carfentanil binding after BUP doses of 2 mg and 16 mg corresponds to fractional receptor occupancies of 36% to 50% and 79% to 95%, respectively. To compare the effects of buprenorphine doses used in these separate studies, the data have been transformed into parametric images that show [^{11}C]carfentanil binding potential (Bmax/K$_d$) on a pixel-by-pixel basis throughout brain. The pseudocolor scale on the right side represents the binding potential values that range from 1 to 4.7, with red being the highest. Images are scaled so that the occipital cortex binding potential, an area devoid of mu-opioid receptors, is equal to 1. In each study, five anatomical levels are shown, from superior, (*left*), to inferior, (*right*), for each set of cross-sectional images. (Reprinted with permission from Zubieta et al.[69])

Other

Although the use of ^{11}C to label organic compounds is limited by its short half-life (20 min), an advantage is that tracers can be prepared which retain the chemical structure and activity of the original compound (i.e., replacing ^{12}C with ^{11}C). These [^{11}C]tracers can be used to assess pharmacokinetic and pharmacodynamic properties of the corresponding pharmacological drug. Traditionally, drug efficacy studies have been conducted in animals and animal models of disease, but those results require careful interpretation because of interspecies differences in pharmacokinetics and how well the animal replicates human disease. With PET, the pharmacology of drugs can be studied *in vivo* directly in the human, obviating extrapolation of results from corresponding animal studies. Initial pharmacokinetic studies can often be safely performed in humans because of the subpharmacologic mass of drug present in typical doses of radiotracers. For example, a pharmacokinetic study with PET was conducted in humans with deprenyl, which is used for treating Parkinson's disease. Deprenyl binds irreversibly to MAO-B. The subsequent enzyme inactivation that occurs at pharmacologic doses of the drug is thought to enhance dopaminergic function by decreasing oxidation of released dopamine and, thus, increasing the concentration of dopamine available for neurotransmission. To determine the distribution and concentration of MAO-B in the brain, [11C]deprenyl was synthesized for use as a PET tracer.[71,72] The results showed that the regional MAO-B distribution in the human brain was ~60% higher in the thalamus and basal ganglia relative to cortical regions and cerebellum.[72] Further, it was demonstrated that age-related increases in MAO-B levels occurred (Figure 7-10).[71] A subsequent study[72] showed that the extent of deprenyl binding to MAO-B after pharmacologic doses could be quantitatively examined by obtaining [11C]deprenyl scans before and after drug administration (5 mg/d for 7 d). The [11C]deprenyl binding was reduced by 90% relative to pretreatment scan values, indicating near complete inactivation of the enzyme. Further, multiple scans performed during the 2 months after the last pharmacologic dose of deprenyl revealed a protracted recovery of MAO-B binding. Because recovery of MAO is generated only by synthesis of new enzyme, that time course was used to calculate a half-time for MAO-B synthesis of 40 days—representing a combined measure of whatever time may have been required to signal an upward shift in gene expression, followed by appropriate transcription, translation, and redeployment of enzyme to where its activity could again be measurably bound by [11C]deprenyl. This study provided the first measurement of the gene expression-based synthetic rate of a specific protein in human brain *in vivo*.[72] These results are of clinical interest, as they raise the possibility that the standard recommended frequency of dosage of deprenyl (5 mg twice a day) may exceed that necessary for maximal therapeutic efficacy.

PET has also been used to quantify the relationship between the dose of a particular drug and the proportion of receptors it occupies. In this paradigm, a PET tracer is used that binds to the same sites as the drug under study. A PET scan is first obtained with the tracer only, followed by subsequent studies in which pharmacological doses of the drug are administered (Figure 7-9). The degree to which binding of the PET tracer in the subsequent studies is competitively inhibited can then be measured. For example, this approach has been applied to studies of antipsychotic drugs. At pharmacologically effective doses, those drugs appear to occupy between 60% and 90% of dopamine D2 receptors, with drug occupancy greater than 80% being associated with extrapyramidal side effects.[73] In contrast, the atypical antipsychotic clozapine at therapeutic doses usually does not induce extrapyramidal side effects, in part due to its D2R occupancy of only 20% to 60% at doses needed to yield therapeutic responses, while its 5HT^{2A} receptor occupancy at those doses is greater than 80% (Figure 7-11).[74]

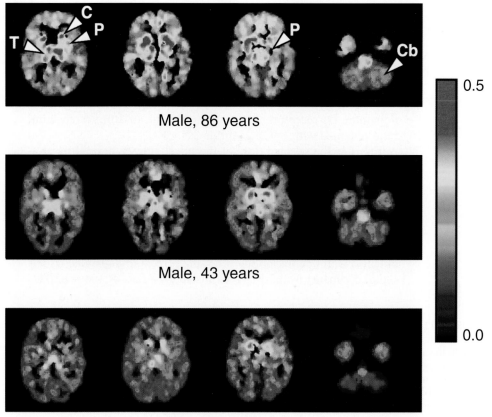

Male, 86 years

Male, 43 years

Male, 27 years

0.5

0.0

FIGURE 7-10. MAO B concentrations in adult human brain increase throughout life. In contrast to general decreases in metabolic markers associated with aging, concentrations of the enzyme monoamine oxidase B (MAO-B) show increases. Because MAO-B functions as an oxidative enzyme, increases in its activity may promote oxidative stress and, possibly, neurotoxicity. In these cross-sectional images, MAO-B is imaged by the binding of the labeled ligand, [^{11}C]L-deprenyl-D2, a selective MAO-B inhibitor with deuterium substituting for two of the hydrogen atoms to yield enzyme kinetics more favorable to imaging in this time-frame.[71] The imaging data have been transformed into parametric images that express on a pixel-by-pixel basis the values of the model term, k_3, which is a function of MAO-B concentration. The color scale ranges from 0—low (black) to 0.5—high (red). As the age of the subject increases from 27 to 43 to 86 years, corresponding increases in [^{11}C]L-deprenyl-D2 binding are detected in the thalamus (T), caudate (C), putamen (P), pons (Pn), and cerebellum (Cb). For example, the k_3 binding values for thalamus increase from 0.25 to 0.35 to 0.43 cc$_{brain}$ (ml$_{plasma}$)$^{-1}$min^{-1}, respectively, between the three subjects. (Reprinted Fowler et al.,[260] with permission from Elsevier.)

EXAMPLE 7-4

Using [^{11}C]raclopride, devise an experiment to determine the percent of dopamine D_2 receptor occupancy *in vivo* (the fraction of the receptors that is occupied by the unlabeled drug) in the human striatum by a novel antipsychotic drug at a given dosage.

ANSWER

1. In the absence of the drug, conduct a $[^{11}C]$raclopride imaging study. Determine the specific binding value in the striatum using an appropriate kinetic model or, under equilibrium conditions, obtain the ratio of total radioactivity in the striatum to that in cerebellum. The cerebellum is considered a reference region with negligible dopamine D_2 receptors. In this example, the striatum/cerebellum ratio obtained with $[^{11}C]$raclopride is 4.

2. Administer the selected dose of the novel antipsychotic drug at a frequency to achieve steady-state conditions, that is, the plasma concentration remains relatively constant; it is assumed that the brain concentration is in equilibrium with that in plasma.

3. Repeat the imaging study with $[^{11}C]$raclopride. The specific binding in striatum will be reduced due to receptor occupancy by the novel antipsychotic drug. For example, if the striatum to cerebellum ratio obtained with $[^{11}C]$raclopride is 1.5, the percent of dopamine D_2 receptor occupancy by the drug is estimated to be $1.5/4 \times 100 = 62.5\%$.

FIGURE 7-11. Characterizing the receptor binding profile of antipsychotic drugs. Many antipsychotic drugs act as antagonists at dopamine D_2 and serotonin 5-HT_2 receptors in brain. In this example, subjects receive multiple-dose regimens of an antipsychotic drug (either haloperidol, risperidone, olanzapine, or clozapine) to achieve steady-state concentrations in plasma and brain. At steady state, the fraction of receptors in brain that is occupied by the drug remains constant. This fractional occupancy by the drug is shown in a subsequent imaging study by the reduction in the normal extent of labeled ligand binding. In this example, the distribution of dopamine D_2 and 5-HT_2 receptors is imaged by the binding of $[^{11}C]$raclopride, a dopamine D_2 receptor antagonist, and by $[^{18}F]$setoperone, 5-HT_2 receptor antagonist. *Upper:* $[^{11}C]$raclopride binding is markedly reduced after haloperidol administration, indicating the high level of D_2 receptor occupancy with haloperidol. Other antipsychotic drugs, particularly clozapine, have less effect on $[^{11}C]$raclopride binding, indicating their low level of D_2 receptor occupancy. *Lower:* The same drugs are now evaluated for their binding affinity to 5-HT_2 receptors. Following administration of either risperidone, olanzapine, or clozapine, $[^{18}F]$setoperone binding is markedly reduced, indicating significant 5-HT_2 occupancy with these drugs. In contrast, haloperidol has minimal effect on $[^{18}F]$setoperone binding, indicating its low 5-HT_2 receptor occupancy. (Reprinted with permission from Verhoeff et al.[40])

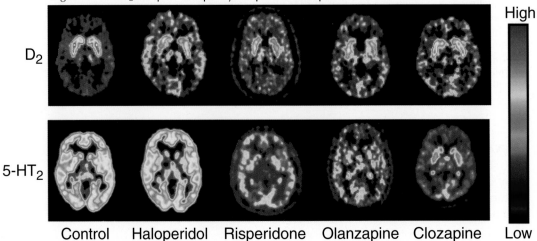

Functional development and aging

How PET-based measurements of normal brain function can be expected to change during the course of development and healthy aging is an important issue. It becomes especially pertinent in the clinical interpretation of scans (where no age-matched explicit control group typically exists) in deciding whether scan findings fall beyond the bounds of what is to be expected for a patient of a given age, in addition to being an issue of intrinsic scientific interest.

Because of understandable ethical concerns surrounding experimental radiation exposure of healthy children, few PET data are available to address normal changes at the young end of the developmental spectrum. Much of what we know in this regard comes from the seminal work of Chugani and colleagues.[75–77] Based on measurements of regional CMRglc in infants who had suffered transient neurologic events—but who were judged to be nearly normal at the time of PET and neurodevelopmentally normal throughout a subsequent followup period—the following picture has emerged. In the newborn, glucose metabolism is highest in primary sensorimotor cortex, cingulate cortex, hippocampal region, thalamus, cerebellar vermis, and midbrain. During the first 3 months of life, the most prominent increases occur in cerebellar cortex, basal ganglia, and parietal, temporal and primary visual cortical areas. In later infancy, increases in glucose utilization are most noticeable in frontal cortex, such that by the end of the first year, the relative distribution of glucose metabolism approximates that of the adult brain. It is interesting to note that this temporal sequence parallels the chronology of evolutionary advancement in mammalian brain structure, with the prefrontal cortex being the last to develop—a vivid illustration of the old biological concept of ontogeny recapitulating phylogeny—and also parallels the emergence of the expanding repertoire of behaviors dependent upon the structures in which CMRglc is increasing.

In terms of absolute rates of glucose utilization, however, developmental changes occur throughout childhood (Figure 7-12, top). Initially lower than in adults, the absolute rate increases throughout the first 3 to 4 years of life, at which time global glucose utilization by the cerebral cortex is actually 2 to 3 times greater than the adult level. This level remains near-constant until age 8 to 10 years, after which a gradual decline subsequently occurs, over approximately 10 years, when adult levels are reached. Autopsy-based studies, involving microscopic analysis of neuritic development, have identified an analogous pattern, except changes in the histopathologically defined density of processes (dendrites, axons, and synapses) precede changes in glucose utilization by about a year. This finding is consistent with a developmental model of anatomic formation of processes, followed by establishment of their capacity to function normally with respect to synaptic transmission. This, in turn, is associated with high demand for energy generated from hydrolysis of ATP, and, therefore, an increased requirement for glucose transport and metabolism, which declines along with the decline in the density of neuritic processes during cerebral maturity (Figure 7-12, middle). A similar developmental course has been observed with respect to glucose metabolism in other mammalian species (Figure 7-12, bottom).

The above developmental pattern has also been observed in measurement of human cerebral blood flow and oxygen metabolism.[78] In absolute terms, those rates are lower at birth than in adults and increase significantly during early childhood. The highest levels of cerebral blood flow throughout the brain are reached by 8 years; they then decline towards adult levels, while the developmental time course

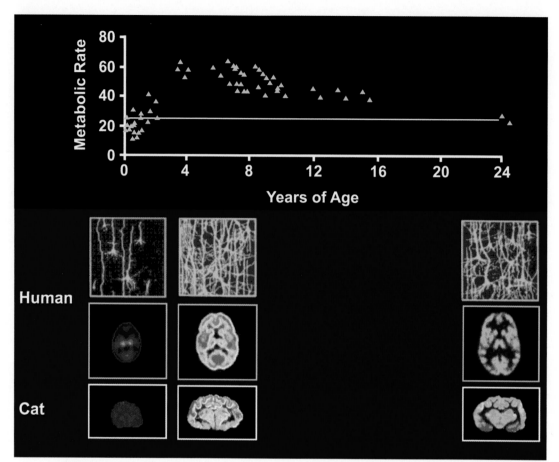

FIGURE 7-12. Time course of early cerebral development, with respect to metabolism and neuronal density, in humans and cats. (See text for details.)

of oxygen utilization shows more variation among regions. Serotonin synthesis capacity has also been reported to be greatest in early childhood years, and subsequently to decline to adult levels,[79] though this remains controversial.[55]

At the other end of the age spectrum, effects of normal aging on brain function of adults have also been examined with PET. In a recent study of 37 healthy adults ranging in age from 19 to 50,[80] the most significant age-related decline in cerebral blood flow was found in the mesial frontal cortex, encompassing the anterior cingulate cortex and extending rostrally into the supplementary motor area. In an independent study of 27 healthy adults ranging from 19 to 76 years old,[24] the most significant age-related decline in cerebral blood flow was found in the medial orbito-frontal cortex; this was the only regional effect to remain significant after correction for partial volume effects of cerebral atrophy, Likewise, recent measures of metabolism using FDG have also identified an age-related decline in healthy adults,[20] most consistently in frontal cortex; nevertheless, as previously reviewed,[81] studies of carefully selected subjects (i.e., generally healthy and with no history of neuropsychiatric disease or drug or alcohol abuse) find declines to be minimal in glucose metabolism throughout most of the brain in normal aging (Figure 7-13).

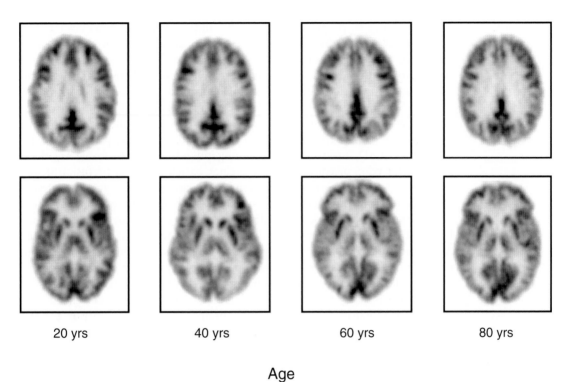

20 yrs   40 yrs   60 yrs   80 yrs

Age

FIGURE 7-13. Normal evolution in regional metabolic pattern of the healthy adult human brain. Normal aging is associated with some generalized cortical atrophy (evidenced here by gradual widening of the separation between the two cerebral hemispheres and between the left and right sides of the thalamus and heads of the caudate nuclei). The general pattern of regional cerebral metabolism otherwise tends to be quite stable throughout the life span of a healthy adult, apart from the mild decline found in the medial prefrontal cortex (seen here in the brain images of the 60- and 80-year-old patients).

STUDIES OF PATHOLOGIC HUMAN BRAIN FUNCTION

Alzheimer's disease and other dementing illnesses

Decreasing mortality, with consequent progressive aging of our mature adult population, has led to a rising prevalence of senile dementia. The condition is tremendously costly to patients, their families, and society in general. In 2000, Alzheimer's disease (AD) in the United States alone affected over 4 million people, who incur associated yearly expenses of nearly $70 billion. When indirect costs such as the lost productivity of caregivers are taken into account, total annual expenditures approximate $100 billion. As the baby boomers approach senior citizen status in the 21st century, it is estimated that over 14 million Americans will suffer from Alzheimer's disease by 2050.[82–85]

PET studies of dementia, and of brain disorders in general, can be grouped into two broad categories: 1) those aimed at elucidating neurologic substrates, either of fundamental pathophysiology or of associations observed between disease and genetic or environmental factors; and 2) those directly aimed at improving diagnosis, prognostic assessment, and/or therapeutic management of neurologically based disorders. With respect to dementia, examples of studies belonging to the first group include those that have examined associations of such factors with the presence or later development of Alzheimer's disease. Epidemiologic studies indicate that lack of education is a major risk factor for AD.[86,87] Several studies using functional brain imaging have shed light on the effect of education on the clinical expression of AD. Using the ^{133}Xe technique to quantify regional cerebral blood flow and approximate the pathophysiological severity of AD, it was shown that among individuals with probable AD, those with several years of education have greater parietotemporal perfusion deficit than those with few years of education.[88] Similarly, it has been demonstrated that individuals with occupations associated with higher interpersonal skills experience greater parietal perfusion deficit for a given level of cognitive function.[89] Using PET to assess cerebral glucose metabolism, Alexander et al.[90] compared AD patients matched for demographic characteristics and dementia severity but differing in estimated pre-AD intellectual ability, as defined by demographics-based intelligent quotient (IQ) estimates, as well as by performance on a test of reading words. They found that estimated IQs were inversely correlated with cerebral metabolism in the prefrontal, premotor, and left superior parietal regions.

In addition to few years of education, genetic risk factors for AD have been identified (Figure 7-14). Recent investigations have revealed that asymptomatic

FIGURE 7-14. Effects of a single apolipoprotein E (apoE) ε4 allele on cerebral glucose metabolism. All subjects (n = 34) were nondemented; Mini-Mental State Examination (MMSE) avg ± SD = 29.2 ± 0.7, of 30 total possible points. In this image (left), highlighted regions in the left hemisphere have significantly lower glucose metabolism (as imaged with FDG) in those subjects having apoE ε4/ε3 genotype, than those with ε3/ε3, in allelic groups well-matched with respect to age, sex, handedness, and years of formal education. In this image (right), highlighted regions demonstrate areas where metabolic activity is correlated with performance on a verbal memory test (on which subjects with ε4 allele score slightly but significantly lower). The correlation is shown after adjusting for each subject's age, MMSE, and nonverbal memory test scores (which do not significantly differ between allelic subject groups). Cerebral metabolism, which is decreased in the parietal and temporal regions in subjects with the ε4 allele, thus correlates with the diminished verbal memory performance of those subjects.[96]

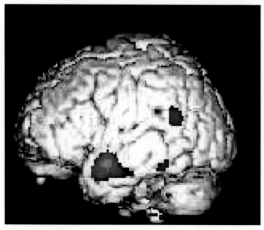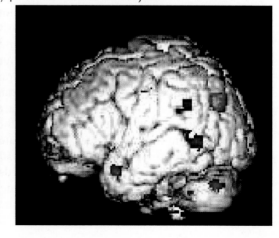

members of families in which familial AD has been observed also have significant parietal and temporal deficits relative to control subjects.[91] Other studies have looked at this relationship with the ε4 allele of the apolipoprotein E gene which is associated with a significantly increased risk of developing AD of senile onset; overall, those with the ε4/ε3 or ε4/ε4 genotype are more than twice as likely to have AD compared to individuals with the ε3/ε3 genotype.[92] FDG–PET studies have linked the ε4 allele to hypometabolism in posterior cingulate, parietal, and temporal cortex, and have identified greater metabolic asymmetry in the parietotemporal cortex of nondemented relatives of individuals with probable AD.[93–96] Furthermore, significant metabolic decline in these regions has been longitudinally observed in those who have inherited the ε4 allele as measured by repeating PET in the same subjects over a 2-year interval.[95]

With regard to the second broad category, investigations into *clinical* applications of PET with dementia patients stem from numerous studies which have found that many neurodegenerative diseases produce significant alterations in brain function detectable with PET even when structural images with CT or MRI reveal no abnormality. The utility of PET in evaluation of dementia has been under study since the early 1980s,[97–100] and has been extensively reviewed in recent years.[91,101–105] The best studied application of this type is the use of FDG–PET to evaluate AD. Assessment of the diagnostic accuracy of PET even for this application, however, has been hindered by the paucity of such studies involving patients who undergo longterm clinical followup[106] and/or subsequent pathologic diagnosis[91,107,108]; the approach used in most previous clinical series has been the comparison of PET findings to clinical assessments performed near the time of PET. The ability of the latter approach to assess diagnostic accuracy is unfortunately limited by the fact that clinical diagnosis can be inaccurate, particularly for patients presenting in the earliest stages of disease—a time when the opportunity for effective therapy, and for meaningful planning, is greatest.

Studies comparing neuropathologic examination with imaging are thus most informative in assessing the diagnostic value of PET. In the largest such single-institution series, Hoffman and coworkers[107] studied 22 patients with various types of dementia (including 64% with Alzheimer's disease alone, and 9% with Alzheimer's plus additional neurologic disease, identified with pathologic diagnosis). Visual interpretations of PET scans yielded estimates of sensitivity and specificity for identifying the presence of Alzheimer's disease of 0.88 to 0.93 and 0.63 to 0.67, respectively. Recently, a multicenter study was organized to compare dementia diagnosis using FDG–PET with diagnosis from autopsy confirmation.[108] The investigators collected data from an international consortium of clinical facilities which acquired both brain FDG–PET and histopathologic data for 138 patients undergoing evaluation for dementia. PET images and pathologic data were independently classified as being positive or negative for: 1) the presence of a progressive neurodegenerative disease in general, and 2) AD, specifically. The PET results identified patients with AD and patients with any neurodegenerative disease with a sensitivity of 0.94 in both cases, specificities of 0.73 and 0.78, respectively, and overall accuracies of 0.88 and 0.92, respectively.

FDG–PET may also serve explicitly as a prognostic tool to determine likelihood of deterioration of mental status in the period following the time of scanning. Relative hypometabolism of associative cortex can be accurately used to predict whether cognitive decline will occur at a rate faster than would be ex-

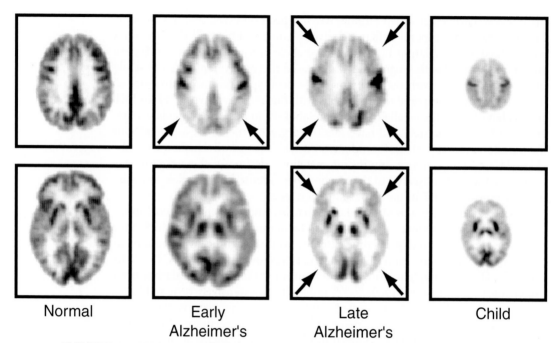

Normal   Early   Late   Child
Alzheimer's   Alzheimer's

FIGURE 7-15. PET images with FDG in early and late Alzheimer's disease. Typical patterns of cerebral metabolism are shown for a normal adult (*far left*), normal newborn (*far right*) and a patient with early (*middle left*) and late (*middle right*) Alzheimer's disease. Image planes are shown at superior (top row) and middle (*bottom row*) horizontal levels. Notice the striking similarity between the metabolic patterns of the advanced Alzheimer's patient and the newborn infant.

pected for normal aging over the several years following a PET evaluation.[108,109] Moreover, the *magnitude* of decline over a 2-year period for some standardized measures of memory correlates with the initial degree of hypometabolism of inferior parietal, superior temporal and posterior cingulate cortical regions.[95] As cognitive impairment caused by a neurodegenerative disease progresses, associated progression of regions of hypometabolism also occurs (Figure 7-15).

Table 7-5[21,107,108,111–118] represents published studies aimed at assessing the diagnostic value of FDG–PET in the evaluation of dementia. The typically high sensitivity of FDG–PET, even in patients with mild impairment, suggests that by the time a patient presents with symptoms of a neurodegenerative dementia, substantial alteration of cortical metabolic function generally has occurred. The associated decreases in glucose metabolism in certain brain areas are readily detectable on FDG images.[110] Table 7-6 summarizes scan findings pertinent to distinguishing between several causes of dementia. Some visually evident differences between scans of patients with different dementing illnesses are seen in Figure 7-16.

EXAMPLE 7-5
Sensitivity refers to the correctly diagnosed proportion of people who have a given disease (true positive cases ÷ the total number of subjects tested who actually have the disease; i.e., [true positives]/[true posi-

tives + false negatives]). Specificity refers to the correctly diagnosed proportion of people who do not have the disease (true negative cases ÷ the total number of subjects tested who actually do not have the disease; i.e., [true negatives]/[true negatives + false positives]).

Assume a clinical workup for the diagnosis of early AD has a sensitivity of 83% and a specificity of 55% and that incorporation of PET into the diagnostic algorithm increases sensitivity and specificity to 94% and 75%, respectively. In evaluating 1000 people for dementia, how many more patients would be correctly diagnosed by including PET in the workup, if the prevalence of AD in the patient population were:

1. 50% ?
2. 70% ?
3. 10% ?

ANSWER

1. 155 more patients will be accurately diagnosed. Given a prevalence of 50%, 500 patients will have AD, and the higher sensitivity achievable with PET will allow $[(0.94 - 0.83) \times 500 = 55]$ additional cases to be correctly identified. Similarly, 500 patients will not have AD, and the higher specificity achievable with PET will prevent $[(0.75 - 0.55) \times 500 = 100]$ people from being falsely diagnosed with AD.
2. 137 more patients will be accurately diagnosed. Given a prevalence of 70%, 700 patients will have AD, and the higher sensitivity achievable with PET will allow $[(0.94 - 0.83) \times 700 = 77]$ additional cases to be correctly identified. Similarly, 300 patients will not have AD, and the higher specificity achievable with PET will prevent $[(0.75 - 0.55) \times 300 = 60]$ people from being falsely diagnosed with AD.
3. 191 more patients will be accurately diagnosed. Given a prevalence of 10%, 100 patients will have AD, and the higher sensitivity achievable with PET will allow $[(0.94 - 0.83) \times 100 = 11]$ additional cases to be correctly identified. Similarly, 900 patients will not have AD, and the higher specificity achievable with PET will prevent $[(0.75 - 0.55) \times 900 = 180]$ people from being falsely diagnosed with AD.

Parkinson's disease and other motor disorders

A major goal of PET imaging for clinical brain applications is the early detection of neurological disease and the monitoring of neuroprotective/neurorestorative interventions. Both of these aims have been demonstrated for Parkinson's disease (PD). In PD, the progressive loss of nigrostriatal neurons results in striatal dopamine system deficits that can be readily detected with PET. The majority of PD studies have been conducted with FDG,[119] raclopride (RAC),[120] and FDOPA.[121] These PET tracers have revealed different aspects of PD biochemical pathology despite the absence of structural abnormalities in the caudate and putamen identified by MR imaging (Figure 7-17).

TABLE 7-5. Use of PET for Differential Diagnosis of Alzheimer's Disease

Radiopharmaceutical(s)	Diagnostic standard	Subjects	Major findings	Comments	Ref
[18]FDG	C	69 AD 48 Non-AD	Sens = 93%, Spec = 58%.Accu = 79% (Spec = 80%, when patients with Parkinson's dementia are excluded. Severity-stratified analysis shows for mild AD (av.MMSE = 26) Sens = 87.5%; for mod./severe AD (av. MMSE = 10) Sens = 96%.	AD av. age = 66.av. duration = 2.5yrs. Groups well-matched for level of severity (AD av. CDR = 2.1, Non-AD av. CDR = 2.1). Visual analysis.	111
[18]FDG	P	13 AD 7 Non-AD	Sens = 92%.Spec = 71%.Accu = 85%	Pooled analysis[91] across three studies providing small groups of pathologically confirmed cases.	111 112 113
[18]FDG	C	20 AD 12 Non-AD 13 NI	PET Accu = 90%,SPECTAccu = 67% A stratified analysis to look at early AD, shows that for subjects with MMSE > 20, PETAccu = 87%,SPECTAccu = 63%	Receiver operator characteristics (ROC) area-under-curve analysis was performed for both SPECT and PET on same 45 patients to determine each method's accuracy.	114
99mTc-HMPAO					
[18]FDG	L	66 AD 23 MI 22 NI	Group analysis shows significant differences for very early AD (av. MMSE = 25) vs. N1(av.MMSE = 28) Posterior cingulate significantly fell (by 21–22%, p = 0.0007), as did parietal and temporal areas.	To obtain very early AD cases, minimally impaired patients were scanned, and then followed longitudinally to determine whether they developed NINCDS criteria for probable AD.	115
[18]FDG	C	9 AD 9 Non-AD	Group analysis by statistical mapping demonstrates significant PET differences between AD and Parkinson's dementia. (See Table 7-2.)	Groups well-matched for level of levels of severity (AD av. CDR = 1.2, Non-AD av. CDR = 1.3).	116
[18]FDG	C	19 AD 19 Non-AD	Group analysis by statistical mapping demonstrates significant PET differences between AD and dementia with Lewy bodies. (See Table 7-2.)	Groups well-matched for level of severity and duration (AD av. MMSE = 18, 24 mos., Non-AD av. MMSE = 18, 24 mos.)	117

Tracer	Design	Groups	Results	Notes	Ref
^{18}FDG	C	21 AD 21 Non-AD 21 NI	Group analysis by region-of-interest method demonstrates significant differences between AD and frontotemporal dementia. (See Table 7-2.)	Groups well-matched for fairly mild level of severity (AD av. MMSE = 20 Non-AD av. MMSE = 19). All subjects had normal MRI studies	21
^{18}FDG	P	16 AD 6 NI	AD identified in 13/14 (Sens = 93%) of AD-only and 1 of 2 AD+ cases (overall Sens = 88%). Absence of AD confirmed in 4/6 cases (Spec = 67%)	14 patients had AD as the only pathological diagnosis, 1 had AD+ Lewy bodies, 1 had AD + PSP	107
^{18}FDG	P	97 AD 41 Non-AD	AD identified in 85/89 (Sens = 96%) of AD-only and 6 of 8 AD+ cases (overall Sens = 94%). Absence of AD confirmed in 30/41 cases (Spec = 73%), including 23 cases with other neurodegen. dementias. Absence of neurodegen. disease confirmed in 14/18 cases (Spec = 78%).	Relatively early dementia group, with 70% having mild or questionable dementia. 89 patients had AD as the only pathological diagnosis, 5 had AD+ Lewy bodies; 1 each had AD + PSP, +Parkinson's disease, or +cerebrovascular disease	108
$H_2^{15}O$ ^{15}O	C	16 AD 10 NI	Scans with $H_2^{15}O$ show decreased perfusion for AD in parietal and lateral temporal regions. Scans with $C^{15}O$ reveal no cerebral blood volume differences between AD and NI groups.	Relatively mild AD group, having av. MMSE = 21.	118

Abbreviations: Accu, overall accuracy; AD, cognitively impaired secondary to Alzheimer's disease; C, diagnosis based on clinical evaluation near time of scan; CDR, Clinical Dementia Rating; L, diagnosis based on longitudinal clinical followup of at least 2 years' duration; MI, isolated memory impairment; MMSE, Mini-Mental State Examination; NI, cognitively normal; Non-AD, cognitively impaired, not secondary to Alzheimer's disease; P, diagnosis based on histopathology; Sens, sensitivity with respect to correctly identifying presence of Alzheimer's disease; Spec, specificity with respect to correctly specifying that Alzheimer's disease is absent.

TABLE 7-6. FDG–PET Findings Pertinent to Differential Diagnosis in Dementia

Etiology of dementia	Regional hypometabolism identified by FDG–PET
Alzheimer's Disease	Parietal, temporal, and posterior cingulate cortices affected early; relative sparing of primary sensorimotor and primary visual cortex; sparing of striatum, thalamus, and cerebellum. In early stages, deficits often appear asymmetric, but degeneration eventually is evident bilaterally.
Vascular Dementia	Hypometabolic foci affecting cortical, subcortical, and cerebellar areas.
Frontotemporal Dementia (e.g., Pick's disease)	Frontal cortex, anterior temporal, and mesiotemporal areas affected earlier and/or with greater initial severity than parietal and lateral temporal cortex; relative sparing of primary sensorimotor and visual cortex.
Huntington's Disease	Caudate and lentiform nuclei affected early, with gradual development of diffuse cortical hypometabolism.
Parkinson's Dementia	Similar to Alzheimer's Disease but more sparing of mesiotemporal area and less sparing of visual cortex.
Dementia with Lewy Bodies	Similar to Alzheimer's Disease but less sparing of occipital cortex and cerebellum.

FIGURE 7-16. PET images with FDG of human brains with different dementing illnesses. Typical patterns of cerebral metabolism are shown for a normal subject and for 4 patients with dementia at superior (top row) and middle (bottom row) horizontal levels. Conventional magnetic resonance imaging (MRI) studies of all brains were read as normal, except in the case of the patient with multiple infarcts.

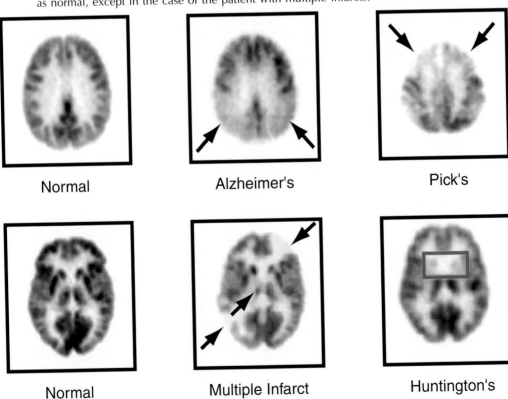

Normal　　　　　　Alzheimer's　　　　　　Pick's

Normal　　　Multiple Infarct Dementia　　　Huntington's

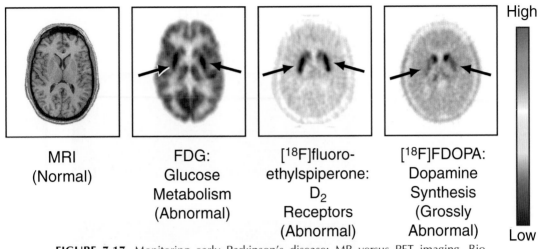

MRI	FDG:	[18F]fluoro-	[18F]FDOPA:
(Normal)	Glucose	ethylspiperone:	Dopamine
	Metabolism	D2	Synthesis
	(Abnormal)	Receptors	(Grossly
		(Abnormal)	Abnormal)

FIGURE 7-17. Monitoring early Parkinson's disease: MR versus PET imaging. Biochemical dysfunction can exist in Parkinson's disease without corresponding deficits in brain structure. A comparison of PET and magnetic resonance (MR) images of an individual with Parkinson's disease shows the sensitivity of PET to detect biochemical pathology in the putamen (arrows) under conditions of normal structure. In the FDG image, an abnormality in putamen glucose metabolic rates is detected, that is, 10% over normal values. Alterations in selective striatal dopamine system parameters can also be imaged. A 15% increase in dopamine D2 receptors is imaged by the binding of the labeled ligand, [18F]fluoroethylspiperone, a dopamine D2 antagonist, and a 70% decrease in dopamine synthesis capacity is imaged with FDOPA (see Figure 7-1 legend for description of FDOPA metabolism). For this series of cross-sectional PET images, a white-black (low-high) scale represents the relative values for the distribution of each tracer. (Reprinted with permission from Phelps[264].)

Staging of PD disease progression can be determined through longitudinal studies, commencing with the detection of reduced striatal dopamine synthesis with FDOPA even prior to the manifestation of behavioral symptoms. In the early phases of PD, unilateral motor deficits are paralleled by a contralateral decrease in striatal dopamine synthesis. As the disease progresses, bilateral symptoms and dopamine synthesis deficits are observed.[122] These reductions show a pronounced selectivity for putamen, with much less deficit seen in the caudate nuclei.

In addition to functional measures of dopamine system activity with FDOPA, reductions in binding to the striatal dopamine transporter are also used to index dopaminergic deficits. As with FDOPA, the transporter ligand [18F]FP-βCIT shows binding deficits greater in putamen relative to those in caudate (Figure 7-18).[123]

FDG has been used to evaluate alterations in glucose metabolic rates consequent to the primary dopamine system deficit and to contribute to the evaluation of those patients suffering from both cognitive and motor symptoms. Combined FDG and FDOPA studies provide a complementary assessment of PD pathology[124] that has been used to differentiate it from related movement disorders such as multiple system atrophy and corticobasal degeneration (Table 7-7).

With regard to *post*-synaptic striatal dopamine system assessment, subregional alterations in striatum have been detected, showing larger compensa-

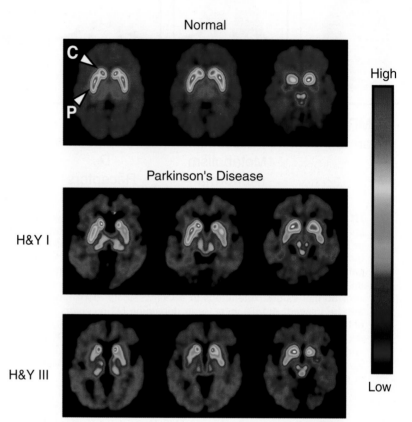

FIGURE 7-18. Monitoring the evolution of Parkinson's disease (PD). The density of dopamine terminals can be estimated by the binding of a labeled ligand such as [^{18}F]FP-βCIT which binds to the dopamine transporter located on dopaminergic axons. *Upper:* In this example, cross-sectional images of [^{18}F]FP-βCIT binding are shown at the level of the caudate and putamen for a normal subject. Two PD patients, at different stages of the disease, are also shown. *Middle:* Initially, unilateral PD deficits are observed (Hoehn and Yahr Stage I, hemi-PD) and appear in the putamen, with sparing of the caudate. *Lower:* As the disease worsens, the deficits become bilateral, with further deterioration in putamen and some caudate involvement (Hoehn and Yahr Stage III). (Reprinted with permission from Kazumata et al.[261])

tory increases in D2R binding in the putamen relative to the caudate.[123] These relative differences in receptor density are paralleled by corresponding increases in FDG metabolism, that is, metabolic rates in putamen being greater than in caudate, reflecting the loss of regulated function in the nigrostriatal pathway.

Although decreases in presynaptic dopamine terminal activity are often associated with corresponding increases in postsynaptic receptor density, the functional significance of these neuroadaptations is unclear. Such increases in D1 receptor (with ^{11}C-SCH23390) and D2 receptor (with ^{11}C-RAC) binding have not been consistently seen in PD.[125] These results suggest that the motor abnormalities may not be directly related to alterations in receptor availability but pos-

TABLE 7-7. PET Findings Pertinent to Differential Diagnosis of Parkinsonian Syndromes

	Parkinson's disease (PD) (nondemented)	*Parkinson's disease with Parkinson's dementia*	*Multiple system atrophy (Shy–Drager)*	*Progressive supranuclear palsy (PSP)*	*Corticobasal degeneration (CBD)*
[18]FDG	Normal or increased in putamen	Low parietal, temporal	Low striatal, frontal, and cerebellar	Low striatal, thalamic, posterior frontal ± cerebellar	Low striatal, posterior-frontal, thalamic, inferior parietal, superior temporal[a]
[18]F-dopa	Low putamen	Low putamen	Low putamen Caudate comparably affected in 70% of all cases	Low putamen and caudate Uniform depression (90% specificity vs. PD)	
Striatal dopamine receptor (D$_2$) sites	Normal or up (untreated) Normal or low (treated)		Normal or low	Normal or low	(?)
Symmetry	Mild asymmetry common	Mild asymmetry common		Typically symmetric	Both F-dopa and FDG are typically strikingly asymmetric

[a]PSP vs. CBD: group comparisons reveal more FDG decrease in CBD in the inferior parietal cortex, sensorimotor cortex, lateral temporal cortex, and striatum.

sibly to alterations in striatal second messenger systems or to downstream neuronal firing patterns within basal ganglia circuitry.[126]

Transplantation strategies for PD have focused on the use of fetal mesencephalon cells to provide dopamine within the striatum. FDOPA–PET studies have been conducted in these patients to monitor the survival and activity of the dopaminergic cells containing AAAD. FDOPA studies have shown longterm increases in AAAD activity (Figure 7-19), clearly demonstrating cell survival and functional AAAD activity in patients with symptomatic improvement.[127,128]

Characteristic alterations in cerebral metabolism associated with central motor disorders can be identified with PET even before those alterations lead to symptoms. Huntington's disease provides an excellent model for studying presymptomatic biological expression with molecular imaging methods. The disease is caused by a genetic defect with a dominant pattern of inheritance, leading to a 50% risk of inheriting the condition. Huntington's disease can be identified in individuals by genetic testing and, when present, is associated with a phenotypic penetrance of nearly 100% (i.e., if you have the mutated gene, you get the disease) by the time the patient's fifth decade is reached. The presymptomatic detection of metabolic abnormalities has specifically been shown for Huntington's disease using PET. Abnormalities are identified by PET with FDG about 7 years before symptoms emerge.[129] In contrast, there are generally no structural abnormalities evident on computerized tomography (CT) or MRI scans preclinically or even during the

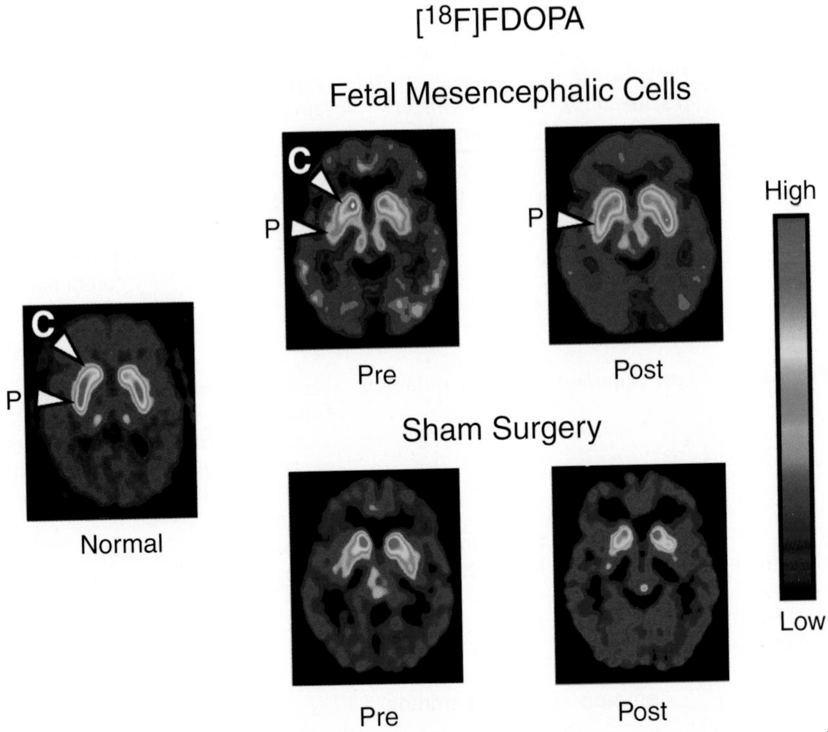

FIGURE 7-19. Monitoring dopamine cell transplantation therapy for Parkinson's disease. Transplantation of fetal mesencephalic dopamine cells is designed as a replacement strategy for the dopamine-depleted striatum of patients with Parkinson's disease. The increases in dopamine synthesis capacity attributable to the transplanted cells can be imaged with FDOPA-PET by measuring the accumulation of [18F]fluorodopamine synthesized from [18F]FDOPA (see legend for figure 7-4 for description of FDOPA metabolism). *Upper:* Cross-sectional FDOPA images show that aromatic acid decarboxylase-mediated synthesis of dopamine is successfully reconstituted in putamen (P) at 15 months after bilateral cell transplantation. *Lower:* In a sham-surgery study, postoperative increases over the same time period are not apparent and, moreover, a further decline in residual dopamine synthesis in putamen (P) is observed. (Reprinted with permission from Freed et al.,[128] copyright © 2001 Massachusetts Medical Society. All rights reserved.)

symptomatic stages. PET scanning thus offers a noninvasive yet sensitive method to detect the disease when the actual pathologic changes in the brain, destined to result from inheritance of the Huntington's gene, first become functionally manifest at the neuronal level, illustrating how molecular errors of disease can be present and produce changes in biological systems for some time before detectable symptomatic changes occur. This hindrance to detection most likely occurs because the brain has reserves and compensatory responses to maintain its function within normal limits. When the reserves or compensatory responses are exceeded due to progression of disease, symptoms appear.

Epilepsy

Epilepsy affects 1% of Americans over the course of their lifetimes.[130] Although the majority of these patients are successfully treated with antiepileptic medications, approximately 10% to 20% of cases are inadequately controlled with pharmacotherapy.[131,132] Surgical intervention is an effective and widely accepted form of treatment for some forms of intractable seizure.[132,133] Successful neurosurgery has two important effects: 1) decreasing or eliminating seizure episodes and 2) reducing neurologic damage due to recurrent seizures and/or the higher doses of anticonvulsants otherwise used in treating them. In an analysis of 3,579 patients who underwent anterior temporal lobe resections for temporal lobe epilepsy, 68% were seizure-free postsurgery and 92% experienced significant improvement with respect to seizure frequency.[130] Extratemporal cortical resections performed for seizure foci in the frontal, parietal, or occipital lobes were somewhat less successful in decreasing seizure frequency.

Many patients with complex partial seizures (epilepsy that leads to temporary impairment but not loss of consciousness), particularly those who have EEG evidence of a temporal lobe focus but inconclusive MRI findings, may be referred for functional brain imaging, generally to assess ictal perfusion by single-photon emission computerized tomography (SPECT) or interictal metabolism by PET.[134] The clinical utility of the former technique is compromised by logistical difficulty in attaining properly timed radiotracer injection and acquisition of images with respect to ictal episodes. There is also a concern that more than one epileptogenic site could be actually present in the patient's brain, even though for a given ictal episode, only one of them might be captured by the ictal imaging study. Furthermore, ambiguity can result in the planning of surgical resections using ictal localization data, which may not only identify primary sites of epileptogenesis but also sites of secondary generalization (i.e., brain tissue to which the initial seizure activity has quickly spread but is not epileptogenic). PET studies, on the other hand, using FDG, can be performed as a straightforward outpatient procedure between seizure episodes to identify cerebral hypometabolism characterizing epileptogenic zones[134,135] (Figure 7-20), without the potential difficulties and ambiguities described above. Introduction of PET imaging has significantly reduced the need for invasive monitoring which requires implantation of sensors (depth electrodes) into the brain or its tightly surrounding meninges.[135,136]

Multiple studies have found FDG–PET to be as useful for presurgical planning in most temporal lobe epilepsy patients as depth electrode monitoring (the method generally held to be the presurgical evaluative gold standard) both by direct comparison with depth electrode findings and by correlation of presurgical PET findings with postsurgical clinical outcomes. Concordant structural abnormalities on MRI or temporal hypometabolism on FDG–PET are comparably predictive of good surgical outcome with respect to seizures among patients who have typical symptoms of mesial temporal lobe epilepsy and a focal scalp/sphenoidal ictal EEG onset without other conflicting findings. Only one of these imaging tests needs to be positive in order to recommend anteromesial temporal lobe resection without invasive studies. FDG–PET appears to be approximately 15% more sensitive in identifying mesial temporal sclerosis (the most common cause of temporal lobe epilepsy), while MRI is more sensitive for identifying rarer small focal lesions.

Thus, a population of patients with surgically remediable mesial temporal lobe epilepsy can be easily defined noninvasively and treated surgically with an excellent outcome. An important clinical implication of this situation is that pa-

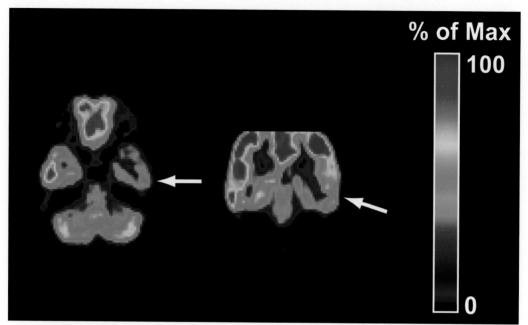

FIGURE 7-20. Asymmetric glucose metabolism in temporal lobes of a patient with epilepsy. The patient underwent PET to assist with neurosurgical planning. The left side of the image corresponds to the right side of the patient's brain. The arrow in each image points to moderately decreased metabolism of the left temporal lobe, evident on cross-sectional (*left*) and coronal (*right*) views. The other portions of the brain are symmetric. The study thus identifies a left temporal zone of epileptogenesis in this interictal study and is indicative of the patient's candidacy for successful neurosurgery to resect the abnormal focus.

tients who will otherwise not meet the usual criteria for surgery without depth electrode evaluation due to a negative MRI scan should be evaluated with FDG–PET, as positive concordant temporal hypometabolism with PET will obviate the need for placement of intracranial electrodes and any attending morbidity of that procedure.

Stroke

Application of PET to the study of cerebrovascular diseases enjoys a long history, extending back two decades.[137,138] PET has been used to directly quantify several parameters pertinent to the status of cerebral perfusion—not only the rate of blood flow through a unit of tissue but also cerebral blood volume, rate of oxygen metabolism, and glucose utilization. The relevance of these measures is evident from the definition of cerebral ischemia and the etiology of stroke, that is, CBF insufficient to meet metabolic demands. This methodology has allowed estimation of further relevant parameters through calculations based on the values derived from those measurements, including cerebrovascular mean transit time, cerebral perfusion pressure, oxygen extraction fraction, and stoichiometry of oxygen and glucose utilization. Each of these have been reported to change, in different ways, under circumstances stemming from the pathophysiological events that occur during cerebrovascular compromise and the evolution of stroke as well as its aftermath. To briefly summarize the most consistently reported findings from PET studies on stroke:

1. In the early phase of cerebrovascular compromise, blood flow is maintained through autoregulated vasodilation, leading to an increase in blood volume.
2. As the compensatory capacity of autoregulation is exceeded, blood flow falls, while oxygen metabolism is maintained, corresponding to an increase in oxygen extraction fraction (the beginning of miserly perfusion, i.e., perfusion that is less than would normally be expected given the level of metabolic demand on the perfused tissue).
3. Once oxygen extraction fraction has increased maximally, continued decline in blood flow leads to a decline in oxygen delivery and metabolism (the onset of ischemia, i.e., inadequate CBF to meet the tissues metabolic demand).
4. Severe and prolonged compromise in blood flow results in infarction of brain tissue, with decreased demand for oxygen metabolism, while vasodilation persists, leading to a decline in oxygen extraction fraction (and onset of luxury perfusion, i.e., perfusion in excess of what would normally be expected given the diminished metabolic demand). As revascularization occurs, blood flow to the region increases, and the infarcted area typically remains in a state of luxury perfusion for days to weeks with the end result that some normal tissue recovers, while other tissue develops a fixed defect in CBF and metabolism (completed infarct).

While there is a wealth of data supporting the sequence of events described above, there have been relatively few investigations directly assessing the clinical utility of PET in the setting of cerebrovascular disease. The prognostic value of oxygen extraction fraction data, calculated from PET measures of regional oxygen metabolism and blood flow using [^{15}O]oxygen gas and [H_2^{15}O]water, was recently demonstrated in patients having a history of stroke or transient ischemic attack in the distribution of an occluded carotid artery.[139] The investigators divided 81 such patients studied with PET into two groups—39 with elevated oxygen extraction fractions (operationally defined by asymmetry, through reference to a control group, approximately corresponding to exceeding the contralateral region by more than 8%), and 42 with normal (symmetric) oxygen extraction fractions. After adjusting for age, those in the first group had a 6-fold higher risk of suffering a stroke (all but one occurring ipsilateral to the side with higher oxygen extraction fraction) than those in the second group.

Similar findings, documenting prognostic value in PET measurements of oxygen extraction fraction, have been found by others. Shortly after the study described above, it was independently reported[140] that among 40 patients followed for 5 years after PET, increased hemispheric oxygen extraction (defined by a reference value derived from the mean and variance of the extraction fraction of a control group) was associated with a 7-fold higher risk of suffering a stroke. A less significant difference was found between groups categorized according to left/right asymmetry of oxygen extraction fraction within each patient.

In the setting of acute stroke, Heiss and his colleagues[141] measured cerebral blood flow with [^{15}O]water in 12 patients before and after therapy with tissue plasminogen activator, a drug that breaks apart the blood clot causing the stroke. Reperfusion, as documented by PET on the day of therapy, predicted clinical improvement assessed 3 weeks later. Marchal et al[142] found that for 19 patients undergoing PET within 5 to 18 h of onset of middle cerebral artery stroke, that extent of abnormally low cerebral blood flow or oxygen metabolism (but not blood volume, perfusion pressure, or oxygen extraction fraction) correlated with final infarct size and longterm clinical outcome. Beyond investigation of these relatively well-studied hemodynamic parameters measurable with PET, recent studies with newer tracers (e.g., those recognizing activated microglial cells or benzodiazepine receptors) are also showing promise of contributing clinically meaningful information to the assessment of patients with cerebrovascular disease.

Pain perception

Until recently, surprisingly little was known concerning the processing of pain information in the human brain. One reason for this penury of knowledge in an area so obviously central to health and well-being has been the inherent limitation of animal models for studying a perceptual process profoundly influenced by cognitive and emotional components relatively specific to the human experience.

In the last few years, functional neuroimaging methods have been successfully applied to provide a window through which to look at processes occurring in living human brain tissue associated with the perception of somatic (body wall) and visceral (internal organ) pain. Table 7-8[143–166] provides a summary of studies applying this general approach. The vast majority of such studies have

TABLE 7-8. Brain Regions with Increased Activity During Perception of Pain, as Identified by PET Studies of CBF

Type of pain	Subjects	Regional activations (increases in CBF)[a]	References
Evoked Somatic Pain			
Capsaicin on skin	Normals: 13, 6, 7	*thalamus, insula*, lent. nuc., *pgACC, mACC, S1, S2*, PFC	143–145
Heat on skin, tonic	Normals: 12, 10, 8, 9	*thalamus, insula*, lent. nuc., *pgACC, mACC, S1, S2*, PFC	146–149
Heat on skin, phasic	Normals: 20, 10, 12, 11, 6, 7, 6, 9, 8, 6	*thalamus, insula*, lent. nuc., *pgACC, mACC, S1, S2, PFC*	150–158
Heat on skin, phasic	Dental patients: 6	*insula*, lent. nuc., *PFC*	159
Heat on skin, phasic	Atypical facial pain: 6	*thalamus, insula*, lent. nuc., *mACC*	155
Intramuscular	Normals: 11	*thalamus, insula*, lent. nuc., *mACC, S1, S2, PFC*	152
Clinical and Evoked Visceral Pain			
Angina	Cardiac patients: 12	*thalamus, pgACC, PFC*	160
Intestinal pressure	Normals: 6	*pgACC*	161
Intestinal pressure	Irritable bowel syndrome patients: 6	*PFC*	161
Esophageal pressure	Normals: 8	*insula, pgACC, S1*	162
Headache	Chronic headache patients: 9, 7, 9	thalamus, *insula*, lent. nuc, PFC, pgACC, mACC,	163–165
Neuropathy	Chronic pain patients: 8	*insula, mACC, PFC*	166

[a]Italicized regions indicate that activation was confirmed in more than half of the studies listed for a given pain/subject category (and for pain/subject categories with a single study).

Abbreviations: CBF, cerebral blood flow; lent. nuc., lentiform nucleus; mACC, mid-(supragenual) anterior cingulate cortex; PET, positron emission tomography; PFC, prefrontal coretx; pgACC, perigenualanterior cingulate cortex; S1, primary somatosensory cortex; S2, secondary somatosensory cortex.

focused on somatic pain, especially pain involving a heat stimulus, largely because of the relative ease with which it can be induced and controlled in an experimental situation. Increased insula activity as assessed by increases in CBF using $H_2^{15}O$-PET has been found for all forms of somatic pain, and activity of the lentiform nucleus has consistently exhibited increased CBF during evoked phasic somatic pain. In studies of normal subjects, somatic pain has also been consistently associated with increased CBF in the thalamus and the midportion of the anterior cingulate cortex. In contrast, studies of headache and evoked visceral pain have most consistently revealed increased CBF of the perigenual anterior cingulate cortex, with the remaining pattern of CBF activation varying with the particular type of pain and subject studied. The rest of the discussion that follows will concentrate on those studies elucidating mechanisms involved in visceral pain, as it represents a common complaint of patients seeking medical care, which frequently precipitates an extensive (and expensive) diagnostic workup.

Abdominopelvic pain

Visceral discomforts, such as the pain of hunger or the sensation of bladder fullness, are universally experienced daily. In healthy humans, they are associated with normal regulation of bodily functions and are generally not unduly distressing. Visceral pain also commonly occurs as a manifestation of disease involving the internal organs, for example, angina (chest pain) from coronary arteriosclerosis, dyspepsia (gastric upset from duodenal ulcer), and even more commonly as a focus of medical complaints in the absence of any identifiable visceral disease.

The most common diagnosis made in patients referred to gastroenterologists for abdominal pain is irritable bowel syndrome (IBS). This disorder is in fact among the most frequently seen in patients by physicians in general, accounting for 12% of all patient visits to primary care physicians.[167] IBS is characterized by chronic intermittent abdominal discomfort and frequently disturbed bowel habits in the absence of any detectable structural, inflammatory, or infectious etiology.

As recently reviewed,[168,169] chronic visceral hyperalgesia (i.e., an increased tendency to feel pain coming from internal organs) has been implicated in many common pain disorders which occur in the absence of other definable disease. These include IBS, nonulcer dyspepsia, noncoronary chest pain, chronic urinary urgency, and chronic pelvic pain. The first direct evidence for the existence of aberrant neocortical function, related to the processing of visceral pain information in patients with such a disorder, was provided by a comparison of brain activity in healthy volunteers and IBS patients utilizing CBF studies with $H_2^{15}O$-PET.[161] The relative distribution of regional CBF was monitored in subjects at rest, and during administration of various levels of lumenal pressure in their distal intestine (Figure 7-21). In healthy subjects, activity of the perigenual anterior cingulate cortex (ACC) in Brodmann's areas 24 and 32 correlated positively with perceived stimulus intensity, and the strength of this correlation exceeded that for all other regions examined. In patients with IBS, that correlation was not observed by these[161] or subsequent investigators,[170] using a similar paradigm.

This area of the brain has extensive connections to amygdala and periacqueductal gray matter, regions involved in processing aversive stimuli. The peri-

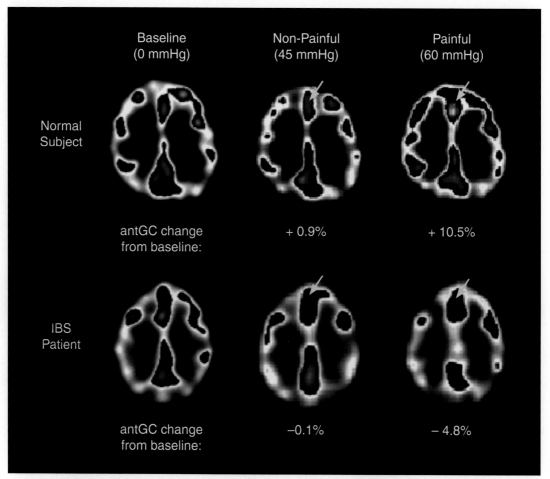

FIGURE 7-21. Response of the anterior cingulate cortex to nonpainful and painful intestinal pressure in healthy and irritable bowel syndrome subjects. Arrows indicate location of the anterior cingulate gyrus (antGC) at this axial level. PET scans of CBF with [O-15]water were obtained at baseline and at pressures that subjects reported as nonpainful or painful. The top row of scans show CBF responses in the brain of a 35-year-old healthy subject. A significant increase in anterior cingulate activity was seen during delivery of painful, but not nonpainful, intestinal pressure. The bottom row of scan shows, under identical stimuli conditions, the CBF patterns in the brain of a 39-year-old, medication-free patient with irritable bowel syndrome (IBS). No increases in anterior cingulate activity occurred during delivery of nonpainful or painful stimuli. These effects were found consistently across 56 studies, half obtained in each subject group.[161]

genual portion of the ACC is a site of dense opiate binding,[171,172] and blood flow in this region has been shown to significantly increase in response to analgesia inducing doses of morphine.[173] Thus, the failure of correlated activation of ACC in patients with IBS expecting or receiving a painful visceral stimulus may represent failure of a central pathway for descending pain inhibition.

Chest pain

Heart disease constitutes the single highest cause of death in the United States, and chest pain is the most common symptom with which it presents. The relationship between heart disease and chest pain is, nevertheless, not straight-forward. Some patients with coronary artery disease, even severe enough to lead to a heart attack, do not experience typical chest pain. Other patients have typical anginal symptoms despite the absence of significant cardiac disease. The two visceral organs from which chest pain signals most commonly arise are the heart and the esophagus, together accounting for the majority of emergency room presentations in which myocardial infarction is suspected.[174] Noncoronary chest pain contributes to more than 25% of hospital admissions for suspected unstable coronary artery disease (CAD) which, except for the need to exclude CAD as the cause of pain, would be unnecessary.[175] Among those in whom diagnostic workup demonstrates their chest pain to originate from a noncardiac source—the largest such group having pain arising from the esophagus—over 80% continue to suffer from pain of undiminished severity throughout several years of followup and over 50% are limited in their ability to work.[174,176] Chest pain syndromes, whether cardiac or noncardiac in origin, thus represent a particularly costly and debilitating problem for patients, and for the health care system which serves them.

Regional brain activity associated with cardiac pain in humans has been assessed with CBF studies of $H_2^{15}O$-PET. Rosen et al[160] found that ischemic pain, induced by intravenous administration of dobutamine in patients with documented CAD, was associated with transient regional cerebral blood flow increases in the periacqueductal gray substance, hypothalamus, thalamus, prefrontal, and cingulate cortices.[160] Those investigators subsequently made an elegant comparison of brain activation patterns associated with ischemia in patients with CAD who did or did not experience angina pectoris.[177] Neither group suffered from diabetes or other known systemic or neurologic abnormality, and the threshold for EKG-documented myocardial ischemia was similar for the two groups. PET scans of CBF were acquired with patients at rest, during placebo infusion, and during infusions of low-dose and high-dose dobutamine. During angina, patients had an increase in regional CBF in anterior/ventral cingulate cortex (Brodmann areas 24, 32 and 25) encompassing the perigenual ACC, as well as in mesial orbitofrontal and basal frontal cortex (Brodmann areas 10 and 11) and the left temporal pole (Brodmann area 28). Patients with silent ischemia demonstrated significantly less cortical activation, especially in the anterior and ventral cingulate and basal frontal cortices. Those regions were proposed to specifically represent central representation of pain signals emanating from the heart.

Cerebral representation of esophageal signals has also been recently examined.[162] In a CBF study using $H_2^{15}O$-PET carried out by Aziz et al,[162] healthy subjects, without a medical history of chest pain or other esophageal symptoms, were studied. Scans were acquired at rest, during administration of a nonpainful pressure stimulus via an intraesophageal balloon, and during painful distension. As previously described for intestinal and myocardial pain stimuli, esophageal pain was associated with activation of perigenual ACC in Brodmann area 32. Other regions for which the authors reported activation associated with pain included right insula and supplementary motor cortex. As the criterion used for statistically significant activation, however, did not include adequate correction for multiple comparisons, conclusions concerning esophageal-directed activation in the latter regions must await confirmation from independent analyses.

Depression and obsessive-compulsive disorder

Much of our understanding of psychopharmacology is based on principles of neurotransmission originally developed from studies on the autonomic nervous system. Current studies seek to link brain activity to behavior by way of chemical manipulation of biochemical processes that result in behavioral changes. Collectively, this knowledge base has provided the conceptual framework within which PET studies can be designed and interpreted. PET tracers can be used to provide measures of activity or quantify regional concentrations of substances in the brain. Tracer kinetic models necessarily restrict defining the temporal and spatial characteristics of the neuronal system under analysis, however, and this constraint likewise limits interpretation of PET studies using these methods. Also, aspects of study design, small sample sizes, and image analysis methods often lead to further limitations on what can be interpreted from these studies. Moreover, individual variability in brain morphology can necessitate MRI coregistration with the PET images for accurate delimitation of brain regions. A comprehensive critique of these issues has been reviewed elsewhere.[178] Despite those caveats, studies with PET have provided the most quantitatively accurate means to investigate the neurochemical bases of normal and abnormal behavior *in vivo*.

The alterations in metabolism and neurochemical systems detected with PET in psychiatric disorders and drug exposure illustrate the present productivity of this imaging approach and the neurochemical insights for interpreting aspects of human central nervous system (CNS) pharmacology and behavior. The fundamental question for clinical PET applications in psychiatry is to what extent can the characterization of biochemical states, as observed with imaging methods, differentiate normal and pathologic brain states. Although this question largely remains to be answered on a subject-by-subject basis, a rapidly increasing number of studies that present group-based analyses are defining and localizing significant associations between the neuropsychologic and neurochemical realms.[56,179]

Depression

Research studies in depression across a wide range of subject groups and assessment protocols have indicated that specific brain regions are affected (Table 7-9).[180–200] In FDG–PET studies of the alterations in CMRglc in primary depression, hypometabolism in the prefrontal cortex and caudate nucleus has been consistently observed.[201] Similar patterns of hypometabolism in the frontal cortex have also been observed in depression secondary to Parkinson's disease, Huntington's disease, obsessive–compulsive disorder (OCD) and epilepsy. This general pattern of prefrontal cortical deficits is sometimes accompanied by hypometabolism in the cingulate and temporal cortex. In light of the heterogeneous etiologies underlying depressive symptoms, FDG–PET could potentially serve as a diagnostic tool to differentiate subclasses of depression based on regional brain patterns of CMRglc.[202] Resultant algorithms could then be generated to guide pharmacotherapy decisions, evaluate therapeutic efficacy, and monitor changes in the illness.

Distinctions between depressive states might also be obtained by assessing the integrity of neurotransmitter systems. Several PET studies have recently explored alterations in the serotonin neurotransmitter system associated with depression and have shown decreases in the serotonin transporter and 5HT2 receptor densities in frontal cortex.[56]

TABLE 7-9. Studies of Regional Cerebral Activity in Patients with Depression

Disorder	PET method	Subjects (N)	Controls (N)	Findings	Reference
Primary Depression					
	[18F]FDG	5	9	Hypometabolism: caudate; bilateral prefrontal cortex	Baxter et al[180]
	[18F]FDG	20	12	Hypometabolism: reductions in anteroposterior gradient	Buchsbaum et al[181]
	[18F]FDG	13	18	Hypometabolism: right temporal lobe	Post et al[182]
	[18F]FDG	10	12	Hypometabolism: dorsolateral prefrontal cortex/hemisphere ratio	Baxter et al[183]
	[18F]FDG	6	6	Hypometabolism: dorsolateral prefrontal cortex; right hemisphere	Hurwitz et al[184]
	[18F]FDG	10	10	Hypometabolism: bilateral prefrontal cortex (L < R); whole cortex	Martinot et al[185]
	[18F]FDG	10	10	Hypometabolism: anterior and right prefrontal cortex, left anterior cingulate	Bench et al[186]
	[18F]FDG	12	12	Hypermetabolism: orbital part of frontal lobe; Hypometabolism: frontal dorsal, and parietal cortex	Biver et al[187]
	[18F]FDG	10	10	Hypometabolism: frontal cortical regions	Drevets et al[188]
	[15O]H$_2$O	10	10	CBF decrease: insular regions, cerebellar regions	Dolan et al[189]
	[15O]H$_2$O	13	33	CBF increase: left prefrontal cortex, amygdala; CBF decrease: caudate; CBF increase: medial thalamus	Drevets et al[190]
	[15O]H$_2$O	40 / 33	23 / 23	CBF reduction: left dorsolateral prefrontal cortex; anterior cingulate	Bench et al[185,191]
	[15O]H$_2$O	13	11	CBF decrease: caudate; anterior cingulate; temporal regions	Mayberg et al[192]
	[15O]H$_2$O	5 / 7	15 / 12	CBF decrease: frontal cortical regions, cingulate,	Drevets et al[188]
Secondary Depression					
Parkinson's disease	[18F]FDG	5 PD	4 + PD / 6-PD	Hypometabolism: caudate orbitofrontal region	Mayberg et al[193]
Huntington's disease	[18F]FDG	4HD	5HD	Hypometabolism: orbitofrontal and inferior parietal region	Mayberg et al[194]
Complex partial seizure	[18F]FDG	5	5	Hypometabolism: inferior frontal region	Bromfield et al[195]
Seasonal affective disorder	[18F]FDG	7	38	Hypometabolism: global; lower superior frontal regions	Cohen et al[196]
	[18F]FDG	9	45	Hypometabolism: orbitofrontal and left anterior parietal regions	Goyer et al[197]
Bipolar (manic mood vs depressed mood)	[18F]FDG	5 unipolar / 5 bipolar / 5 manic	9	Whole brain hypometabolism in bipolars	Baxter et al[180]

Abbreviations: CBF, cerebral blood flow; HD, Huntington's Disease; N, number of subjects; PD, Parkinson's Disease; PET, positron emission tomography.

Source: Data used with permission and adapted from Staley et al,[198] Kennedy et al,[199] and Videbach.[200]

CBF studies have also been conducted in patients with depression. In this paradigm, the coupling of neural activity and CBF allows for indirect assessment of localized changes in metabolism. Study results have shown both relative increases (amygdala and orbital cortex) and decreases (subregions of cingulate and prefrontal cortex) in depression. Additionally, activation studies, in which a particular cognitive or emotional task is performed during the time of the scan, have also been used to reveal alterations not manifested under baseline conditions. For both types of studies, however, interpretation of these differences remains problematic because of the wide range of metabolic- and neurotransmission-related factors that summatively affect CBF regulation.[203]

Obsessive-compulsive disorder

OCD is a condition characterized by obsessions (recurrent and persistent unwanted thoughts, impulses, or images) and/or compulsions (repetitive behaviors or mental acts that the person feels driven to perform), which are associated with marked anxiety or distress. PET studies of untreated, nondepressed subjects with OCD have reported elevated resting CMRglc or CBF variously in orbitofrontal cortex, caudate nuclei, thalamus, and anterior cingulate cortex.[204–207] Interventions that provoke OCD symptoms have also been reported to be associated with increased CBF to these structures[208] and therapies (both pharmacologic and behavioral) that improve symptoms have been reported to produce a relative decrease in caudate CMRglc.[209] It has been proposed that the symptomatic expression of OCD is mediated by abnormally high activity occurring through neuropathways running between frontal cortical structures (anterior cingulate and orbitofrontal cortex, in particular) and subcortical structures (basal ganglia and medial dorsal nucleus of thalamus).[210,211] The literature in this field has not been entirely consistent, however. For example, the caudate hypermetabolism reported in early studies[204,212] has not been found in several subsequent investigations.[206,207,213] The reason for such discrepant results remains unclear but could relate to biological and clinical heterogeneity of patients carrying the diagnosis of OCD.

Recently, patients were examined with PET who were suffering from both major depression and OCD.[214] Their patterns of regional CMRglc were compared with those of three control groups—patients with major depression alone, patients with OCD alone, and normal subjects, all in an unmedicated state. It was found that regardless of the presence of OCD, the severity of depression was associated with severity of hypometabolism in the left hippocampal region. In addition, the increased thalamic metabolism characteristic of OCD was diminished by the concomitant presence of major depression. The group reporting this study failed to replicate in this investigation their own prior reports of hypermetabolism in orbitofrontal cortex and caudate, despite the large number of subjects they included (N = 88), further raising questions, along the lines alluded to above, of the generalizability of such findings across the patients carrying the diagnosis of OCD—even when that diagnostic category is assigned with the systematic caution typically found in research settings, and even within the established practices of a single institution. The possibility is thus raised that PET could be used to noninvasively shed light upon the biological substrates of interindividual heterogeneity, and the information thus gleaned might then help in directing patients towards therapies from which they would be likely to benefit most, as suggested by results of group-based analyses (e.g., Mayberg et al[192]). At present, however, it remains to be established what clinical roles PET may play in the evaluation and management of OCD and major depression.

Schizophrenia

Because the first class of effective antipsychotic drugs were antagonists selective for dopamine D2 receptors, the radiolabeled D2 receptor antagonists, [^{11}C]N-methylspiperone (NMS) and [^{11}C]raclopride (RAC), were synthesized to assess those receptors in striatum. Although a number of studies have been conducted with these tracers, the results have been inconsistent: For example, increases with NMS but not with RAC.[216] These apparent discrepancies may be related to methodological issues across different subject samples (naïve or drug-treated) and the different pharmacology of the two tracers *in vivo.*[120]

The effective use of FDOPA for detection of Parkinson's disease provided the rationale for its use to assess alterations in dopamine synthesis capacity of schizophrenics. In the few studies that have been conducted, increased dopamine synthesis has been reported in patients, compared with control subjects.[217]

Alterations in serotonergic function also likely contribute to schizophrenic symptomatology and may be related to regional differences in 5HT receptor subtypes. For example, the newer class of effective antipsychotic drugs have relatively high affinity for the 5HT2 receptor. The PET analog tracers, [^{18}F]setoperone[218] and [^{18}F]altanserin,[219] have been synthesized to assess this serotonin receptor subtype. Similarly, the 5-HT$_{1A}$ PET tracers [^{11}C]carbonyl WAY 100635[220] and [18F]MPPF[221] can be used to assess alterations in that receptor subtype. It is apparent that each of these receptor subtypes has markedly different distribution profiles in the brain (Figure 7-22). Further, the selectivity of antipsychotic drugs for both serotonergic and nonserotonergic receptor subtypes as imaged by PET can provide insights into drug efficacy and side-effect profiles (Figure 7-11).

Addiction and drug effects

Prior to PET, data on the effects of drugs on human brain function were primarily obtained from postmortem studies. With PET, both the pharmacology of the drugs as well as the consequences of drug exposure can be evaluated. Also, the pharmacokinetic and pharmacodynamic effects of drugs can be assessed in vivo. The following examples highlight these types of paradigms for assessing commonly used addictive drugs.

Alcohol

The acute consequences of alcohol abuse on motor and cognitive skills are well known. Chronic alcohol consumption can induce alterations in the function and morphology of many brain systems, including the frontal cortex, thalamus, medial temporal lobe structures and cerebellum, as has been determined by numerous methods in animal studies, and by neuroimaging and postmortem examinations in humans. The neural circuitry that is affected in those regions has not been precisely defined but several changes in regional activity have been associated with chronic ethanol exposure. For example, FDG studies in chronic alcoholic persons have shown decreased CMRglc in frontal regions, particularly, the mediofrontal and left dorsolateral prefrontal cortex—brain regions associ-

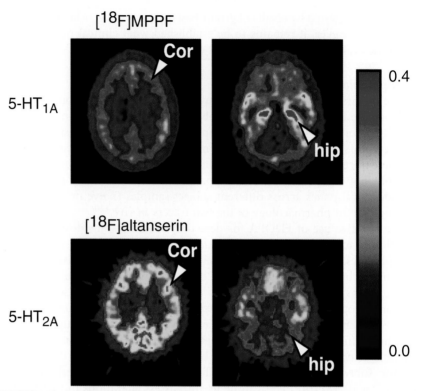

FIGURE 7-22. Regional distribution of serotonin 5-HT$_{1A}$ and 5-HT$_{2A}$ receptors. The serotonin system in brain modulates many aspects of behavior, in part, through its actions on 14 subtypes of 5-HT receptors. The characterization of these receptor subtypes in brain is important because abnormal distribution profiles may be related to psychiatric disease processes. Images of the 5-HT$_{1A}$ and 5-HT$_2$ receptor subtypes are shown here for comparison. 5-HT$_{1A}$ receptors are imaged by the binding of the labeled ligand, 4-(2′-methoxyphenyl)-1-[2′-[N-(2″-pyridinyl)-p-[^{18}F]fluorobenzamido]ethyl]piperazine, ([^{18}F]MPPF), a 5-HT$_{1A}$ antagonist. *Upper:* The [^{18}F]MPPF binding has been transformed into parametric images showing the binding potential on a pixel by pixel basis. The 5-HT$_{1A}$ receptor distribution is highest in the hippocampus (hip) and lower in the caudate and putamen. *Lower:* In contrast, the 5-HT$_{2A}$ receptor distribution is highest in cortex (Cor), and lower in putamen, thalamus, and cerebellum as shown by the binding of the labeled ligand, [^{18}F]altanserin, a 5-HT$_{2A}$ antagonist. (Images courtesy of A. Plenevaux, MD, and A. Luxen, MD.)

ated with general and executive functioning.[222,223] Yet, there remains plasticity within some of these systems; for example, recovery of metabolic deficits in the frontal cortex and of associated behaviors has been demonstrated in longitudinal studies on alcoholic persons during detoxification and longterm abstinence.[224,225]

Tobacco

The cholinergic actions of nicotine affect dopaminergic systems which contribute to the reinforcing properties and dependency related to tobacco smoking. Additionally, hundreds of other volatile compounds are contained in tobacco, many of which are poorly characterized with respect to effects on the brain.[226] Recent PET studies revealing significant differences in neurochemistry between smokers and nonsmokers lend support to the hypothesis that molecules contained in tobacco smoke may augment neurotransmission associated with changes in mood state. For example, brain levels of an enzyme that intracellularly degrades dopamine, MAO (see Figure 7-4) are decreased in smokers. MAO-A, as examined with a selective inhibitor [11C]chlorgyline, was found to be approximately 25% lower in smokers relative to nonsmokers[227]; MAO-B, as examined by the selective inhibitor analog [11C]L-deprenyl-D2, was found to be approximately 40% lower in smokers relative to nonsmokers. The magnitude of the former reduction was approximately 50% of that obtained after a 3-day administration to nonsmokers of pharmacologic dosages of tranylcypromine, a MAO inhibitor antidepressant in clinical use (Figure 7-23). These results suggest MAO inhibition may represent a molecular mechanism contributing to smoking-related elevations in mood state, due to increases in dopamine resulting from decreases in enzymatic degradation of the neurotransmitter. A common neurochemical theme that has emerged over the past several years is that drugs which produce elevations in mood often amplify transmission through dopaminergic pathways. The alterations in the dopamine system observed with PET in smokers could contribute to the powerful addiction and withdrawal syndromes associated with smoking.

Cocaine

The pharmacokinetics of cocaine in the central nervous system have been studied with ^{11}C-labeled cocaine. Its binding ranges from high levels in the striatum to low levels in the orbital cortex and cerebellum, and intermediate levels in the thalamus, amygdala, and hippocampus.[228] The time course of [^{11}C]cocaine kinetics in striatum parallels that of the associated sense of feeling high following intravenous cocaine, providing correlative *in vivo* evidence in support of the notion that the kinetics of cocaine occupancy of the dopamine transporter mediates the duration of subjective effect (Figure 7-24, left).[229] In a corresponding study with [^{11}C]methylphenidate, the rate of its binding to the dopamine transporter also correlated with the onset and magnitude of the subjective high. Different clearance rates for the two drugs suggested, however, that it is the uptake rate and not the transporter occupancy *per se* that mediates the time frame of the subjective effects.

Similarly, studies with [^{11}C]cocaine have been used to determine the level of cocaine occupancy of the dopamine transporter necessary to produce a subjective effect. In this study design, [^{11}C]cocaine PET images in each individual are acquired in the presence and absence of a pharmacologic cocaine dose. The receptor occupancy by cocaine is quantified from the difference observed in [^{11}C]cocaine binding under these two conditions.[230] These studies showed that cocaine dosages that result in greater than 50% of the transporter occupancy are generally required to achieve subjective effects.

The extent of cocaine-induced dopamine release can also be assessed by PET scans measuring displacement of the D2 receptor PET tracer, [^{11}C]raclopride (RAC). Cocaine-induced increases in extracellular dopamine concentrations compete with RAC for the D2 receptor, resulting in lower RAC binding relative to baseline values. This protocol has also been used to show a blunted response to intravenous methylphenidate in cocaine-dependent subjects, suggesting that dopamine-release mechanisms in those subjects have become less sensitive.[231]

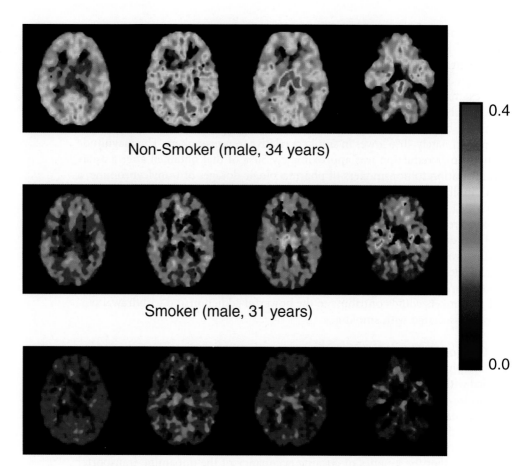

Non-Smoker (male, 34 years)

0.4

Smoker (male, 31 years)

0.0

Tranylcypromine Treatment (male, 34 years)

FIGURE 7-23. Monitoring the effects of tobacco smoke on MAO-A in the human brain. *Top row:* MAO-A concentrations in brain regions can be imaged by binding the labeled ligand, [^{11}C]chlorgyline, a selective MAO-A inhibitor. *Bottom row:* To provide evidence that [^{11}C]chlorgyline binds selectively to MAO, a study was conducted in which nonsmoker-control subjects first receive an MAO inhibitor, tranylcypromine (10 mg/d for 3 d). Essentially, all MAO binding sites were occupied at this tranylcypromine dosage. When [^{11}C]chlorgyline was subsequently administered, its binding was markedly reduced, indicating the specificity of [^{11}C]chlorgyline-MAO binding. In another application, [^{11}C]chlorgyline binding imaged the effects of smoking on MAO-A. *Middle row:* Smokers showed a 30% reduction in [^{11}C]chlorgyline binding relative to nonsmokers, indicating that components in tobacco smoke decrease MAO-A concentrations in brain. The color scale represents the values of the tracer kinetic modeled binding constant k_3, which is a function of MAO-A concentration and affinity of chlorgyline for MAO-A. (Reprinted from Fowler et al.,[227] with permission form National Academy of Sciences, U.S.A., Copyright 1996.)

These studies provide powerful evidence of neuroadaptations in the striatal dopamine system consequent to chronic cocaine exposure.

Methylphenidate

For several decades, the primary pharmacotherapy for attention-deficit hyperactivity disorder (ADHD) has been methylphenidate.[232,233] It binds to dopamine transporter, inhibiting the reuptake of dopamine from the synaptic

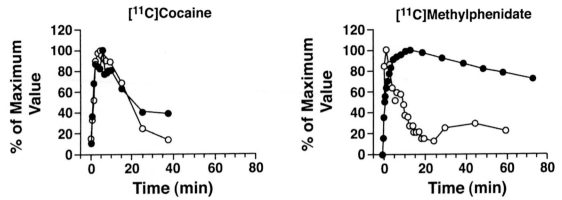

FIGURE 7-24. Monitoring the pharmacokinetics of psychotropic drugs. Cocaine and methylphenidate are both dopamine reuptake inhibitors and their similar molecular mechanisms of actions imply similar behavioral profiles. The durations of what is known as the high produced with each drug show parallel time courses (open circles in each graph). Left: For cocaine, the drug concentration-response relationship is observed when imaging the striatum of a normal subject with the labeled ligand, [¹¹C]cocaine (solid circles). That is, relative changes in brain concentrations of [¹¹C]cocaine, which are a function of its binding and clearance, parallel the changes in the subjective high time course induced by the pharmacological dose. *Right:* In contrast, imaging with the labeled ligand, [¹¹C]methylphenidate (solid circles), shows that its uptake and binding parallel the 0 to 10-minute period of pharmacological dose/high time course but not that between 10 minutes to 70 minutes when brain concentrations of [¹¹C]methylphenidate remain elevated. These results show that two dopamine reuptake inhibitor drugs with similar time courses for their subjective high have markedly different brain pharmacokinetics, suggesting that factors other than drug concentration also modulate the duration of the behavioral response. (Reprinted from Fowler et al.,[234] by courtesy of Marcel Dekker, Inc.)

cleft into the presynaptic neuron, a mechanism of action similar to that for cocaine, with paradoxical reduction of hyperactivity in patients with ADHD. With intravenous administration, it can produce a high in normal adult subjects similar to that produced by cocaine. The two drugs, however, have different kinetic profiles: although both [¹¹C]methylphenidate and [¹¹C]cocaine rapidly enter the brain, the clearance from the brain of methylphenidate proceeds much more slowly (Figure 7-24, right).[234]

RAC displacement by pharmacological dosages of methylphenidate has been used to estimate the extent of methylphenidate-induced increases in extracellular dopamine. For example, oral (~0.8 mg/kg) and intravenous (0.5 mg/kg) methylphenidate doses resulted in similar decreases in RAC binding potential values.[235] Studies such as these have led Volkow et al.[235] to postulate possible mechanisms for the efficacy of methylphenidate in patients with ADHD. Noting that dopamine normally decreases background firing rates and that ADHD patients have abnormally high striatal dopamine transporter levels, one possibility they raise is that methylphenidate amplifies synaptic extracellular dopamine and thereby reduces distracting neuronal activity. They also consider an alternative, though not mutually exclusive, hypothesis that the increased dopaminergic signal enhances interest in task performance through the effects of dopamine on the reward pathway of the brain (which cocaine is also thought to potently modulate).

Methamphetamine

The neurotoxicity of high-dose methamphetamine exposure has been extensively documented across a wide range of study protocols in both rodents and nonhuman primates.[236] Yet, the extrapolation of these results to humans had remained tenuous in the absence of corresponding observations in people. Recent data in humans from both postmortem[237] and PET studies have now shown that there are striatal dopaminergic deficits associated with chronic methamphetamine exposure. In separate PET studies of methamphetamine-dependent subjects after 2 weeks to 5 months of abstinence, both [11C]methylphenidate[238] and [11C]WIN 35,428[239] showed 20% to 30% reductions in striatal dopamine transporter binding, suggestive of long-term alterations of the dopaminergic terminals. Yet, in subsets of these subjects, significant recovery of dopamine transporter binding by [11C]methylphenidate was observed upon protracted abstinence, indicating the reversibility of some neurotoxic effects of methamphetamine (Figure 7-25). Methamphetamine-induced alterations in regional CMRglc, as measured with FDG–PET, have also been examined. Relative to control subjects, the methamphetamine-dependent subjects have reduced metabolism in the striatum and thalamus but higher metabolism in the parietal cortex, indicating that effects of methamphetamine extend beyond areas of high concentration of dopaminergic terminals.[240]

STUDIES OF OTHER MAMMALIAN BRAINS

Research involving PET in humans represents the culmination of prior studies in which the chemistry and radiochemistry, pharmacokinetics, drug metabolism, and safety of PET tracers have been characterized. Additionally, a range of preclinical testing in animals is often necessary to evaluate issues of tracer specificity and sensitivity *in vivo*. Animal studies can be structured to include evaluations with PET and corresponding neurochemical analysis of tissue *in vitro*. This use of animal models also provides a valuable experimental paradigm in which to design, test, and evaluate potential therapeutic strategies prior to their consideration for human applications. Those data can then support a biochemical interpretation for the results of subsequent human PET studies. As our insights into disease processes evolve, both early detection of neurological disease and assessment of intervention strategies have emerged as key objectives for further preclinical PET research.

Primates

Models for studying Parkinson's disease

The etiology of PD remains unknown and, consequently, animal models only approximate aspects of the disease process and pathology. Nonetheless, the use of the dopamine neurotoxin 1-methyl-4-phenyl-1,2,5,6-tetrahydropyridine (MPTP)[241,242] has provided significant insights into basal ganglia circuitry and function.[243] In particular, MPTP administration to monkeys results in extensive nigrostriatal degeneration and behavioral deficits resembling PD. A less debilitating symptomatology can be produced by intracarotid MPTP administration that produces predominantly unilateral nigrostriatal dopamine deficits.[244] In this unilateral MPTP-lesioned PD model, the effects of MPTP on striatal dopamine function can be evaluated with FDOPA assessments of dopamine synthesis,[245]

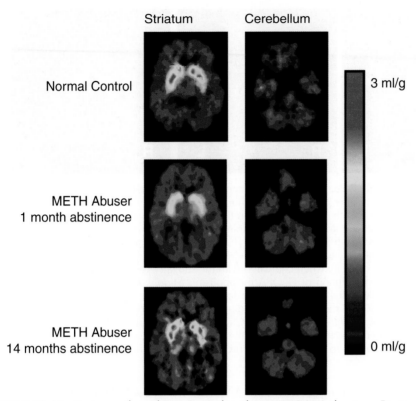

FIGURE 7-25. Monitoring methamphetamine-induced neurotoxicity in humans. Presynaptic dopamine transporter (DAT) availability is imaged by the binding of the labeled ligand, [^{11}C]methylphenidate, an inhibitor of DAT activity. After 4 weeks of abstinence, the striatum of a chronic methamphetamine abuser (drug use > 2 y) shows a loss of DAT as measured by a 25% reduction in the distribution volume of [^{11}C]methylphenidate binding (*middle*) when compared to that of a nonuser (*top*). When this methamphetamine-dependent subject was reevaluated at 14 months of abstinence, a significant recovery in [^{11}C]methylphenidate binding was observed (*bottom*). These results show that chronic methamphetamine abuse results in striatal dopamine system deficits that are reversible with protracted abstinence. (Reprinted from Volkow et al.,[263] with permission from the Society for Neuroscience, copyright 2001.)

while alterations in dopamine transporter density can be evaluated with WIN 35,428 (Figure 7-26, left and middle). Additionally, increases in ipsilateral D2 receptor binding to [^{11}C]raclopride indicate that postsynaptic alterations have occurred (Figure 7-26, right).

In squirrel monkeys lesioned with graded doses of MPTP, FDOPA studies showed that in individual subjects, decreases in kinetic measures of striatal AAAD activity measured with PET *in vivo* were significantly correlated with AAAD enzymatic activities that were measured *in vitro*.[246] Absolute rates measured *in vivo*, however, differed significantly from the corresponding measurements made *in vitro*. Additionally, the extent of substantia nigra cell loss was not paralleled by

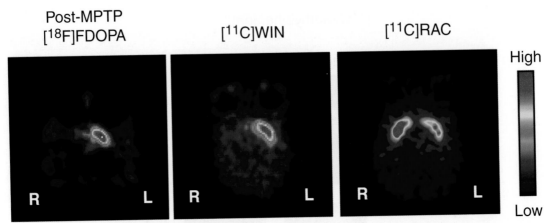

FIGURE 7-26. Monitoring parameters of pre- and postsynaptic striatal dopamine system integrity after MPTP administration. The dopamine system neurotoxin, MPTP, was injected into the right internal carotid artery of a vervet monkey to produce a unilateral nigrostriatal dopamine lesion (unilateral deficits are often the first manifestation of PD). *Left:* After MPTP, imaging with [^{18}F]FDOPA shows a significant reduction in [^{18}F]fluorodopamine accumulation in the right striatum, indicating a decrease in dopamine synthesis capacity when compared with the subject's left striatum (see legend for Figure 7-4 for description of FDOPA metabolism). *Middle:* In the same subject, imaging with [^{11}C]WIN35,428, ([^{11}C]WIN), a labeled ligand that binds selectively to the dopamine transporter, shows reduced binding, indicating a corresponding loss of dopamine terminals. *Right:* Imaging with [^{11}C]raclopride, a dopamine D2 antagonist, shows an increased binding in right striatum, suggesting an apparent upregulation of D2 receptors in response to the reduction in presynaptic dopamine terminals.

corresponding decreases in AAAD activity. The AAAD activity is thus not a simple function of dopamine cell number: Compensating increases in residual AAAD levels can occur after partial nigrostriatal degeneration.

ASSESSMENT OF INTERVENTION STRATEGIES IN PARKINSON'S DISEASE

MPTP-induced alterations in the nonhuman primate have provided an excellent model to assess the sensitivity of PET tracers for detection of dopaminergic deficits and the efficacy of neurorestoration strategies. Recent studies that have combined *in vivo* PET assessment with corresponding *in vitro* measurments highlight the benefits of animal research for the interpretation of human PET studies. Such studies in experimental animals can provide proof of principle of a novel therapy. In animal studies designed for that purpose, the potential therapy should be modeled as closely as possible to the clinical application. These therapies can then be quantitatively assessed with PET tracers that have been designed to monitor specific aspects of neuronal function. For example, the use of gene therapies to alter neurotransmitter activity within the brain will likely be incorporated into therapeutic options in the coming years. In a preclinical gene transfer study in unilaterally MPTP-lesioned monkeys, the gene for AAAD was inserted into an adeno-associated virus that had been stripped of its replicative functions but was still capable of infecting cells.[247] With injection of the virus into the striatum, the subsequent expression of AAAD within striatal cells would then provide a local source of decarboxylase activity. The AAAD substrate 6-[F-18]fluoro-L-m-tyrosine (FMT) was used as a probe to demonstrate the effects of this therapy over time. At 2 months, FMT–PET showed significant restoration of striatal FMT decarboxylation by AAAD, thus providing evidence that this potentially therapeutic AAAD gene was properly expressed—that is, it led to the transcription of mRNA that was translated into a protein, which, in turn, led to reconstitution of enzymatic function (Figure 7-27).

FIGURE 7-27. Monitoring gene therapy in an animal model of Parkinson's disease. Experimental evidence of gene therapy efficacy is required before gene therapy can be used to treat Parkinson's disease (PD) patients. These data can be acquired from animal studies that mimic aspects of the PD disease process. For example, a right-striatum dopamine lesion was produced in a nonhuman primate by injecting the dopamine system neurotoxin, MPTP, into its right-internal carotid artery. The resultant deficit was imaged with the labeled ligand, FMT. The pharmacokinetics of FMT are similar to those of FDOPA (see legend for Figure 7-4 for description of FDOPA metabolism). Following FMT administration, it was converted to [18F]fluoro-m-tyramine in striatum by aromatic amino acid decarboxylase (AADC) which is contained primarily in dopaminergic terminals. The extent of [18F]fluoro-m-tyramine accumulation is then used to estimate dopamine synthesis capacity. For this gene therapy study, a preintervention FMT coronal image (*upper left:* A) shows a significant unilateral reduction in dopamine synthesis capacity in the striatum lesioned by MPTP. Subsequently, an adeno-associated virus (AAV) that was genetically engineered to express the AADC enzyme was stereotactically injected into the lesioned striatum. Approximately 2 months later, a postintervention FMT image (*upper right:* B) shows a unilateral increase in dopamine synthesis capacity, indicating both gene expression of the AADC protein and establishment of its enzymatic activity. In postmortem immunohistochemical studies of this subject, coronal sections of the anterior striatum show a unilateral decrease in tyrosine-hydroxylase immunoreactivity (*lower left*), indicating the persistence of the dopamine terminal deficit induced by MPTP. In contrast, increases in AADC immunoreactivity are evident throughout the lesioned striatum (*lower right*), showing selective expression of the AADC-AAV enzyme. (Reprinted from Rankiewicz et al.,[247] with permission from Elsevier.)

[18F]FMT Binding in Striatum

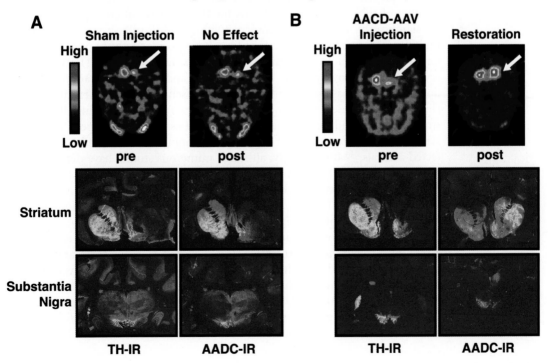

Models for studying drug abuse

Human studies on the effects of drug abuse are often difficult to interpret because of confounding factors, such as inaccurate drug histories, polydrug abuse, and uncertainties regarding total drug exposure. In animal models of drug abuse, the effects of a particular quantity of drug can be studied in isolation to determine its contribution, if any, to neuroadaptations associated with acute and chronic drug intake. One can further dissect the evolution of those changes through examination of a developmental time course of drug effects. Also, upon removal of the drug, the effects of the withdrawal state as well as the extent of reversible and irreversible deficits can be determined. For those types of studies, PET can be used to assess the time course of alterations in individual subjects in a within-subject study design. This approach allows for high accuracy in measurement of longitudinal changes and a concomitant reduction in the large number of subjects usually required in cross-sectional studies in which wide interindividual biological variability predominates as an experimental variable. The following examples demonstrate how these principles are applied in PET studies with nonhuman primates.

EFFECTS OF PSYCHOSTIMULANT EXPOSURE

The psychostimulants (e.g., cocaine, amphetamine, and methamphetamine) have potent effects on the striatal dopamine system. Postmortem studies in rodents and nonhuman primates have generally shown that high dosages of the class of amphetamines, *d*-amphetamine and *d*-methamphetamine produce longterm deficits in striatal dopaminergic markers.[236] Such effects were generally considered irreversible, based predominantly on rodent studies that incorporated a cross-sectional design and relatively shortterm recovery periods. Corresponding studies in nonhuman primates in vitro, conducted at multiple time points and with appropriate subject numbers, are not feasible in terms of the number of subjects that would be required to achieve differences with statistical significance. In contrast, protocols with a within-subject study design and multiple PET imaging studies over time have been effectively used to show a longterm time-course of dopaminergic deficits. Longitudinal PET studies have revealed that recovery from amphetamine- and methamphetamine-induced dopamine deficits is possible,[248] even in the absence of any further intervention (Figure 7-28). These findings have been further corroborated in vitro by demonstrating corresponding presynaptic abnormalities (e.g., of transport, enzymatic synthesis, and degradation of dopamine) in brain tissue resected from the affected animals.[248] Interestingly, although numerous studies have demonstrated neurotoxicity associated with high-dose methamphetamine exposure,[249] similar deficits have not been observed following high-dose chronic cocaine exposure. Thus, broad generalizations regarding the toxicity of the psychostimulant class of drugs even at relatively high dosages have become less tenable.

This pre- and post-treatment assessment paradigm can also be extended to assess the effects of neuroprotective strategies. For example, pretreatment with glial cell line derived growth factor (GDNF) in the striatum was evaluated for its effects on subsequent neurotoxic methamphetamine exposure.[250] Individual variation in reactivity to GDNF and sensitivity to methamphetamine would be expected to lead to effects of different magnitude and rates of recovery. However, by conducting multiple WIN–PET studies over time in each subject, the

Pre-Amphetamine Control

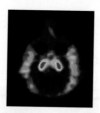

Chronic Amphetamine (10 days)

High

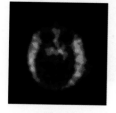 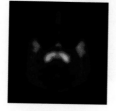 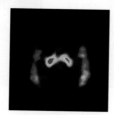 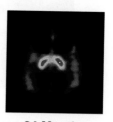

| 1 Month | 6 Months | 12 Months | 24 Months | Low |

Post-Amphetamine   Recovery of Dopamine Synthesis ⟶

Recovery of Dopamine Synthesis Capacity

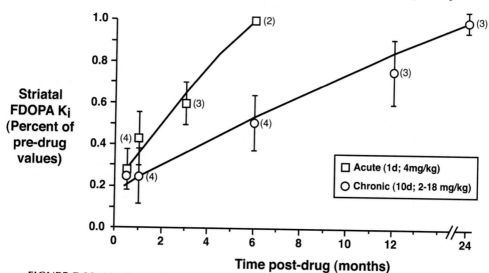

Striatal FDOPA K_i (Percent of pre-drug values)

□ Acute (1d; 4mg/kg)
○ Chronic (10d; 2-18 mg/kg)

Time post-drug (months)

FIGURE 7-28. Monitoring longterm neurotoxic effects of amphetamine on the striatal dopamine system. Dosages of *d*-amphetamine that increase from 4 mg/kg/d to 18 mg/kg/d over 10 days result in a profound deficit in dopamine synthesis capacity at 1 month, using FDOPA, relative to its pre-amphetamine-control image. Without any further intervention, subsequent PET studies with FDOPA at 6 months, 12 months, and 24 months in the same subject show a protracted recovery of dopamine synthesis. In other subjects, a lower amphetamine dosage (1 dose of 4 mg/kg, i.m.) also produced similar striatal dopamine deficits but the recovery was faster and occurred over a period of only 6 months. The graph plots FDOPA influx rate constant (FDOPA K_i), a model parameter used to quantitate [^{18}F]fluorodopamine synthesis for each amphetamine dosage. Results indicate that the adult primate brain retains endogenous repair mechanisms. Elucidation of the molecular pathways underlying this recovery process may provide new targets for the design of therapies to treat neurodegenerative diseases in the brain. (Reprinted from Melega et al.,[265] with permission from Elsevier.)

[^{11}C]WIN Binding in Striatum

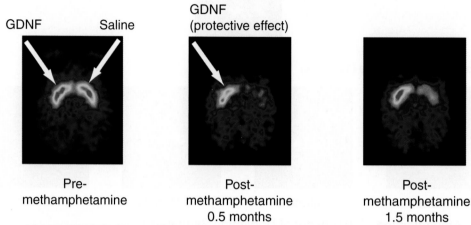

GDNF   Saline

GDNF
(protective effect)

Pre-
methamphetamine

Post-
methamphetamine
0.5 months

Post-
methamphetamine
1.5 months

FIGURE 7-29. Monitoring the neuroprotective effects of a neurotrophic factor. The use of neurotrophic factors has been proposed as a protective and restorative therapy to reduce the progressive loss of dopamine terminals associated with Parkinson's disease (PD). In this experimental study on a vervet monkey, glial cell line-derived neurotrophic factor (GDNF) is injected into the right striatum to stimulate the activity of the dopamine system. Saline is injected into the left striatum in order to determine any effects due to the injection procedure. One week later, d-Methamphetamine (2 doses of 2 mg/kg, i.m., 24 h apart) is administered to produce striatal dopamine deficits similar to those observed in PD and illustrated in Figure 7-28. The longterm efficacy of the GDNF therapeutic approach is then assessed in multiple imaging studies using the labeled ligand, [^{11}C]WIN 35,428, ([^{11}C]WIN). [^{11}C]WIN binds selectively to the dopamine transporter in striatum as shown in the preintervention image (left). Decreases in [^{11}C]WIN binding resulting from the methamphetamine-induced neurotoxicity indicate a reduction in dopamine transporter availability, suggesting terminal loss. At 2 weeks after methamphetamine exposure, the saline-injected striatum shows a greater loss of [^{11}C]WIN relative to the GDNF-injected striatum (middle), indicating partial neuroprotection by GDNF. At 1.5 months as the dopamine system gradually recovers bilaterally, the GDNF-injected striatum shows an accelerated improvement (right). These results suggest that the use of GDNF may provide similar benefits in PD. (Reprinted from Melega et al.,[250] with permission from Synapse © 2000.)

results clearly showed that despite variable time courses, GDNF pretreatment provided partial neuroprotection and accelerated recovery of the striatal dopamine system (Figure 7-29).

Rodents

Until recently, it has only been possible to use PET for imaging brains as large as those in humans and nonhuman primates. The development of PET systems for small animals (Chapter 1) has now created opportunities to image the brains of animals as small as rat and mouse (Figure 7-30). Many new therapies to treat disease are first tested in small animals before consideration of human applications. Also, models of human diseases have been developed in rats and mice, with the mouse as the primary animal used for models involving genetic manipulation. A variety of *in vitro* methods have been developed to quantify various biological parameters in these animals that can facilitate validation of new PET methodologies. Many of those procedures would be prohibitively expensive and technically difficult in nonhuman primates. With PET, longitudinal studies can be conducted in an individual animal. Therapeutic strategies for central nervous system intervention can be modeled in the rodent and evaluated with PET imaging prior to further evaluation in nonhuman primate models and, eventually, humans.

The rodent imaging systems that have now been developed by different research groups share a common set of challenges, e.g., sensitivity, spatial resolution, and partial volume effects,[251,252] as discussed in Chapter 1. For this section, the current state and future prospects are described for rodent studies conducted with a microPET system that was developed at the University of California, Los Angeles.[253] It is a 3-D scanner and uses lutetium oxyorthosilicate

FIGURE 7-30. Imaging the striatal dopamine system of a human, monkey, rat, and mouse. The striatal dopamine system is imaged in humans and other animal species with the labeled ligand, [^{11}C]WIN35,428, ([^{11}C]WIN). [^{11}C]WIN binds selectively to the dopamine transporter located on dopaminergic axons. The extent of its binding provides an estimate of dopamine terminal density. In animal studies, combined PET and postmortem studies establish the correlation between *in vivo* and *in vitro* [^{11}C]WIN binding. Those results provide critical biochemical data to interpret PET images obtained in humans. The coronal images show clear delineation of [^{11}C]WIN binding to dopaminergic axons in the left and right striatum, across species from rodents (rat and mouse) to humans. Rodents do not have anatomically separate structures of caudate and putamen as do primates (monkey and human). In rodents, these two structures are fused into a single structure, the striatum.

[^{11}C]WIN 35, 428 Binding in Striatum

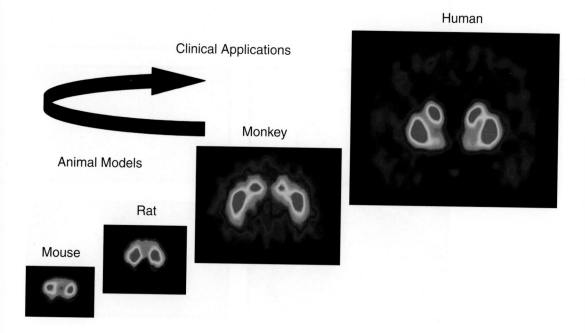

Human

Clinical Applications

Animal Models

Monkey

Rat

Mouse

(LSO) for its scintillation crystal in place of the usual Bismuth Germanate (BGO). LSO has a shorter decay time and a higher light output than BGO. An iterative reconstruction algorithm, 3-D Maximum A Posteriori (MAP),[254] has been adapted for use with microPET, resulting in volumetric spatial resolution of 1.5 mm in all directions.[255] Images of the rat brain acquired with this system allow for the visualization of major structures, as shown with FDG (Figure 7-31A). More recently, a second generation instrument (microPET II) has been developed with approximately eight times better volume resolution and higher efficiency compared to microPET I (Chapter 1).

To give an example of the power of this approach, assessments of the striatal dopamine system have now been conducted in rodents, with WIN as a

FIGURE 7-31. Imaging the rat brain with microPET. The development of high-resolution PET technology has led to production of a microPET system that can image the brains of smaller animals, such as rats and mice. In this series of studies, labeled ligands were used to image different aspects of rat brain neurochemistry. The excellent resolution of microPET for imaging small brain regions is evident by comparing the coronal PET images to corresponding sections from a cryosectioned rat brain atlas (Brain atlas—courtesy of A. Toga, University of California, Los Angeles). The use of microPET generates new possibilities for the development of imaging applications and small animal research. A: Assessment of cerebral glucose metabolic rates with FDG. Proceeding from anterior to posterior planes of the rat brain atlas (*left*), the relative differences in glucose metabolic rates for cortex, thalamus and cerebellum as imaged with FDG are shown in corresponding coronal planes.

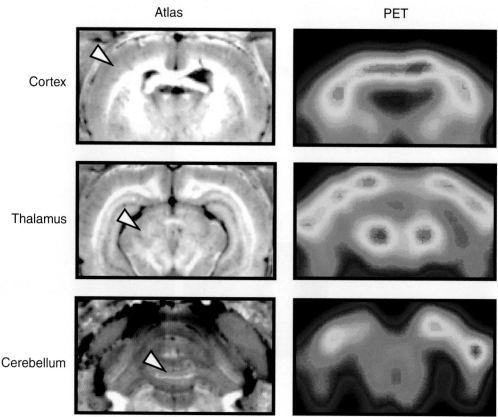

A.

[¹¹C]WIN

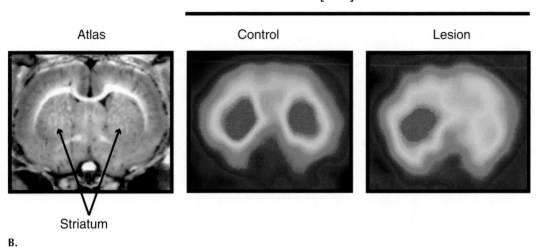

Atlas   Control   Lesion

Striatum

B.

Rat Brain Atlas   [¹⁸F]MPPF Binding

Cortex   Hippocampus   Cortex   Hippocampus

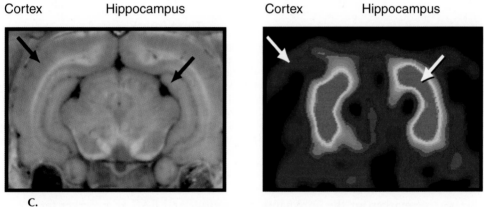

C.

FIGURE 7-31. *Continued.* B: Monitoring the effects of neurotoxin exposure on the striatal dopamine system. Estimates of dopamine terminal density in striatum are obtained by imaging the binding of [¹¹C]WIN 35,428 ([¹¹C]WIN) to the dopamine transporter located on dopaminergic axons (*middle*). Following a unilateral injection of the dopamine system neurotoxin, 6-hydroxydopamine, into the substantia nigra of the rat, the resultant striatal dopamine terminal loss is imaged in a coronal plane by the reduction in [¹¹C]WIN binding (*right*). To quantitate the extent of the lesion, the corresponding plane of the atlas can be used to accurately define the area of the striatum. C: Assessment of 5-HT$_{1A}$ receptors in the hippocampus. *Left:* The hippocampus contains more 5-HT$_{1A}$ receptors than adjacent cortical brain regions. This relative distribution is shown in the rat by the binding of the labeled ligand, 4-(2′-methoxyphenyl)-1-[2′-[N-(2″-pyridinyl)-p-[¹⁸F]fluorobenzamido]-ethyl]piperazine, ([¹⁸F]MPPF), a 5HT$_{1A}$ receptor antagonist. *Right:* The resolution of microPET for imaging small brain regions such as the hippocampus can be verified by comparing the coronal PET image to a corresponding plane from the rat brain atlas.

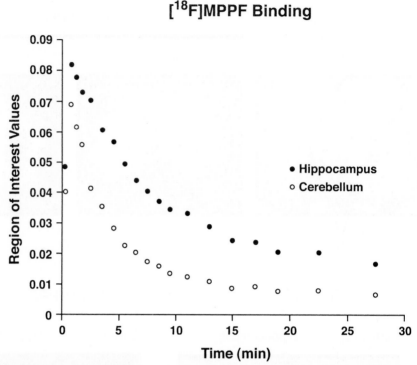

FIGURE 7-31. *Continued.* D: Hippocampus and cerebellum pharmacokinetics for [^{18}F]MPPF, a 5-HT$_{1A}$ receptor antagonist. [^{18}F]MPPF time-activity curves for the hippocampus and cerebellum of the rat reflect the transport, binding, and clearance of [^{18}F]MPPF from these two selected tissues. To generate these profiles, regions of interests (ROIs) are drawn on coronal images that contain the hippocampus and cerebellum to obtain kinetic data throughout the study. The higher concentration of 5-HT$_{1A}$ receptors in hippocampus relative to cerebellum is shown by the differences in [^{18}F]MPPF binding between the two regions. These data can then be fitted to an appropriate kinetic model for quantitative analysis of specific binding of [^{18}F]MPPF.

marker for the presynaptic transporter and RAC as a marker for D2 receptor. In normal and 6-hydroxydopamine unilaterally lesioned animals, multiple studies with WIN have been used to monitor longterm alterations. In the latter set of animals, the presynaptic terminal loss was reflected by significant decreases in WIN binding relative to control animals (Figure 7-31B). This lays the foundation for studies with interventions designed to restore normal function in which these same subjects can then be assessed for behavioral recovery.

The approach has also been applied to other molecules important to neuronal function in other brain regions. For example, studies have been done to measure aspects of the serotonergic system, as illustrated by images obtained with the radiotracer [^{18}F]MPPF, an antagonist of the 5-HT$_{1A}$ receptor (Figure 7-31C). Its distribution profile is clearly shown. The postsynaptic density of this receptor subtype is highest in the hippocampus. As with conventional PET analysis, a ROI can be placed on the hippocampal region to generate a time activity curve for kinetic model fitting and analysis (Figure 7-31D).

NEW DIRECTIONS

Both normal biology and disease processes are increasingly coming to be understood at the molecular level in the brain and other organ systems. As reviewed in this chapter, many phenomena previously studied at only the psychological level, such as human mood states, pain perception, and substance abuse, are now being explored in terms of their underlying neuroanatomical and neurochemical substrates, in living human beings. Many diseases that have no gross structural abnormalities on CT and MRI have been revealed with biological studies with PET. Neurodegenerative processes that previously only became apparent when sufficient brain tissue was decimated to lead to overt symptoms can now be detected and studied years—sometimes decades—in advance of symptomatic expression through molecular imaging with PET.

The past decade has seen fruition of the increasingly molecular approach to biology and medicine, not only in terms of expanding our understanding of complex biological systems, but in terms of direct clinical benefit through development of rationally designed effective therapeutic strategies. Imaging with PET allows microstructures and processes in the brain and elsewhere to be localized within an accuracy of a few millimeters with continuing efforts to improve spatial resolution and expand the diversity of molecular imaging probes. It also allows for quantification of image data from molecular probes both in absolute (molar) terms of concentration or rates of reactions (moles/min/g of tissue), as well as in terms of relative spatial distribution patterns. Moreover, the drive for development of ultra-high resolution PET scanners for small animals is producing innovative new detector, scanner, and image reconstruction technologies that will likely lead to major advances in resolution and image quality in human PET scanners.

The biomedical sciences are headed towards a future of accelerating translation of research activity that moves from bench to bedside with the help of such imaging approaches: biologic and pathologic processes that may be first characterized *in vitro* or in tissue culture are explored in animal models *in vivo* with correlations made between invasive gold standard methods of bioassay and noninvasive image-based measurements. Once those correlations are established, the imaging methods can be used to noninvasively follow the processes longitudinally in nonhuman animals and people. In some instances, through studying in patients those disease processes that will lead to invasive procedures on clinical grounds alone, it is practically and ethically possible to obtain gold standard validation by transitioning directly from the research laboratory to the laboratory of the human body. Finally, these validated imaging methods can then contribute information that serves to improve routine clinical care by impacting upon: 1) accuracy of diagnosis, 2) assessment of prognosis, 3) individualization of treatment approaches, including (but not limited to) selection and dose titration of specific pharmacotherapies, and 4) monitoring a patient's course during and following therapy.

Molecular imaging of the biology of disease will move medical imaging from the lesion classification to the molecular classification that is more informative in diagnosis and in selection of the most effective treatment. This is particularly important in the era of molecular medicine, which is focused on defining molecular targets of diseases for designating effective and increasingly specific molecular therapies. Success in this arena is continually prompting the development of new imaging probes with which to explore the molecular intricacies of those disease processes.

Virtually any biochemical that exists in the body, or any drug that is used for research or therapeutic purposes, can in principle be labeled with a positron-emitting nuclide, and thereby visualized with PET *in vivo*. PET is proving valuable in facilitating the movement forward from the research laboratory to the clinical practice setting and holds promise for becoming even more valuable in that regard, in part because of this great versatility. Examples of the research value and clinical utility of several kinds of tracers have been illustrated in the preceding sections of this chapter, as well as other chapters in this text. Maximizing the usefulness of PET in the future will depend upon concomitant development of new radiopharmaceuticals with which to probe at the molecular level those biologic and pathologic activities occurring in the living body.

ACKNOWLEDGMENTS

We are indebted to Dana Marseille and Shanna Kim for their assistance with manuscript preparation.

REFERENCES

1. Phelps ME. Positron emission tomography provides molecular imaging of biological processes. *Proc Natl Acad Sci.* 2000;97:9226–9233.
2. Huang SC. Anatomy of SUV. Standardized uptake value. *Nucl Med Biol.* 2000;27:643–646.
3. Gottstein U, Held K. Effects of aging on cerebral circulation and metabolism in man. *Acta Neurol Scand.* 1979;72(Suppl 60):54–55.
4. Dastur DK, Lane MH, Hansen DB, et al. Effects of aging on cerebral circulation and metabolism in man. In: J.E. Birren, R.N. Butler, et al., eds. *Human Aging: A Biological and Behavioral Study*, U.S. Government Printing Office, Washington, DC; 1963;59–78.
5. Kety SS. Circulation and metabolism of the human brain in health and disease. *Am J Med.* 1950;8:205–217.
6. Kety SS, Schmidt CE. Human cerebral blood flow and oxygen consumption as related to aging. *J Chronic Dis.* 1956;3:428–486.
7. Smith CB, Sokoloff L. The energy metabolism of the brain. In: *The Molecular Basis of Neuropathology*. Arnold, London; 1981;104–131.
8. Sokoloff L. The metabolism of the central nervous system in vivo. In: J Field, HW Magoun, VE Hall, eds. *Handbook of Physiology—Neurophysiology* Vol. 3. American Physiological Society, Washington, DC; 1960;1843–1864.
9. Kety SS, Schmidt CE. The nitrous oxide method for the quantitative determination of cerebral blood flow in man: Theory, procedure and normal values. *J Clin Invest.* 1948;27:476–483.
10. Alexander SG, Smith TC, Stroble G, et al. Cerebral carbohydrate metabolism of man during respiratory and etabolic alkalosis. *J Appl Physiol.* 1968;24:66–72.
11. Takeshita H, Okuda Y, Sari A. The affects of ketamine on cerebral circulation of metabolism in man. *Anesthesiology.* 1972;36:69–75.
12. Sokoloff L, Reivich M, Kennedy C, et al. The [^{14}C]deoxyglucose method for the measurement of local cerebral glucose utilization: Theory, procedure and normal values in the conscious and anesthesized albino rat. *J Neurochem.* 1977;28:897–916.
13. Huang S-C, Phelps ME, Hoffman EJ, et al. Noninvasive determination of local cerebral metabolic rate of glucose in man. *Am J Physiol.* 1980;238:E69–E82.

14. Kuhl DE, Phelps ME, Kowell AP, Metter EJ, Selin C, Winter J. Mapping local metabolism and perfusion in normal and ischemic brain by emission computed tomography of [18]FDG and [13]NH$_3$. *Ann Neurol*. 1980;8:47–60.

15. Mazziotta JC, Phelps ME, Miller J. Tomographic mapping of human cerebral metabolism: Normal unstimulated state. *Neurology*. 1981;31:503–516.

16. Phelps ME, Huang SC, Hoffman EJ, Selin C, Sokoloff L, Kuhl DE. Tomographic measurement of local cerebral glucose metabolic rate in humans with (F-18)2-fluoro-2-deoxyglucose: Validation of method. *Ann Neurol*. 1979;6:371–388.

17. Reivich N, Kuhl D, Wolf A, Greenberg J, Phelps M, Ido T, Casella V, Hoffman E, Alavi A, Sokoloff L. The [^{18}F]fluorodeoxyglucose method for the measurement of local cerebral glucose utilization in man. *Circ Res*. 1979;44:127–137.

18. Kuhl DE, Phelps ME, Markham C, et al. Local cerebral glucose metabolism in Huntington's disease determined by emission computed tomography of ^{18}F-flurodeoxyglucose. *J Cereb Blood Flow Metab*. 1981;I(Suppl. 1):S459–S460.

19. Minoshima S, Frey KA, Burdette JH, Vander Borght T, Koeppe RA, Kuhl DE. Interpretation of metabolic abnormalities in Alzheimer's disease using three-dimensional stereotactic surface projections (3D-SSP) and normal database. *J Nucl Med*. 1995;36:237P.

20. Moeller JR, Ishikawa T, Dhawan V, et al. The metabolic topography of normal aging. *J Cereb Blood Flow Metab*. 1996;16:385–398.

21. Ishii K, Sakmoto S, Sasaki M, et al. Cerebral glucose metabolism in patients with frontotemporal dementia. *J Nucl Med*. 1998;39:1875–1878.

22. Law I, Iida H, Holm S, et al. Quantitation of regional cerebral blood flow corrected for partial volume effect using O-15 water and PET: II. Normal values and gray matter blood flow response to visual activation. *J Cereb Blood Flow Metab*. 2000;20:1252–1263.

23. Huang SC, Carson RE, Hoffman EJ, et al. Quantitative measurement of local cerebral blood flow in humans by positron computed tomography and ^{15}O-water. *J Cereb Blood Flow Metab*. 1983;3:141–153.

24. Meltzer CC, Cantwell MN, Greer PJ, et al. Does cerebral blood flow decline in healthy aging? A PET study with partial-volume correction. *J Nucl Med*. 2000;41:1842–1848.

25. Phelps ME, Huang SC, Hoffman EJ, et al. Validation of tomographic measurement of cerebral blood volume with C-11 labeled carboxyhemoglobin. *J Nucl Med*. 1979;20:328–334.

26. Celesia GG, Polcyn RE, Holden JE, et al. Visual evoked potentials and positron emission tomographic mapping of regional cerebral blood flow and cerebral metabolism: Can the neuronal potential generators be visualized? *Electroencephalogr Clin Neurophysiol*. 1982;54:243–256.

27. Heiss WD, Kloster G, Vyska K, et al. Regional cerebral distribution of ^{11}C-methyl-D-glucose compared with CT perfusion patterns in stroke. *J Cereb Blood Flow Metab*. 1981;1(Suppl. 1):S506–S507.

28. Yamamoto YL, Little S, Thompson C, et al. Positron emission tomography following EC-IC bypass surgery. *Acta Neurol Scand*. 1979;60(Suppl. 72):522–523.

29. Alpert NM, Ackerman RH, Correia JA, et al. Measurement of rCBF and rCMRO$_2$ by continuous inhalation of ^{15}O-labeled CO$_2$ and O$_2$. *Acta Neurol Scand*. 1977;56(Suppl. 72):186–187.

30. Frackowiak R, Lenzi G, Jones T, et al. Quantitative measurement of regional cerebral blood flow and oxygen metabolism in man using [15]O and positron emission tomography: Theory, procedure and normal values. *J Comput Assist Tomogr*. 1980; 4:727–736.

31. Jones T, Chesler DA, Ter-Pogossian MM. The continuous inhalation of oxygen-15 for assessing regional oxygen extraction in the brain of man. *Br J Radiol*. 1976;49:339–343.

32. Lenzi GL, Frackowiak RS, Jones T, et al. CMRO$_2$ and CBF by the oxygen-15 inhalation techniques: Results in normal volunteers and cerebrovascular patients. *Eur Neurol*. 1981;20:285–290.

33. Lenzi GL, Frackowiak RS, Jones T. Cerebral oxygen metabolism and blood flow in human cerebral ischemic infarction. *J Cereb Blood Flow Metab*. 1982;2:321–335.

34. Hoyer S. Normal and abnormal circulation and oxidative metabolism in the aging human brain. *J Cereb Blood Flow Metab*. 1982;2(Suppl. 1):S10–S13.

35. Huang SC, Phelps ME, Carson RE, et al. Tomographic measurement of local cerebral blood flow in man with 0–15 water. *J Cereb Blood Flow Metab*. 1981;1(Suppl. 1):S31–S32.

36. Lammertsma AA, Frackowiak RS, Lenzi GL, et al. Accuracy of the oxygen-15 steady state technique for measuring CBF and $CMRO_2$: Tracer modeling, statistics and spatial sampling. *J Cereb Blood Flow Metab.* 1981;1(Suppl. 1):S3–S4.

37. Frackowiak RS, Jones T, Lenzi GL, et al. Regional cerebral oxygen utilization and blood flow in normal man using oxygen-15 and positron emission tomography. *Acta Neurol Scand.* 1980;62:336–344.

38. Vallone D, Picetti R, Borrelli E. Structure and function of dopamine receptors. *Neurosci Biobehav Rev.* 2000;24:125–132.

39. Volkow ND, Fowler JS, Gatley SJ, et al. PET evaluation of the dopamine system of the human brain. *J Nucl Med.* 1996;37:1242–1256.

40. Verhoeff NP. Radiotracer imaging of dopaminergic transmission in neuropsychiatric disorders. *Psychopharmacology (Berl)* 1999;147:217–249.

41. Cho S, Neff NH, Hadjiconstantinou M. Regulation of tyrosine hydroxylase and aromatic L-amino acid decarboxylase by dopaminergic drugs. *Eur J Pharmacol.* 1997;323:149–157.

42. Cumming P, Kuwabara H, Ase A, Gjedde A. Regulation of DOPA decarboxylase activity in brain of living rat. *J Neurochem.* 1995;65:1381–1390.

43. Volkow ND, Fowler JS, Ding YS, Wang GJ, Gatley SJ. Positron emission tomography radioligands for dopamine transporters and studies in human and nonhuman primates. *Adv Pharmacol.* 1998;42:211–214.

44. Soucy JP, Mrini A, Lafaille F, Doucet G, Descarries L. Comparative evaluation of [3H]WIN 35428 and [3H]GBR 12935 as markers of dopamine innervation density in brain. *Synapse.* 1997;25:163–175.

45. Brownell A, Elmaleh DR, Meltzer PC, et al. Cocaine congeners as PET imaging probes for dopamine terminals. *J Nucl Med.* 1996;37:1186–1192.

46. Morris ED, Alpert NM, Fischman AJ. Comparison of two compartmental models for describing receptor ligand kinetics and receptor availability in multiple injection PET studies. *J Cereb Blood Flow Metabol.* 1996;16:841–853.

47. Farde L, Hall H, Pauli S, Halldin C. Variability in D2-dopamine receptor density and affinity: a PET study with [11C]raclopride in man. *Synapse.* 1995;20:200–208.

48. Meyer JH, Ichise M. Modeling of receptor ligand data in PET and SPECT imaging: a review of major approaches. *J Neuroimag.* 2001;11:30–39.

49. Piggott MA, Marshall EF, Thomas N, et al. Dopaminergic activities in the human striatum: rostrocaudal gradients of uptake sites and of D1 and D2 but not of D3 receptor binding or dopamine. *Neuroscience.* 1999;90:433–445.

50. Laruelle M. Imaging dopamine transmission in schizophrenia. A review and meta-analysis. *Quart J Nucl Med.* 1998;42:211–221.

51. Laruelle M. Imaging synaptic neurotransmission with in vivo binding competition techniques: a critical review. *J Cereb Blood Flow Metabol.* 2000;20:423–451.

52. Murphy DL, Andrews AM, Wichems CH, et al. Brain serotonin neurotransmission: an overview and update with an emphasis on serotonin subsystem heterogeneity, multiple receptors, interactions with other neurotransmitter systems, and consequent implications for understanding the actions of serotonergic drugs. *J Clin Psychiatry.* 1998;59:4–12.

53. Chugani DC, Muzik O, Chakraborty P, Mangner T, Chugani HT. Human brain serotonin synthesis capacity measured in vivo with alpha-[C-11]methyl-L-tryptophan. *Synapse.* 1998;28:33–43.

54. Chugani DC, Niimura K, Chaturvedi S, et al. Increased brain serotonin synthesis in migraine. *Neurology.* 1999;53:1473–1479.

55. Shoaf SE, Carson RE, Hommer D, et al. The suitability of [11C]-alpha-methyl-L-tryptophan as a tracer for serotonin synthesis: studies with dual administration of [11C] and [14C] labeled tracer. *J Cereb Blood Flow Metabol.* 2000;20:244–252.

56. Staley JK, Malison RT, Innis RB. Imaging of the serotonergic system: interactions of neuroanatomical and functional abnormalities of depression. *Biol Psychiatry.* 1998;44:534–549.

57. Szabo Z, Scheffel U, Mathews WB, et al. Kinetic analysis of [11C]McN5652: a serotonin transporter radioligand. *J Cereb Blood Flow Metab.* 1999;19:967–981.

58. Gündisch D. Nicotinic acetylcholine receptors and imaging. *Curr Pharmaceut Design.* 2000;6:1143–1157.

59. Muzic RF Jr, Berridge MS, Friedland RP, Zhu N, Nelson AD. PET quantification of specific binding of carbon-11-nicotine in human brain. *J Nucl Med.* 1998;39:2048–2054.

60. Ding YS, Molina PE, Fowler JS, et al. Comparative studies of epibatidine derivatives [18F]NFEP and [18F]N-methyl-NFEP: kinetics, nicotine effect, and toxicity. *Nucl Med Biol.* 1999;26:139–148.

61. Zubieta JK, Koeppe RA, Mulholland GK, Kuhl DE, Frey KA. Quantification of muscarinic cholinergic receptors with [11C]NMPB and positron emission tomography: method development and differentiation of tracer delivery from receptor binding. *J Cereb Blood Flow Metab.* 1998;18:619–631.

62. Knapp FF Jr, McPherson DW, Luo H, Zeeburg B. Radiolabeled ligands for imaging the muscarinic-cholinergic receptors of the heart and brain. *Anticancer Res.* 1997;17:1559–1572.

63. Mehta AK, Ticku MK. An update on GABAA receptors. *Brain Res Rev.* 1999;29:196–217.

64. Koepp MJ, Hammers A, Labbé C, et al. 11C-flumazenil PET in patients with refractory temporal lobe epilepsy and normal MRI. *Neurology.* 2000;54:332–339.

65. Delforge J, Pappata S, Millet P, et al. Quantification of benzodiazepine receptors in human brain using PET, [11C]flumazenil, and a single-experiment protocol. *J Cereb Blood Flow Metab.* 1995;15:284–300.

66. Koepp MJ, Hand KS, Labbé C, et al. In vivo [11C]flumazenil-PET correlates with ex vivo [3H]flumazenil autoradiography in hippocampal sclerosis. *Ann Neurol.* 1998;43:618–626.

67. Cohen RM, Andreason PJ, Doudet DJ, Carson RE, Sunderland T. Opiate receptor avidity and cerebral blood flow in Alzheimer's disease. *J Neurol Sci.* 1997;148:171–180.

68. Schadrack J, Willoch F, Platzer S, et al. Opioid receptors in the human cerebellum: evidence from [11C]diprenorphine PET, mRNA expression and autoradiography. *Neuroreport.* 1999;10:619–624.

69. Zubieta J, Greenwald MK, Lombardi U, et al. Buprenorphine-induced changes in mu-opioid receptor availability in male heroin-dependent volunteers: a preliminary study. *Neuropsychopharmacology* 2000;23:326–334.

70. Burn DJ, Rinne JO, Quinn NP, et al. Striatal opioid receptor binding in Parkinson's disease, striatonigral degeneration and Steele-Richardson-Olszewski syndrome, A [11C]diprenorphine PET study. *Brain.* 1995;118:951–958.

71. Fowler JS, Wang GJ, Logan J, et al. Selective reduction of radiotracer trapping by deuterium substitution: comparison of carbon-11-L-deprenyl and carbon-11-deprenyl-D2 for MAO B mapping. *J Nucl Med.* 1995;36:1255–1262.

72. Fowler JS, Volkow ND, Logan J, et al. Slow recovery of human brain MAO B after L-deprenyl (Selegeline) withdrawal. *Synapse* 1994;18:86–93.

73. Kapur S, Zipursky R, Jones C, Remington G, Houle S. Relationship between dopamine D(2) occupancy, clinical response, and side effects: a double-blind PET study of first-episode schizophrenia. *Am J Psychiatry.* 2000;157:514–520.

74. Kapur S, Zipursky RB, Remington G. Clinical and theoretical implications of 5-HT2 and D2 receptor occupancy of clozapine, risperidone, and olanzapine in schizophrenia. *Am J Psychiatry.* 1999;156:286–293.

75. Chugani HT, Phelps ME. Maturational changes in cerebral function in infants determined by 18FDG positron emission tomography. *Science.* 1986;231:840–843.

76. Chugani HT, Phelps ME, Mazziotta JC. Positron emission tomography study of human brain functional development. *Ann Neurol.* 1987;22:487–497.

77. Chugani HT. A critical period of brain development: Studies of cerebral glucose utilization with PET. *Preven Med.* 1998;27:184–188.

78. Takahashi T, Shirane R, Sato S, Yoshimoto T. Developmental changes of cerebral blood flow and oxygen metabolism in children. *AJNR.* 1999;20:917–922.

79. Chugani DC, Muzik O, Behen M, et al. Developmental changes in brain serotonin synthesis capacity in autistic and nonautistic children. *Ann Neurol.* 1999;45:287–295.

80. Schultz SK, O'Leary DS, Boles Ponto LL, et al. Age-related changes in regional cerebral blood flow among young to mid-life adults. *NeuroReport.* 1999;10:2493–2496.

81. Mazziotta JC, Phelps ME. Positron emission tomography studies of the brain. In: Phelps M, Mazziotta, J, Schelbert H, eds. *Positron Emission Tomography and Autoradiography: Principles and Applications for the Brain and Heart*, Raven Press: New York; 1986; 493–579.

82. Evans DA. Estimated prevalence of Alzheimer's disease in the US. *Milbank Q.* 1990;68: 267–289.

83. Carr DB, Goate A, Phil D, Morris JC. Current concepts in the pathogenesis of Alzheimer's disease. *Am J Med.* 1997;103:3S–10S.

84. Ernst RL, Hay JW. The U.S. economic and social costs of Alzheimer's disease revisited. *Am J Pub Health.* 1994;84:1261–1264.

85. National Institute of Aging. Progress Report on Alzheimer's disease. NIH Publication No. 96-4137. Bethesda, M.D.: National Institute of Aging. 4137. 1996.

86. Zhang MY, Katzman R, Salmon D, et al. The prevalence of dementia and Alzheimer's disease in Shanghai, China: impact of age, gender, and education. *Ann Neurol.* 1990;27: 428–437.

87. Katzman R. Education and the prevalence of dementia and Alzheimer's disease. *Neurology.* 1993;43:13–20.

88. Stern Y, Alexander GE, Prohovnik I, Mayeux R. Inverse relationship between education and parietotemporal perfusion deficit in Alzheimer's disease. *Ann Neur.* 1992;32:371–375.

89. Stern Y, Alexander GE, Prohovnik I, et al. Relationship between lifetime occupation and parietal flow: Implications for a reserve against Alzheimer's disease pathology. *Neurology.* 1995;45:55–60.

90. Alexander GE, Furey ML, Grady CL, et al. Association of premorbid intellectual function with cerebral metabolism in Alzheimer's disease: Implications for the cognitive reserve hypothesis. *Am J Psychiatry.* 1997;154:165–172.

91. Silverman DHS, Small GW, Phelps ME. Clinical value of neuroimaging in the diagnosis of dementia: sensitivity and specificity of regional cerebral metabolic and other parameters for early identification of Alzheimer's Disease. *Clin Positron Imag.* 1999;2:119–130.

92. Evans DA, Beckett LA, Field TS, et al. Apolipoprotein E epsilon-4 and incidence of Alzheimer disease in a community population of older persons. *JAMA.* 1997;277:822–824.

93. Small GW, Mazziotta JC, Collins MT, et al. Apolipoprotein E type 4 allele and cerebral glucose metabolism in relatives at risk for familial Alzheimer disease. *JAMA.* 1995;273: 942–947.

94. Reiman EM, Caselli RJ, Yun LS, Chen K, Bandy D, Minoshima S. Preclinical evidence of Alzheimer's disease in persons homozygous for the e4 allele for apolipoprotein E. *New Engl J Med.* 1996;334:752–758.

95. Small GW, Ercoli LM, Silverman DHS, et al. Cerebral metabolic and cognitive decline in persons at genetic risk for Alzheimer's disease. *PNAS.* 2000;97:6037–6042.

96. Silverman DHS, Hussain SA, Ercoli LM, et al. Detection of differences in regional cerebral metabolism associated with genotypic and educational risk factors for dementia. *Proc Intl Conf Math Eng Tech Med Biol Sci.* 2000;2:422–427.

97. Farkas T, Ferris SH, Wolf AP, et al. ^{18}F-2-deoxy-2-fluoro-D-glucose as a tracer in the positron emission tomographic study of senile dementia. *Am J Psychiatr.* 1982;139: 352–353.

98. Benson DF, Kuhl DE, Phelps ME, Cummings JL, Tsai SY. Positron emission computed tomography in the diagnosis of dementia. *Trans Am Neurol Assoc.* 1981;106:68–71.

99. Frackowiak RS, Pozzilli C, Legg NJ, et al. Regional cerebral oxygen supply and utilization in dementia. A clinical and physiological study with oxygen-15 and positron tomography. *Brain.* 1981;104:753–778.

100. Foster NL, Chase TN, Fedio P, Patronas NJ, Brooks RA, Di Chiro G. Alzheimer's disease: focal cortical changes shown by positron emission tomography. *Neurology.* 1983;33: 961–965.

101. Friedland RP, Jagust WJ. Positron and single photon emission tomography in the differential diagnosis of dementia. In: Duara R, ed. *Positron Emission Tomography in Dementia.* New York: Wiley–Liss, Inc; 1990;161–177.

102. Haxby JV. Resting state regional cerebral metabolism in dementia of the Alzheimer type. In: Duara R, ed. *Positron Emission Tomography in Dementia.* New York: Wiley–Liss, Inc; 1990;93–116.

103. Mazziotta JC, Frackowiak RSJ, Phelps ME. The use of positron emission tomography in the clinical assessment of dementia. *Sem Nucl Med.* 1992;22:233–246.

104. Herholz K. FDG PET and differential diagnosis of dementia. *Alzheim Dis Assoc Disord.* 1995;9:6–16.

105. Pietrini P, Alexander GE, Furey ML, Hampel H, Guazzelli M. The neurometabolic landscape of cognitive decline: in vivo studies with positron emission tomography in Alzheimer's disease. *Int J Psychophysiol.* 2000;37:87–98.

106. Smith GS, de Leon MJ, George AE, et al. Topography of cross-sectional and longitudinal glucose metabolic deficits in Alzeimer's disease. Pathophysiologic implications. *Arch Neurol* 1992;49:1142–1150.

107. Hoffman JM, Welsh-Bohmer KA, Hanson M, et al. FDG PET imaging in patients with pathologically verified dementia. *J Nucl Med.* 2000;41:1920–1928.

108. Silverman DH, Small GW, Chang CY, et al. Positron emission tomography in evaluation of dementia. *JAMA.* 2001;286:2120–2127.

109. Silverman DH, Lu CS, Czernin J, Small GW, Phelps ME. Prognostic value of brain PET in patients with early dementia symptoms, treated or untreated with anticholinesterase therapy. *J Nucl Med.* 2000;41:64P.

110. Herholz K. FDG PET and differential diagnosis of dementia. *Alzheim Dis Assoc Disord.* 1995;9:6–16.

111. Salmon E, Sadzot B, Maquet P, et al. Differential diagnosis of Alzheimer's disease with PET. *J Nucl Med.* 1994;35:391–398

112. Tedeschi E, Hasselbach SG, Waldemar G, et al. Heterogeneous cerebral glucose metabolism in normal pressure hydrocephalus. *J Neurol Neurosurg Psychiatr.* 1995;59:608–615.

113. Mielke R, Schröder R, Fink GR, Kessler J, Herholz K, Heiss WD. Regional cerebral glucose metabolism and postmortem pathology in Alzheimer's disease. *Acta Neuropathol.* 1996;91:174–179.

114. Mielke R, Heiss WD. Positron emisssion tomography for diagnosis of Alzheimer's disease and vascular dementia. *J Neural Transm.* 1998;53 [Suppl]:237–250.

115. Minoshima S, Giordani B, Berent S, Frey K, Foster NL, Kuhl DE. Metabolic reduction in the posterior cingulate cortex in very early Alzheimer's disease. *Ann Neurol.* 1997;42:85–94.

116. Vander Borght T, Minoshima S, Giordani B, et al. Cerebral metabolic differences in Parkinson's and Alzheimer's diseases matched for dementia severity. *J Nucl Med.* 1997; 38:787–802.

117. Imamura T, Ishii K, Sasaki M, et al. Regional cerebral glucose metabolism in dementia with Lewy bodies and Alzheimer's disease: a comparative study using positron emission tomography. *Neurosci Lett.* 1997;235:49–52.

118. Ishii K, Sasaki M, Yamaji S, Sakamoto S, Kitagaki H, Mori E. Paradoxical hippocampus perfusion in mild-to-moderate Alzheimer's disease. *J Nucl Med.* 1998;39:293–298.

119. Eidelberg D, Moeller JR, Dhawan V, et al. The metabolic anatomy of Parkinson's disease: complementary [18F]fluorodeoxyglucose and [18F]fluorodopa positron emission tomography. *Mov Disord.* 1990;5:203–213.

120. Kaasinen V, Ruottinen HM, Nagren K, et al. Upregulation of putaminal dopamine D2 receptors in early Parkinson's disease: a comparative PET study with [11C] raclopride and [11C]N-methylspiperone. *J Nucl Med.* 2000;41:65–70.

121. Morrish P, Sawle G, Brooks D. An [18F]dopa-PET and clinical study of the rate of progression in Parkinson's disease. *Brain.* 1996;119:585–591.

122. Morrish PK, Rakshi JS, Bailey DL, Sawle GV, Brooks DJ. Measuring the rate of progression and estimating the preclinical period of Parkinson's disease with [18F]dopa PET [see comments]. *J Neurol Neurosurg Psychiatry.* 1998;64:314–319.

123. Ilgin N, Zubieta J, Reich SG, et al. PET imaging of the dopamine transporter in progressive supranuclear palsy and Parkinson's disease. *Neurology.* 1991;52:1221–1226.

124. Eidelberg D, Moeller JR, Dhawan V, et al. The metabolic anatomy of Parkinson's disease: complementary [18F]fluorodeoxyglucose and [18F]fluorodopa positron emission tomographic studies. *Mov Disord.* 1990;5:203–213.

125. Brooks DJ, Piccini P, Turjanski N, Samuel M. Neuroimaging of dyskinesia. *Ann Neurol.* 2000;47:S154–S158; discussion S158–S159.

126. Lozano AM, Lang AE, Hutchison WD, Dostrovsky JO. New developments in understanding the etiology of Parkinson's disease and in its treatment. *Curr Opin Neurobiol.* 1998;8:783–790.

127. Wenning GK, Odin P, Morrish P, et al. Short- and long-term survival and function of unilateral intrastriatal dopaminergic grafts in Parkinson's disease. *Ann Neurol.* 1997;42:95–107.

128. Freed CR, Greene PE, Breeze RE, et al. Transplantation of embryonic dopamine neurons for severe Parkinson's disease. [Comment In: N Engl J Med. 2001 Mar 8;344(10): 762–3 UI: 21115012]. *New Engl J Med.* 2001;344:710–719.

129. Mazziotta JC, Phelps ME, Huang S-C, et al. Cerebral glucose utilization reductions in clinically asymptomatic subjects at risk for Huntington's disease. *New Engl J Med.* 1987;316:357–362.
130. Engel JJ. Surgery for seizures. *New Engl J Med.* 1996;334:647–652.
131. Engel J Jr, Wieser H-G. Mesial temporal lobe epilepsy. In: Engel J Jr, ed. *Epilepsy: A Comprehensive Textbook.* Philadelphia: Lippincott-Raven; 1997;2417–2426.
132. Bailey P. The surgical treatment of psychomotor epilepsy. *J Am Med Assoc.* 1951;145: 365–370.
133. Engel J Jr. Overview: who should be considered a surgical candidate? In: Engel EJ Jr, ed. *Surgical Treatment of the Epilepsies.* New York: Raven Press; 1993;23–34.
134. Henry TR, Engel J, Mazziotta JC. Clinical evaluation of interictal fluorine-18-fluorodeoxyglucose PET in partial epilepsy. *J Nucl Med.* 1993;34:1892–1898.
135. Engel JJ, Henry TR, Risinger MW, et al. Presurgical evaluation for partial epilepsy: Relative contributions of chronic depth electrode recordings versus FDG-PET and scalp-sphenoidal ictal EEG. *Neurology.* 1990;40:1670–1677.
136. Risinger MW, Engel J Jr, Van Ness PC, Henry TR, Crandall PH. Ictal localization of temporal lobe seizures with scalp/sphenoidal recordings. *Neurology.* 1989;39:1288–1293.
137. Ackerman RH, Correia JA, Alpert NA, et al. Positron imaging in ischemic stroke disease using compounds labeles with oxygen-15. *Arch Neurol.* 1981;38:537–543.
138. Baron JC, Rey A, et al. Reversal of focal "misery-perfusion syndrome" by extra-intracranial arterial bypass in hemodynamic cerebral ischemia: A case study with ^{15}O positron tomography. *Stroke.* 1981;12:454–459.
139. Grubb RL, Derdeyn CP, Fritsch SM, et al. Importance of hemodynamic factors in the prognosis of symptomatic carotid occlusion. *JAMA.* 1998;280:1055–1060.
140. Yamauchi H, Fukuyama H, Nagahama Y, et al. Significance of increased oxygen extraction fraction in five-year prognosis of major cerebral arterial occlusive diseases. *J Nucl Med.* 1999;40:1992–1998.
141. Heiss W-D, Grond M, Thiel A, et al. Tissue at risk of infarction rescued by early reperfusion: A positron emission tomography study in systemic recombinant tissue plasminogen activator thrombolysis of acute stroke. *J Cereb Blood Flow Metab.* 1998;18: 1298–1307.
142. Marchal G, Benali K, Iglesias S, Viader F, Derlon J-M, Baron J-C. Voxel-based mapping of irreversible ischaemic damage with PET in acute stroke. *Brain.* 1999;122:2387–2400.
143. Iadarola MJ, Berman KF, Zeffiro TA, et al. Neural activation during acute capsaicin-evoked pain and allodynia assessed with PET. *Brain.* 1998;121:931–947.
144. Andersson JLR, Lilja A, Hartvig P, et al. Somatotopic organization along the central sulcus, for pain localization in humans, as revealed by positron emission tomography. *Exper Brain Res.* 1997;117:192–199.
145. May A, Kaube H, Buchel C, et al. Experimental cranial pain elicited by capsaicin: A PET study. *Pain.* 1998;74:61–66.
146. Derbyshire SWG, Jones AKP. Cerebral responses to a continual tonic pain stimulus measured using positron emission tomography. *Pain.* 1998;76:127–135.
147. Svennson P, Jensen TS, et al. Cerebral blood-flow changes evoked by two levels of painful heat stimulation: a positron emission tomography study in humans. *Eur J Pain.* 1998;2: 95–107.
148. Rainville P, Duncan GH, Price DD, et al. Pain affect encoded in human anterior cingulate but not somatosensory cortex. *Science.* 1997;277:968–971.
149. Casey KL, Minoshima S, Morrow TJ, Koeppe RA. Comparison of human cerebral activation patterns during cutaneous warmth, heat pain, and deep cold pain. *J Neurophysiol (Bethesda).* 1996;76:571–581.
150. Paulson PE, Minoshima S, Morrow TJ, Casey KL. Gender differences in pain perception and patterns of cerebral activation during noxious heat stimulation in humans. *Pain.* 1998;76:223–229.
151. Derbyshire SVG, Jones AKP, Gyulai F, Clark S, Townsend D, Firestone LL. Pain processing during three levels of noxious stimulation produces differential patterns of central activity. *Pain.* 1997;73:431–445.
152. Svennson P, Minsohima S, Beydoun A, et al. Cerebral processing of acute skin and muscle pain in humans. *J Neurophysiol.* 1997;78:450–460.

153. Xu X, Fukuyama H, Yazawa S, et al. Functional localization of pain perception in the human brain studied by PET. *Neuroreport.* 1997;8:555–559.

154. Vogt BA, Derbyshire S, Jones AKP. Pain processing in four regions of human cingulate cortex localized with co-registered PET and MR imaging. *Eur J Neurosci.* 1996;8:1461–1473.

155. Derbyshire SWG, Jones AKP, Devani P, et al. Cerebral responses to pain in patients with atypical facial pain measured by positron emission tomography. *J Neurol Neurosurg Psychiatry.* 1994;57:1166–1172.

156. Coghill RC, Talbot JD, Evans AC, et al. Distributed processing of pain and vibration by the human brain. *J Neurosci.* 1994;14:4095–4108.

157. Talbot JD, Marrett S, Evans AC, Meyer E, Bushnell MC, Duncan GH. Multiple representations of pain in human cerebral cortex [see comments]. *Science.* 1991;251:1355–1358.

158. Jones AK, Brown WD, Friston KJ, Qi LY, Frackowiak RS. Cortical and subcortical localization of response to pain in man using positron emission tomography. *Proc Roy Soc Lond. Series B: Biol Sci.* 1991;244:39–44.

159. Derbyshire SWG, Jones AKP, Collins M, et al. Cerebral responses to pain in patients suffering acute post dental extraction pain measured by positron emission tomography (PET). *Eur J Pain.* 1999;3:103–113.

160. Rosen SD, Paulesu E, Jones T. Central nervous pathways mediating angina pectoris. *Lancet.* 1994;344:147–150.

161. Silverman DHS, Munakata JA, Enne H, et al. Regional cerebral activity in normal and pathologic perception of visceral pain. *Gastroenterology.* 1997;112:64–72.

162. Aziz D, Andersson JLR, Valind S, et al. Identification of human brain loci processing esophageal sensation using positron emission tomography. *Gastroenterology.* 1997;13:50–59.

163. May A, Bahra A, Buchel C, Frackowiak RSJ, Goadsby PJ. Hypothalamic activation in cluster headache attacks. *Lancet (North American Edition).* 1998;352:275–278.

164. Hsieh J-C, Hannerz J, Ingvar M. Right-lateralised central processing for pain of nitroglycerin-induced cluster headache. *Pain.* 1996;67:59–68.

165. Weiller C, May A, Limmroth V, et al. Brain stem activation in spontaneous human migraine attacks. *Nat Med.* 1995;1:658–660.

166. Hsieh J-C, Belfrage M, Stone-Elander S, Hansson P, Ingvar M. Central representation of chronic ongoing neuropathic pain studied by positron emission tomography. *Pain.* 1995;63:225–236.

167. Drossman DA, Whitehead WE, Camilleri M. Irritable bowel syndrome: a technical review for practice guideline development. *Gastroenterology.* 1997;112:2120–2137.

168. Mayer EA, Silverman DHS. Gastrointestinal and genitourinary pain. In: *Joint/Muscle and Visceral Pain: Basic Mechanisms with Implications for Assessment and Management.* Seattle: IASP Press; 1996;361–368.

169. Mayer EA, Naliboff B, Munakata J, Silverman DHS. Brain-gut mechanisms of visceral sensitivity. In: Corazziari E, ed. *NeuroGastroenterology.* New York: Walter de Gruyler and Co.; 1996;17–31.

170. Mertz H, Morgan V, Tanner G, et al. Regional cerebral activation in irritable bowel syndrome and control subjects with painful and nonpainful rectal distention. *Gastroenterology.* 2000;118:842–848.

171. Jones AKP, Derbyshire SWG. Positron emission tomography as a tool for understanding the cerebral processing of pain. In: Boivie HP, Lindblom U, eds. *Touch, Temperature, and Pain in Health and Disease: Mechanisms and Assessments. Progress in Pain Research and Management,* Seattle: IASP Press; 1994;491–520.

172. Jones AKP, Qi LY, Fujirawa T. In vivo distribution of opioid receptors in man in relation to the cortical projections of the medial and lateral pain systems measured with positron emission tomography. *Neurosci Lett.* 1991;126:25–28.

173. Jones AKP, Friston KJ, Qi LY. Sites of action of morphine in the brain. *Lancet.* 1991; 338:825.

174. Davies HA. Anginal pain of esophageal origin: clinical presentation, prevalence, and prognosis. *Am J Med.* 1992;92:5S–10S.

175. Aisenberg J, Castell DO. Approach to the patient with unexplained chest pain. *Mount Sinai J Med.* 1994;61:476–483.

176. Lichtlen P, Bargheer RK, Wenzlaff P. Long-term prognosis of patients with anginalike chest pain and normal coronary angiographic findings. *J Am Coll Cardiol.* 1995;25:1013–1018.

177. Rosen SD, Paulesu E, Nihoyannopoulos P. Silent ischemia as a central problem: regional brain activation compared in silent and painful myocardial ischemia. *Ann Intern Med.* 1996;124:939–949.

178. Drevets WC. Neuroimaging studies of mood disorders. *Biol Psychiatry* 2000;48:813–829.

179. Drevets WC. Functional anatomical abnormalities in limbic and prefrontal cortical structures in major depression. *Progr Brain Res.* 2000;126:413–431.

180. Baxter LR Jr, Phelps ME, Mazziotta JC, et al. Cerebral metabolic rates for glucose in mood disorders. Studies with positron emission tomography and fluorodeoxyglucose F 18. *Arch Gen Psychiatry.* 1985;42(5):441–447.

181. Buchsbaum MS, Wu J, DeLisi LE, et al. Frontal cortex and basal ganglia metabolic rates assessed by positron emission tomography with [18F]2-deoxyglucose in affective illness. *J Affect Disord.* 1986;10(2):137–152.

182. Post RM, DeLisi LE, Holcomb HH, Uhde TW, Cohen R, Buchsbaum MS. Glucose utilization in the temporal cortex of affectively ill patients: positron emission tomography. *Biol Psychiatry.* 1987;22(5):545–553.

183. Baxter LR Jr, Schwartz JM, Phelps ME, et al. Reduction of prefrontal cortex glucose metabolism common to three types of depression. *Arch Gen Psychiatry.* 1989;46(3):243–250.

184. Hurwitz TA, Clark C, Murphy E, Klonoff H, Martin WR, Pate BD. Regional cerebral glucose metabolism in major depressive disorder. *Can J Psychiatry.* 1990;35(8):684–688.

185. Martinot JL, Hardy P, Feline A, et al. Left prefrontal glucose hypometabolism in the depressed state: a confirmation. *Am J Psychiatry.* 1990;147(10):1313–1317.

186. Bench CJ, Friston KJ, Brown RG, Scott LC, Frackowiak RS, Dolan RJ. The anatomy of melancholia—focal abnormalities of cerebral blood flow in major depression. *Psychol Med.* 1992;22(3):607–615.

187. Biver F, Goldman S, Delvenne V, et al. Frontal and parietal metabolic disturbances in unipolar depression. *Biol Psychiatry.* 1994;36(6):381–388.

188. Drevets WC, Price JL, Simpson JR Jr, et al. Subgenual prefrontal cortex abnormalities in mood disorders. *Nature.* 1997;386(6627):824–827.

189. Dolan RJ, Bench CJ, Brown RG, Scott LC, Friston KJ, Frackowiak RS. Regional cerebral blood flow abnormalities in depressed patients with cognitive impairment. *J Neurol Neurosurg Psychiatry.* 1992;55(9):768–773.

190. Drevets WC, Videen TO, Price JL, Preskorn SH, Carmichael ST, Raichle ME. A functional anatomical study of unipolar depression. *J Neurosci.* 1992;12(9):3628–3641.

191. Bench CJ, Friston KJ, Brown RG, Frackowiak RS, Dolan RJ. Regional cerebral blood flow in depression measured by positron emission tomography: the relationship with clinical dimensions. *Psychol Med.* 1993;23(3):579–590.

192. Mayberg HS, Lewis PJ, Regenold W, Wagner HN Jr. Paralimbic hypoperfusion in unipolar depression. *J Nucl Med.* 1994;35(6):929–934.

193. Mayberg HS, Starkstein SE, Sadzot B, et al. Selective hypometabolism in the inferior frontal lobe in depressed patients with Parkinson's disease. *Ann Neurol.* 1990;28(1):57–64.

194. Mayberg HS, Starkstein SE, Peyser CE, Brandt J, Dannals RF, Folstein SE. Paralimbic frontal lobe hypometabolism in depression associated with Huntington's disease. *Neurology.* 1992;42(9):1791–1797.

195. Bromfield EB, Altshuler L, Leiderman DB, et al. Cerebral metabolism and depression in patients with complex partial seizures. *Arch Neurol.* 1992;49(6):617–623.

196. Cohen RM, Gross M, Nordahl TE, et al. Preliminary data on the metabolic brain pattern of patients with winter seasonal affective disorder. *Arch Gen Psychiatry.* 1992;49(7):545–552.

197. Goyer PF, Schulz PM, Semple WE, et al. Cerebral glucose metabolism in patients with summer seasonal affective disorder. *Neuropsychopharmacology.* 1992;7(3):233–240.

198. Staley JK, Malison RT, Innis RB. Imaging of the serotonergic system: interactions of neuroanatomical and functional abnormalities of depression. *Biol Psychiatry.* 1998;44(7):534–549.

199. Kennedy SH, Javanmard M, Vaccarino FJ. A review of functional neuroimaging in mood disorders: positron emission tomography and depression. *Can J Psychiatry.* 1997;42(5):467–475.

200. Videbech P. PET measurements of brain glucose metabolism and blood flow in major depressive disorder: a critical review. *Acta Psychiatr Scand.* 2000;101(1):11–20.
201. Fowler JS, Volkow ND, Wang GJ, et al. Inhibition of monoamine oxidase B in the brains of smokers. *Nature.* 1996;379:733–736.
202. Fowler JS, Volkow ND, Wang GJ, et al. Neuropharmacological actions of cigarette smoke: brain monoamine oxidase B (MAO B) inhibition. *J Addict Dis.* 1998;17:23–34.
203. Grafton ST. PET: activation of cerebral blood flow and glucose metabolism. *Adv Neurol.* 2000;83:87–103.
204. Baxter LR, Phelps ME, Mazziotta JC, et al. Local cerebral glucose metabolic rates in obsessive-compulsive disorder—a comparison with rates in unipolar depression and in normal control subjects. *Arch Gen Psychiatr.* 1987;44:211–218.
205. Nordahl TE, Benkelfat C, Semple WE, et al. Cerebral glucose metabolic rates in obsessive-compulsive disorder. *Neuropsychopharmacol.* 1989;2:23–28.
206. Perani D, Colombo C, Bressi S, et al. [18F]FDG-PET study in obsessive-compulsive disorder: a clinical/metabolic correlation study after treatment. *Br J Psychiatr.* 1995;166: 244–250.
207. Swedo S, Schapiro MG, Grady CL, et al. Cerebral glucose metabolism in childhood onset obsessive-compulsive disorder. *Arch Gen Psychiatr.* 1989;46:518–523.
208. Rauch SL, Jenicke MA, Alpert NM, et al. Regional cerebral blood flow measured during symptom provocation in obsessive-compulsive disorder using oxyen-15-labeled carbon dioxide and positron emission tomography. *Arch Gen Psychiatr* 1994;51:62–70.
209. Baxter LR, Schwartz JM, Bergman KS, et al. Caudate glucose metabolic rate changes with both drug and behavior therapy for obsessive-compulsive disorder. *Arch Gen Psychiatry.* 1992;49:681–689.
210. Modell JG, Mountz JM, Curtis GC, et al. Neurophysiologic dysfunction in basal ganglia/limbic striatal and thalamocortical circuits as a pathogenetic mechanism of obsessive-compulsive disorder. *J Neuropsychiatr Clin Neurosci.* 1989;1:27–36.
211. Alexander GE, Delong MR, Strick PL. Parallel organization of functionally segregated circuits linking basal ganglia and cortex. *Ann Rev Neurosci.* 1986;9:357–381.
212. Baxter LR, Schwartz JM, Mazziotta JC, et al. Cerebral glucose metabolic rates in nondepressed obsessive-compulsives. *Am J Psychiatr.* 1988;145:1560–1563.
213. Sawle GV, Hymas NF, Lees AJ, et al. Obsessional slowness: functional studies with positron emission tomography. *Brain.* 1991;114:2191–2202.
214. Saxena S, Brody AL, Ho ML, et al. Cerebral metabolism in major depression and obsessive-compulsive disorder occurring separately and concurrently *Biol Psychiatr.* 2001;50:159–170.
215. Saxena S, Brody AL, Maidment KM, et al. Localized orbitofrontal and subcortical metabolic changes and predictors of response to paroxetine treatment in obsessive-compulsive disorder. *Neuropsychopharmacol.* 1999;21:683–693.
216. Tarazi FI, Florijn WJ, Creese I. Differential regulation of dopamine receptors after chronic typical and atypical antipsychotic drug treatment. *Neuroscience.* 1997;78:985–96.
217. Hietala J, Syvalahti E, Vilkman H, Vuorio K, Rakkolainen V, et al. Depressive symptoms and presynaptic dopamine function in neuroleptic-naive schizophrenia. *Schizophr Res.* 1997;35:41–50.
218. Lewis R, Kapur S, Jones C, DaSilva J, Brown GM, et al. Serotonin 5-HT2 receptors in schizophrenia: a PET study using [18F]setoperone in neuroleptic-naive patients and normal subjects. *Am J Psychiatry.* 1999;156:72–78.
219. Smith GS, Price JC, Lopresti BJ, et al. Test-retest variability of serotonin 5-HT2A receptor binding measured with positron emission tomography and [18F]altanserin in the human brain. *Synapse.* 1998;30:380–392.
220. Gunn RN, Lammertsma AA, Grasby PM. Quantitative analysis of [carbonyl-(11)C]-WAY-100635 PET studies. *Nucl Med Biol.* 2000;27:477–482.
221. Passchier J, van Waarde A, Pieterman RM, et al. Quantitative imaging of 5-HT(1A) receptor binding in healthy volunteers with [(18)f]p-MPPF. *Nucl Med Biol.* 2000;27: 473–476.
222. Adams KM, Gilman S, Koeppe RA, et al. Neuropsychological deficits are correlated with frontal hypometabolism in positron emission tomography studies of older alcoholic patients. *Alcohol Clin Exp Res.* 1993;17:205–210.

223. Dao-Castellana MH, Samson Y, Legault F, et al. Frontal dysfunction in neurologically normal chronic alcoholic subjects: metabolic and neuropsychological findings. *Psychol Med.* 1998;28:1039–1048.

224. Volkow ND, Wang GJ, Hitzemann R, et al. Recovery of brain glucose metabolism in detoxified alcoholics. *Am J Psychiatry* 1994;151:178–183.

225. Johnson-Greene D, Adams KM, Gilman S, et al. Effects of abstinence and relapse upon neuropsychological function and cerebral glucose metabolism in severe chronic alcoholism. *J Clin Exp Neuropsychol.* 1997;19:378–385.

226. Rodgman A, Smith CJ, Perfetti TA. The composition of cigarette smoke: a retrospective, with emphasis on polycyclic components. *Hum Exp Toxicol.* 2000;19:573–595.

227. Fowler JS, Volkow ND, Wang GJ, et al. Brain monoamine oxidase A inhibition in cigarette smokers. *PNAS.* 1996;93:14065–14069.

228. Volkow ND, Fowler JS, Logan J, et al. Carbon-11-cocaine binding compared at subpharmacological and pharmacological doses: a PET study. *J Nucl Med.* 1995;36:1289–1297.

229. Volkow ND, Wang GJ, Fischman MW, et al. Relationship between subjective effects of cocaine and dopamine transporter occupancy. *Nature.* 1997;386:827–830.

230. Logan J, Volkow ND, Fowler JS, et al. Concentration and occupancy of dopamine transporters in cocaine abusers with [11C]cocaine and PET. *Synapse* 1997;27:347–356.

231. Volkow ND, Wang GJ, Fowler JS, et al. Decreased striatal dopaminergic responsiveness in detoxified cocaine-dependent subjects. *Nature.* 1997;386:830–833.

232. Zuddas A, Ancilletta B, Muglia P, Cianchetti C. Attention-deficit/hyperactivity disorder: a neuropsychiatric disorder with childhood onset. *Eur J Paediatr Neurol* 2000;4:53–62.

233. Sagvolden T, Sergeant JA. Attention deficit/hyperactivity disorder—from brain dysfunctions to behaviour. *Behav Brain Res.* 1998;94:1–10.

234. Fowler JS, Volkow ND. PET imaging studies in drug abuse. *J Toxicol Clin Toxicol.* 1998; 36:163–174.

235. Volkow ND, Wang G, Fowler JS, et al. Therapeutic doses of oral methylphenidate significantly increase extracellular dopamine in the human brain. *J Neurosci.* 2001;21: RC121.

236. Seiden LS, Sabol KE. Methamphetamine and methylenedioxymethamphetamine neurotoxicity: possible mechanisms of cell destruction. *NIDA Res Monogr.* 1996;163:251–276.

237. Wilson JM, Kalasinsky KS, Levey AI, et al. Striatal dopamine nerve terminal markers in human, chronic methamphetamine users. *Nat Med.* 1996;2:699–703.

238. Volkow ND, Chang L, Wang GJ, et al. Association of dopamine transporter reduction with psychomotor impairment in methamphetamine abusers. *Am J Psychiatry.* 2001;158: 377–382.

239. McCann UD, Wong DF, Yokoi F, et al. Reduced striatal dopamine transporter density in abstinent methamphetamine and methcathinone users: evidence from positron emission tomography studies with [11C]WIN-35,428. *J Neurosci.* 1998;18:8417–8422.

240. Volkow ND, Chang L, Wang GJ, et al. Higher cortical and lower subcortical metabolism in detoxified methamphetamine abusers. *Am J Psychiatry.* 2001;158:383–389.

241. Langston JW. MPTP neurotoxicity: an overview and characterization of phases of toxicity. *Life Sci.* 1985;36:201–206.

242. Snyder S, D'Amato R. MPTP: a neurotoxin relevant to the pathophysiology of parkinson's disease. *Neurology.* 1986;36:250–258.

243. Bergman H, Feingold A, Nini A, et al. Physiological aspects of information processing in the basal ganglia of normal and parkinsonian primates. *Trends Neurosci.* 1998;21: 32–38.

244. Bankiewicz K, Oldfield E, Chiueh C, et al. Hemiparkinsonism in monkeys after unilateral internal carotid artery infusion of 1-methyl-4-phenyl-1,2,3,6-tetrahydropyridine (MPTP). *Life Sci.* 1986;39:7–16.

245. Melega WP, Raleigh MJ, Stout DB, et al. Longitudinal behavioral and 6-[18F]Fluoro-L-DOPA-PET assessment in MPTP-hemiparkinsonian monkeys. *Exp Neurol.* 1996;141: 318–329.

246. Yee RE, Huang SC, Stout DB, et al. Nigrostriatal reduction of aromatic L-amino acid decarboxylase activity in MPTP-treated squirrel monkeys: in vivo and in vitro investigations. *J Neurochem.* 2000;74:1147–1157.

247. Bankiewicz KS, Eberling JL, Kohutnicka M, et al. Convection-enhanced delivery of AAV vector in parkinsonian monkeys; in vivo detection of gene expression and restoration of dopaminergic function using pro-drug approach. *Exp Neurol.* 2000;164:2–14.

248. Melega WP, Raleigh MJ, Stout DB, et al. Recovery of striatal dopamine function after acute amphetamine- and methamphetamine-induced neurotoxicity in the vervet monkey. *Brain Res* 1997;766:113–120.

249. Kleven MS, Woolverton WL, Seiden LS. Lack of long-term monoamine depletions following repeated or continuous exposure to cocaine. *Brain Res Bull.* 1988;21:233–237.

250. Melega WP, Lacan G, Desalles AA, Phelps ME. Long-term methamphetamine-induced decreases of [(11)C]WIN 35,428 binding in striatum are reduced by GDNF: PET studies in the vervet monkey. *Synapse.* 2000;35:243–249.

251. Weber S, Terstegge A, Herzog H, et al. The design of an animal PET: flexible geometry for achieving optimal spatial resolution or high sensitivity. *IEEE Trans Med Imag.* 1997; 16:684–689.

252. Pichler B, Lorenz E, Mirzoyan R, et al. [Readout of lutetium oxyorthosilicate crystals with avalanche photodiodes for high resolution positron emission tomography]. *Biomed Tech (Berl).* 1997;42:37–38.

253. Chatziioannou AF, Cherry SR, Shao Y, et al. Performance evaluation of microPET: a high-resolution lutetium oxyorthosilicate PET scanner for animal imaging. *J Nucl Med.* 1999;40:1164–1175.

254. Qi J, Leahy RM, Cherry SR, Chatziioannou A, Farquhar TH. High-resolution 3D Bayesian image reconstruction using the microPET small-animal scanner. *Phys Med Biol.* 1998;43:1001–1013.

255. Chatziioannou A, Qi J, Moore A, et al. Comparison of 3-D maximum a posteriori and filtered backprojection algorithms for high-resolution animal imaging with microPET. *IEEE Trans Med Imag.* 2000;19:507–512.

256. Halldin C, Foged C, Chou YH, et al. Carbon-11-NNC 112: a radioligand for PET examination of striatal and neocortical D1-dopamine receptors. *J Nucl Med.* 1998;39: 2061–2068.

257. Breier A, Su TP, Saunders R, et al. Schizophrenia is associated with elevated amphetamine-induced synaptic dopamine concentrations: evidence from a novel positron emission tomography method. *PNAS.* 1997;94:2569–2574.

258. Parsey RV, Kegeles LS, Hwang DR, et al. In vivo quantification of brain serotonin transporters in humans using [11C]McN 5652. *J Nucl Med.* 2000;41:1465–1477.

259. Ryvlin P, Bouvard S, Le Bars D, et al. Clinical utility of flumazenil-PET versus [18F]fluorodeoxyglucose-PET and MRI in refractory partial epilepsy. A prospective study in 100 patients. *Brain.* 1998;121:2067–2081.

260. Fowler JS, Volkow ND, Wang GJ, et al. Age-related increases in brain monoamine oxidase B in living healthy human subjects. *Neurobiol Aging.* 1997;18:431–435.

261. Kazumata K, Dhawan V, Chaly T, et al. Dopamine transporter imaging with fluorine-18-FPCIT and PET. *J Nucl Med.* 1998;39:1521–1530.

262. Plenevaux A, Lemaire C, Aerts J, et al. [(18)F]p-MPPF: A radiolabeled antagonist for the study of 5-HT(1A) receptors with PET. *Nucl Med Biol.* 2000;27:467–471.

263. Volkow ND, Chang L, Wang GJ, et al. Loss of dopamine transporters in methamphetamine abusers recovers with protracted abstinence. *J Neurosci.* 2001;21:9414–9418.

264. Phelps ME. PET: The merging of biology and imaging into molecular imaging. *J Nucl Med.* 2000;41:661–681.

265. Melega WP, Raleigh MJ, Stout PB, et al. Ethological and 6-[18F]fluoro-L-DOPA-PET profiles of long term vulnerability to chronic amphetamine. *Behav Brain Res.* 1997;84: 259–268.

GLOSSARY

6-[¹⁸F]fluoro-L-m-tyrosine: A tyrosine analog used to assess dopamine synthesis.

6-hydroxydopamine: A neurotoxin that is taken up into dopamine and norepinephrine nerve terminals. Inside the terminal, it is oxidized to a quinone, which reacts with proteins, causing neurotoxicity and cell death.

AAAD: *See* Aromatic amino acid decarboxylase.

Aromatic amino acid decarboxylase: An enzyme that catalyzes the synthesis of the neurotransmitters norepinephrine, dopamine, and serotonin, from their amino acid precursors.

Accelerator: A device that produces a well-defined high energy beam of charged particles with a high beam intensity for producing radioactive isotopes.

Acycloguanosine derivatives: Analogs of the natural nucleoside guanosine where the D-ribose has been replaced by an aliphatic chain, conserving their ability to be phosphorylated by Herpes Simplex virus thymidine kinase (HSV1-TK) but with very low affinity for mammalian TK.

AD: *See* Alzheimer's disease.

Adenoma: A benign epithelial tumor in which the cells form recognizable glandular structures or in which the cells are clearly derived from glandular epithelium.

Adenosine 5′-diphosphate: An energy-rich phosphate compound in cells.

Adenosine 5′-triphosphate: An energy-rich phosphate compound in cells that is a product of oxidative phosphorylation.

ADHD: *See* Attention deficit hyperactivity disorder.

ADP: *See* Adenosine 5′-diphosphate.

Adrenergic: Referring to nerve fibers that release norepinephrine from their synapse when a nerve impulse passes, i.e., the sympathetic fibers.

Affinity: A measure of the strength of binding of a ligand to another molecule. The reciprocal of affinity is called K_d—the equilibrium dissociation constant. Thus, the higher the affinity that the ligand has for a receptor, the lower its K_d will be. *See also* K_d.

Agonist: A molecule that binds to a receptor and activates it.

Akinesis: Absent inward systolic motion of the left ventricular wall, i.e. the myocardium.

Alzheimer's disease: A progressive, degenerative disease of the brain. It is characterized by diffuse cortical atrophy and distinctive extracellular lesions called senile plaques, as well as intracellular clumps of fibrils called neurofibrillary tangles. Deficits in cholinergic and other neurotransmitter systems also occur. Symptoms commonly include memory loss, personality changes, and gradual progression to severe impairment of general cognitive and motor functions.

AMP: Adenosine 5′-monophosphate.

Amphetamine and **methamphetamine:** Potent stimulant drugs. Their primary mechanisms of action are to stimulate the release of catecholamines (norepinephrine and dopamine) and serotonin, and to block their reuptake into the nerve terminal. The net effect of both of these processes is to increase extracellular concentrations of the neurotransmitters, which is typically accompanied by an elevation of mood. At high doses, monoamine oxidase activity is also inhibited by the amphetamines to further increase dopamine. For both amphetamine and methamphetamine, the d-isomer is more potent than the l-isomer.

Anaerobic glycolysis: Metabolic pathway for glucose to lactate with net production of 2 molecules of ATP per molecule of glucose. *See also* Glycolysis.

Angiogram, angiographic: Radiological visualization of blood vessels using a radio-opaque contrast material.

Antagonist: A molecule that binds to a receptor but does not activate it but rather blocks its normal activation by agonists.

Assay: An approach for the quantitative estimation of a specific molecular (biochemical) and/or biological process.

ATP: *See* Adenosine 5′-triphosphate.

Attention deficit hyperactivity disorder: A common behavioral syndrome frequently diagnosed in childhood, and characterized by inability to adequately focus on tasks, as well as a tendency to engage in excessive physical activity.

Autoradiogram: An image made from placing an object containing a radioactive substance or substances on a photographic plate or film, or by coating the object with photographic emulsion. The image is formed by exposure of the plate, film, or emulsion to radiation emitted from the object. The radiation is typically beta particles.

Basal ganglia: Includes the caudate, putamen, globus pallidus (external and internal segments), subthalamic nucleus, and substantia nigra (pars compacta, pars reticulata). The basal ganglia is involved in the regulation of posture and movement initiated by the cerebral cortex, in support of motor, cognitive, and emotive functions.

BBB: *See* Blood-brain-barrier.

Beam: The continuous stream of high energy particles produced by the cyclotron.

Becquerel: The unit of radioactivity defined in Standard International Units (SI) as one nuclear decay per second. The more common unit for radioactivity is still the Curie (1 Curie = 3.700 × 10^{10} Bq).

Beta-amyloid plaques: Extra-neuronal beta-amyloid peptide aggregates typically present in the brain of Alzheimer's disease patients.

Beta-oxidation: Oxidation of a fatty acid by the beta carbon atom, the second carbon from the carboxyl, with the result that the two end carbons are split off as acetic acid and with the formation of a fatty acid containing two less carbon atoms.

BGO: *See* Bismuth germanate oxyrthosilicate.

Bismuth germanate oxyrthosilicate: Traditional PET detector material.

Blood-brain-barrier: Typically described as the tight endothelial junctions at the capillary wall that restrict transport and diffusion from blood to brain and brain to blood.

B_{max}: The maximum number of receptor binding sites in a given preparation.

Bone scanning: Conventional whole body scan utilizing the adsorption of radiolabeled diphosphonates to hydroxyapatite crystals in bones. Used for staging of bone involvement in cancer patients

Bq: *See* Becquerel.

Bronchoscopy: A visual examination of the bronchial tree through a bronchoscope.

Buprenorphine: A partial mu opioid agonist.

Carcino-embryonic antigen: Serves as a tumor marker. Often referred to as CEA.

Carcinoma: A malignant growth made up of epithelial cells tending to infiltrate the surrounding tissues and giving rise to metastases.

Cardiomyopathy: Diagnostic term referring to primary disease of the myocardium, often of unknown or uncertain etiology. Can be associated with thickening of the left ventricular wall or myocardium (hypertrophic cardiomyopathy), or an enlargement of the left ventricle (idiopathic dilated cardiomyopathy). Also frequently associated with or caused by coronary artery disease (ischemic cardiomyopathy).

Carrier-added radioisotope: Its preparation refers to a radioactive production during which a known amount of the corresponding stable isotope (generally termed as carrier) has been added.

CBF: Cerebral blood flow.

CBV: Cerebral blood volume.

CEA: *See* Carcino-embryonic antigen.

Cerebellum: A posterior part of the brain, behind the brain stem and below the cortex, in large part concerned with the coordination of movements.

Chemo-embolization: A process by which a chemotherapeutic agent is administered via an arterial catheter into the region of a tumor. Carries the advantage of very limited systemic effects and side effects of chemotherapeutic agents.

CMRglc: Cerebral metabolic rate of glucose.

CMRO$_2$: Cerebral metabolic rate of oxygen.

Coincidence Imaging: Based on the near simultaneous detection of two events such as the annihilation photons by two detectors. Typically the events fall within 0.5–20 nanoseconds of each other. The coincidence event helps to position the location of the annihilation event during the process of image reconstruction.

Collateral blood vessels: Small side branches of a blood vessel or vessels connecting different vascular territories.

Colonoscopy: An endoscopic examination of the colon.

Combinatorial chemistry: A technology for synthesizing and characterizing large collections of compounds (chemical libraries) and screening them for useful properties (e.g., in drug discovery).

Compartment: A space or form in which substances/tracers are distributed uniformly. The amount of substance/tracer transported out of a compartment is proportional to the amount in the space or form.

Compartmental model: A mathematical description of the transport/reaction pathways of tracers in terms of interconnected compartments.

Computed tomography: X-ray technique that measures the spatial distribution of attenuation of x-ray by tissue. Transmission of x-rays through the body are recorded at multiple angles around a subject to compute tomographic images of x-ray attenuation by tissue.

Conventional imaging: Includes anatomical imaging techniques such as computed tomography, MRI, X-ray techniques, and ultrasound, and conventional nuclear medicine imaging procedures other than PET.

Coronary angiogram: Visualization of the coronary arteries using x-rays and contrast material injection in arteries.

Coronary flow reserve: The ratio of maximum coronary flow (after a maximum vasodilation stimulus) to resting coronary blood flow.

Coronary flow: Blood flow through coronary arteries (ml/min); phasic with maximum during ventricular diastole.

Coronary perfusion pressure: Driving pressure (mmHg) for flow of blood through coronary circulation usually determined as pressure in the aorta or the pressure differences between the aorta (inflow pressure) and the right atrium (outflow pressure) of coronary circulation.

Coronary resistance: Resistance to blood flow through the coronary arteries, estimated from the ratio of the mean arterial blood pressure/coronary blood flow (mmHg/ml/min).

Coronary sinus: Terminal segment of the great cardiac vein, emptying into the right atrium.

Correlation: A dimensionless measure of the linear relationship between two random variables. The covariances of a vector of random variables can be condensed into a correlation matrix.

Coulomb barrier: The minimum energy that a charged particle should possess to overcome the repulsive electrostatic force as it approaches a target nucleus.

Cross section: A measure of the probability of a particular nuclear reaction to occur.

Curie (Ci): A unit of activity equal to 3.700×10^{10} nuclear decays per second or 3.700×10^{10} Becquerel ($1 \text{ Ci} = 10^3 \text{ mCi} = 10^6 \text{ }\mu\text{Ci} = 10^9 \text{ nanoCi}$).

D1, D2, D3, D4, D5: Dopamine receptors; presently, five dopamine receptor subtypes have been identified. Stimulation of D1 and D5 receptors increases adenylyl cyclase activity; stimulation of D2, D3, and D4 receptors inhibits adenylyl cyclase activity.

DAT: *See* Dopamine transporter.

Decision tree sensitivity analysis: Mathematical means to analyze the cost-effectiveness of medical procedures. Takes into consideration downstream costs of medical decisions (correct and incorrect ones).

Deoxyribonucleic acid (DNA): The fundamental hereditary material of all living organisms composed of four kinds of nucleotides (adenine, thymine, guanine, cytosine) creating a long double-helical molecule.

Differential equation: An equation in which there is at least one term that involves a variable that changes with respect to a second variable (e.g., d/dt).

Differential uptake ratio: Ratio of glucose metabolic activity within a tumor to the glucose metabolic activity in the non-affected site.

Digital rectal examination: Standard physical examination of the rectum.

Distant metastases: The shifting of cancer from one location in the body to a distant site. It usually involves movement of tumor cells by the lymphatic system or blood vessels to the organ system.

Distribution centers: Commercial radiopharmacy centers for distribution of PET molecular probes, typically within a radius compatible with the half-life of the radioisotope used for labeling the molecular imaging probe.

Distribution volume: *See* Volume of distribution.

DNA: *See* Deoxyribonucleic acid.

Dopamine transporter: A protein located on dopamine-releasing axons that takes dopamine from the extracellular space back into the nerve terminal.

DUR: *See* Differential uptake ratio.

Dyskinesis: Paradoxical, inward motion of the ventricular wall or myocardium during systole.

Electronic generators: Automated synthesis systems integrated with new, compact cyclotron technology for the preparation of molecular imaging probes for use in animals or humans with positron emission tomography and controlled by personal computer.

Embryonal carcinoma: Carcinoma consisting of highly undifferentiated cells.

Endocardium; endocardial: Inner layer of the myocardium or ventricular wall.

Endogenous substrate: Typically refers to the main substrate for a given enzyme present in body tissues.

Endoscopic techniques: Diagnostic tools utilizing optical instruments advanced into the body.

Endothelium: Layer of cells lining the lumen of blood vessels.

Energy of activation: In a chemical reaction, refers to the difference between the free energy of the re-

actants and the free energy that the reactants will have to achieve before their transformation into products.

Enzyme catalysis: Specific chemical reaction facilitated by an enzyme, without being consumed, by lowering the energy of activation of that reaction.

Enzymes: Specific proteins that catalyze myriad of chemical reactions in body tissues producing rate enhancements for these reactions of many orders of magnitude.

Enzyme specificity: Refers to the property of enzymes that restricts its substrates to one or very few structurally nuclear compounds.

Epicardium; epicardial: Outer layer of the myocardium or ventricular wall.

Epithelial cancers: Cancers arising from epithelial cells.

Excitation function: A graphical relationship between cross section and the energy of the incident particle for a nuclear reaction.

Extraction fraction (single pass): Fraction of substrate or tracer extracted from blood to tissue during the first passage through the organ.

[F-18]fluorodihydroxyphenylalanine: an analog of L-DOPA (dopamine precursor), used to image dopamine transporters in PET studies.

False negative findings: Presence of abnormality or disease undetected by diagnostic technique.

False positive findings: Absence of abnormality or disease falsely considered abnormal by a diagnostic technique.

FDG: *See* Fluorine-18 labeled fluorodeoxyglucose.

FDOPA: *See* [F-18]fluorodihydroxyphenylalanine.

Fecal occult blood testing: Colorimetric technique to determine hemoglobin in fecal matter.

FFA: Free fatty acids, as opposed to esterified fatty acids.

Fick method: Technique for determining consumption of a substance by an organ. It is calculated from the product of the arteriovenous concentration difference of the substance and blood flow. An expression of mass conservation (i.e., mass of a substance entering an organ minus the mass of the substance leaving the organ equals the mass of substance retained in the organ).

Flow: Volume of fluid passing a certain observation point in a certain time interval (ml/min). Not the same as perfusion which is in units of ml/min/g tissue.

Fluorine-18 labeled fluorodeoxyglucose: A tracer, 2-deoxy-2-[F-18]fluoro-D-glucose (FDG) for PET imaging. FDG is a derivative of glucose, the predominant energy source for most cells of the body and for tumors. After intracellular phosphorylation via hexokinase, FDG-6-phosphate is not significantly metabolized and remains trapped in the tumor cells.

Flux: The amount of tracer or substance through a transport or reaction step per unit of time. In a first order reaction, flux $= k[C]$ where k is a rate constant, typically in units of time $^{-1}$ and $[C]$ is the concentration of the tracer in units of μCi/volume or substance in units of moles/volume. In a second order reaction, flux $= k[C_1][C_2]$, where $[C_1]$ and $[C_2]$ are the concentrations of the two reactants.

FMT: *See* 6-[^{18}F]fluoro-L-m-tyrosine.

GABA: *See* Gamma-aminobutyric acid.

Gamma-aminobutyric acid: The predominant inhibitory transmitter in the brain. The GABA-chloride channel complex (GABA-A receptor) is a member of the ligand-gated ion channel family of receptors. Activation of the GABA receptor opens a chloride channel, leading to enhanced chloride flux across the membrane. The increase in chloride conductance results in hyperpolarization of the membrane, leading to neuronal inhibition.

GDNF: *See* Glial cell line-derived neurotrophic factor.

Glucose 6-phosphatase: An enzyme that reverses the phosphorylation of glucose.

Glial cell line-derived neurotrophic factor: GDNF in the brain is relatively selective for the dopaminergic system. GDNF was initially characterized as a neurotrophic factor, based on its actions on dopaminergic neurons in culture that included extension of neurites, increases in dopamine uptake and cell size. Numerous other studies in rodents and monkeys subsequently showed that GDNF increases the expression of dopaminergic phenotypic proteins, prevents neurotoxic drug-induced nigrostriatal degeneration, and increases the residual activity of a lesioned nigrostriatal dopamine system.

Glycolysis: The metabolic pathway from glucose to pyruvate with a net production of 2 molecules of ATP per molecule of glucose. Pyruvate can then be converted to lactate or enter the tricarboxylic acid cycle (TCA cycle for glucose oxidation). Complete oxidation of glucose through glycolysis and the TCA cycle yields a net production of 38 molecules of ATP, 6 molecules of CO_2 and 6 molecules of H_2O per molecule of glucose.

Half-life (general): Time during which the amount of substance decreases to half its original value.

Half-life (radioactive): For a single radioactive decay process, the time required for the activity to decrease to half its original value.

Hematocrit: The volume percentage of erythrocytes (red blood cells) in whole blood.

Hexose monophosphate shunt: Pentose phosphate pathway. Provides ribose for purine and pyrimidine synthesis, which are required for providing the carbon backbone for DNA and RNA synthesis.

Huntington's disease: An autosomal dominant, neurodegenerative disorder, manifested by progressive chorea (abnormal uncontrollable movements) and dementia. Its most pronounced changes are related to striatal cell loss (mainly GABAergic) of medium spiny neurons. Each child of an affected parent has 50% probability of receiving the pathologic gene and nearly 100% of those who do will develop the disease before the age of 50.

Hyperalgesia: Abnormally heightened sense of pain.

Hyperemia: Increased or excessive blood supply or tissue perfusion.

Hypokinesis: Diminished inward motion of the myocardium during systole.

Hypoxia: Diminished or reduced tissue oxygenation frequently resulting from inadequate oxygen content of blood.

Identifiability: A property of a parameter. An identifiable parameter can be uniquely determined from noise-free data.

Infarction, myocardial: Gross necrosis of the myocardium, caused by cessation of blood supply to the affected myocardium as, for example, caused by coronary thrombosis.

Inotropic: Affecting the force or energy of muscular contraction. Negatively inotropic weakens the force and positively inotropic increases the strength of muscle contraction.

Ischemia: Inadequate supply of tissue with blood and oxygen, caused by reduction of blood flow or increase in demand for blood and oxygen in excess of what can be delivered. Frequently the result of vascular disease or emboli lodged in vasculature.

k: Rate constant.

k_a: The rate constant for association, the rate of the forward direction of a molecular reaction.

k_d: The rate constant for dissociation of one molecule from another.

K_D: Equilibrium dissociation constant, usually in reference to a ligand-receptor complex. K_D corresponds to the concentration of ligand that results in binding of half of the total number of specific binding sites. K_D is also equal to the ratio of the rate of offset to that of onset for the ligand's interaction with those sites.

K_{eq}: Equilibrium constant of chemical reactions, the value of which is determined by the molar ratio of reactants to products at equilibrium, when concentrations of reactants and products are not changing with time.

K_m: Michaelis-Menten constant.

Lactic acid: Metabolic end product of anaerobic glycolysis.

LAD: Left anterior descending coronary artery.

Laparoscopy: Examination of the interior of the abdomen by means of an optical instrument, such as the laparoscope.

Laparotomy: A surgical incision through the abdominal wall.

Left ventricular ejection fraction: Fraction of the left ventricular volume at end diastole that is ejected from the left ventricle during systole. It is calculated from the difference between end-diastolic and end-systolic volume, also called stroke volume (ml) divided by the end-diastolic volume(ml).

Ligand: Any compound or drug (either agonist or antagonist) that binds to the receptor.

LSO: *See* Lutetium oxyorthosilicate.

Lutetium oxyorthosilicate: New PET detector material with higher light output and reduced scintillation decay time.

LV: Left ventricle.

LVEF: *See* Left ventricular ejection fraction.

Magnetic resonance imaging: Commonly referred to as MRI and provides images of the body from the magnetic properties of hydrogen.

Mathematical model: A set of equations used to describe a system and predict a set of measurements in terms of independent variables and parameters.

MBF: *See* Myocardial blood flow.

MBq: *See* Mega Becquerel.

mCi: milliCurie. $Ci = 3.7 \times 10^{10}$ Bq.

Mean transit time: The average time for tracer molecules to pass through a flow system. It is equal to the first moment of the transit time distribution curve.

Mediastinoscopy: Examination of the mediastinum by means of a tubular instrument permitting direct inspection of the tissues in the area.

Mediastinum: The mass of tissues and organs separating the two lungs, between the sternum in front and the vertebral column behind, and from the thoracic inlet above the diaphragm below.

Mega Becquerel: Measure of activity defined as disintegrations of radioactive material/second $\times$ 1000.

Messenger RNA: In protein biosynthesis, the genetic message is enzymatically transcribed by formation of a ribonucleic acid, called mRNA, whose nucleotide sequence is complementary to that of the DNA in the gene. After transcription, the mRNA moves to the ribosomes where it serves as a template for the specific sequence of amino acids during protein biosynthesis.

Metabolic rate of glucose utilization: Units are μmoles/min/g (units of mg/min/g are also commonly used).

Metabolism: The sum of all the physical and chemical processes by which living organized substance is produced and maintained (anabolism), and also the transformation by which energy is made available for the uses of the organism (catabolism).

Metastasis: The transfer of disease from one organ or part to another not directly connected with it due to the transfer of cells, as in malignant tumors.

Methylphenidate: A stimulant drug that acts as a dopamine reuptake inhibitor causing reductions in—attention deficit disorder and elevation of—in normal subjects.

Michaelis-Menten constant (Km): It is equal to the concentration of a substrate at which the rate of an enzyme-catalyzed reaction is one-half its maximal velocity (V_m).

Michaelis-Menten equation: An equation used to describe a reaction rate as a function of substrate concentration in an enzyme-catalyzed reaction.

Mitochondrium: Small, spherical, rod-shaped component in the cytoplasma of cells that is enclosed in a double membrane, the inner one having infoldings called cristae. They are the principal sites of the generation of energy in the form of ion gradients and adenosine triphosphate (ATP) synthesis resulting from the oxidation of substrates; contain the enzymes of the Krebs or tricarboxylic acid cycles in the respiratory pathway.

Molar (M): Unit of concentration of 1 mole/liter. 1 Molar $= 10^3$ millimoles $= 10^6$ micromoles $= 10^9$ nanomoles $= 10^{12}$ picomoles.

Mole (m): Defined as Avogadro's number (N) of atoms or molecules (6.023×10^{23} atoms or molecules/mole). Mole $= 10^3$ millimoles $= 10^6$ micromoles $= 10^9$ nanomoles $= 10^{12}$ picomoles.

Molecular imaging probes: A molecule with specific labeling (e.g., radioactive atom or fluorophor) that allows for the distinction of specific molecular components of biochemical processes for in vitro or in vivo biological assays.

MPTP: 1-methyl-4-phenyl-1,2,3,6-tetrahydropyridine, a neurotoxin that has been shown to induce Parkinsonism in humans and monkeys by killing dopaminergic cells in the substantia nigra of the brain.

MRglc: *See* Metabolic rate of glucolization.

MRNA: *See* Messenger RNA.

MVO$_2$: Myocardial oxygen consumption in units of μmoles/min/g (units of ml/min/g are also commonly used). LMVO$_2$ and RMVO$_2$ refer to local and regional values, respectively.

Myocardial blood flow (MBF): RMBF and LMBF refer to regional and local values respectively. Strict definition is blood flow in units of ml/min but conventionally defined as blood flow per gram of tissue (i.e., perfusion) in units of ml/min/g.

Myocardial flow resistance: Resistance of the myocardium to blood flow; derived as the ratio of the mean arterial blood pressure over myocardial blood flow; (ml/min/g); serves as a means of relating myocardial blood flow to the coronary perfusion pressure.

Myocyte: Cell of muscular tissue, specifically the heart muscle.

Necrosis: Death of tissue, usually as individual cells, groups of cells, or in small, localized areas.

Negative-ion cyclotron: A device in which negatively charged particles (e.g., H^-) are accelerated in circular paths to several million electron volts (MeV) in a magnetic field. The high energy, negatively charged hydrogen atom, upon passage through a thin foil of carbon, loses two electrons and is converted to a positively charged particle (i.e. H^+). This polarity change from H^- to H^+ under the influence of the magnetic field causes the proton to curve outward for extraction from the cyclotron for the production radioisotopes.

Negative predictive value: Number of true negative findings divided by number of all negative findings.

Neocortex: The most recently evolved portion of the brain, comprising much of the thin covering of gray matter surrounding the outside surfaces of the cerebral hemispheres.

Net extraction: Fraction of a substance or tracer taken up by tissue when system and tracer are in steady state.

Neurofibrillary tangles: Intraneuronal tau-protein aggregates present in the brain of Alzheimer's disease patients and other dementias.

No-carrier-added radioisotope: Preparation involves no intentional or otherwise addition of the corresponding stable isotope during the production.

Non-small cell lung cancer: Most frequent histological type of lung cancer. Consists of a variety of different tumor types.

Nonspecific binding: Binding to tissue (or filters, glassware, etc.) components other than the receptor and is usually measured by incubating the tissue in a high concentration (100 times the K_D concentration at the specific binding site) of unlabeled ligand.

Nuclear reaction energy: Represents the release or absorption of energy during a nuclear reaction. It is customarily called the Q value.

OEF: *See* Oxygen extraction fraction.

OER: *See* Oxygen extraction ratio.

Oncogenes: A gene whose protein product is involved in inducing cancer.

Opiate: Any drug that mimics the actions of morphine.

Oxidation: The act of oxidizing or state of being oxidized. Consists chemically in an increase of positive charges on an atom or the loss of negative charges. Most biological oxidations are accomplished by removal of a pair of hydrogen atoms from a molecule. Such oxidations must be accompanied by a reduction of an acceptor molecule.

Oxidative metabolism: Refers to breakdown of molecules (e.g., sugars, fatty acids, etc.) by oxidation. Complete oxidation of glucose through the tricarboxylic acid cycle. Yields 38 molecules of ATP.

Oxygen equivalent: Moles of oxygen required for complete oxidation of a mole of substrate. For example, this value for glucose is 6.

Oxygen extraction fraction: A measure of the quantity of oxygen delivered to tissue. Defined as(A-V)/A where A and V are the arterial and venous concentrations of oxygen. LOEF refers to local value.

Oxygen extraction ratio: Defined as the ratio of the net oxygen equivalent of substrate extracted by tissue, assuming substrate is completely oxidized to CO_2 and H_2O, to the net oxygen extraction by tissue. *See also* Oxygen equivalent.

Parameter (of a model): A numerical quantity whose value affects the response of a model. In tracer kinetic models, the parameters usually are the rate constants of transfer between the model's compartments. The meaning of these parameters is usually related to physiological or biochemical processes (e.g., blood flow, PS product, metabolic rate, and so on) in tissue and characteristics of a substance/tracer.

Parameter estimate: A random variable based on measured data used to estimate the value of an underlying parameter.

Parkinson's disease: A progressive neurodegenerative disease, involving especially dopaminergic neurons projecting from the brainstem into the cerebral hemispheres which are essential for motor control. Symptoms typically include resting tremor, slowness of voluntary movements, and muscular rigidity. The disease is marked by the appearance of intracellular inclusions known as Lewy bodies, in the pars compacta of the brainstem substantia nigra. Dopaminergic cell depletion reaches 60–70% in the substantia nigra, before clinical symptoms become evident.

Partial agonist: A molecule that binds to a receptor and activates it, but not as strongly as does a full agonist. Thus, in the presence of a full agonist, a partial agonist can act effectively as an antagonist by blocking binding sites for an agonist.

Partial volume effect: When a structure is smaller, in any dimension, than twice the FWHM of an imaging system, the structure does not fill the sensitive volume of one resolution element of the system and due to this partial volume effect, the measured activity concentration is less than the true concentration.

Partition coefficient: Experimentally determined or calculated distribution of a given molecule between hydrophobic solvents and water, typically between 1-octanol and water for molecules used in living systems. The partition coefficient is also the equilibrium ratio of concentrations of a solute in two immiscible solvents. For example, the ratio of the concentration of a tracer in tissue to that in blood, assuming tracer distributes uniformly in blood and tissue. The partition coefficient is unitless because it is a ratio of concentrations. The unit of ml/g frequently used originates from tracer measurements of tissue/blood partition coefficient determined by amount/g in tissue divided by amount/ml in blood.

PD: *See* Parkinson's disease.

Perfusion: Blood flow per mass of tissue in units of ml/min/g tissue.

Peripheral metabolism: The metabolic transformation that a given molecule experiences in various body organs and is commonly assayed by the presence of plasma metabolites.

Peritoneum: The serous membrane lining the abdomino-pelvic walls and investing the viscera.

PET: *See* Positron emission tomography.

Pharmacological agents: Substances that, when administered in vivo, produce specific pharmacological activity.

Pixel: A unit of graphical information that represents a small area in 2-D space.

Polar map: Cartographic approach for displaying the three dimensional shape of the earth in the form of a two dimensional map. Typically, the north or south pole serves as the center of the map with the periphery of the map represented by the equator. Used routinely for displaying the three dimensional distribution of tracer activity in the myocardium with the apex representing the pole and the base of the left ventricle the equator; also referred to as "bull's eye."

Portography: Roentgenography of the portal vein after injection of the opaque material.

Positive-ion cyclotron: A device in which positively charged particles such as protons, deuterons, α-par-ticles, etc. are accelerated in circular paths in a magnetic field to very high energies. These high energy particles are then extracted from the cyclotron using a negatively charged electrode called deflector for radioisotope production.

Positive predictive value: True positive findings divided by all positive findings.

Positron emission tomography: Imaging technique that uses coincidence detection and molecules labeled with positron emitting isotopes, such as glucose labeled with fluorine 18, to probe molecular processes of biology in vivo.

Positron emitter labeled precursor: Refers to chemically distinct radioactive reagent that is used in the preparation of a PET radiotracer.

Predictive accuracy: Number of all correct findings divided by number of all findings.

Probability distribution: A mathematical description of the relative likelihood of all possible outcomes of a random variable.

Prodrug: A precursor of a drug which is converted to the drug in vivo. For example, drugs attached to another molecule that acts to transport or protect an active form of a drug but dissociates in vivo to the drug and the carrier is a prodrug.

PS (permeability-surface) product: Product of the permeability ($ml/min/cm^2$) of a substance or tracer across a capillary wall and the capillary surface area per unit weight of tissue (cm^2/g). It determines the rate at which a substance or tracer is transported from the vascular to tissue space. Note that PS has same units as blood flow (i.e., ml/min/g).

Pyrimidine analogs: In the context of in vivo gene expression determinations, these are radiolabeled pyrimidines structurally related to the natural nucleoside thymidine that are substrates of Herpes Simplex virus thymidine kinase (HSV1-TK).

Rate coefficient A model parameter similar to a rate constant except that it incorporates flow and is in units of ml/min/g.

Rate constant: Term denoting a rate constant. Units depend on the order of the reaction and are $[conc]^{1-n}$ $[time]^{-1}$, where n is the order of the reaction. Rate constant tells the fractional rate at which a process proceeds. For example, for a first order reaction the units are time^{-1}, and a rate constant of 0.1 min^{-1} indicates that reaction proceeds at 10% per min or that 10% of the precursor pool turns over in a minute.

Rate pressure product: Used as index of cardiac work (mmHg/min), represents the product of heart rate (beats per minute) and systolic blood pressure (mmHg).

RCA: Regional cerebral activity.

RCf: Regional cerebral function.

Receptor: A molecule within the cell membrane (or in some cases within the cytoplasm) that recognizes and binds an agonist or antagonist hormone, transmitter, or drug, thereby activating or deactivating a biological response.

Receptor binding affinity: The ability of a given molecule or ligand to bind to a specific receptor system, frequently expressed as the dissociation constant K_D of the ligand-receptor complex.

Recovery coefficient: The ratio of the measured isotope concentration of a structure in an image to the true radioisotope concentration in the structure. The recovery coefficient is a measure of the ability of the system to make a quantitative measurement of the radioisotope concentration in specific structures.

Receptor occupancy: Proportion of receptors that are bound to an endogenous neurotransmitter or exogenous drug at a given time under the experimental conditions and often related to pharmacological effects.

Regional metastases: The transfer of disease from one organ, to another one, due to the transfer of cells. For example, in cancer the migration of malignant cells from the primary site to distant ones.

Regression: A common set of methods used in parameter estimation. These methods are divided into two classes: linear and nonlinear.

Residuals: The difference between the measured data and the predictions of a model using the estimated parameters.

Response function: The measured time-activity function of a dynamic system, when the input func-

tion is an impulse (a bolus whose time duration at the input of the organ is shorter than the minimum vascular transit time through the organ).

Restaging: The process of determining the presence and extent of cancer at any time after treatment.

Retention fraction: Fraction of the total tracer delivered to an organ (or region of an organ) that is extracted into and retained by the tissue. This fraction is the residual after clearances of the vascular component and the portion of tracer that rapidly back diffuses from tissue to blood. Usually this fraction of tracer is sequestered in more slowly turning over metabolic or membrane binding processes.

RMBF: *See* Myocardial blood flow.

Roentgenography: Photography by means of roentgen rays.

RV: Right ventricle.

Sarcolemma: Plasma membrane that invests striated muscle fiber.

Sarcoma: Malignant tumors not arising from epithelial cells. Sarcomas are divided into two groups—bone and soft tissue—according to the type of tissue they arise from.

Saturation yield: The theoretical maximum rate of production of a radioisotope from a nuclear reaction for a given accelerator beam energy condition.

Scintillation cameras: Cameras that detect gamma rays from radioactive decay by the production of light when the gamma ray hits the detector of the camera.

Second look surgery: Exploratory surgery to rule out the presence of residual or recurrent disease. It is most frequently performed in women with gynecological malignancies.

Self-shielded cyclotron: A low energy ($\sim$11 MeV) negative ion cyclotron in which the steel frame or yoke serves as primary radiation shield and hydraulically driven movable blocks made of specially formulated concrete surround the cyclotron for complete radiation protection.

Seminoma: A malignant tumor of the testis thought to arise from primitive gonadal cells, which is considered to be quite radiosensitive.

Sensitivity analysis: A mathematical technique generally used to assess the effects of parameters of complex models or functions. It evaluates the amount of change in the observations/measurements due to a small variation in the value of each combination of the model parameters.

Sensitivity: Accuracy of a test, usually expressed in terms of percent correctly diagnosed, among those tested who actually have the condition of interest.

Serotonin transporter: A protein located on serotonin-releasing axons that takes serotonin from the extracellular space back into the nerve terminal.

SERT: *See* Serotonin transporter.

Sigmoidoscopy: Inspection of a portion of the bowel with an optical instrument.

Specific activity: The amount of radioactivity of a specific radionuclide divided by the mass of the radionuclide or labeled compound into which it has been incorporated (i.e., mCi/g or mCi/mmole).

Specific binding: The difference between total binding to the tissue and binding that occurs in the presence of an excess concentration of unlabeled ligand (i.e., 100 times the K_D concentration of the specific binding site). Binding of a compound to a specific receptor as opposed to general solubility or nonspecific binding of a compound in tissue.

Specificity: Accuracy of a test, usually expressed in terms of percent correctly diagnosed, among those tested who actually do not have the condition of interest.

Spillover: Radioactivity recorded in a region of interest due to spillage of radioactivity from a nearby object. The spillage occurs due to finite spatial resolution of imaging systems.

Standard deviation: The square root of the variance of a random variable. For Gaussian distributions, 68% of the outcomes lie within one standard deviation of the expected value and 95% lie within two standard deviations.

Standard error of the mean: Standard deviation divided by $n^{1/2}$ where n is the number of observations. It is a measure of the estimated mean from n observations.

Standardized Uptake Value (SUV):
Ratio of concentration of tracer activity in a region of interest (ROI) to mean tracer concentration throughout the body and estimated by

$$\frac{\text{ROI tracer concentration (mCi/cc)}}{\text{tracer dose (mCi)/patient weight (g)}}$$

Starting energy: The starting energy of a nuclear reaction includes the energy of charged particle needed to transmit momentum to the reaction system during collision along with the energy required to overcome the Coulomb barrier of electrostatic repulsion.

Steady state: Rate of a transport or reaction sequence is not changing with time and concentrations are constant with time.

Steady state extraction fraction: Net fraction of substrate extracted from blood into tissue under steady state conditions (i.e., when extraction fraction is not changing with time). Commonly measured for whole organs as the arteriovenus differences divided by the arterial concentration of the substrate or tracer of interest during steady state.

Stoichiometric binding: Refers to the quantitative relationship between a small molecule (e.g. ligand) and a larger molecule (e.g. receptor) in molecular binding interactions.

Stoichiometry: The numerical mass balance in chemical and physiological processes.

Striatum: The caudate, putamen, and nucleus accumbens, which are major components of the basal ganglia (see basal ganglia).

Substantia nigra: The main group of dopaminergic cell bodies located in the midbrain.

Substrate analogs: Molecules structurally related to the principal substrate of a given enzyme that can participate in reactions catalyzed by the enzyme.

SUV: *See* Standardized uptake value.

Target body: An ancillary unit of a cyclotron wherein irradiation of target material (liquid or gas) takes place to generate radioisotopes.

Target specificity: In a biological assay, refers to the sensitivity of a molecular probe to detect the desired target system resulting in high signal-to-noise ratios.

TCA cycle: Tricarboxylic acid cycle (also referred to as citric acid or Krebs cycle). Cycle through which acetyl CoA from glycolytic pathway or from beta oxidation of free fatty acids can be fully oxidized to CO_2 and H_2O by transferring electrons stepwise to coenzymes.

Teratocarcinoma: malignant Teratoma. *See also* Teratoma.

Teratoma: A true neoplasm made up of a number of different types of tissue, none of which is native to the area in which it occurs; most often found in the ovary and testis.

Theoretical maximum specific activity: The maximum specific activity that a radioisotope can attain when every atom of the element is identically radioactive (i.e., entirely free from any nonradioactive forms of the element).

Thick target: One in which the energy of the incident particle beam is completely stopped within the target material or degraded to an energy less than the threshold for the nuclear reaction.

Thick target yield: The radioactive disintegration rate (in mCi), at saturation, divided by the beam current (in μA). The thick target yield data are generally obtained from integration of the corresponding excitation function.

Threshold energy: The minimum kinetic energy that a charged particle must possess for a nuclear reaction to be energetically possible.

TNM stage: Standardized system to determine the extent of cancer. T describes tumor size, N depicts lymph node involvement, and M evaluates presence of metastatic disease.

Tracer: A measurable substance used to mimic, follow, or trace a chemical compound or process without significantly disturbing the process under study.

Tracer kinetic modeling: The use of mathematical description/formulation to incorporate a priori information about the behavior of a tracer in a dynamic system in order to calculate properties of the system from the kinetics of tracer.

Transmission scan: Using an external radiation source, transmission images are obtained to correct for photon attenuation in tissues localized between the radiation source and the radiation detectors.

True negative findings: Absence of abnormalities on images are confirmed by normal histology, other imaging findings, and/or normal clinical outcome.

True positive findings: Imaging findings are verified by histology, other imaging techniques, or clinical outcome.

Unit operation principle: An approach in which a multi-step synthetic process is broken down into several unit operations such as addition of reagent, removal of solvent, chromatography and sterilization, etc. These simple unit operations are performed in sequence where standard laboratory glassware and equipment are used in conjunction with solenoid values.

Variable: Usually represented by letters (e.g., y, z), signify an empty space into which an arbitrary element (or its symbol) form a fixed set that can be substituted.

Vesicular monoamine transporter: A protein that transports amines from the cytosol into biogenic amine storage vesicles of nerve terminals in brain. It is located on the vesicle membrane.

V_m: The maximal velocity of an enzyme catalyzed reaction. Value is achieved when the substrate steady state is high enough that essentially all the enzyme is in the form of the enzyme/substrate complex.

VMAT: *See* Vesicular monoamine transporter.

Volume of distribution: The equivalent hypothetical volume that a tracer can distribute in tissue with the same concentration as in blood. It has the unit of ml/g and is often denoted by the variable V_d.

Voxel: A unit of graphical information that represents a small volume in 3-D space.

Weighted nonlinear regression: A modified version of ordinary least squares estimation involving the determination of parameters by minimizing the weighted sum of squared deviations between the data and the model.

Index

597